Volume 1

ANALYSIS OF ROENTGEN SIGNS

IN GENERAL RADIOLOGY

INTRODUCTION / SKELETAL SYSTEM
(Including Joints, Skull and Spine)

ISADORE MESCHAN, M.A., M.D.

Professor and Director of the Department of Radiology
at the Bowman Gray School of Medicine of Wake Forest
University, Winston-Salem, North Carolina; Consultant,
Walter Reed Army Hospital; Member Committee on Radiology,
National Research Council, National Academy of Sciences

with the assistance of

R. M. F. FARRER-MESCHAN, M.B., B.S. (Melbourne, Australia), M.D.

Clinical Assistant Professor, Department of Obstetrics and Gynecology and
Associate in Radiology, Bowman Gray School of Medicine of
Wake Forest University, Winston-Salem, North Carolina

W. B. SAUNDERS COMPANY *Philadelphia · London · Toronto*

W. B. Saunders Company: West Washington Square
Philadelphia, PA 19105

1 St. Anne's Road
Eastbourne, East Sussex BN21 3UN, England

1 Goldthorne Avenue
Toronto, Ontario M8Z 5T9, Canada

Analysis of Roentgen Signs in General Radiology — Volume 1   ISBN 0-7216-6305-2

Print No.:   9   8   7   6   5

To the memory of our parents

"If we shadows have offended,
Think but this, and all is mended,
That you have but slumbered here
While these visions did appear. . . ."
Shakespeare

A Midsummer Night's Dream

V, ii, 54

PREFACE

This is our third text concerning roentgen signs. In the previous two, the emphasis was on compilation and illustration of *major* roentgen signs in general radiology, their classification and correlation with clinical diagnosis and practice.

In this text, there is a greater emphasis on inclusion of as many signs as space (and imagination) allow; on an appropriate standardized classification which could apply throughout diagnostic roentgenology; and on optimum illustration and explanation of the signs in general diagnostic radiology, omitting special procedures.

The correlation with the clinical practice has been reduced and the narrative presented almost in outline form.

It has been our further purpose to review the literature more completely with respect to roentgen signs, along with their statistical significance for diagnosis where feasible.

We have continued to utilize the "midget exhibit" concept, with summarized data and important article reviews set off from the rest of the text in enclosures. These "boxes" are, indeed, to be regarded as additional illustrations, amplifying the truly pictorial. In order to provide as much space as possible for these, the narrative text has had to be doubly succinct and abbreviated — and yet repetitive at times of that which is illustrated.

Our audience, we hope, will be those who desire a ready reference to an illustrated and organized amalgamation of roentgen signs and the literature pertaining thereto. Our choices were purposeful to conserve space; unfortunately, there must be omissions. I would hope that the students, residents, practitioners, and radiologists who may use this text will find in it the stimulation and resources for further study of *roentgen signs*.

I. Meschan, M.D.

March 30, 1973

CREDITS AND ACKNOWLEDGMENTS

My indebtedness to many people involved in this endeavor is very great.

My wife, Rachel Farrer Meschan, M.D., M.B., B.S., has been an "assistant author." She has given unstintingly of her time throughout the entire production. She has herself labeled most of the new illustrations, compiled the index, and her criticism throughout this enterprise has been most valuable. These volumes would not have been possible without her assistance.

To Mrs. Edna Snow, my secretary, and to Mrs. Betty Stimson, who assisted her, I owe a great debt of gratitude. Mrs. Snow has conscientiously and patiently typed each draft of the manuscript without complaint and with great perseverance. She has been responsible for the typing of the index and the great load of correspondence that is incumbent on such an endeavor as this book. Again, this text would have been impossible without her tremendous assistance.

My associates also, both past and present, have been extremely helpful. They have substituted for me from time to time in my regular duties so that I might pursue this one. Moreover, when given sections of the text to read, they have done so conscientiously, directly and without stint of favor. Their suggestions were always received appreciatively and have been most helpful in the course of this production. To name a few of these (in alphabetical order): Dr. Frank Farrell, Dr. Laurence Leinbach, Dr. James Martin, Dr. Nitaya Suwanwela (who is now in Thailand), Dr. Joseph Whitley, and Dr. Nancy Whitley.

Mr. Doug Shiflett, soon to be Dr. Shiflett, was of great help in library and literature search. As a medical student he was able to help me greatly, particularly in the checking of bibliography. At times I am certain this was a tedious task and for this I am extremely grateful.

Mr. Glenn Foy, artist, was responsible for many of the new drawings. He was assisted in this by members of our Audiovisual Aid Department — Mr. George Lynch, artist; Mr. Joe Roselli, artist; Mr. Jack Dent, photographer, and my daughter, Joyce Meschan.

At times, when special photographic assistance was necessary, Dr. Thomas Thompson put at our disposal his Logetronic facility, which gave us an additional dimension in our photographic reproductions.

I owe a further debt of gratitude to present and past Residents who helped me throughout this endeavor. When called upon, they searched the literature for me, reviewed special sections of the text critically, and helped organize and seek out many illustrations—and this, too, made this text feasible. The men particularly responsible for this were (in alphabetical order): Dr. Richard Bird, Dr. James Crowe (now a member of our faculty), Dr. Robert Davis, Dr. James Fagan, Dr. David Gaillard, Dr. John Harrill, Dr. William Harriss, Dr. William Hines, Dr. Mitchell Russ, Dr. John Scott, Dr. John Stevenson, and Dr. Kyle Young.

From time to time, special technical assistance was offered by Mrs. Polly Story, one of our Chief Technicians, who supplied a number of the illustrations necessary for this purpose.

To the many physicians who have allowed me to borrow illustrations or use their material, I hope all due credit has been given. If perchance, omission has occurred, my humble apologies.

Last but not least, I am particularly grateful to the W. B. Saunders Company, Publishers, and their very helpful personnel. They offered their services beyond the usual call of duty in providing excellent reproductions of radiographs, very superior editorial assistance, and rapidity and accuracy of production.

To all of these and many others too numerous to name, I owe a great debt of gratitude, credit, and acknowledgment. Ultimately, however, I must assume full responsibility for what appears in this text. I can only hope that it will have fulfilled its purposes.

I. MESCHAN, M.D.

March 30, 1973

TABLE OF CONTENTS

VOLUME 1

SECTION ONE. INTRODUCTION

1

Background Fundamentals for Diagnostic Radiology 3

2

Protective Measures in X-Ray Diagnosis 21

3

General Terms and Concepts Regarding Diagnostic Radiology 39

SECTION TWO. MUSCULOSKELETAL SYSTEM

4

Basic Concepts Regarding the Radiographic Study of Bones and Joints 49

5

Fractures and Dislocations of the Extremities 116

6

Fracture Healing, Complications From Fractures, and Methods of
Treatment From the Radiologic Standpoint 167

7

Congenital and Hereditary Abnormalities of the Skeletal System 182

8

Radiolucent Bone Diseases of Multiple Extremities or Regions 230

9

Radiolucent Bone Diseases of a Single Extremity 274

10
Bone Diseases of the Extremities Characterized by Increased Density,
Expansion, or Enlargement 323

11
Radiology of Joints 380

12
Roentgenology of the Skull 433

13
Radiology of Special Areas of the Skull and Space-Occupying Lesions
Within the Cranium 524

14
The Radiology of the Vertebral Column 602

VOLUME 2

SECTION THREE. RESPIRATORY SYSTEM

15
Introduction to Roentgenologic Analysis of the Chest 701

16
Radiology of the Diaphragm, Pleura, Thoracic Cage, and Upper Air Passages ... 748

17
Diffuse, Poorly Defined, Homogeneous Shadows of the Lung Parenchyma 799

18
Radiology of Nodular Lesions of the Lung Parenchyma 890

19
Radiology of Lesions of the Lungs Characterized by Increase in
Linear Markings 938

20
Radiology of Lung Lesions Characterized by Increased Radiolucency
in the Lung Fields—Either Localized or Generalized 987

SECTION FOUR. MEDIASTINUM AND HEART

21
Radiology of the Mediastinum, Excluding the Heart..................................... 1011

22
Roentgenology of the Heart (Exclusive of Congenital Heart Disease) 1067

23
Congenital Heart Disease: Plain Film Interpretation 1165

VOLUME 3

SECTION FIVE. ABDOMEN AND URINARY TRACT

24
Radiologic Study of the Abdomen Without Added Contrast Media.................. 1217

25
Radiology of the Urinary Tract and Suprarenal Glands 1310

SECTION SIX. ALIMENTARY TRACT

26
Roentgenology of the Biliary System... 1479

27
Upper Alimentary Tract: Oropharynx, Laryngopharynx, and Esophagus 1522

28
Stomach, Duodenum, and Pancreas.. 1582

29
Radiology of the Small Intestine Beyond the Duodenum............................. 1689

30
Radiology of the Colon 1754

SECTION SEVEN. OBSTETRICS AND GYNECOLOGY

31
Roentgen Diagnosis in Obstetrics and Gynecology...................................... 1863

SECTION ONE

INTRODUCTION

1

Background Fundamentals for Diagnostic Radiology

HISTORICAL INTRODUCTION

In 1895, while working with a Hittorf-Crookes type light-proof cathode ray tube. Wilhelm Konrad Röntgen discovered that a cardboard covered with barium platinocyanide crystals would fluoresce whenever a charge of cathode rays passed through the tube. He further noted that this fluorescence would occur despite the placement of certain materials between the tube and the phosphorescent surface, and he collected a variety of materials and showed that these materials varied somewhat in their permeability. Even aluminum sheeting was permeable, but a thin sheet of lead was not. The fingers of the hand, when interposed, would reveal the bones. He also noted that these new rays, which he called "x-rays," would affect a photographic plate encased in a light-tight cassette. The rays were unlike the cathode rays of the tube in that they could not be deflected by a magnet.

Röntgen, with these simple experiments, laid the foundation for the science of medical and industrial radiology, and in a matter of months, there were hundreds of other papers published relating to this remarkable discovery. Within several years, the far-reaching biological effects of these rays on the skin and blood vessels were also known, but the accumulated information along these lines left a trail of martyrs who had exposed themselves in one way or another to these powerful and penetrating rays.

A summary discussion of the biological effects of these rays is being deferred to Chapter 2. In this chapter, we shall briefly review the manner in which x-rays are produced for medical diagnostic purposes, and describe some of the important ancillary materials which enhance the utilization of x-rays in diagnostic radiology.

PRODUCTION OF X-RAYS (Figures 1–1, 1–2)

Within the X-ray Tube

Important Components of the X-ray Tube. The x-ray tube is a *glass-encased bulb,* from which the air has been removed, creating a *vacuum;* an electrode is at either end.

THE X-RAY TUBE

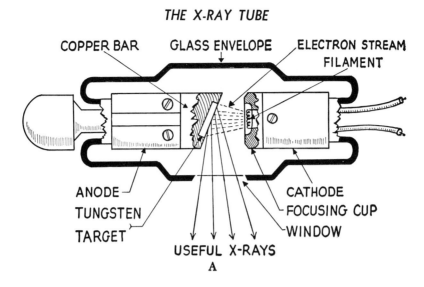

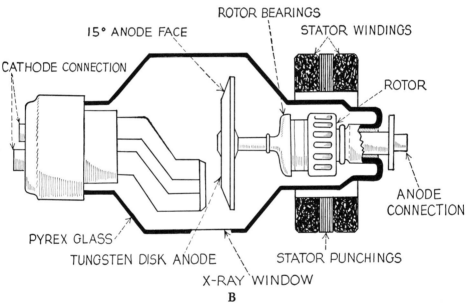

Figure 1–1   The x-ray tube. *A.* Stationary anode. *B.* Rotating anode.

The cathode is the *tungsten filament,* which is provided with a separate electrical circuit (high amperage, low voltage) for heating the filament and thereby producing electrons.

The anode is the *target,* usually tungsten in medical x-ray tubes, annealed to a copper bar to facilitate heat conduction.

Anodes may be *stationary* or *rotating.* The rotating anode is in essence a disk with the target material annealed to the rim at a sufficient angle to provide the desired angle of reflection of the x-rays (Fig. 1–1B). The cathode rays strike this rim as the disk rotates, permitting heat dissipation. A motor and its appropriate circuit are mounted in continuum with the anode, so that the target is rotated prior to the production of the cathode rays.

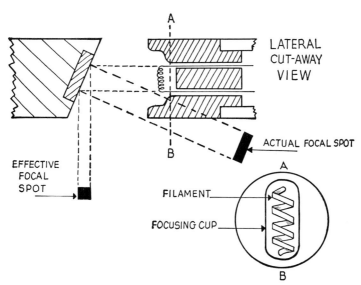

Figure 1–2 Diagram of focusing cup and filament of x-ray tube. The average size of "small" focal spot is 0.6 to 1 mm. A large focal spot is ordinarily 2 mm. in size.

The *major electrical circuit* (low milliamperage, high voltage) between the anode and the cathode, creates a large potential difference, and a stream of electrons, known as cathode rays, passes from one to the other.

When the cathode rays strike the target *tremendous heat* evolves and some x-rays are produced, but the cross-sectional area of the x-rays so produced is controlled both by the area of the anode and by the angle of reflection of the rays. The cross-sectional area at the site of origin of the rays is called the *"effective focal spot size"* and usually ranges between 0.5 mm. and 2.0 mm., although some special tubes are now made with effective spot sizes of 0.12 mm. which are useful in magnification techniques.

The size of the effective focal spot is responsible for the detail of the roentgen image produced. The smaller the effective focal spot, the better the detail, since there is a lesser "shadow effect" (penumbra and umbra) around the image (see the section on the "Geometry of the X-ray Image").

Other ancillary components of the x-ray tube are the *focusing cup*, which helps direct the stream of electrons, and the *special grid devices* which facilitate extremely short exposure times. Most x-ray tubes come equipped with two anodes, each of a different size, since the smaller the target, the greater the problem of heat dissipation; and when an abundance of x-rays is required to penetrate large anatomic parts the larger target may be necessary.

Outside the X-ray Tube

Heat Dissipation from the X-ray Tube. The various mechanisms for cooling the x-ray tube include: (1) fins, which are attached to the copper anode bar; (2) circulating oil; (3) circulating water; (4) combinations of circulating oil and water by conjoined circulation systems; and (5) the rotating anode previously described.

Other Ancillary Circuits

1. *Rectification Circuits.* These are incorporated to provide a steady stream of electrons in one direction, since the alternating current source of the major x-ray

circuit would otherwise cause either an alternation of direction or an intermittence of the cathode rays in the x-ray tube.

2. *Timing Circuits.* These provide accurate control of the bursts of cathode rays, and thus, x-rays.

3. *Automatic Stabilization Circuits* supply milliamperage and voltage control.

4. *External Circuitry* is used in connection with image amplification and closed circuit television for fluoroscopy and rapid-film sequencing.

SPECIAL PROPERTIES OF X-RAYS WHICH PERTAIN TO DIAGNOSTIC RADIOLOGY

The special properties of x-rays which make them so very useful to diagnostic radiology are: (1) their *ability to penetrate* organic matter; (2) their ability to produce a *photographic effect* on photosensitive film surfaces; and (3) their ability to produce a *phosphorescence* (fluorescence) in certain crystalline materials.

Penetrability of Tissues and Other Substances by X-rays. Tissues and other substances with medical applications may be classified into the categories indicated in Figure 1–4 on the basis of their density and atomic structure. At one end of the spectrum are the *radiolucent* materials, through which the x-rays pass readily; at the other end are the *radiopaque* substances in which the x-rays are absorbed to a considerable degree in their passage so that little radiation escapes.

The x-rays which penetrate an anatomic part may be spoken of as the "remnant rays." These are the rays which ultimately affect the x-ray film or fluorescent screen and are responsible for the gradations of black and white on the image. Thus, in Figure 1–5, x-rays are shown diagrammatically to be traversing the cross-section of a forearm. The gradations of black, gray, and white as shown on the film beneath the forearm are due to the "remnant radiation" after the rays have been absorbed by the interposed tissues such as subcutaneous fat, muscles, and bone.

Unfortunately, in the process of passage through an anatomic structure the x-rays (and the secondary electrons produced within the anatomic part) are scattered in all directions, depending upon the energy of the primary x-ray beam. Such *scattered radiation* causes a loss of detail. Special devices must be interposed between the x-ray source and the film to eliminate the scattered rays from the ultimate image. *Coning devices, stationary and moving grids (Potter-Bucky diaphragm),* which help eliminate such scattered radiation will be described later.

Photographic Effect of X-rays. Just as visible or ultra-violet rays alter light sensitive photographic emulsion, so do roentgen rays, so that when appropriately "developed," "fixed," and "washed," a permanent image is produced. The film

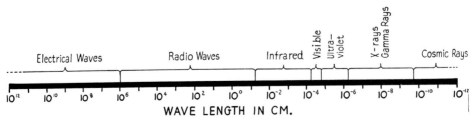

Figure 1–3 Diagram of the electromagnetic spectrum, illustrating the part of this spectrum occupied by x-rays.

VERY RADIOLUCENT	MODERATELY RADIOLUCENT	INTERMEDIATE	MODERATELY RADIOPAQUE	VERY RADIOPAQUE
Gas	Fatty tissue	Connective tissue Muscle tissue Blood Cartilage Epithelium Cholesterol stones Uric acid stones	Bone Calcium salts	Heavy metals

Figure 1–4 Classification of tissues and other substances with medical application in accordance with five general categories of radiopacity and radiolucency.

employed for this purpose is ordinarily made with a thicker emulsion, although this is not absolutely necessary. The utilization of intensifying fluorescent screens (to be described below) has largely obviated such "direct radiography," since less x-irradiation is necessary for radiography by intensification techniques. However, when the body part under study (such as an extremity) is not large, when optimum detail is required, and when it is desired to allow no possibility for the interposition of an artefact on the roentgen image, such direct radiography is employed.

Fluorescent Effect of X-rays. When roentgen rays strike certain crystalline materials, a phosphorescence results. The spectrum of light so produced will vary with the crystalline substance—at times, it is largely ultraviolet, at other times, largely visible light. The ultraviolet light has proved to be most advantageous in respect to x-ray film emulsion. Intensifying screens consist mostly of a thin coating of such crystals on a cardboard surface. Their function is to provide a brighter image than would be provided by the direct photographic effect of the x-rays alone.

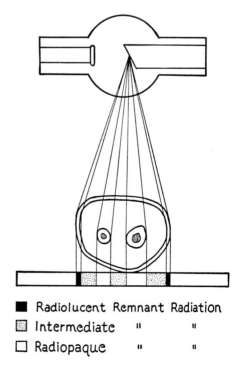

Figure 1–5 Diagram showing x-rays passing through the cross-section of the forearm to illustrate the varying degrees of lucency and opacity of the "remnant rays" which strike the film.

■ Radiolucent Remnant Radiation
▨ Intermediate   "   "
☐ Radiopaque   "   "

Intensifying screens are categorized with respect to "brightness," (called "speed") and "detail," one being inverse in respect to the other, thus requiring some compromise.

Prior to the advent of image amplification, which has replaced conventional fluoroscopy, the crystalline substance chosen for its fluorescence produced light in the visible light range. In image amplification requiring electromagnetic enhancement, the "input phosphorescent" and "output phosphorescent" screens are similarly constructed.

ACCESSORIES NECESSARY FOR THE RECORDING OF THE X-RAY IMAGE

The accessories which make radiography and fluoroscopy possible are:

1. The x-ray film;
2. The x-ray cassette, with its enclosed intensifying screens;
3. The x-ray film which does not require an intensifying screen or conventional cassette, but is placed in a plastic or cardboard folder;
4. The stationary and moving grids, such as the Potter-Bucky diaphragm;
5. Various cones, apertures and adjustable diaphragms for delimiting the x-ray beam to the body part in question;
6. Body-section radiographic equipment;
7. Stereoscopic radiographic accessories;
8. The fluoroscopic screen and the fluoroscope;
9. Image amplifiers used in conjunction with fluoroscopy and radiography;
10. Equipment for television fluoroscopy and radiography with television tape recording;
11. Accessories for spot film radiography;
12. Devices for photographing the output phosphor of an image amplifier (the radiographs may be miniature in size, such as 16 mm., 35 mm., 70 mm., 90 mm., or 100 mm., or cineradiographic sequences);
13. Rapid sequence film changers for either roll film or cut film, or rapid sequence cassette changers for recording rapidly changing x-ray images;
14. Magnification accessories;
15. Contrast media.

Each of these devices will now be briefly illustrated and discussed.

X-ray Film.   X-ray film consists of a transparent cellulose acetate or plastic base coated on each side with a photosensitive emulsion, such as silver bromide crystals. Rarely, single emulsion films are employed. The emulsion is designed to be most efficiently photosensitized in an ultraviolet radiation range by the light rays emitted by the intensifying screens, when these latter structures are activated by x-rays. X-ray film, with a somewhat different emulsion, is utilized when the film is contained in a light-proof folder without intensifying screens, in which case the film is photosensitized by the x-rays directly. X-ray film is developed in a special developing solution which precipitates the exposed crystals; the unused developing solution clinging to the film is rapidly washed away, and the precipitated silver halide crystals are "fixed" in "hypo" solution. The film is then washed and dried prior to

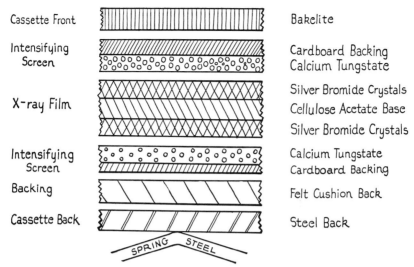

Cassette Front		Bakelite
Intensifying Screen		Cardboard Backing Calcium Tungstate
X-ray Film		Silver Bromide Crystals Cellulose Acetate Base Silver Bromide Crystals
Intensifying Screen		Calcium Tungstate Cardboard Backing
Backing		Felt Cushion Back
Cassette Back		Steel Back

SPRING STEEL

Figure 1–6 Diagrammatic cross-section illustrating an x-ray film contained within an x-ray cassette.

viewing and interpretation. Film processing may now be carried out very efficiently in 90 seconds or even less with appropriate automated equipment.

The X-ray Cassette (Figures 1–6 and 1–7). An open x-ray cassette is shown in Figure 1–7, and its cross-sectional diagram in Figure 1–6. It is a light-proof container for the film, designed to permit easy loading and unloading, while near perfect contact is maintained with the intensifying screens. When the x-ray beam strikes the intensifying screen, ultra-violet and visible light rays are produced and the film is photosensitized. A suitable "x-ray" image is thereby produced employing fewer x-rays. Unfortunately, any dirt particles upon the film or intensifying screen or defects in either film or screen will also produce an image on the film, so that the x-ray cassette must be cleaned and handled with extreme care.

ACCESSORIES NECESSARY FOR RECORDING OF THE X-RAY IMAGE

THE CASSETTE AND ITS CARE

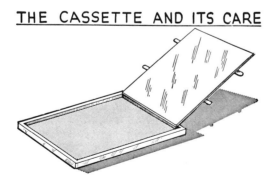

1. AVOID INJURY OR DROPPING.
2. AVOID CHEMICAL CONTACT WITH SCREENS.
3. HANDLE ON DRY BENCH.
4. AVOID STORAGE OF ITEMS ABOVE LOADING BENCH.
5. DO NOT LEAVE CASSETTE OPEN.
6. INSPECT FREQUENTLY TO DETECT WEARING OF FELT OR BENDING OF HINGES.
7. TEST SCREEN FILM CONTACT WITH FLAT WIRE MESH.

Figure 1–7 Diagram illustrating an open x-ray cassette with tabulated emphasis upon its proper care.

THE POTTER-BUCKY DIAPHRAGM

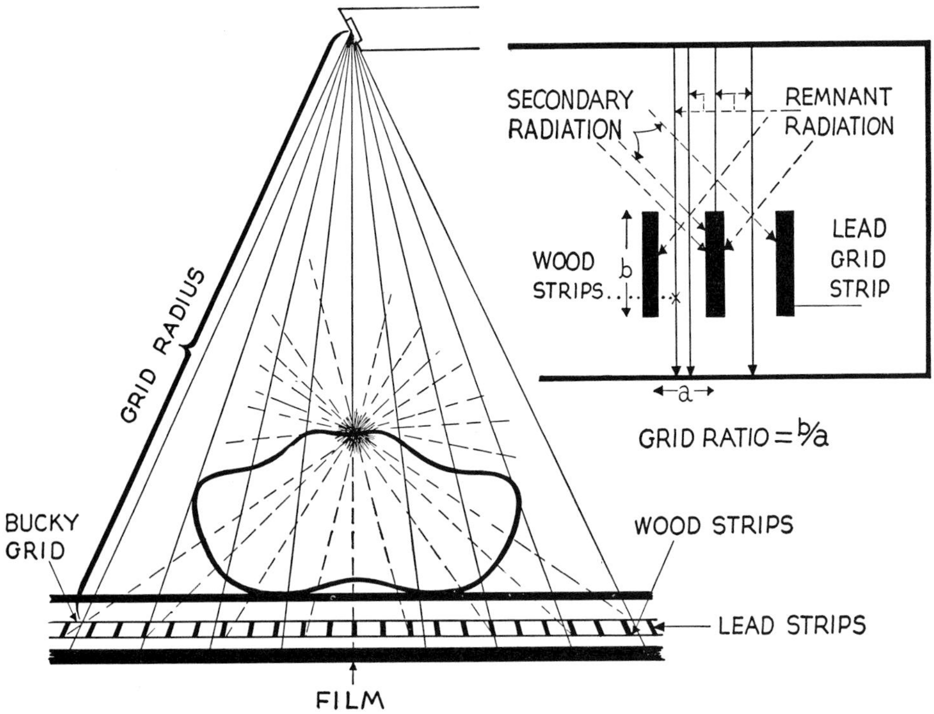

Figure 1–8 Diagram of a Potter-Bucky diaphragm and how it is used.

X-Ray Film in a Cardboard or Plastic Holder. When it is desirous to detect minute foreign bodies by x-ray examination, the x-ray film in a cardboard or plastic holder is utilized wherever possible to avoid potential artefacts.

The Stationary and Moving Grids (Figure 1–8). The x-rays are scattered in all directions when they strike an object. The grid is a device for collimating the x-rays after transmission through the patient so that the image on the film is formed by "orderly" rays which have penetrated the body part. The grid is composed of alternating strips of lead with intervening pieces of wood, bakelite, or plastic. It is placed between the part to be radiographed and the film, usually under the table top.

When a focused grid is employed, only the rays in direct radial alignment with the target can pass through the grid, since the scattered rays are absorbed by the lead strips. When the lead strips are parallel with one another, the grid is described as "unfocused" and the target must then be at a distance of at least 40 inches from the grid. The diaphragm moves or oscillates during the exposure and thus no lines related to the lead strips are visible on the film. Grids are further characterized by their "grid ratio" as shown in the insert, and also by the number of "lines" per square unit of area.

If the grid is stationary, the lead lines will be visible on the film unless it is an extremely fine grid. Stationary grids usually have very fine lead lines, so that these are barely detectable. Moving grids (the Potter-Bucky diaphragms) are used whenever possible. These are usually oscillating types in modern equipment.

Stationary grids may be incorporated into the cassette front, in which case a "grid-cassette" is obtained.

X-RAY CONING DEVICES

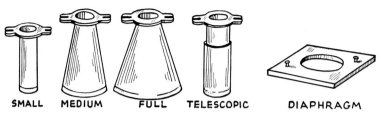

SMALL   MEDIUM   FULL   TELESCOPIC   DIAPHRAGM

Figure 1–9   Various accessories used to delimit secondary irradiation. Adjustable collimators are also available. The diaphragm is ordinarily fixed to the x-ray tube housing over the window, and the cones lock into position over the diaphragm.

Cones, Apertures, and Adjustable Diaphragms for Delimiting the X-ray Beam (Figures 1–9 and 1–10).   Cones and aperture diaphragms are applied to the x-ray tube window in order to delimit the x-ray beam and reduce the secondary radiation. There are various designs of these coning devices, so it is desirable to choose the cone best suited both to the anatomic part and to the size of the film being exposed. Adjustable cones equipped with light localizers are also available for this purpose; these may be cylindrical as shown, or rectangular in cross-section.

Cones have the additional advantage of reducing the stray radiation toward the operator, and thus furnish a very important protective mechanism as well.

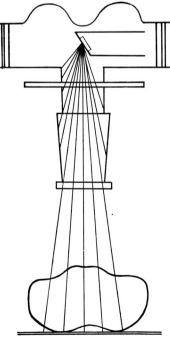

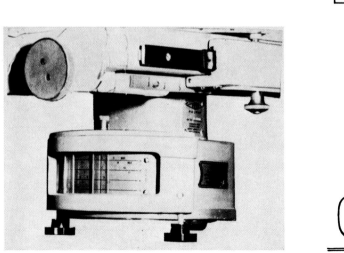

Figure 1–10   *A*. An adjustable cone for various field sizes with a light localizer and centering device. *B*. Diagram illustrating effect of cone in delimiting scattered radiation.

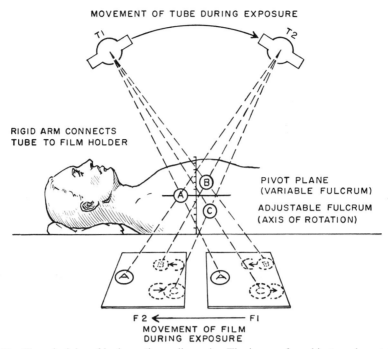

MOVEMENT OF TUBE DURING EXPOSURE

RIGID ARM CONNECTS
TUBE TO FILM HOLDER

PIVOT PLANE
(VARIABLE FULCRUM)

ADJUSTABLE FULCRUM
(AXIS OF ROTATION)

F 2 ← ——————— F I
MOVEMENT OF FILM
DURING EXPOSURE

Figure 1–11   The principles of body section radiography. The image of an object, such as *A*, located on the pivot plane remains in focus during movement of tube and film. An object above the pivot plane, *B*, or below, *C*, blurs due to its realignment between tube and film as they move during exposure.

Body Section Radiographic Equipment (Figure 1–11).   The body section radiograph is known by various names, depending on slightly different operating principles (i.e., polytome, laminograph, stratograph, tomograph). The main factor in each of these is the movement of the x-ray tube and the x-ray film around a fixed axis or center of rotation, so that all images are blurred except in the chosen axis or center. By this means a planar surface or small area of the anatomy is brought into clear perspective while adjoining areas are "blurred." In the radiography of the middle ear or larynx the "cuts" are usually no more than 1 mm. apart, whereas in larger body volumes, such as the chest, the usual "cuts" are 1 cm. or more apart.

Stereoscopic Radiographic Accessories (Figure 1–12).   To obtain radiographs that can give a true stereoscopic effect, two slightly different views are obtained — the first is the view as seen by one eye; and the second is that seen by the other eye. This is done by taking two radiographs from two separate tube positions; the amount of tube shift is in a definite ratio to the normal interpupillary distance. These two radiographs are then placed in a stereoscope or viewed with special prismatic lenses or mirrors, so that each eye will see the separate image. The brain fuses the two images into one and the correct spatial, three dimensional relationship is reconstructed.

The Fluoroscopic Screen and the Fluoroscope (Figure 1–13).   Fluoroscopy is the study of the x-ray image after its transformation into visible light. By it the physician may study an anatomic part in motion. After passing through the patient, the remnant rays strike a special screen composed of fluorescent crystals which transform the x-rays into visible light. Leaded glass protects the observer's head and eyes.

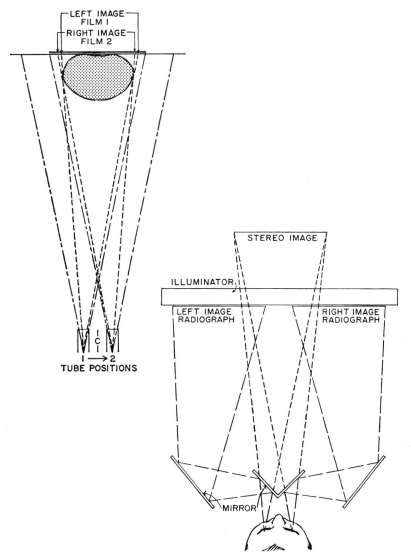

Figure 1–12 The principles of roentgen stereoscopy.

Electronic Amplification of the Fluoroscopic Image is now almost universally employed (Figure 1–14). Instead of the image being seen directly after it strikes the fluoroscopic screen, it is electronically amplified and directed toward an "output phosphor," which may then be viewed through appropriate lens and mirror systems, or by a

Television Camera.   The image may thus be projected by closed circuit television systems to appropriately placed monitors.

Spot Film Radiography.   This refers to instantaneous radiography while the patient is being examined by fluoroscopy. Spot film radiography is accomplished by storing a cassette in a lead-protected frame on the fluoroscopic screen, or on the frame support of the image tube. When radiography is desired, a rapid spring release brings the cassette over the patient, and the x-ray technique selector switch rapidly and automatically switches from fluoroscopic exposure values to radiographic factors, and the exposure is made. Often photoelectric ion chambers (or cells) are

DIAGRAM OF A FLUOROSCOPE

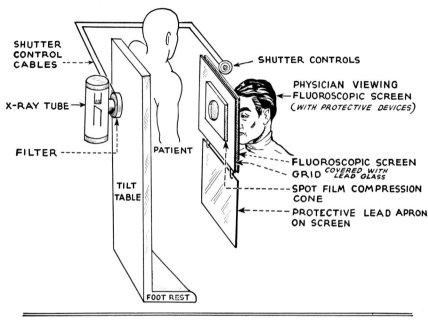

SHUTTER CONTROL CABLES

SHUTTER CONTROLS

PHYSICIAN VIEWING FLUOROSCOPIC SCREEN *(WITH PROTECTIVE DEVICES)*

X-RAY TUBE

FILTER

PATIENT

FLUOROSCOPIC SCREEN

GRID *COVERED WITH LEAD GLASS*

SPOT FILM COMPRESSION CONE

TILT TABLE

PROTECTIVE LEAD APRON ON SCREEN

FOOT REST

Figure 1–13   Diagram of a simple fluoroscope.

interposed, so that the exposure is automatically timed to produce an optimum radiographic image.

Radiography with the Image Amplifier.   When the image amplifier is used, a movie camera or any other suitable still camera may be focused on the output phosphor of the image tube, and the image may be totally or in part transmitted to the camera, even while it is being viewed by the television camera system. It is also possible to photograph the television monitor (called *kineradiography*).

Rapid Sequence Film Changers for Roll Film or Cut Film, or Rapid Sequence Cassette Changers.   The first device allows x-ray films to be interposed between two intensifying screens in rapid sequence, and the second allows cassettes to be changed rapidly and mechanically. Films may be changed as rapidly as 12 per second, and cassettes as fast as two per second, simultaneously in each of two planes if desired. Programmers are provided with changers so that appropriate sequences may be chosen. Long films (as long as three 14- by 17-inch films in tandem) may thus be exposed in one apparatus, and may include, for example, the lower aorta and an entire lower extremity simultaneously and in rapid sequence.

Magnification (Figure 1–15).   Magnification of an anatomic part results when the film is at a considerable distance from it. The degree of magnification is directly related to the square of the distance between the film and the focal spot of the x-ray tube as compared with the anatomic part and the x-ray tube. When the film-to-focal spot distance is equal to the film-to-anatomic part distance, a magnification of four times will result. The limiting factor in this procedure is the size of the focal spot of the x-ray tube. It must be virtually pinpoint in size for optimum detail with magnification. Special high speed fractional focal spot tubes have been manufactured for this purpose, with effective focal spots approaching 0.1 mm. Heat dissipation must be very efficient for x-ray tubes of this design, and magnification of small anatomic parts with films in rapid sequence is becoming available.

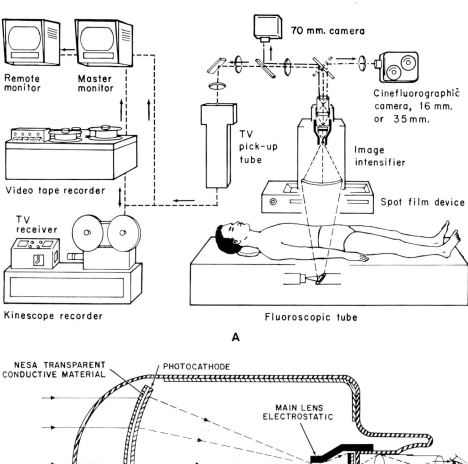

A

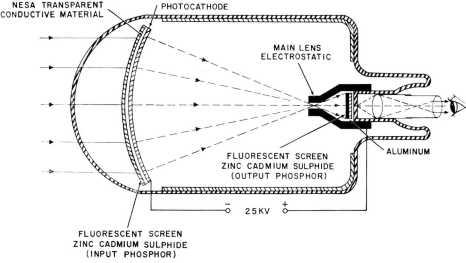

B

Figure 1–14 *A.* Diagram of presently available fluoroscopic equipment, containing image amplification, cinefluoroscopy, cineradiography, and kineradiography. The amplified image from the output phosphor may be conducted through a lens and mirror system directly to the human eye, directly to a stationary or movie camera device, through a television camera to a television receiver, or through a television camera to a television tape recorder. The image on the television screen may be viewed by the human eye or by an additional camera. *B.* Diagram of image intensifier tube. X-rays which pass through an object form an image on the input phosphor screen emitting visible light proportional to the impinging radiation. The photocathode in contact with this screen is an alkali metal layer that emits electrons proportional to the brightness of the fluorescing screen. This electron image is focused by electrostatic lenses on the output phosphor screen. The electrons are also accelerated by a potential difference of 25,000 volts, and a further increase in brightness results. The proper optical system permits the eye to view the brilliant image. To obtain cineradiography or television fluoroscopy one needs only to substitute a movie or television camera for the eye, or a mirror system, to obtain simultaneous viewing and filming.

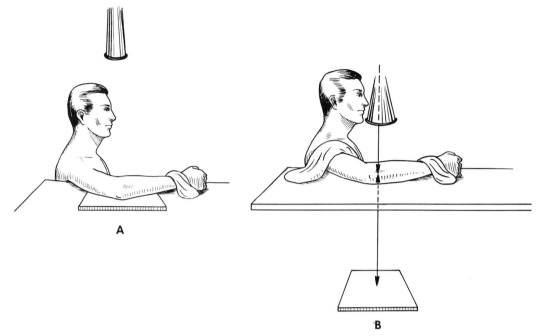

Figure 1–15 *A.* When the film is in close contact with the part being radiographed, and the x-ray tube target is 36 to 40 inches from the film, very little magnification of the part ensues. *B.* When the film is at a considerable distance from the part being radiographed, and the target-to-film distance is 24 to 30 inches, considerable magnification results.

Contrast Media. A body part may be visualized radiographically on the following bases:

1. By its delineation with naturally occurring fatty envelope (or fascia);
2. By its naturally occurring gaseous content (lungs; gastrointestinal tract);
3. By its naturally occurring mineral salts, such as the calcium salts of bone;
4. By abnormally occurring gas, fat, or calcium salts;
5. By the introduction of a contrast agent, which may be either *radiolucent* or *radiopaque*, into or around the body part. Such contrast agents should be physiologically inert and harmless.

Commonly Used Radiopaque Contrast Media

BARIUM SULFATE is particularly useful in studies of the gastrointestinal tract. It is inert, is not absorbed, and does not alter the normal physiologic function. At times it is used in colloidal suspension to obtain a particular type of coating of the mucosa, more effective for demonstration of small filling defects.

ORGANIC IODIDES, which are *predominantly excreted by the liver* and concentrated in the biliary tract, include: Telepaque, Priodax, Teridax, and Monophen, which may be given orally; and Cholografin (Biligrafin), which may be given intravenously.

ORGANIC IODIDES, which are *predominantly excreted or secreted selectively by the kidneys,* include: Hypaque (sodium diatrizoate), Renografin (Meglumine diatrizoate), and Iothalamates, such as Conray or Angioconray. These compounds are also widely favored for visualization of blood vessels. In low concentrations, they may be used for visualization of hepatic and biliary radicles by T-tube and operative cholangiography.

ORGANIC IODIDES *in suspension* may be particularly useful in visualization of oviducts (hysterosalpingography) or the urethra (Salpix, Skiodan Acacia, Cystokon, and Thixokon).

IODIZED OILS, *slowly absorbable,* are used in myelography (Pantopaque); or in bronchography (Dionosil Oily).

Radiolucent Contrast Substances are *gases:* air, oxygen, helium, carbon dioxide, nitrous oxide and nitrogen. These are commonly used for visualization of the brain (pneumoencephalograms and ventriculograms), joints (arthrograms), and occasionally the subarachnoid space surrounding the spinal cord (myelograms). Air may also be used in the pleural space, peritoneal cavity, and pericardial space. Carbon dioxide is of particular value since it is well tolerated and very rapidly absorbed.

FUNDAMENTAL GEOMETRY OF IMAGE FORMATION AND INTERPRETATION

Penumbra Formation, Distortion, Magnification.   The manner in which an object placed in the path of the x-ray beam is projected depends on five factors: (1) the size of the light source (effective focal spot size); (2) the alignment of the object with respect to the focal spot of the x-ray tube and the screen or films; (3) the distance of the object from the focal spot; (4) the distance of the object from the screen or film; and (5) the plane of the object with respect to the screen or film.

When an image is projected from a pinpoint light source or focal spot, its borders are sharp. However, if the light source is a larger surface, the image is ill-defined at its periphery owing to "penumbra" formation (Figure 1–16).

In order to reduce the penumbra as much as possible the following measures must be taken: (1) the focal spot must be as small as possible; (2) the object-to-film distance must be as short as possible; (3) the object-to-focal-spot distance must be as distant as is practicable (Figure 1–17).

When the object is not centrally placed with respect to the central ray its image will be distorted, sometimes considerably (Figure 1–18). At times this distortion is unavoidable if one is to visualize an anatomic part (Figure 1–19), and in some of the radiographic positions this distortion brings into view a part which otherwise would be hidden. The phenomenon of projection may therefore be utilized to good advantage.

The problems of magnification, already described, must also be taken into consideration. Teleroentgenograms are "long distance radiographs," which diminish magnification. A minimum target-to-film distance of 6 feet is utilized for this purpose and even under these circumstances magnification of 10 to 15 per cent may be obtained for structures at a considerable distance from the film.

Developing a Three-Dimensional Concept.   The obvious method of examining an anatomic part is to look at it from several different aspects. This allows a three-dimensional concept of the entire structure. In x-ray studies usually a minimum of two different views are employed for this purpose. Even under these circumstances, the student must develop the ability to reconstruct the isometric viewpoint and the three-dimensional view for himself. In looking at a chest radiograph the student would do well at first to train himself to picture in his mind's eye the position of the various lobes of the lung and the ribs of the thoracic cage, the diaphragm and the interlobar fissures. The liberal use of transparent models and articulated skeletons

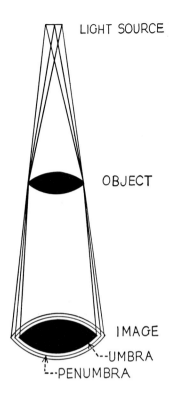

LIGHT SOURCE

OBJECT

IMAGE
--UMBRA
---PENUMBRA

Figure 1–16 Penumbra and umbra formation from a "surface" light source rather than a "point" source. Most x-ray targets are surface sources even though they are a fraction of a millimeter in size. A 0.12 mm. focal spot if available is useful in some magnification procedures, since it has virtually no penumbra. Most x-ray images are made with effective focal spot sizes of 0.6 mm. to 2 mm.

Figure 1–17 Effect of focal-object distance and object-film distance on magnification.

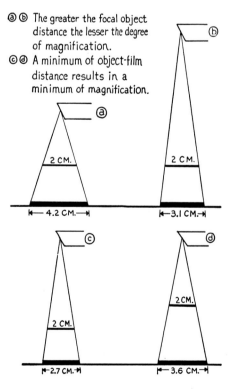

ⓐ ⓑ The greater the focal object distance the lesser the degree of magnification.
ⓒ ⓓ A minimum of object-film distance results in a minimum of magnification.

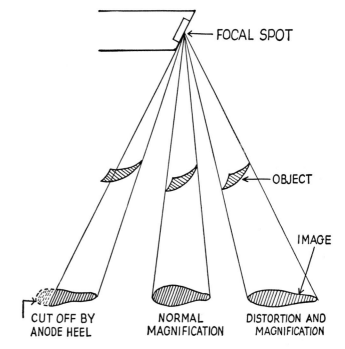

Figure 1–18 Effect of position of object with respect to the central ray on distortion, magnification, and anode heel effect.

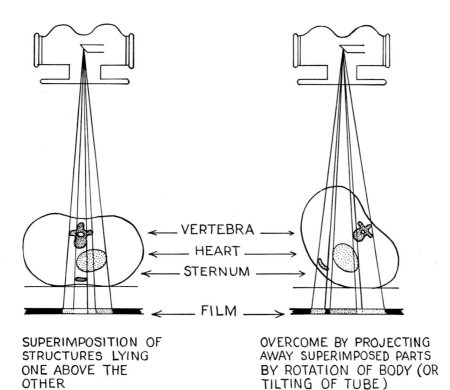

Figure 1–19 Utilization of projection to overcome superimposition of anatomic parts.

is very helpful in these exercises. Another simple exercise, the drawing of a vertebral body while studying the articulated spine, will do much to teach this three-dimensional perspective.

Questions—Chapter 1

1. Draw a diagram of the basic components of an x-ray tube labeling the following:
   a. Filament.
   b. Electron stream.
   c. Target.
   d. Cooling mechanism of target.
   e. Effective focal spot.
   f. Useful x-ray.
2. What is the main purpose of rectification of the x-ray circuit?
3. Draw a table with five columns with the following terms at the head of each column in sequence: Very radiolucent; moderately radiolucent; intermediate radiolucency; moderately radiopaque; very radiopaque. Under each column list as many substances as you know that are appropriate for the column. Define the terms radiopaque and radiolucent.
4. Draw a diagram illustrating how radiation affects a film when it passes through various anatomic parts differing in radiolucency and/or radiopacity.
5. Draw a simplified block diagram of an x-ray circuit explaining the various component parts.
6. Why does a cassette need special care? Why is it so easy to introduce artefacts on x-ray film when an x-ray cassette is employed?

References

Altschule, M. D.: The use of urographic agents to measure renal clearances and blood flow. Medical Science, 15:50, 1964.

Barnhard, H. J., and Barnhard, F. M.: The emergency treatment of reactions to contrast media. Radiol. Clin. N. A., 3:51–64, 1965.

Cahoon, J. B.: Formulating X-ray Techniques. Fifth Edition. Durham, N. C., Duke University Press, 1961.

Etter, L.: Glossary of Words and Phrases Used in Radiology. The Fundamentals of Radiography. Medical Division, Eastman Kodak Co., Rochester, New York. Springfield, Ill., Charles C Thomas, 1960.

Hildreth, E. A., Pendergrass, H. P., Tondreau, R. L. and Ritchie, I.: Reactions associated with intravenous urography; discussion of mechanisms of therapy. Radiology, 74:246–254, 1960 (36 references).

Marshall, T. R., and Ling, J. T.: Clinical evaluation of two new contrast media: Conray and Angioconray. Am. J. Roentgenol., 89:423–431, 1963.

Meschan, I., Deyton, W. N., Schmid, H. E., and Watts, F. C.: The utilization of ^{131}I-labelled Renografin as an inulin substitute for renal clearance rate determination. Radiology, 81:974–979, 1963.

Meschan, I., Hosick, T. A., Schmid, H. E., and Watts, F. C.: Variability in renal clearance rate studies using fresh O^{131}IHA, purified product and stored product. J. Nuclear Med., 4:70–77, 1963.

Meschan, I., Schmid, H. E., Watts, F. C., and Witcofski, R. L.: The utilization of radioactive iodinated Hippuran for determination of renal clearance rates. Radiology, 81:438–446, 1963.

Peterson, H. O.: The radiologist and the special procedures. Amer. J. Roentgenol., 88:4–20, 1962.

Potsaid, M. S.: Iodinated organic contrast agents. Medical Science, 15:40–49, 1964.

Schmorl, G., and Junghanns, H.: Die Gesunde und Kranke Wirbelsäule in Roentgenbild und Klinik. Stuttgart, Germany, Georg Thieme, 1951.

Weigen, J. F., and Thomas, S. F.: Reactions to intravenous organic iodine compounds and their immediate treatment. Radiology, 71:21–27, 1958.

2

Protective Measures in
X-Ray Diagnosis

INTRODUCTION

Great benefits have accrued to mankind by the proper utilization of ionizing radiation, both in the diagnosis and in the treatment of disease. Those who would utilize ionizing radiation for its benefits, however, must be thoroughly cognizant of its hazards.

An understanding of the balance of benefit vs. hazard requires the following considerations:

1. Definitions of quantities and qualities of ionizing radiation.
2. The systemic effects of ionizing radiation on the body, as well as the organ-specific effects and their dose relationships.
3. Concepts of "safe," "acceptable," and "tolerance" doses. The differentiation of those occupationally exposed from those who are in an "uncontrolled" population.
4. Protection of the patient from excessive exposure to ionizing radiation.
5. Representative radiation doses to patients in the various diagnostic examinations.
6. Protection of the radiologist and technician (radiographer).
7. Electrical hazards in relation to handling of equipment.

DEFINITION OF PHYSICAL TERMS

Quality of Ionizing Radiation. The quality of ionizing radiation is dependent in great part on the *kilovoltage* applied and the so-called *"filters"* inserted in the beam.

X-rays produced by low voltage cathode ray tubes are ordinarily referred to as *"soft"* and do not penetrate the body part for great distances. X-rays produced by high voltage (*"hard"*) cathode rays penetrate more deeply.

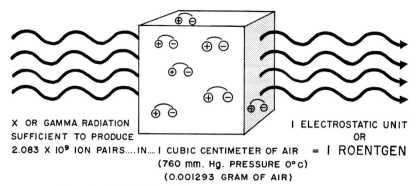

X OR GAMMA RADIATION
SUFFICIENT TO PRODUCE
2.083 X 10⁹ ION PAIRS....IN....I CUBIC CENTIMETER OF AIR   = I ROENTGEN
(760 mm. Hg. PRESSURE 0°C)
(0.001293 GRAM OF AIR)

I ELECTROSTATIC UNIT
OR

Figure 2–1   Definition of the "roentgen" in diagrammatic form.

The term "filters" with respect to radiation refers to a layer of absorbing medium, usually a metal such as aluminum, copper, tin or lead. This absorbing medium *diminishes* the soft rays relative to the hard ones, but, unlike chemical filters, does not eliminate all soft rays.

Generally, radiation produced by kilovoltages below 60 is considered soft, and 120 and 150 kilovolts moderately penetrating. Hard radiation derived from kilovoltages higher than 150 Kv. are not utilized in conventional diagnostic radiology.

In diagnostic radiology, at least 2 to 4 mm. of aluminum are ordinarily added as filtration at the open diaphragm of the tube to produce an optimum quality of radiation.

Quantification of Ionizing Radiation.   Ionizing radiations are radiations consisting of alpha, beta, gamma, neutron rays (or particles) and x-rays which produce biological effects because they ionize, or separate, electrons from their parent atoms in compounds in the body. The *roentgen* (Figure 2–1) is the internationally accepted

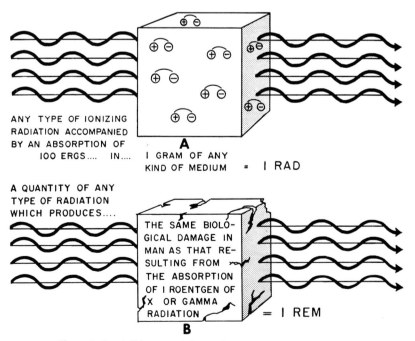

ANY TYPE OF IONIZING
RADIATION ACCOMPANIED
BY AN ABSORPTION OF
100 ERGS....   IN....

A

I GRAM OF ANY
KIND OF MEDIUM   = I RAD

A QUANTITY OF ANY
TYPE OF RADIATION
WHICH PRODUCES....

THE SAME BIOLO-
GICAL DAMAGE IN
MAN AS THAT RE-
SULTING FROM
THE ABSORPTION
OF I ROENTGEN OF
X OR GAMMA
RADIATION   = I REM

B

Figure 2–2   *A.* Diagram of the "rad." *B.* Diagram of the "rem."

unit for quantity of ionizing radiation. It is defined as *"the quantity of x- or gamma radiation such that the associated corpuscular emission per 0.001293 grams of air produces, in air, ions carrying one electrostatic unit of quantity of electricity of either sign."* In everyday radiological practice it requires approximately 200 to 300 roentgens of x-radiation in the diagnostic quality range to produce a skin erythema. This occurs usually after a latent period of several days. Although the long term hazards of repeated exposure to x-rays are great for the technician and the physician, exposures of this order are seldom necessary for patients; hence, an erythema resulting from a diagnostic roentgenologic procedure is almost never observed in a patient.

The *rad* (a word derived from "*r*oentgen *a*bsorbed *d*ose") (Figure 2–2A) *is the dose of any type of ionizing radiation accompanied by an absorption of 100 ergs of energy per gram of absorbing material.* In contrast to the roentgen, which is a measure of "ionization in air," the rad is a measure of absorbed dose in terms of ergs of energy. Wherever feasible the *rad* is a more meaningful unit of quantification of ionizing radiation, since it is the absorbed dose which is most significant in the ultimate analysis of biological effect.

The *rem* (derived from "*r*oentgen *e*quivalent *m*an") (Figure 2–2B) *is that quantity of any type of ionizing radiation which produces the same biological*

TABLE 2–1 RADIATION DOSE RECEIVED BY THE SKIN AND GONADS IN RADIOGRAPHIC EXAMINATIONS (per film)

Examination	kV.	mAs.	Focus-film distance	Added filtration	Dose per exposure (with back scatter)		
					SKIN DOSE (MR)	MALE GONAD DOSE (MR)	FEMALE GONAD DOSE (MR)
Sinuses	80	40	27 in.	3 mm. Al	1040	0.1	0.05
Hand and wrist, postero-anterior	46	50	27 in.	3 mm. Al	100	0.04	0.01
Chest, postero-anterior	90	3	27 in.	3 mm. Al	8	0.01	0.02
Chest, tomogram (apices) antero-posterior	85	12B	100 cm.	3 mm. Al	110	0.01	0.02
Dorsal spine, antero-posterior	75	80B	110 cm.	3 mm. Al	480	1.0	1.3
Lumbar spine, antero-posterior	75	80B	110 cm.	3 mm. Al	480	0.5*	95.0
Lumbar spine, lateral	85	300B	110 cm.	3 mm. Al	2000	2.25	270.0
Lumbar sacral joint, lateral	90	400B	110 cm.	3 mm. Al	3000	2.0	350.0
Pelvis, antero-posterior	75	80B	110 cm.	3 mm. Al	480	20.0*	80.0
Abdomen, antero-posterior	75	60B	110 cm.	3 mm. Al	360	0.5*	75.0
Abdomen, B meal, prone (H.V.)	90	20B	110 cm.	3 mm. Al	130	1.5	20.0
I.V.P. renal, antero-posterior	75	80B	110 cm.	3 mm. Al	480	0.5*	95.0
I.V.P. bladder, antero-posterior	75	80B	110 cm.	3 mm. Al	480	10.0*	80.0
Knee, antero-posterior	82	25B	110 cm.	3 mm. Al	180	1.25	0.4
Ankle, antero-posterior	70	30B	36 cm.	1 mm. Al	200	0.1	0.025
Duodenal cap series, postero-anterior (H.V.)	90	15G	18 in.	5 mm. Al + TT	130	0.05	0.05
Fluoroscopy chest (I.I.)	75	90G (3 min.)	18 in.	5 mm. Al + TT	900	3.0	3.0
Fluoroscopy B meal (I.I.)	75	150G (5 min.)	18 in.	5 mm. Al + TT	1500	5.0	5.0

* Lead rubber protection.
B—Bucky.
G—Stationary grid.
H.V.—High voltage screen–Ilford Red Seal film. Other examinations Par Speed screens and Red Seal film extremities.
Ilfex film.
I.I.—Image intensifier, tube current, 0.5 to 1.0 Ma.
From Ardran, G. M., and Crooks, H. E.: Gonad Radiation Dose from Diagnostic Procedures. Brit. J. Radiol., *30*:295–297, 1957.

damage in man as that resulting from the absorption of 1 roentgen of medium energy x-rays. This, too, is a measure of biological dose, and *is obtained by multiplying the dose in rads by the relative biological effectiveness (RBE) of the irradiation.*

The *RBE is a measure of absorbed radiation,* but is *the ratio of the absorbed dose in rads of x-rays or gamma rays to the number of rads of a particular radiation producing the same biological effect.* Thus, the RBE for cobalt-60 radiation as compared with 250 KvP x-ray radiation is ordinarily given as approximately 0.8 to 0.9.

Radiation Dose Received by the Skin and Gonads in Radiographic Examinations. Table 2–1 summarizes interesting dose data in relation to commonly employed diagnostic radiologic procedures, with usual exposure times and numbers of films. The estimated dose to the ovaries ranges between 0.1 and 0.3 roentgens for the examination of the upper gastrointestinal tract, and 0.1 to 0.8 roentgens for barium enema study of the colon. It is important to know the physical factors employed: thus, in comparing a fluoroscopic technique with a target-to-tabletop distance of 30 inches without added filtration and one with a distance of 46 inches and 3 mm. added filtration, it becomes evident that a dosage ratio of almost 10:1 exists at the surface. At 10 cm. depth, however, this difference is minimized.

The dose range for single abdominal films to the mid-pelvis was found to fluctuate between 0.05 and 0.1 R for each exposure.

It is apparent from study of the accompanying table that the exposure most important for consideration is that related to the lumbar spine, the pelvis, the abdomen, excretory urography, and fluoroscopy.

EFFECTS OF IRRADIATION ON THE BODY

Systemic Effects

Although the biological effects of whole body irradiation must be understood, it is important to realize that in diagnostic radiology relatively small dose levels are utilized, and the whole body effects to be described are usually of academic interest only. *There is little chance for the occurrence of observable deleterious effects with the small doses employed in diagnostic roentgenology.* Effects from whole body irradiation begin to be observable at approximately the 100 rad level. These whole body levels are not obtained in diagnostic radiology. Whole body radiation which exceeds 125 rads may produce severe illness; 250 rads may produce severe illness with loss of hair temporarily, nausea, and even a persistent skin erythema after an initial delay. The person exposed to 250 rads will usually regain his hair and recover fully in a matter of a few months with no *observable* consequences. Very much later in life he may become susceptible to some secondary illness or perhaps even cancer in one form or another. If whole body irradiation of 500 rads occurs, approximately one-half of those exposed will not survive beyond 21 days. The major effects of doses of this order are related to alterations in the bone marrow and reticuloendothelial apparatus. As the whole body exposure level increases to 1500 or 2000 rads, additional effects occur in the gastrointestinal tract, where glandular functions are suppressed, mucosa eroded, and hemorrhage encountered. In doses exceeding 3000 or 4000 rads, additional deleterious effects upon the central nervous system occur.

Fortunately, *dramatic protection is afforded the body by shielding even a part of it from ionizing radiation.* For example, if only one leg is thoroughly shielded, the chance of survival is markedly increased; and of course, irradiation of only a small part of the body has far less dramatic effects. In therapeutic radiology, it is not uncommon to administer 5000 to 6000 rads over a period of five to six weeks to a given small area of the body in treatment of a malignant tumor, with only moderate or negligible systemic effects.

Organ, Tissue, and Cellular Effects

Radiation Effects on Cells.   These effects may be summarized for present purposes as follows:

1. *Radiation suppresses the ability of cells to multiply and reproduce themselves.*

2. *Cells are most sensitive to radiation just before DNA synthesis is well established in their reproductive cycle.* This cycle consists of a resting state, a synthesis period during which DNA is synthesized rapidly, and a third phase when growth continues but DNA synthesis has largely stopped. Division takes place after this third phase.

3. There is a measure of recovery in irradiated cell populations which is not purely physical. Recovery is enhanced by reducing the temperature.

4. Hypoxic tissues are less subject to the damaging effects of radiation as compared with normally oxygenated tissues. This difference in sensitivity is called the *"oxygen effect."*

5. Generally speaking, *at elevated temperatures* nearly unbearable in the living system, *radiation sensitivity is high.*

6. If the body or the cells being irradiated contain a high concentration of *sulfhydryl (−SH) radicals,* there is a sharp *reduction in radiation sensitivity.* Substances like cysteine and glutathione fall into this category of protective substances.

Superficial Injuries from Ionizing Radiation.   Superficial injuries include: (1) Epilation, (2) Skin damage, (3) Brittleness of nails with ultimate destruction of nail bed, (4) Lenticular cataracts of the eye, and (5) Mucous membrane ulceration of the lips, mouth and oropharynx. In practically no instance is an immediate effect noted. Depending upon the dose, however, the effects may be seen in days or weeks. If the initial delay period is approximately one week, complete repair usually does not ensue for a period of four to six weeks. Skin carcinomas may result from superficial injury by ionizing radiation after several years.

Hematopoietic Injury.   Injury to the reticuloendothelial system results not only in a deprivation of the primordial cells but in thrombocytopenia, lymphopenia, leukopenia, anemia, and loss of specific immune response. Repeated exposure over a prolonged period of time in certain susceptible persons may result in malignant transformation, such as leukemia.

Variability of Tissue or Organ Radiosensitivity.   The different tissues, organs, or organ systems throughout the body vary in their *radiation sensitivity.* To a great extent, this *depends upon the relative numbers of undifferentiated, immature, and unspecialized cells as against the number of cells which are highly differentiated.* This relationship was noted very early in the history of radiation biology and has been called the "law of Bergionér and Tribondeau," which states: ". . . that radiosensitivity of tissues depends upon the number of undifferentiated cells which the tissue contains, the degree of mitotic activity in the tissue, and the length of time that the cells of the tissue stay in active proliferation. . . ."* Ordinarily there is a continuous equilibrium between the rate of reproduction of new cells and the disappearance of older, more highly differentiated cells. Radiation interferes with cell division by suppression of DNA synthesis, chromosome breaks, recombinations, and bridging. A tissue with a high rate of mitotic activity may be expected to be radiosensitive. *The hematopoietic system is the most radiosensitive, and the central nervous system the most radioresistant; the respiratory and gastrointestinal systems occupy intermediate positions.*

A detailed description of the various effects of radiation on the several systems is not included in this text since the *dose levels in diagnostic radiology would not, if properly carried out, induce any detectable change in any of the organ systems of the body.*

Genetic Aberrations and Sterility.   Radiation may produce *chromosome breaks, recombinations, bridging, and other alterations in chromosomal constitution.* Radiation *interferes with mitosis* through its effects on the centromeres, resulting in an unequal distribution of chromosomes on the spindle at anaphase. There is also a *high probability of direct gene mutation.*

Apart from the genetic aberrations, the embryo itself is probably in a most sensitive stage in respect to radiation and will be profoundly affected by radiation at any stage of its development. If the embryo is irradiated the reactions induced will depend upon those organ systems which happen to be in a high stage of differentiation at the time. This in turn will determine the kind of abnormality which ultimately could be manifest. In mammals, irradiation of a developing embryo before it becomes implanted in the uterus often results in the death of the embryo. It is here that *exposures in diagnostic radiology can be highly significant,* since it has been shown that "even with doses as low as 200 r, up to 80 per cent of early preimplantation embryos of mice are killed."† In the mouse, neonatal death may result from irradiation seven to twelve days after fertilization; in humans this is probably equivalent to the second through the sixth week of pregnancy. Even doses as low as 25 roentgens in the seven and one-half day mouse will greatly increase the incidence of skeletal anomalies.

In general, *it is during the first trimester of pregnancy that the embryo is most vulnerable,* and exposure of the embryo during this period should be avoided if at all possible. Irradiation of women of child-bearing age after the first ten days following the onset of menstruation or during the first trimester of pregnancy should also be avoided if at all possible. Exposure of the pelvis under these circumstances should be limited to emergency procedures. *However, whether or not abnormalities are produced in human embryos during any roentgenologic diagnostic procedure is as yet uncertain.*

Inferences regarding the induction of sterility in man are largely made from comparable data in experimental animals, with full knowledge that this data cannot always be extrapolated. Exposure to radiation in males does not appear to affect sexual capacity or libido, but with sufficient exposure *fertility* may be at least temporarily impaired. Permanent sterility can be produced if sufficiently high doses of radiation are given to the gonads in isolated fashion. *Sterility would not be likely to result from whole body exposure* since the doses required to produce this result would be so high as to bring about one or another of the death-producing radiation syndromes. Sterility may be produced if the number of sperm is sufficiently reduced so that the probability of fertilization of an egg is reduced to unlikely levels. *It is*

---

*Pizzarello, D. J., and Witcofski, R. L.: Basic Radiation Biology. Philadelphia, Lea & Febiger, 1967, p. 226.
†Pizzarello and Witcofski, p. 260.

probable that at doses in the diagnostic range of roentgenology there is no clear-cut period of complete sterility or even of functional sterility since doses well below 200 or 300 rads would have been administered. It is possible that "a single dose of about 250 rads" might "bring about sterility for about one year."*

In females, a similar situation obtains. Permanent sterilization varies with the age of the individual because older females require smaller doses to be made sterile than do younger ones. Again, the radiation would have to be given directly to the ovaries to bring about sterility—otherwise the dose required for whole body radiation for sterility would cause one or another of the death-producing radiation syndromes. "Induced menopause" may result in individuals nearing the menopause with doses as little as 1000 to 1500 rads. In females thirty years of age or younger, a permanent induced menopause may not result even with doses of 3000 rads.

Reduction in Life Span. Exposure of the entire body to radiation of significant degree shortens the life span. This is true whether the exposures are given over short or long periods of time. Irradiated animals also develop malignant tumors more frequently than do nonirradiated ones. However, even if all deaths due to malignant disease are excluded, the life of an irradiated animal is shorter by statistically significant amounts than that of a nonirradiated one. There are some experiments in rodents, however, where very small doses of irradiation, accumulated over periods of time, actually produced a life-lengthening effect.

In general, it may be concluded that the amount of shortening of life of small animals after total body irradiation appears to be dependent upon dose, but it is not known whether or not a threshold dose response in respect to this does exist. *Hence, it is doubtful that a life-shortening effect at the usual dose ranges employed in diagnostic roentgenology can ever be demonstrated.*

COMMON SENSE APPROACH TO THE PROBLEM OF HAZARDS DUE TO DIAGNOSTIC RADIOLOGY

The dose levels administered to the skin and gonads in radiographic examinations are usually so low that general effects of irradiation such as superficial injuries, hematopoietic injury, induction of malignant tumors, reduction in life span, or other effects such as lenticular cataract and sterility, are not observed. This is true, assuming that appropriate precautions are employed. However, the genetic aspects of roentgen exposure are important for consideration (Meschan; Norwood).

If one accepts the age of 30 to 35 years as the age by which most people have produced the majority of their children, we need take into account only this younger population when considering the genetic aspects. Presumably, if the entire population is at risk, the average individual dose must be reduced to 4.8 rads for the total span prior to the 30 to 35 year age limit.

A higher dose (ten times this amount) is permitted for people whose occupation requires a risk exposure to radiation. This is permitted because of the great genetic dilution afforded by the unirradiated public.

Although diagnostic procedures have increased in frequency, (Gitlin and Lawrence; Stein) technical improvements have correspondingly diminished exposure.

By present standards, it is estimated that, even though the individual dose is limited to 4.8 rads during the first 30 to 35 years of life, it is probable that a dose of

---

*Pizzarello and Witcofski, p. 250.

approximately 14 rads to the gonads from *all* sources during the first 30 years of life, would not upset the genetic milieu of mankind.

Webster has calculated that the saving of lives by discovery of tuberculosis and cancer by routine chest radiology far exceeds the hazards of the irradiation encountered when good technique is employed. **So long as physicians have proper indication for the examinations chosen in a given patient, and so long as physicians who handle radiation use this valuable tool with the greatest of precision and precaution to themselves and their patients and personnel, the medical usage of radiation in the future is not likely to be deleterious to mankind.**

PROTECTION OF THE PATIENT IN X-RAY DIAGNOSIS

Exposure of the patient in x-ray diagnosis may be considered from the standpoint of protection against the acute and chronic effects of overexposure, each being dealt with in relation to fluoroscopy on the one hand, and radiography on the other.

Safety Recommendations for Fluoroscopy
(Figure 2–3)

1. *The target-to-tabletop distance, minimum 18 inches.*
2. *Added filtration, 2.5 to 4 mm. of aluminum.*

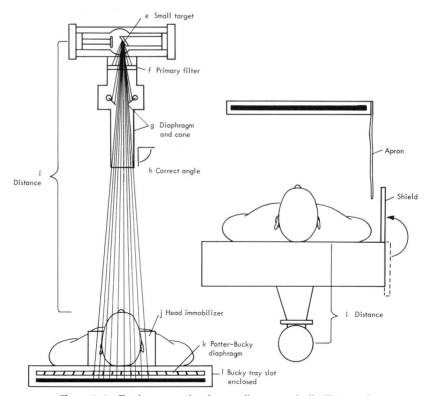

Figure 2–3 Further protection factors diagrammatically illustrated.

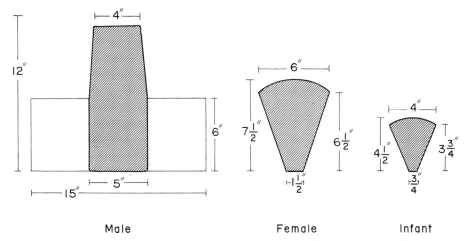

Male   Female   Infant

Figure 2–4 Design of lead gonad shields useful in radiography. These should be 1/8 inch lead (or equivalent) in thickness. They should be placed over the patient's gonads whenever such exposure is not required as part of the diagnostic test.

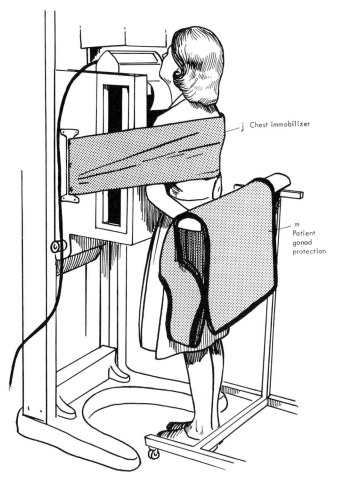

Figure 2–5 Further radiation protection factors diagrammatically illustrated.

3. *Whenever possible, protective equipment such as lead rubber should be utilized over the gonads* (Figure 2–4).

4. *The dosage rate measured in air at the tabletop should be measured frequently, and if possible, kept at a minimum of 5 roentgens per minute (or less).*

5. *The field size should be as small as possible* to cover the anatomic part being studied. In patients under 40 years of age, the gonads should be covered with leaded shielding as protection against scattered radiation (Figure 2–5).

6. A *self-limiting fluoroscopic timer* should be placed in the circuit and this will automatically shut off the fluoroscope after an appropriate time interval. In general, the timer may be set anywhere between three and five minutes (Figure 2–6).

7. *High kilovoltage techniques* with milliamperage settings as low as possible, not to exceed 5 milliamperes, and dial setting appropriately modified to deal with different body thicknesses of infants, children, and adults should be employed. The examination should be conducted as rapidly as warranted.

8. *To diminish exposure, films should be employed whenever feasible rather than fluoroscopy.*

9. *Image intensifiers should be employed in fluoroscopy* (Figure 2–7).

10. *Hand fluoroscopes should never be employed.*

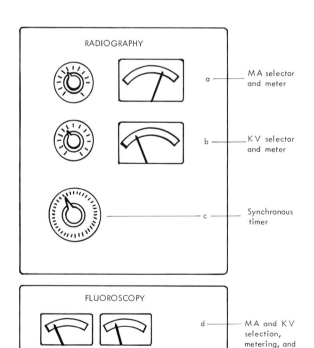

Figure 2–6 Diagram of x-ray control panel to emphasize control of physical factors in radiation protection.

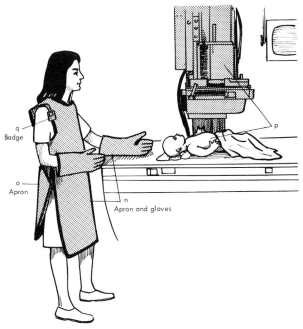

Figure 2–7   Further radiation protection factors diagrammatically illustrated.

Safety Recommendations for Radiography

1. Whenever possible, *fast film-screen combinations* should be used if they are suitable for a given purpose *without sacrifice of detail.*
2. *Added filtration,* up to 3 or 4 mm. of aluminum, should almost invariably be used. A minimum of 0.5 mm. of aluminum must be added for beryllium window x-ray tubes for mammography.
3. An adequate range of *adjustable or fixed cones* and *diaphragms* for limiting the useful beam to the smallest dimension necessary in any given examination ought to be available and used.
4. Tests should be made to *insure that leakage of radiation from the tube housing to cones is limited to the degree recommended* by the National Bureau of Standards Handbook 60.
5. For diagnostic examinations in general: (a) *Gonadal exposure must be minimized.* With suitable cones and diaphragms and special lead protective devices, the gonads can be kept out of the direct beam in most cases. In particular, shielding of the testes can be practiced without much difficulty or inconvenience. (b) *Expert assistance and calibration should be sought for every x-ray machine installation.* Dosage factors should be established at tabletop, and the maximum permissible fluoroscopic time posted; tests must ascertain that there is no radiation leakage from the x-ray tube housing. The equipment should be designed to afford a maximum of shielding for the operator.
6. There are *three basic factors* to consider always: (*a*) *time of exposure,* (*b*) *distance from the radiation source,* and (*c*) *shielding* provided.
7. It is recommended that, prior to the examination of all females *under 45 years of age* who could conceivably be pregnant, a brief *menstrual history be obtained.* Rapid immunologic type tests are now available which may, if desired, be performed in minutes prior to radiation exposure. Where impregnation is a possibility, radiation exposure of the

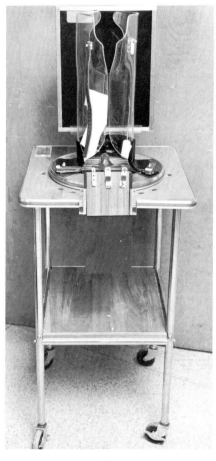

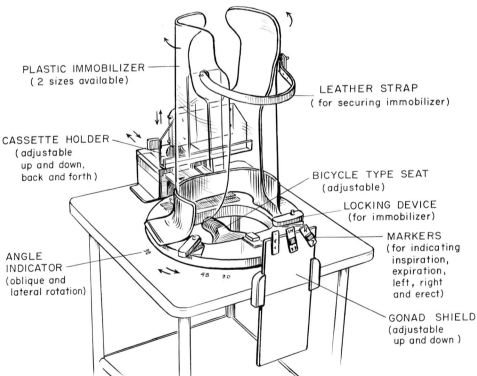

PLASTIC IMMOBILIZER
(2 sizes available)

LEATHER STRAP
(for securing immobilizer)

CASSETTE HOLDER
(adjustable
up and down,
back and forth)

BICYCLE TYPE SEAT
(adjustable)

LOCKING DEVICE
(for immobilizer)

MARKERS
(for indicating
inspiration,
expiration,
left, right
and erect)

ANGLE
INDICATOR
(oblique and
lateral rotation)

GONAD SHIELD
(adjustable
up and down)

Figure 2–8 Pigg-o-stat infant immobilization device for erect radiography (made by Modern Way Immobilizers, Memphis, Tennessee).

embryo should be avoided except in dire emergencies. If pregnancy is known to exist, radiation should be avoided in the first trimester and as much as possible in pregnancy thereafter. When feasible, diagnostic x-ray examinations should be scheduled during the first 10 days following the onset of menstruation.

8. Patients should be immobilized as much as is comfortably possible to avoid movement during the radiographic exposure. (For chest immobilizer in children see Figure 2–8).

9. During petrous bone tomography especially, the dose to the eye can be as high as 10 roentgens (Chin et al.). When simple lead shields are placed over the cornea this dose may be reduced to about 1 roentgen. (For tables see Chin et al.).

PROTECTION OF PERSONS OCCUPATIONALLY EXPOSED TO RADIATION

In this discussion special emphasis is placed on the protection of physicians and radiologic technicians.

The International Commission on Radiological Protection (ICRP) has made separate regulations for three types of personnel: (1) those occupationally exposed, (2) those near controlled areas or atomic energy establishments, and (3) the population at large. The ICRP has also made separate regulations for different tissues of the body (Johns).

Persons Occupationally Exposed

The blood-forming organs, gonads, and lenses of the eyes:
The maximum permissible total dose (D) accumulated in these tissues shall be governed by the formula:

$$D = 5 (N - 18) \text{ rems}$$
$$N = \text{age in years}$$

This formula implies a constant dose rate not exceeding 5 rems per year or 0.1 rem per week. In any period of 13 weeks, a dose rate of 3 rems must not be exceeded.

The ICRP allows for an accidental exposure of 25 rems once in a lifetime, and this accidental dose may be additive to that allowed by the above formula.

For single organs other than the gonads, blood-forming organs, and eyes:
A higher dose for these other organs is permitted as follows: skin and thyroid: 8 rems every 13 weeks; hands, forearms, feet and ankles: 20 rems every 13 weeks; other internal organs not mentioned above: 4 rems every 13 weeks.

For whole body exposure from the uptake of several isotopes:
The same limitations are applied as for blood-forming organs, gonads, and lenses of the eyes.

For Persons Near Controlled Areas of Atomic Energy Establishments

The yearly adult dose to the gonads, the blood-forming organs and the lenses of the eyes must be limited to 1.5 rems or less and 3 rems to the skin and thyroid.

For children who live near controlled areas, the yearly dose is limited to 0.5 rems per year (one-tenth of the value for those occupationally exposed).

Public at Large

Here the main concern is the genetic hazard. The dose for those below age 30 must not exceed 5 rems plus the lowest possible contribution from medical procedures. Since the background varies in different parts of the country, this is excluded from consideration. Also, the dose of 5 rems is actually an average figure which includes those who are occupationally exposed — and thus the average for the rest of the population is less. It is estimated that the general population is exposed to about 3 rems from background radiation and about 3 rems from diagnostic procedures.

In order to comply with these rules, physicians and technicians are advised as follows:

1. Personnel must never allow themselves to be exposed to a direct beam of radiation. Immobilization devices must be devised and used. Anesthesia must be employed if immobilization is not feasible.

2. Lead protective gloves and aprons must be worn at all times when the possibility of exposure to scattered radiation exists. These leaded flexible materials must have a lead equivalency of 0.5 mm. (Figure 2–7). Roentgenoscopic screens with lead rubber drapes also diminish radiation exposure.

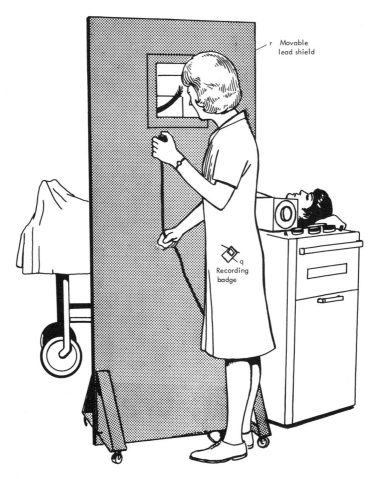

Figure 2–9   Further radiation protection factors diagrammatically illustrated.

3. The physician's unprotected hands, wrists, arms, or other parts should never be exposed to the x-ray beam (Figure 2–9).

4. Avoid fluoroscopy if films can suffice.

5. Suitable kilovoltage and milliamperage settings at fluoroscopy should be adopted as follows (with image amplifier):

Abdomen	95 KvP.	2–3 Ma. or less
Chest	70 KvP.	2 Ma. or less
Thick extremities	60 KvP.	2 Ma. or less
Thin extremities	50 KvP.	$\frac{1}{2}$–1 Ma.
Children	50–60 KvP.	$\frac{1}{2}$–1 Ma.

6. General *principles of fluoroscopic use:*

a. Shutters must be closed down to no more than 30 to 40 square centimeters.

b. The fluoroscope should be used intermittently, and should be avoided when the patient is not intercepting the beam.

c. The examination should be concluded as quickly as possible, usually within 5 minutes. It is well to have a special timing device in the circuit to turn off the machine automatically when this time is exceeded.

d. When fractures are being set or foreign bodies located, alternation of radiography with manipulation should be used, if possible, rather than fluoroscopy.

e. All x-ray machines should be thoroughly checked before using for (1) electrical shock properties, (2) radiation leakage around tube housing, (3) roentgen output at the tabletop, (4) scattered irradiation dose pattern around the table with a phantom in place, (5) safe operating voltages and times, and (6) safe continuous fluoroscopic times from the standpoint of the x-ray tube and thermal capacity.

f. All lead protective equipment should be checked frequently for possible leakage (aprons and gloves).

7. It is well for the physician and his personnel to have frequent blood counts (at least at six month intervals), and if there is any opportunity for absorption of internal emitters, frequent urinary assays should also be performed. *A radiation monitoring device should be worn at all times and frequent assays noted in a permanent record.* The film badge or pocket chamber measurement device is ordinarily considered adequate for this purpose, unless there is a single opportunity for excessive exposure, in which case an accurately calibrated milliroentgen pocket chamber would be more accurate and should be employed (Figure 2–9). Metabolic changes are perhaps incurred by physicians even though sufficient protection is worn. The high incidence of leukemia in radiologists, and even among nonradiologists, has already been alluded to; it is possible that when certain susceptible individuals receive even the minimal exposure allowed for in the above methods, they may ultimately develop this form of malignancy.

8. When the mobile x-ray unit is employed, a movable lead shield should also be used to protect the technician or radiologist during the x-ray exposure.

PROTECTION AGAINST ELECTRICAL HAZARD

In addition to the radiation hazard, an electrical hazard may also be present, particularly in the presence of explosive anesthetic gases. It is well under these circumstances to employ only explosion-proof procedures with explosion-proof apparatus. No switch devices should be permissible below 5 feet above the floor, and all switches should be explosion-proof. Provision should be made to protect all exposed cables from mechanical damage, and these should be periodically inspected for defects or abrasions. Low voltages and currents also present a hazard during intracardiac catheterization by inducing ventricular fibrillation (Barry et al.). All the exposed noncurrent-carrying parts of the apparatus should be permanently grounded in acceptable fashion with good ground leads. It is well to bear in mind first aid practices, such as artificial respiration and emergency treatment for burns, in the event the need for these should arise.

Although the high tension does not extend to the darkroom, the hazard of electrical shock in the darkroom is great. Lighting fixtures form the greatest potential hazard in this regard and must be carefully installed with every attention to proper insulation and grounding.

Questions — Chapter 2

1. Define the following terms:
    a. "Soft" x-rays.
    b. "Hard" x-rays.
    c. X-ray filters.
    d. The roentgen.
    e. The rad.
    f. The rem.

2. Describe some of the general effects of irradiation on skin, hair, nails, bone marrow and its constituents, the body's immune mechanisms, genes, chromosomes, the eye, the reproductive organs.

3. What are the rules for protection of a patient in x-ray diagnosis?

4. What are the rules for protection of the physician employing radiation for x-ray diagnosis?

References

Addendum: Maximum permissible radiation exposures to man. Radiology, *71*:263–266, 1958.

Archer, V. W., Cooper, G., Jr., Kroll, J. G., and Cunningham, D. A.: Protection against x-ray and beta radiation; lead glass fabric. J.A.M.A., *148*:106–108, 1952.

Ardran, G. M., and Crooks, H. E.: Gonad radiation dose from diagnostic procedures. Brit. J. Radiol., *30*:295–297, 1957.

Ardran, G. M.: Hazards from increasing use of ionizing radiations: Symposium; The dose to operator and patient in x-ray diagnostic procedures. Brit. J. Radiol., *29*:266–269, 1956.

Aub, J. C., Evans, R. D., and Hempelmann, L. H.: Late effects of internally-deposited radioactive materials in man. Medicine, *31*: 221–239, 1952.

Bacon, J. F., and Leddy, E. T.: Proctection in roentgenoscopy. Med. Clin. N. Amer., *29*: 1036–1041, 1945.

Barry, W. F., Jr., Starmer, C. F., Whalen, R. E., and McIntosh, H. D.: Electrical shock hazards in radiology departments. Amer. J. Roentgenol., *95*:976–980, 1965.

Blair, N. A.: Data pertaining to shortening of life span by ionizing radiation. A.E.C. Documents U.R.-442, April, 1956.

Braestrup, C. B.: Past and present radiation exposure to radiologists from the point of view of life expectancy. Amer. J. Roentgenol., *78*: 988–992, 1957.

Brucer, M.: The clinical story of radiation damage and definition of radiation complex. Conn. Med., *28*, 167–202, 1964.

Brues, A. M., and Sacher, G. A.: Analysis of mammalian radiation injury and lethality; in Nickson, J. J., ed.: *Symposium on Radiobiol-*

ogy: The Basic Aspects of Radiation Effects on Living Systems. New York, John Wiley and Sons, 1952, pp. 441–465.

Chamberlain, R. H.: The medical use of ionizing radiation: Benefits and hazards. Mod. Med., 26:67–73, 1958.

Chin, F. K., Anderson, W. B., and Gilbertson, J. D.: Radiation dose in critical organs during petrous tomography. Radiology, 94:623–727, 1970.

Clark, D. E.: The association of irradiation with cancer of the thyroid in children. J.A.M.A., 159:1007–1009, 1955.

Crow, J. F.: Genetic considerations in establishing maximum radiation doses. Radiology, 69:18–22, 1957.

Dahlgren, S.: Thorotrast tumors: A review of the literature and report of two cases. Acta Path. Microbiol. Scand., 53:147–161, 1961.

Dobzhansky, T.: Genetic loads in natural populations. Science, 126:191–194, 1957.

Dunn, L. C.: Radiation and genetics. Scientific Monthly, 84:6–10, 1957.

Failla, G., and McClement, P.: The shortening of life by chronic whole-body irradiation. Amer. J. Roentgenol., 78:946–954, 1957.

General Electric X-ray Corporation: What You Should Know About X-ray Protection.

Gitlin, J. N., and Lawrence, P. S.: *Population Exposure to X-rays U.S. 1964.* U.S. Department of Health, Education and Welfare. Public Health Service Publication, No. 1519. (Excellent bibliography)

Hatano, H.: III. Short term and long term effect: A. Some aspects of radiation biochemistry. Conn. Med. 28:203–206, 1964.

Henshaw, P. S., and Hawkins, J. W.: Incidence of leukemia in physicians. J. Nat. Cancer Inst., 4:339–346, 1944.

International Commission on Radiological Protection: Recommendations of the ICRP, 1958. Pergamon Press, New York, 1959.

Johns, H. E.: *The Physics of Radiology.* 2nd ed. Charles C Thomas, Springfield, Ill., 1964.

Jones, H. B.: Factors in longevity. Kaiser Found. Med. Bull., 4:329–341, 1956.

Laughlin, J. S., Meurk, M. L., Pullman, I., and Sherman, R. S.: Bone, skin, and gonadal doses in routine diagnostic procedures. Amer. J. Roentgenol., 78:961–982, 1957.

Lewis, E. B.: Leukemia and ionizing radiation. Science, 125:965–972, 1957.

Lincoln, T. A., and Gupton, E. D.: Radiation dose to gonads from diagnostic x-ray exposure. J.A.M.A., 166:233–239, 1958.

Macht, S. H., and Kutz, E. R.: Detection of faulty roentgenoscopic technique by direct radiation measurements. Amer. J. Roentgenol., 68:809–814, 1952.

Macht, S. H., and Lawrence, P. S.: National survey of congenital malformations resulting from exposure to roentgen radiation. Amer. J. Roentgenol., 73:442–446, 1955.

MacKenzie, K. G., Preston, C. D., Stewart, W., and Haggith, J. H.: Thorotrast retention following angiography: A case with postmortem studies. Clin. Radiol., 13:157–162, 1962.

March, H. C.: Leukemia in radiologists in a twenty year period. Amer. J. Med. Sci., 220: 282–286, 1950.

March, H. C.: Leukemia in radiologists, ten years later. Amer. J. Med. Sci., 242:137–149, 1961.

Medical Research Council: Hazards to man of nuclear and allied radiation. Command Paper 9780, London, Her Majesty's Stationery Office, 1956.

Meschan, I.: A common sense approach to the problem of the hazards of radiation fall-out and diagnostic radiology. J. Ark. Med. Soc., 57:488–498, 1961.

Moloney, W. C., and Kastenbaum, M. A.: Leukemogenic effects of ionizing radiation on atomic bomb survivors in Hiroshima City. Science, 121:308–309, 1955.

Muller, H. I.: Genetic damage produced by radiation. Science, 121:837–840, 1955.

Myrden, J. A., and Hiltz, J. E.: Breast cancer following multiple fluoroscopies during artificial pneumothorax treatment of pulmonary tuberculosis. Canad. Med. Ass. J. 100:1032–1034, 1969.

National Research Council.: The biological effects of atomic radiation: Summary reports from the Study by National Academy of Sciences. Washington, D.C., 1956.

Neel, J. Van G., and Schull, W. J.: The effect of exposure to the atomic bomb on pregnancy termination in Hiroshima and Nagasaki (Publication #461). Washington, D.C., National Academy of Sciences, National Research Council, 1956.

Norwood, W. D.: Common sense approach to the problem of genetic hazard due to diagnostic radiology: Report based in part on study of exposures in a small American industrial city. J.A.M.A., 167:1928–1935, 1958.

Pizzarello, D. J., and Witcofski, R. L.: *Basic Radiation Biology.* Philadelphia, Lea & Febiger, 1967.

Proceedings of Health Physics Society, 114–126, New York, Pergamon Press, June, 1956.

Ritter, V. W., Warren, S. R., Jr., and Pendergrass, E. P.: Roentgen doses during diagnostic procedures. Radiology, 59:238–251, 1952.

Russell, L. B., and Russell, W. L.: Radiation hazards to the embryo and fetus. Radiology, 58:369–376, 1952.

Russell, W. L.: Genetic effects of radiation in mice and their bearing on the estimation of human hazards. Proc. of International Conference on Peaceful Uses of Atomic Energy. Geneva, Vol. II, pp. 382–383, 401–402, 1955.

Sanders, A. P., Sharpe, K., Cahoon, J. B., Reeves, R. J., Isley, J. K., and Baylin, G. J.: Radiation dose to the skin in roentgen diagnostic procedures: Optimum KVP and tissue measurement techniques. Amer. J. Roentgenol., 84:359–368, 1960.

Seltser, R., and Sartwell, P. E.: Ionizing radiation and longevity of physicians. J.A.M.A., 166:585–587, 1958.

Seltser, R., and Sartwell, P. E.: The effect of occupational exposure to radiation on the mortality of physicians. J.A.M.A., 190, 1046–1048, 1964.

Simon, N., Muller, H. J., Tessmer, C. F., and Henry, H. F.: Side effects of radiation: Genetics, carcinogenesis, aging, and leukemogenesis. Lippincott's Medical Science, 15:69–77, 1964.

Simpson, C. L., Hempelmann, L. H., and Fuller, L. M.: Neoplasia in children treated with x-rays in infancy for thymic enlargement. Radiology, *64*:840–845, 1955.

Sonnenblick, B. P.: Aspects of genetic and somatic risk in diagnostic roentgenology. J. Newark Beth Israel Hosp., *8*:81–95, 1957.

Sonnenblick, B. P. (Editor): Protection in Diagnostic Radiology. New Brunswick, N. J., Rutgers University Press, 1959.

Sonnenblick, B. P.: X-rays and leukemia. Lancet, *1*:1197–1198, 1957.

Sorrentino, J., and Yalow, R.: A nomogram for dose determinations in diagnostic roentgenology. Radiology, *55*:748–753, 1950.

Stanford, R. S., and Vance, J.: The quantity of radiation received by the reproductive organs of patients during routine diagnostic x-ray examinations. Brit. J. Radiol., *28*:266–273, 1955.

Stein, J. J.: The carcinogenic hazards of ionizing radiation in diagnostic and therapeutic radiology. Ca: A Cancer Journal for Clinicians, *17*, 278–287, 1967. (Excellent compilation of references)

Stern, C.: Genetics in the atomic age. Eugen. Quart., *3*:131–138, 1956.

Stewart, A., Webb, J., Giles, D., and Hewitt, D.: Malignant disease in childhood and diagnostic irradiation in utero; Preliminary communication. Lancet, *2*:447, 1956.

Stone, R. S.: The concept of a maximum permissible exposure. Radiology, *58*:639–660, 1952.

Ulrich, H.: The incidence of leukemia in radiologists. With a review of the pertinent evidence for radiation leukemia. New Eng. J. Med., *234*:45–46, 1946.

U.S. National Bureau of Standards. Protection Against Radiations From Radium, Co-60 and Cedium-137 (issue Sept. 1). Handbook 54. Washington, D.C., Supt. of Documents, 1954.

U.S. National Bureau of Standards. X-ray Protection (issue Dec. 1). Handbook 60. Washington, D.C., Supt. of Doc., 1955.

U.S. National Bureau of Standards. Safe Handling of Bodies Containing Radioactive Isotopes. Handbook 65. Washington, D.C., Supt. of Documents, 1958.

U.S. National Bureau of Standards. Maximum Permissible Body Burdens and Maximum Permissible Concentrations of Radionuclides in Air and in Water for Occupational Exposure. Handbook 69. Washington, D.C., Supt. of Documents, 1959.

Upton, A. C., Furth, J., and Chirstenberry, K. W.: The late effects of thermal neutron irradiation in mice. Cancer Res., *14*:682–690, 1954.

Van Swaay, H.: Aplastic anaemia and myeloid leukaemia after irradiation of the vertebral column. Lancet, *2*:225–227, 1955.

Warren, S.: Longevity and causes of death from irradiation in physicians. J.A.M.A., *162*:464–468, 1956.

Webster, E. W.: Hazards of diagnostic radiology: A physicist's point of view. Radiology, *12*:493–507, 1959.

Weens, H. S., Clements, J. L., and Tolan, J. H.: Radiation dosage to the female genital tract during fluoroscopic procedures. Radiology, *62*:745–749, 1954.

Webster, E. W.: Hazards of diagnostic radiology: A physicist's point of view. Radiology, *72*, 493–507, 1959.

3

General Terms and Concepts Regarding Diagnostic Radiology

DEFINITION OF TERMS WITH SPECIAL RADIOGRAPHIC USAGE

Increased density: denotes a lighter or whiter shadow on the x-ray film or a darker shadow on the fluoroscopic screen, as produced by substances of greater density or thickness.

Decreased density: denotes a darker or blacker shadow on the x-ray film or a lighter one on the fluoroscopic screen. It is produced by substances of low density or slight thickness.

Increased radiolucency (hyperlucency): implies greater penetrability by the x-rays, and has the same connotation as decreased density.

Increased radiopacity: implies diminished penetrability by the x-rays and has the same connotation as increased density.

Antero-posterior and postero-anterior: indicates that aspect of the patient first in contact with the x-ray beam and thereafter the beam exit surface. Thus, the patient is in the postero-anterior position when the x-ray beam strikes the posterior aspect of the patient first and the anterior part of the patient is next to the film. The patient is in the antero-posterior position when the beam strikes the anterior aspect of the patient first.

Laterality: in describing the laterality of the patient relative to the x-ray beam, one always names the lateral or oblique projection according to the side of the patient closer to the film. Thus, a *right lateral film* is one taken with the right side of the patient next to the film. A *left lateral* is the reverse.

Obliquity: the oblique projections are named according to the side of the patient which is closer to the film. Thus, a *right anterior oblique* film is taken with the right anterior aspect of the patient closest to the film. A *right posterior oblique* film is obtained when the right posterior aspect of the patient is closest to the film. There are also the left anterior and left posterior oblique positions. The patient or part is usually at an angle of 45 degrees unless otherwise specified in these oblique views.

Recumbency: indicates that the patient is lying down when the film is taken. He may be either *supine* (on his back) or *prone* (on his abdomen). The beam in these cases is vertical with respect to the patient.

Decubitus films: the patient is in the *decubitus* position when he is lying on either side while an antero-posterior or postero-anterior film is taken. The beam in these cases is always horizontal. Thus, *right lateral decubitus* means that the right side of the patient is uppermost. *Left lateral decubitus* is the reverse. A more accurate terminology is desirable as follows: (1) Horizontal beam study, antero-posterior, with the patient on right (or left) side. (2) Horizontal beam study, postero-anterior, with the patient on right (or left) side. (3) Horizontal beam study, with patient supine (or prone) and right (or left) side nearest film.

Erect position: in this position the patient or the anatomic part is upright and the beam is horizontal. An erect chest film may be obtained with the patient standing or sitting.

Semirecumbent (also called semi-erect):   this term implies that the vertical axis of the part being radiographed is at an angle of approximately 45 degrees with the horizontal.

Filling defect: a space-occupying mass within a hollow organ.

Niche: in the wall of a hollow organ a recess which tends to retain contrast media. This term usually implies ulceration. A niche, in contrast to a diverticulum, has a broad, wide neck fusing imperceptibly with the contour of the lumen of the organ, whereas a diverticulum has a narrow neck.

Fluid level: the interface between fluid and air; it always assumes a horizontal appearance. The air above the fluid level is of diminished density, while the fluid itself is of intermediate density.

Bone sclerosis: an increase in the density of bone so that its radiographic appearance is much whiter than normal.

Eburnation of bone: same as bone sclerosis.

Osteoporosis: a pathologic state in which there is a diminished number of ossified trabeculae, so that the bone appears more radiolucent. The trabeculae which remain are normal bone.

Osteomalacia: a pathologic state characterized by diminished bone density due to loss of bone mineral content. The protein content of the bone is less impaired or may not be impaired at all.

Hyperlucency of bone: a radiographic appearance of either osteoporotic or osteomalacic bone. This term should be utilized in description of the radiographs unless the true pathologic state is known.

Lipping: a small osteophyte formation on the margins of the articular surfaces of bones. This is also called bony spur formation, although the latter term is commonly reserved for nonarticular bone.

Artefacts: changes on the film which do not have an anatomical basis directly related to the part being radiographed but are introduced by some technical fault, such as dirt in the cassette, or static electrical charge. Occasionally artefacts are introduced by items of clothing, immobilization devices, or even hair braids projected over the part.

Comparison films: films taken of the side opposite to the one in question for comparison with the suspected abnormal side. These are very useful, particularly in children, and should be taken whenever possible.

Serial films: films taken in sequence, either during a single study or after longer intervals of time, such as days or weeks.

GENERAL ASPECTS OF RADIOGRAPHIC PATHOLOGY

Introduction and Definition.   The radiograph is a record of the remnant radiation which penetrates the body part and strikes the film (Figure 3–1). It is composed of various gradations of black and white, the blackest portions representing areas of greatest penetrability, and the whitest areas, those of greatest opacity. The interpretation of these gradations of black and white depends upon a careful comparison of normal and abnormal anatomy and physiology, coupled with interpretation of pertinent clinical facts.

Sequence of Study of Radiographs.   The usual sequence in the study of a radiographic examination is as follows:

1. Identification of the *type of examination* and the *views obtained.*
2. Description of the *radiographic pathology in objective terms.*
3. Notation of the available *clinical data* with respect to the problem at hand.
4. *Synthesis* of the objective findings on the radiograph with the significant clinical data.
5. *Designation of disease states* in which both the radiographic and the clinical data would relate together properly.
6. *Recording of a spectrum of possible disease states* beginning with the most probable and ending with the least probable on a statistical basis.
7. *Suggestion of additional radiographic or other studies* which might assist further in the differential diagnosis.

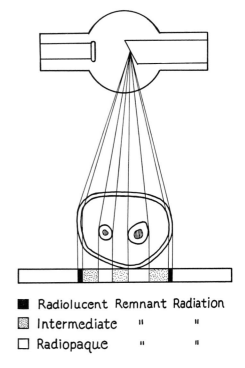

Figure 3–1 Diagrammatic illustration of how remnant radiation will vary in intensity and radiopacity, when x-rays pass through the tissues of the forearm, shown in cross section.

■ Radiolucent Remnant Radiation
▨ Intermediate   "   "
□ Radiopaque   "   "

Identification of Type of Examination and Films Obtained. The student is referred to our related text *Radiographic Positioning and Related Anatomy* for detailed elaboration of these matters. We must assume that the student has acquired a thorough understanding of basic radiographic positioning, the appropriate views to be obtained for specific anatomic problems, and the radiographic anatomy depicted in the views so obtained. The student must recognize "standard" views, when they are indicated, and when specific views may play an appropriate part.

It is best to arrange these views on viewing boxes in tandem with one another so that appropriate comparisons and localizations can be made. Here, the student begins to visualize the "three-dimensional concept" of the disease pattern.

If the patient has had previous similar examinations, these too must be viewed simultaneously so that a temporal concept of the disease process may be understood. Has the disease process changed? Has it remained stationary over a prolonged period of time? Are there new and adjoining densities which must be taken into account? A careful comparison of every aspect of the radiographic pathology on the old as well as the new must be outlined.

Description of Radiographic Pathology. Radiographic pathology can be classified into the following categories in practically all instances: abnormality in (1) *position* of an organ or part; this includes the relationship to adjoining structures; (2) *size;* (3) *contour or shape;* (4) *density;* (5) *architectural pattern,* either a. *"edge"* pattern ("margins of lesion") or b. *internal* pattern; (6) *function;* (7) *number;* (8) *time sequence* (seconds, minutes, days, weeks, months, or even years); (9) *changes in response to treatment.* Additional descriptive categories may be applied in special circumstances to certain regions, organs, or organ systems.

RADIOGRAPHIC PATHOLOGY—ITS GENERAL UNIVERSAL DESCRIPTION

Abnormality in:

Position and positional relationships
Size
Contour or shape
Density (increased or decreased)
Architectural pattern
    Internally
    At margins
Function
Number
Time sequence
Response to treatment

For example, in respect to the skeletal system, *alignment* of bone fragments with respect to one another and to the normal line of weight-bearing is important. Alignment of bones in respect to a joint is also important.

In the skeletal system, as in the lungs, the exact position of the abnormality must be described. In the long bones, is it epiphyseal, metaphyseal, or diaphyseal? In the lungs, is it in the upper lobe, middle lobe, or lower lobe?

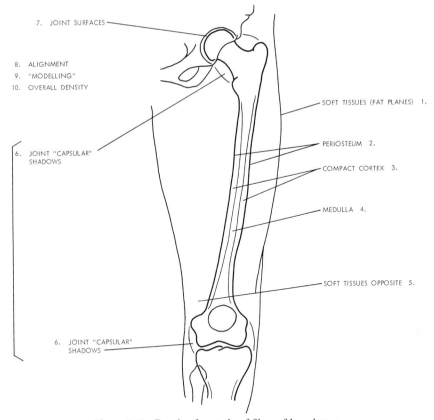

Figure 3-2   Routine for study of films of long bones.

In each area of the body a routine for study will be recommended. In the case of bones, for instance, the following sequence for detecting radiographic pathology is employed (Figure 3-2):

1. Changes in the cutaneous, subcutaneous or muscular tissues, or periosteal layer;

2. Changes in the compact cortex or the medullary sponge bone;

3. Changes which may be diffuse or localized to the epiphysis, metaphysis, or diaphysis.

In the case of joints a slightly different sequence is employed (see also Chapter 11):

1. Pericapsular tissues;

2. Joint surfaces;

3. Joint width;

4. Subarticular bone;

5. Loose bodies within the joints.

All these terms add to a better understanding of the disease process and are important in radiographic description of pathology.

Architectural Description concerns the "edge" or "marginal pattern," and the "internal appearance," in respect to the abnormal anatomic part, or the roentgen pathology per se. If a margin is present, there may or may not be a discrete "white line," suggesting a capsule or reaction in the adjoining bone. The "white line," if present, may be continuous, discontinuous, thin (less than 1 mm. ordinarily), moderately thick (1 to 2 mm.), or thick (approximately 3 mm. or more). Lung lesions may be ill-defined, nodular, linear, or lucent. If circumscribed and lucent, the margin may be thin or thick; if thick, it may be shaggy or regular. Each of these descriptive terms has special significance in relation to probable pathology, since the thin line may suggest a thin-walled cyst, while the thick wall suggests either tumor or abscess. The internal architectural appearance is of equal significance whether it is homogeneous, mottled, reticular, linear, lucent, or has water density, calcific density, or even greater than calcific density. Moreover, if there is a calcific density present, the size, shape, and position of the density are also important.

TERMS OFTEN USED IN ARCHITECTURAL DESCRIPTION

Margin	*Internal Appearance*
Well-defined and sharp	Homogeneous
a. No line of demarcation	Mottled
b. Thin line of demarcation	Reticular
c. Moderately thick demarcation	"Bubble-like"
d. Thick and "shell-like" demarcation	Linear-vertical
Ill-defined	Linear-horizontal
Shaggy	Lucent { gas, fat
Scalloped (or undulating)	
Laminated	
"Lacelike"	Water density
"Hair-on-end" or spiculated	Calcific density
"Maplike" or geographic	Speckled
"Picture-frame-like"	Punctate
"Spadelike"	"Popcorn-like"
"Applecore-like"	Metallic

The study of the architecture of the organ or part will often require the introduction of a contrast agent. Thus, the study of the intricate architecture of the brain may require pneumographic visualization of the ventricles or angiographic visualization of the blood vessels of the brain. A study of the architecture of the kidney, for example, will require not only excretory urography for visualization of the kidney cortex, the kidney calyces, pelves and adjoining ureters, but also renal arteriography and renal venography. The performance and study of these specialized procedures are often outside the scope of the present text, but appropriate mention will be made of them as necessary.

Terms often used in description of radiographic architecture as well as those used in description of contour have been drawn from common daily usage, where their familiarity makes for a natural basis for comparison. In some instances, these terms have become incorporated into the glossary of the radiologic vocabulary, to the extent that they conjure up specific pathology. The purist may take exception to this approach to radiologic pathology, since the application of such terms borrowed from elsewhere in our vocabulary may lead to misunderstanding. Perhaps a better substitute would be the development of a more specific radiologic vocabulary. As long as the limitations of this descriptive technique are understood, and as long as terms are borrowed and used which cannot have diverse or varied interpretations, a useful purpose is served. Care must be exercised, however, that the term employed has a specific definable connotation, preferably in terms of histopathology; and that vague terms making comparisons to items of variable appearance, size, and contour are avoided. Preference must always be given to geometric terms with specific measurements.

TERMS OFTEN USED IN DESCRIPTION OF CONTOUR

Spherical
Conical
Ellipsoid
Triangular
Erlenmeyer flask-like
Coinlike
Discoid
Platelike
Linear
Nodular
Acinar-like
Thumb-printing
Spindling
"Spiderweb-like"

New vistas are also opening up in relation to roentgen studies of *function*. Fluoroscopy, with the aid of image amplification, video tape recording, and cineradiography, now permits us to study flow phenomena in great detail, the coughing response of the bronchi of the lungs, and secretory and motor phenomena in respect to the biliary, urinary, and gastrointestinal tracts. Films in different phases of activity record inhalation, exhalation, positive pressure in the lungs with the Valsalva test, the Mueller test, gastrointestinal peristalsis, and similar phenomena. The Valsalva maneuver is particularly important in a study of the laryngeal and paralaryngeal tissues. These various phases of activity may be recorded in rapidly obtained sequential films, or by cineradiographic study.

Integration of the Radiographic Pathology with the Other Clinical Data. In essence, the various steps in radiologic diagnosis include: (1) *identification of the problem;* (2) *analysis,* to the extent that all facets are objectively separated one from the other and clearly defined; (3) *synthesis of diagnosis* by the integration of the available clinical facts and objective roentgen criteria.

This final synthesis involves a knowledge of disease patterns and of statistical incidence of disease in relation to age, sex, race, geography, familial tendency, occupational history, symptomatology, and clinical signs. The radiologist is in this instance the "complete physician."

Osler has stated that the practice of medicine is the "practice of an art which consists largely in balancing possibilities. . . . It is a science of uncertainty and an art of probability. . . . Absolute diagnoses are unsafe and made at the expense of the conscience."*

---

*Bean, W. B.: Sir William Osler's Aphorisms. New York, Henry Schuman, Inc., 1950.

Questions—Chapter 3

1. Define the following terms:
   a. Increased radiographic density.
   b. Decreased radiographic density.
   c. Increased radiolucency.
   d. Increased radiopacity.
   e. Postero-anterior position.
   f. Antero-posterior position.
   g. Right lateral film.
   h. Right anterior oblique film.
   i. Supine film.
   j. Prone film.
   k. The decubitus position.
   l. Filling defects.
   m. Niche.
   n. Fluid level.
   o. Bone sclerosis.
   p. Eburnation of bone.
   q. Osteoporosis.
   r. Lipping of bone.
   s. Artefacts.
   t. Comparison films.
   u. Serial films.
2. List nine general factors for description of radiographic pathology.
3. What factors enter into the description of "architecture" in radiographic terminology?
4. What is a good systematic approach to the development of an opinion in respect to a radiographic problem?

References

Bean, W. B.: Sir William Osler's Aphorisms. New York, Henry Schuman, Inc., 1950.

Meschan, I.: An Atlas of Normal Radiographic Anatomy. Second Edition. Philadelphia, W. B. Saunders Co., 1959.

Meschan, I.: Radiographic Positioning and Related Anatomy. Philadelphia, W. B. Saunders Co., 1968.

SECTION TWO

MUSCULOSKELETAL SYSTEM

4

Basic Concepts Regarding the Radiographic Study of Bones and Joints

BONE FORMATION

Basic Concepts. Long bones are formed in cartilage by a process known as *endochondral* (or *enchondral*) *ossification*. Flat bones, such as the vault of the skull, are laid down by direct conversion of a fibrous matrix in a process known as *intramembranous ossification*.

Long bones grow in length at the *epiphyseal plates* at either end, and circumferentially under the periosteum and endosteum.

Secondary centers of ossification known as *epiphyses* appear at intervals just outside the epiphyseal plates. That portion of the shaft of the long bone which lies inside the epiphyseal plate is known as the *metaphysis*, and the remainder is the *diaphysis*.

Sequence of Endochondral Ossification (Figures 4–1, 4–2, 4–3). In the various sites where bones are to form, the mesenchyme of each area begins to differentiate into cartilage with a surrounding membrane called the *perichondrium* (Figure 4–1A).

The cartilage cells undergo maturation and vacuolation with the secretion of phosphatase. Intercellular calcification of the cartilaginous matrix then occurs. The cartilage cells then die and the calcified intercellular matrix becomes fragmented. Blood vessels and osteogenic cells, apparently derived from the perichondrium, invade the disintegrating calcific areas (Figure 4–1B).

The osteogenic cells lay down a layer of osteoid around the calcific foci, and the osteoid ultimately becomes calcified, forming bony trabeculae (Figure 4–1C). The perichondrium has thus been transformed to *periosteum*, and the center of chondrification has become a *center for ossification*.

From this centrum, there is a gradual replacement of the chondrified anlage by blood vessels, osteoid, osteoblasts, and new bone formation, until the *epiphyseal plate* or *disk* is reached (Figure 4–1 D to G).

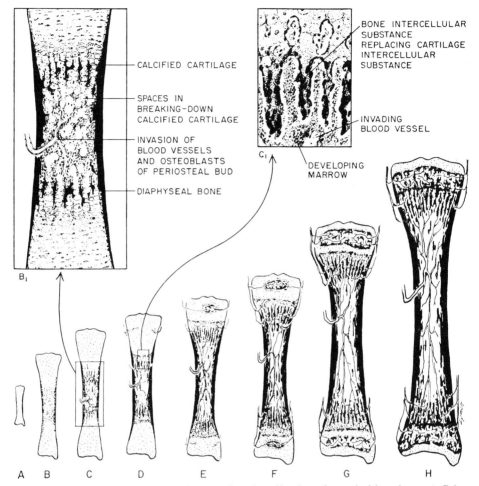

CALCIFIED CARTILAGE

SPACES IN BREAKING-DOWN CALCIFIED CARTILAGE

INVASION OF BLOOD VESSELS AND OSTEOBLASTS OF PERIOSTEAL BUD

DIAPHYSEAL BONE

BONE INTERCELLULAR SUBSTANCE REPLACING CARTILAGE INTERCELLULAR SUBSTANCE

INVADING BLOOD VESSEL

DEVELOPING MARROW

A B C D E F G H

Figure 4–1 Diagram to illustrate the growth and ossification of a typical long bone: *A.* Primary cartilaginous anlage. *B.* Primary center of ossification in shaft with early conversion of perichondrium to periosteum. *C.* Further progression of the perichondrial ossification and extension of the partially calcified cartilage upward toward the metaphysis. *D.* Continued absorption of the inner compact bony wall and new bone deposition beneath the periosteum. Note the bone intercellular substance replacing the cartilage intercellular substance and the invasion of the blood vessels from the region of the marrow. *E, F,* and *G.* Commencement and continued ossification of the epiphyses. Note the demarcation between the metaphysis and epiphyseal plate. *H.* The ossification of the epiphyseal plate and cessation of growth. Note the covering of articular cartilage which remains unossified.

Figure 4–1 continued on opposite page.

In the metaphysis just proximal to the epiphyseal plate occurs a "molding" process which, by resorbing some bone and laying down new bone, gives the metaphysis its proper tapered appearance (Figure 4–3).

Chondrification precedes ossification in a balanced fashion until chondrification ceases, and the epiphyseal plate itself becomes ossified (Figure 4–1 I to K).

In the meantime, a similar center of ossification has appeared in the epiphysis, and growth has proceeded toward the distal end of the bone or toward the adjoining joint (Figure 4–1 E to H).

The periosteum of the bone is normally not detected in the radiograph because it is not calcified, and thus offers no contrast to overlying structures. The outer por-

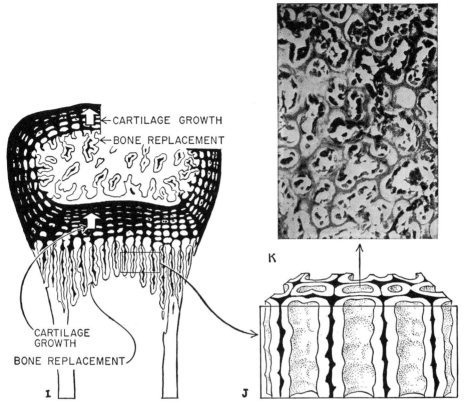

Figure 4–1 (*Continued*). *I.* Diagram which illustrates an end of a growing long bone in longitudinal section. The trabeculae appear stalactite-like in such representations. However, if they could be seen three-dimensionally, as in *J*, it would be seen that close to the plate the structures that appear as trabeculae in a longitudinal section are slices that have been cut through walls that surround spaces; they are slices cut through walls of tunnels. Photomicrograph *K* represents what is seen in a cross section cut through the metaphysis of a growing long bone of a rabbit, close to the epiphyseal disk. In it the trabeculae of bone have cartilaginous cores and they surround spaces. These spaces under the periphery of the disk become filled in to form haversian systems and such compact bone as is present in the flared extremities of bone is built by spaces such as these becoming filled in. (Modified from Ham, A. W.: *Histology,* 3rd Ed. Philadelphia, J. B. Lippincott Co., 1957.)

tions of the bone consist of dense lamellae of bony cortex; in contrast to them, the central portions are spongy and contain bone marrow within these spongy spaces. Yellow marrow consists mainly of fat; red marrow contains the hematogenic elements of the blood, as well as connective tissue, fat, blood vessels, nerve fibers, and osteogenic elements.

The blood supply (Figure 4–4) of a long bone is derived from three sets of vessels: (1) The *nutrient artery* (or arteries) is derived from the original bud to the primary ossification center. (2) The *metaphyseal and epiphyseal vessels* enter these regions directly. Epiphyseal vessels may enter the epiphysis either directly or at the junction of the cartilage covering the articular surface and the epiphyseal end plate. At times, anastomoses between the epiphyseal and metaphyseal vessels occur, and these are referred to as metaphyseal-epiphyseal vessels. (3) The *periosteal vessels* communicate directly with those vessels traversing the haversian systems and Volkmann's canals of the bone.

(*Text continued on page 55*)

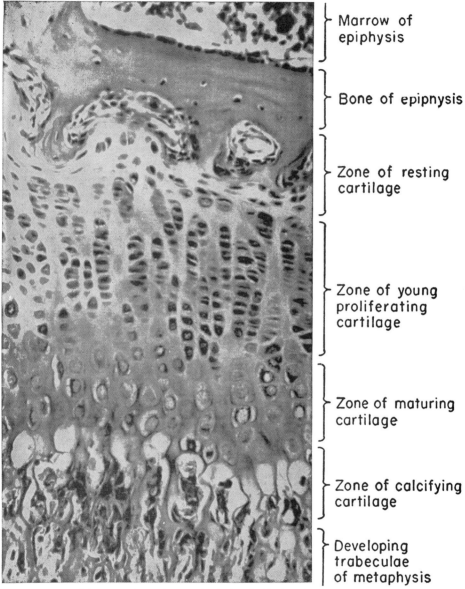

Marrow of epiphysis

Bone of epipnysis

Zone of resting cartilage

Zone of young proliferating cartilage

Zone of maturing cartilage

Zone of calcifying cartilage

Developing trabeculae of metaphysis

Figure 4–2   High-power photomicrograph of a longitudinal section cut through the upper end of the tibia of a guinea pig. Note the different zones of cells in the epiphyseal plate. (Modified from Ham, A. W.: *Histology,* 3rd Ed. Philadelphia, J. B. Lippincott Co., 1957.)

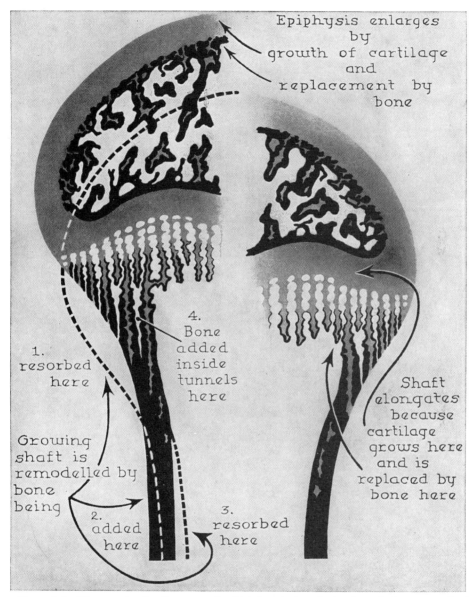

Figure 4–3   Diagram showing the manner in which bone is deposited and resorbed to account for the remodeling that takes place at the ends of growing long bones that have flared extremities. (From Ham, A. W.: J. Bone Joint Surg., *34A*:701–728, 1952.)

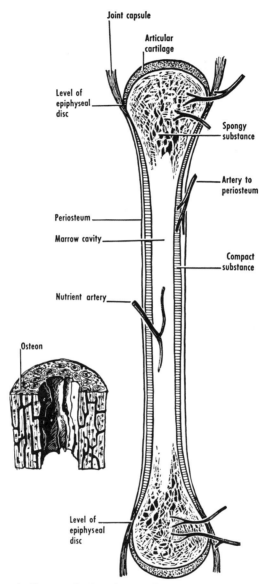

Figure 4–4 Schematic diagram of a long bone and its blood supply. The inset diagram shows the lamellae of the compacta bone arranged into osteons. The blood vessels of long bones are: (1) nutrient artery or arteries; (2) periosteal vessels supplying the compact bone; (3) metaphyseal and epiphyseal vessels arising from arteries supplying the joint. These latter pierce the compact bone and supply the spongy bone and marrow. When the epiphyseal plate fuses and becomes ossified the epiphyseal and metaphyseal vessels anastomose. (From Gardner, E., Gray, D. J., and O'Rahilly, R.: *Anatomy: A Regional Study of Human Structure,* 3rd Ed. Philadelphia, W. B. Saunders Co., 1969.)

The blood supply of the bone marrow is very rich. Originally, it is derived from the nutrient arteries, but ultimately it forms sinusoids and rich anastomoses with the other vessels described.

Afferent veins, as companion veins to the arterial system described earlier, return the blood. Nerves accompany the blood vessels throughout.

BLOOD VESSELS OF BONES

1. Compact bone derives its vessels from the periosteum. The vessels run through canals traversing the periosteal substance (Figure 4–4A).

2. Cancellous tissue is supplied in a similar way.

3. In long bones numerous apertures near the articular surfaces give passage to arteries and veins (Figure 4–4B).

4. The marrow in the body of a long bone is supplied by one or more large arteries which enter at the nutrient foramen (situated usually near the center of the body) and perforate it obliquely through the compact bone.

5. The nutrient artery (usually accompanied by one or two veins) (Figure 4–4C) sends branches upward and downward, ramifies in the marrow, and gives twigs to the adjoining canals. These twigs anastomose with the previously described vessels in the canals of compact and cancellous bone.

6. The veins emerge from the long bones in three places:

    (1) Accompanying the nutrient artery,

    (2) At the articular extremities, and

    (3) Passing out of the compact substance.

7. In the flat bones are tortuous canals in the diploic tissue for veins, with occasional perforating canals.

8. In cancellous tissue the veins have thin walls, supported by thin osseous walls.

BONE PATHOPHYSIOLOGY AND BIOCHEMISTRY

Bone Composition.   Bone is composed of 25 per cent water, 30 per cent organic substances, and 45 per cent inorganic substances. The organic content of bone consists mainly of proteins; the inorganic consists of 85 per cent calcium phosphate and 10.5 per cent calcium carbonate. The latter mineral substances are radiopaque and give bone its radiographic density.

The osteoblast is capable of extracting albumin and forming osteoid as its metabolic product. Osteoid is a collagenous substance which contains specific binding sites for bone minerals.

Factors Affecting Bone Formation (Figure 4–5).   Bone may be laid down in accordance with predetermined congenital pathways (Barnhard and Geyer). It is probable that trabeculae usually develop according to prevailing stress (Feist). Systemic factors which play an essential role in bone formation are shown in Table 4–1.

Phosphatase is found consistently at sites of new bone formation as well as in

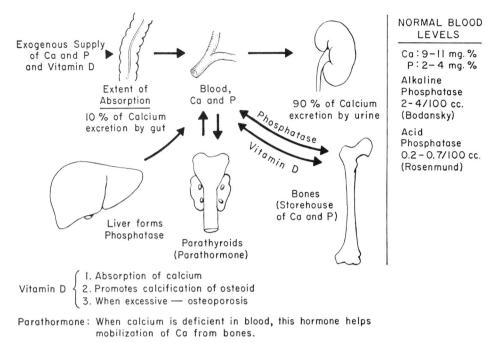

Exogenous Supply
of Ca and P
and Vitamin D

Extent of
Absorption
10 % of Calcium
excretion by gut

Blood,
Ca and P

90 % of Calcium
excretion by urine

Phosphatase

Vitamin D

NORMAL BLOOD
LEVELS

Ca : 9-11 mg. %
P : 2-4 mg. %

Alkaline
Phosphatase
2-4/100 cc.
(Bodansky)

Acid
Phosphatase
0.2-0.7/100 cc.
(Rosenmund)

Liver forms
Phosphatase

Parathyroids
(Parathormone)

Bones
(Storehouse
of Ca and P)

Vitamin D { 1. Absorption of calcium
2. Promotes calcification of osteoid
3. When excessive — osteoporosis

Parathormone: When calcium is deficient in blood, this hormone helps
mobilization of Ca from bones.

Figure 4–5   Factors governing calcium metabolism.

bone osteolysis. In an acid medium, phosphatase splits bone salts and returns the salt into the solution; in an alkaline medium, phosphatase activity promotes osteogenesis by liberating phosphate ions and precipitating calcium salts. Acid phosphatase is otherwise confined within the intact prostate gland, from which it may be released by invasive carcinoma.

Calcitonin is secreted in response to hypercalcemia in the thyroid gland (and possibly parathyroid gland as well), and its function seems to be to depress serum calcium levels by inhibiting bone resorption (Aliapoulios, Berstein and Balodimos; Foster).

Parathyroid hormone functions principally in the maintenance of a proper level of calcium in the blood by mobilization of calcium. A decrease in the level of serum

TABLE 4–1   FACTORS AFFECTING BONE FORMATION

Exogenous	Gastrointestinal Tract		Blood Serum Levels	Bone	Kidneys
Dietary calcium	Acid chyme	Favor absorption	Calcium	Storehouse for calcium and phosphorus	Glomerular function
Phosphorus	Adequate vitamin D		Phosphorus		
Vitamins	Alkaline chyme		Phosphatase*		Tubular function
A, C, D*	Excessive phosphates, fatty acids, soaps and carbonates	Impair absorption	Vitamins		
Proteins			Hormones		
			Pituitary (growth)		
			Calcitonin*		
	Fluoride		Adrenal corticosteroids (anabolic and catabolic)		
			Estrogens		
			Androgens		
			Parathormone*		

*See accompanying text.

calcium causes an increase in parathyroid hormone secretion. Parathormone exerts its effects at three distinct levels:

1. Inhibition of phosphate resorption at the renal tubular level, thus leaving a relative excess of calcium ions in the circulation;

2. Promotion of absorption of calcium and phosphorus at the intestinal mucosa level;

3. Direct stimulation of osteoclasts in bones to mobilize calcium.

Hyperparathyroidism is "primary" if it is due to a functioning adenoma of the parathyroid glands, or to diffuse hyperplasia; it is "secondary" when parathyroid stimulation results from intestinal malabsorption or renal malexcretion. "Autonomous" hyperparathyroidism (also called "tertiary") (Kleeman) is seen in those patients with chronic and overwhelming renal failure without adequate subsidence after institution of adequate treatment by dialysis and correction of electrolyte balance.

Vitamin D has three essential roles:

1. Absorption of calcium from the ileum;

2. Promotion of tubular phosphate excretion much like parathormone in the kidneys;

3. Direct action on bone by potentiating the osteoclastic activity stimulated by parathormone.

As a fourth possible function it may tend to catalyze bone calcification.

THE CORRELATION OF THE BONE RADIOGRAPH WITH THE PHOTOMICROGRAPH

Normal Bone.   In the normal healthy state, bone is a constantly changing organ, and bone formation and bone resorption are in equilibrium with one another except as required by growth and repair.

The accompanying radiograph, low-power photomicrograph (Figure 4–6A) and diagram (Figure 4–6B) show the following:

The dense, white zones (Figure 4–6A) immediately adjoining the epiphyseal plate, shown in (4) and (6), represent zones of compact bone in the former, and calcified cartilage and osteoid in the latter (the zone of provisional calcification). The compact bone (2) is readily differentiated from the spongy bone of the diaphysis (7).

The articular cartilage is of intermediate radiolucency and blends with the surrounding intermediate-density soft tissues; it cannot be seen distinctly on the radiograph unless a contrast agent is introduced into the joint. When this is done, the examination is described as *arthrography*. Positive contrast agents, such as sodium or meglumine diatrizoate (Hypaque or Renografin), may be used, or gases such as air or oxygen, or double contrast techniques involving a combination of both. The epiphyseal plate (5) is similarly of intermediate density.

Bone in Generalized Disease States.   The different appearances of an isolated segment of bone, inclusive of outer cortex and medulla, may be categorized as shown in Figure 4–7 and Table 4–2.

Ectopic Calcifications and Ossifications.   These occur in soft tissues from unknown causes, or in association with hyperparathyroidism, sarcoidosis, and certain neoplasms (Figure 4–9). In *"alteration in soft tissue density"* adjoining bones may take on several different appearances.

(Text continued on page 64)

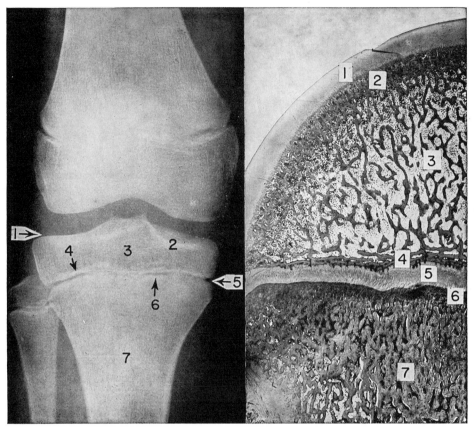

Figure 4–6 *A.* Antero-posterior radiograph of the knee and low-power photomicrograph of the end of a long bone with related areas labeled. (From Pyle, S. I., and Hoerr, N. I.: *Radiographic Atlas of Skeletal Development of the Knee.* Springfield, Charles C Thomas, 1955.)

Radiologic Terms

1. Articular cartilage does not show in a film.
2. White outline of subarticular margin of epiphysis.
3. Epiphysis.
4. Increased density of terminal plate; inner bone margin of epiphysis.
5. Epiphyseal line; strip of lesser density; epiphyseal plate; diaphyseal-epiphyseal gap. Radiographically, these terms exclude the recently calcified cartilage, which appears as part of the metaphysis.
6. Metaphysis; includes both calcified cartilage and newly-formed bone. (Zone of provisional calcification.)
7. Diaphysis or shaft.

Histologic Terms

1. Articular cartilage.
2. Compact bone of subarticular margin.
3. Epiphysis, spongy bone.
4. Terminal plate.
5. Epiphyseal disk; growth cartilage. Histologically, these terms include the calcified cartilage.
6. Metaphysis; includes only newly formed bone of primary ossification.
7. Spongy bone of diaphysis.

Figure 4–6 continued on opposite page.

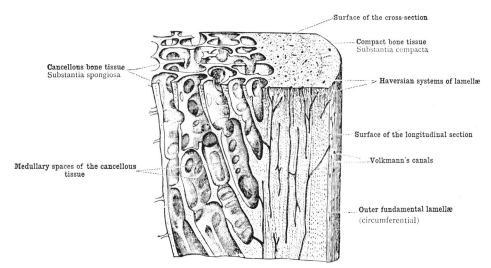

Figure 4–6 *B.*   Diagram to illustrate the structure of bone. (From Toldt, C.: *An Atlas of Human Anatomy for Students and Physicians.* New York, Macmillan Co., © 1926.)

TABLE 4–2   RADIOGRAPHIC PATHOLOGY OF BONES*

Periosteum	Cortex	Trabeculae of Medulla	Disease States
1. Normal	Thin	Thin subnormal	Osteoporosis from multiple diseases
2. Normal	Thin	Trabeculae coarse; demineralization	Osteomalacia, rickets, hypophosphatasia Hypervitaminosis D Vitamin D resistant rickets
3. Normal	Subperiosteal resorption	Demineralization	Hyperparathyroidism
4. Normal	Normal	Trabeculae increased in number, thickness, or even density	Marrow disorders
5. Increased	Increased	Normal	Infantile cortical hyperostosis Treated rickets
6. Normal	Increased thickness	Trabeculae increased in thickness	Osteopetrosis Hypoparathyroidism Hyperphosphatasemia Vitamin D intoxication Idiopathic hypercalcemia
7. Increased	Increased	May be normal	Fluorosis (Adams and Jowsey; Carbone, et al.; Cohen; Rich and Ivanovich)
8. Normal	Increased but mosaic and bizarre	Decreased and increased, intermixed and mosaic	Osteitis deformans (Paget's disease)
9. Normal	Increased in thickness	Increased in number	Acromegaly

*Modified from Feist, J. H.: Radiol. Clin. N. Amer., *8*:182 (No. 2) 1970; and Meschan, I.: Atlas of Normal Radiographic Anatomy, 2nd Ed. Philadelphia, W. B. Saunders Co., 1959.

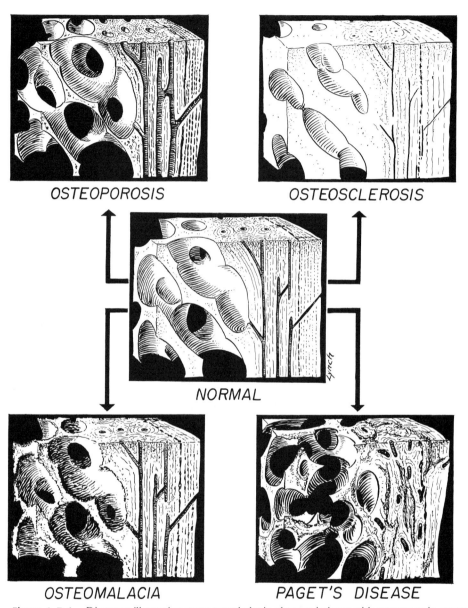

Figure 4–7 *A.*   Diagrams illustrating gross morphologic changes in bone with osteoporosis, osteosclerosis, osteomalacia, and Paget's disease. On each diagram cancellous bone is represented on the left side and compact on the right. The haversian systems are shown to be widened in osteoporosis and osteomalacia, narrowed in osteosclerosis, and bizarre in configuration in osteitis deformans (Paget's disease).

Figure 4–7 continued on opposite page.

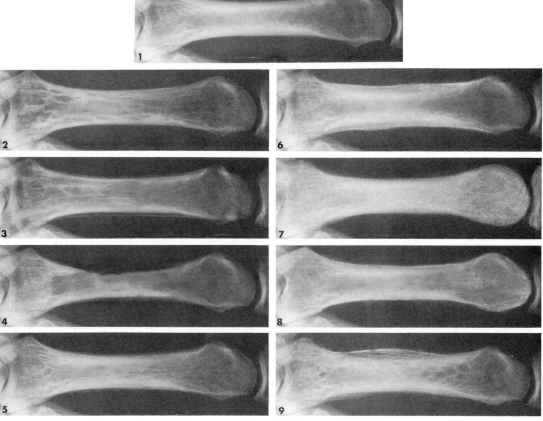

Figure 4–7 *B*

1. Normal cortex and medulla of bone: diagrammatic radiograph.
2. Cortex thin, trabeculae thin and diminished in number; diagrammatic radiograph of osteoporosis.
3. Cortex thin; bony trabeculae coarse and ill-defined; diagrammatic radiograph of rickets.
4. Subperiosteal resorption of cortical bone; diagrammatic radiograph of phalanx in hyperparathyroidism.
5. Cortex unaffected; trabeculae of medulla increased in thickness and number; diagrammatic radiograph of malignant lymphoma.
6. Increased thickness of cortex; medulla relatively unchanged; diagrammatic radiograph of melorheostosis.
7. Increased thickness of both cortex and medullary trabeculae; diagrammatic radiograph of marble bone disease.
8. Cortex thickened by coating of periosteal new bone; medullary trabeculae thickened; diagrammatic radiograph of fluorosis.
9. Increased thickness of cortex and medullary trabeculae which are bizarre in pattern; diagrammatic radiograph of Paget's disease of bone.

TABLE 4–3   LOCAL OR REGIONAL ALTERATIONS IN
ARCHITECTURE OF BONES

Alterations	Disease States
1. Local foci of increased density	Bone infarction
2. Local foci of reactive new bone formation	Fracture repair; response to local inflammation
3. Neoplastic new bone formation	Osteosarcoma
4. Hypertrophic osteoarthropathy (Goldbloom, et al.)	Response to some chronic lung diseases
5. Local decreases in bone density	Bone atrophy

TABLE 4–4   BONE CHANGES IN SPECIFIC AREAS OF THE SKELETON

Alterations	Disease States
1. Phalangeal changes (Figure 4–8)	Scleroderma
	Sarcoidosis
	Hyperparathyroidism
	Acromegaly
	Rheumatoid arthritis
	Dermatomyositis
2. Localized gigantism	Localized gigantism
3. Diminished size of bone	Hypoplasia
	Erosion by contiguous lesion

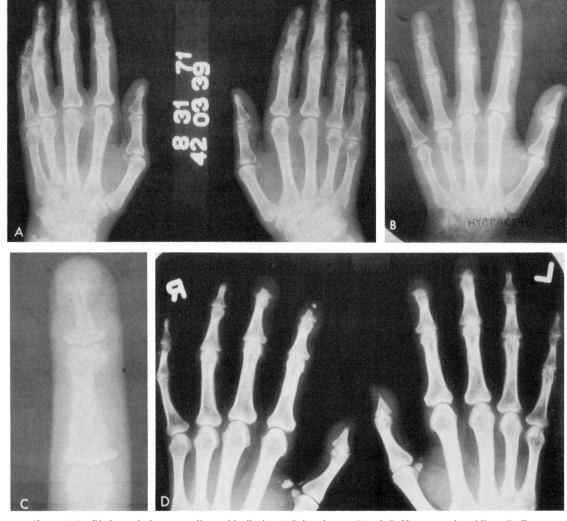

Figure 4–8   Phalangeal changes radiographically in: *A*. Scleroderma. *B* and *C*. Hyperparathyroidism. *D*. Dermatomyositis. (*Figure continued on following page.*)

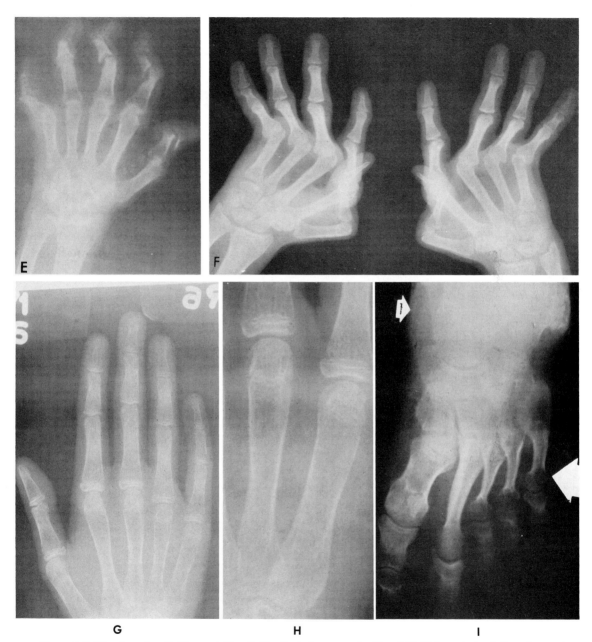

Figure 4–8 (*Continued*).   *E*. Rheumatoid arthritis. *F*. Arthrogryposis. *G* and *H*. Osteomalacia. *I*. Foot in pseudo-hypoparathyroidism. The large arrow points to the shortened third, fourth, and fifth metatarsals. The small arrow points to the calcified interstitial tissues adjoining the medial malleolus extending into the foot.

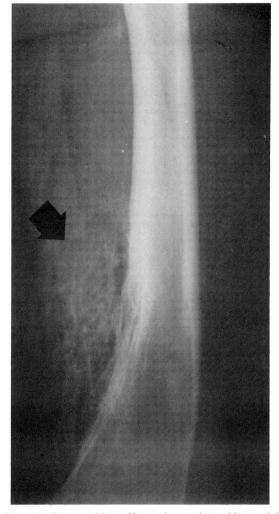

Figure 4–9 Thigh demonstrating myositis ossificans, in a patient with pseudohypoparathyroidism.

1. If diminished in comparison with water density:
   a. It may connote the fatty envelope surrounding muscles, in fascial planes, or in subcutaneous layers.
   b. It may connote the fatty replacement of muscle, which may occur with muscle atrophy. Occasionally, this becomes a "herring-bone pattern."
   c. It may be due to free entry of air through a break in the skin.
   d. It may be gas-produced by gas-producing microbial organisms.
2. If increased in comparison with water density:
   a. It may be *amorphous* interstitial *calcinosis.*
   b. It may be *ossific,* from an ossifying tumor, or myositis ossificans.
   c. It may be *metallic,* owing to penetration by a metallic foreign body.
   d. It may be *faintly opaque,* owing to foreign bodies such as glass or road gravel.

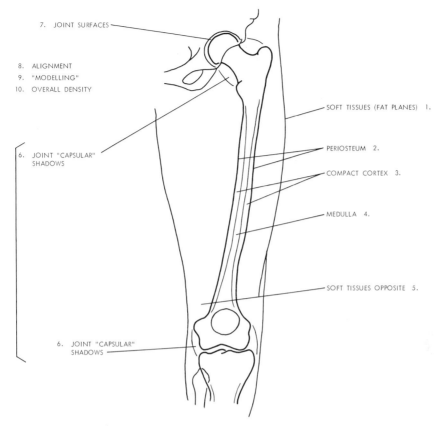

Figure 4–10 Method of roentgen analysis of bones.

METHOD OF ROENTGEN ANALYSIS OF BONES (Figure 4–10)

1. Always have at least *two perpendicular views and one joint view.*
2. Determine whether or not *single or multiple foci* are involved by a bone survey wherever necessary. A *bone survey* consists of: two views of skull; two views of lumbar or thoracic spine; antero-posterior view of pelvis; and antero-posterior views of arms and thighs.
3. Make *comparison studies* of the two comparable sides of the body when appropriate.
4. Know *age and sex* of patient.
5. Know *hereditary factors, occupational history,* and, whenever possible, *clinical and laboratory data.*
6. *Study bones in following sequence* (Figure 4–10):
   a. *Soft tissues* adjoining
   b. *Periosteal region*
   c. *Cortex*
   d. *Medulla*
   e. *Joint capsule and joint*
   f. *Subarticular bone*
   g. *Epiphysis, epiphyseal plate, metaphysis*

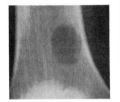 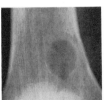 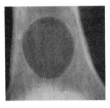 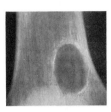 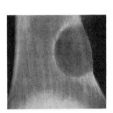

NO "RADIOLOGIC" CAPSULE

MALIGNANT TUMOR METASTASES

MULTIPLE MYELOMA

EOSINOPHILIC GRANULOMA

LIPOID DYSCRASIA

GIANT CELL
TUMOR   USUALLY
                         SOAP-
ANEURYSMAL BONE BUBBLE
CYST   INTERIOR

DISCONTINUOUS THIN
"RADIOLOGIC" CAPSULE

OSTEITIS FIBROSA CYSTICA
("BROWN TUMOR")

GAUCHER'S DISEASE

BRODIE'S ABSCESS

CONTINUOUS THIN
"RADIOLOGIC" CAPSULE

BRODIE'S ABSCESS

THICK "RADIOLOGIC" CAPSULE

CHRONIC GRANULOMA
OR ABSCESS

FIBROUS DYSPLASIA

BRODIE'S ABSCESS

THICK "RADIOLOGIC" CAPSULE
CORTICAL

FIBROUS CORTICAL DEFECT

FIBROMAS (CHONDROMYXOID)

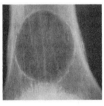

BONE CYST

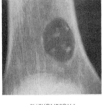

ENCHONDROMA

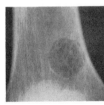

HEMANGIOMA

Figure 4–11   Diagrams demonstrating how roentgen analysis of the margins of a bony lesion and internal architecture can assist in final diagnosis.

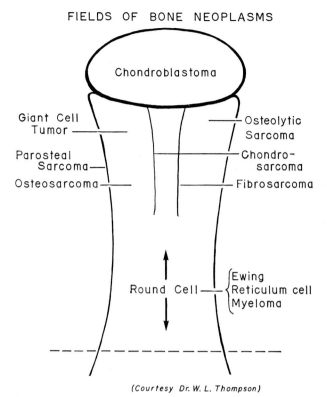

FIELDS OF BONE NEOPLASMS

(Courtesy Dr. W. L. Thompson)

Figure 4–12   Diagram showing how the position of a bony lesion may assist in final diagnosis.

h. Systematically review general roentgen pathology, such as alterations in *position, size, contour, density, architecture* (internal and marginal), *number, function, changes occurring over a period of time, and changes resulting from treatment.*

7. *Classify objective roentgen signs* in respect to:
   a. *Monostotic vs. polyostotic*
   b. *Increased density vs. hyperlucency*
   c. *Overgrowth vs. undergrowth*
   d. *Architecture* of lesion or lesions (1) *internal,* and (2) *marginal* (Figure 4–11)
   e. *Soft tissue and/or periosteal involvement*
   f. *Joint involvement*

Categorization of Bone Abnormalities by Tissue of Origin (Edling).   Edling (1968) categorized bone lesions into three types of disorders: (1) formation of bone, (2) modeling of bone, (3) rebuilding in bone.

The abnormal tissues were classified by their origin: (1) fibrous, (2) chondromatous, (3) osseous, (4) granulation, (5) avascular, (6) fat marrow, (7) fibrous marrow, (8) vasculocellular, (9) hemangiomatous, (10) reticuloendothelial, and (11) cellular.

Congenital disorders are abnormalities in "formation of bone" and "modeling of bone." They fall into the fibrous, chondromatous, and osseous categories.

Disorders in "rebuilding of bone" include: callus, necrosis, hyperparathyroid-dysfibroplasia, inflammation, hemangioma, reticuloses, and metastases.

(*Text continued on page 88*)

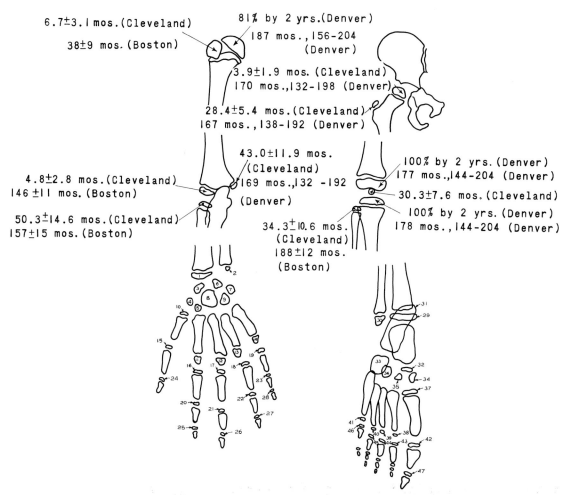

6.7±3.1 mos.(Cleveland)

38±9 mos. (Boston)

81% by 2 yrs.(Denver)

187 mos.,156-204
(Denver)

3.9±1.9 mos. (Cleveland)
170 mos.,132-198 (Denver)

28.4±5.4 mos.(Cleveland)
167 mos.,138-192 (Denver)

43.0±11.9 mos.
(Cleveland)
169 mos.,132 -192
(Denver)

4.8±2.8 mos.(Cleveland)
146 ±11 mos. (Boston)

50.3±14.6 mos.(Cleveland)
157±15 mos. (Boston)

34.3±10.6 mos.
(Cleveland)
188±12 mos.
(Boston)

100% by 2 yrs. (Denver)
177 mos.,144-204 (Denver)

30.3±7.6 mos.(Cleveland)

100% by 2 yrs. (Denver)
178 mos.,144-204 (Denver)

Figure 4–13   *A*. Onset and completion of ossification of secondary centers of ossification of the upper and lower extremities in females, according to the Denver, Cleveland and Boston studies (data compiled from Acheson, 1966). (This data is continued in chart form in Figures 4–13 *B, C, D* and *E.*)

Figure 4–13 continued on opposite page.

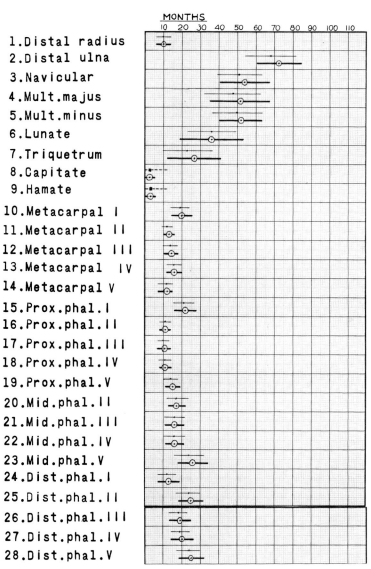

Figure 4–13 *B*. Onset of ossification of the wrist and hand in females. *Thin lines*, Cleveland study; *thick lines*, Boston study.

Figure 4–13 continued on following page.

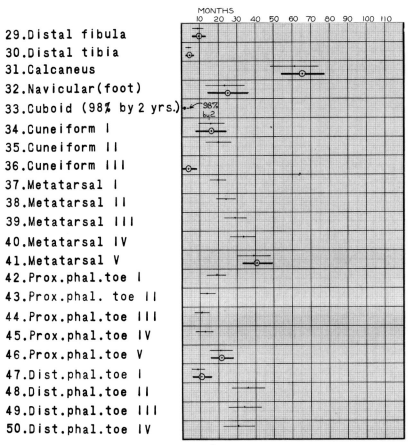

Figure 4–13 *C.* Onset of ossification of secondary centers of the ankle and foot in females, according to the Cleveland and Boston studies. (Data compiled from Acheson, 1966.) *Thin lines,* Cleveland study; *thick lines,* Boston study.

Figure 4–13 continued on opposite page.

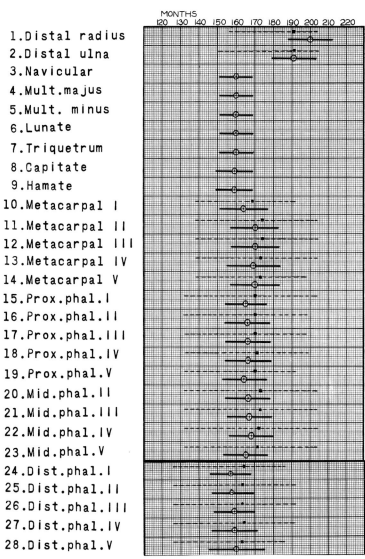

Figure 4–13 *D.* Completion of ossification of the wrist and hands in females, according to the Cleveland and Boston studies. (Data compiled from Acheson, 1966.) *Thin lines,* Cleveland study; *thick lines,* Boston study.

Figure 4–13 continued on following page.

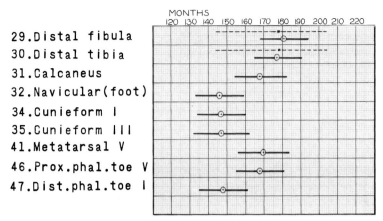

Figure 4–13   E. Completion of ossification of the ankle and foot in females, according to the Cleveland and Boston studies. (Data compiled from Acheson, 1966.) *Thin lines,* Cleveland study; *thick lines,* Boston study.

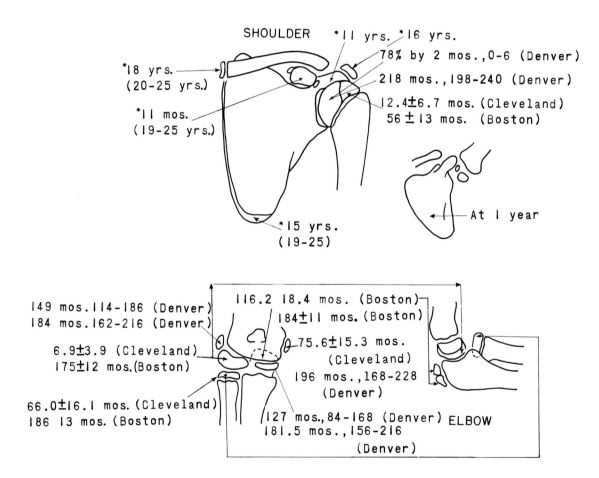

*Schinz-Baensch-Friedl-Uehlinger

Figure 4–13 *F.* Onset and completion of ossification of secondary centers of the shoulder and elbow in males, according to the Denver, Cleveland and Boston studies. (Data compiled from Acheson, 1966.)

Figure 4–13 continued on opposite page.

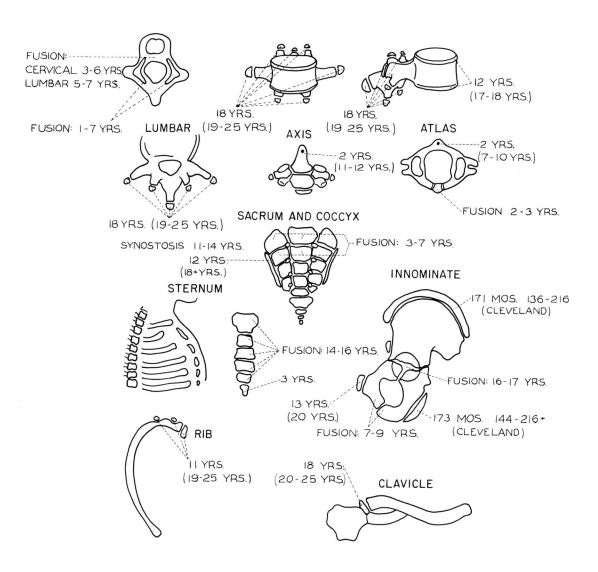

( ) indicate time of fusion

Figure 4–13 *G*. Ossification onset and/or fusion of vertebrae, sternum, innominate bone, ribs and clavicle. (Data modified from Girdany and Golden, 1952.)

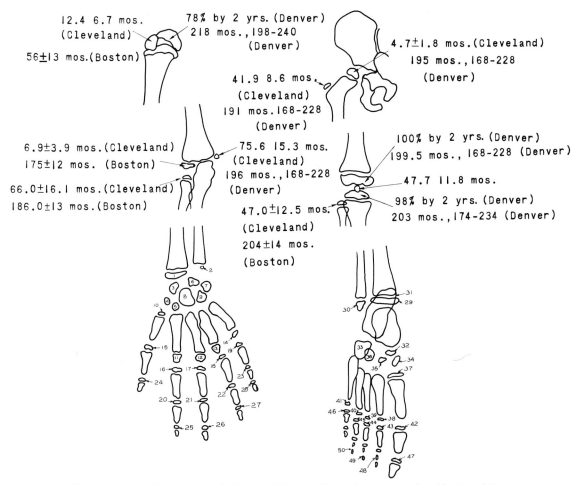

12.4 6.7 mos.
(Cleveland)

56±13 mos.(Boston)

78% by 2 yrs. (Denver)
218 mos.,198-240
(Denver)

4.7±1.8 mos.(Cleveland)
195 mos.,168-228
(Denver)

41.9 8.6 mos.
(Cleveland)
191 mos.168-228
(Denver)

6.9±3.9 mos.(Cleveland)
175±12 mos. (Boston)

66.0±16.1 mos.(Cleveland)
186.0±13 mos.(Boston)

75.6 15.3 mos.
(Cleveland)
196 mos.,168-228
(Denver)

47.0±12.5 mos.
(Cleveland)
204±14 mos.
(Boston)

100% by 2 yrs.(Denver)
199.5 mos., 168-228 (Denver)

47.7 11.8 mos.

98% by 2 yrs. (Denver)
203 mos.,174-234 (Denver)

Figure 4–14 *A*. Onset and completion of ossification of secondary centers of ossification of the upper and lower extremities in males, according to the Denver, Cleveland, and Boston studies. (Data compiled from Acheson, 1966.) (This data is contained in chart form in Figures 4–14 *B, C, D,* and *E.*)

Figure 4–14 continued on opposite page.

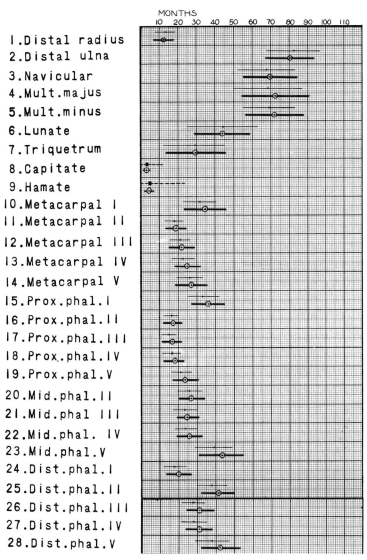

Figure 4–14   *B*. Onset of ossification of secondary centers of the wrist and hands in males according to the Cleveland and Boston studies. (Data compiled from Acheson, 1966.) *Thin lines*, Cleveland study; *thick lines*, Boston study.

Figure 4–14 continued on following page.

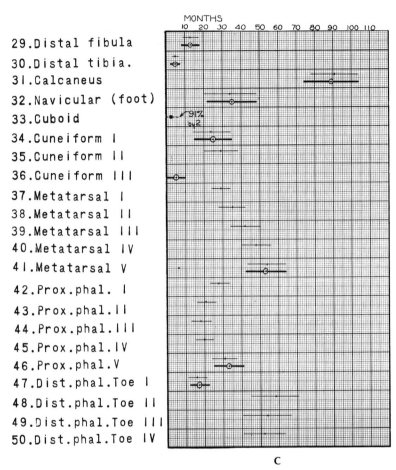

MONTHS

29.Distal fibula
30.Distal tibia.
31.Calcaneus
32.Navicular (foot)
33.Cuboid
34.Cuneiform I
35.Cuneiform II
36.Cuneiform III
37.Metatarsal I
38.Metatarsal II
39.Metatarsal III
40.Metatarsal IV
41.Metatarsal V
42.Prox.phal. I
43.Prox.phal.II
44.Prox.phal.III
45.Prox.phal.IV
46.Prox.phal.V
47.Dist.phal.Toe I
48.Dist.phal.Toe II
49.Dist.phal.Toe III
50.Dist.phal.Toe IV

C

Figure 4–14   *C*. Onset of ossification of secondary centers of the ankle and foot in males, according to the Cleveland and Boston studies. (Data compiled from Acheson, 1966.) *Thin lines*, Cleveland study; *thick lines*, Boston study.

Figure 4–14   *D*. Completion of ossification of the wrist and hands in males, according to the Cleveland and Boston studies. (Data compiled from Acheson, 1966.) *Thin lines*, Cleveland study; *thick lines*, Boston study.

Figure 4–14   *E*. Completion of ossification of the ankle and foot in males, according to the Cleveland and Boston studies. (Data compiled from Acheson, 1966.) *Thin lines*, Cleveland study; *thick lines*, Boston study.

Figure 4–14 continued on opposite page.

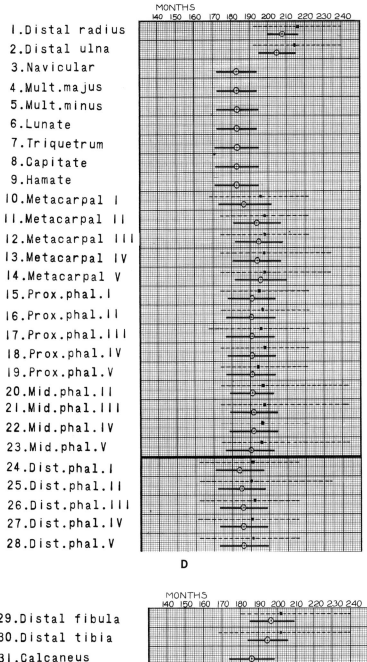

1. Distal radius
2. Distal ulna
3. Navicular
4. Mult.majus
5. Mult.minus
6. Lunate
7. Triquetrum
8. Capitate
9. Hamate
10. Metacarpal I
11. Metacarpal II
12. Metacarpal III
13. Metacarpal IV
14. Metacarpal V
15. Prox.phal.I
16. Prox.phal.II
17. Prox.phal.III
18. Prox.phal.IV
19. Prox.phal.V
20. Mid.phal.II
21. Mid.phal.III
22. Mid.phal.IV
23. Mid.phal.V
24. Dist.phal.I
25. Dist.phal.II
26. Dist.phal.III
27. Dist.phal.IV
28. Dist.phal.V

D

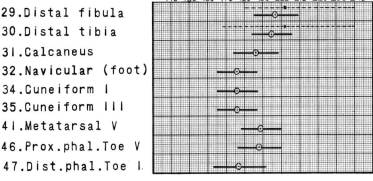

29. Distal fibula
30. Distal tibia
31. Calcaneus
32. Navicular (foot)
34. Cuneiform I
35. Cuneiform III
41. Metatarsal V
46. Prox.phal.Toe V
47. Dist.phal.Toe I

E

Figures 4–14 D and E; see opposite page for legends.

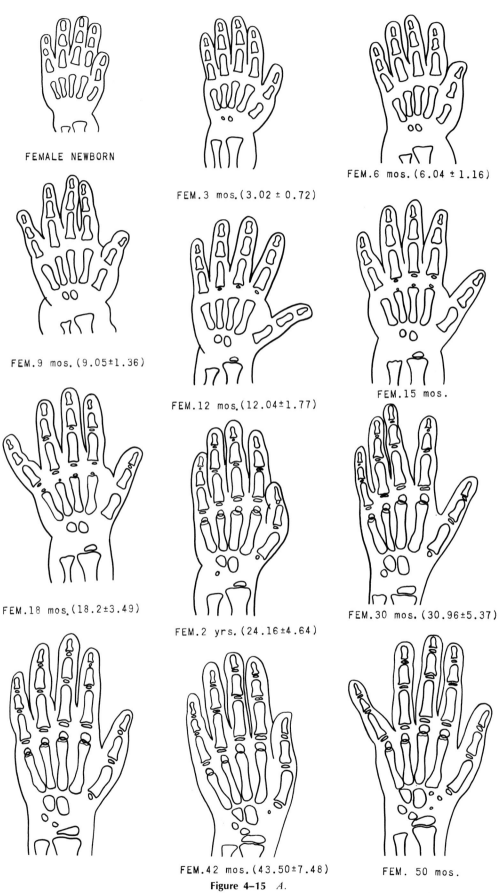

FEMALE NEWBORN

FEM.3 mos.(3.02 ± 0.72)

FEM.6 mos.(6.04 ± 1.16)

FEM.9 mos.(9.05±1.36)

FEM.12 mos.(12.04±1.77)

FEM.15 mos.

FEM.18 mos.(18.2±3.49)

FEM.2 yrs.(24.16±4.64)

FEM.30 mos.(30.96±5.37)

FEM.42 mos.(43.50±7.48)

FEM. 50 mos.

Figure 4–15   *A.*

Figure 4–15   *A. See opposite page for legend.*   *Figure 4–15 continued on opposite page.*

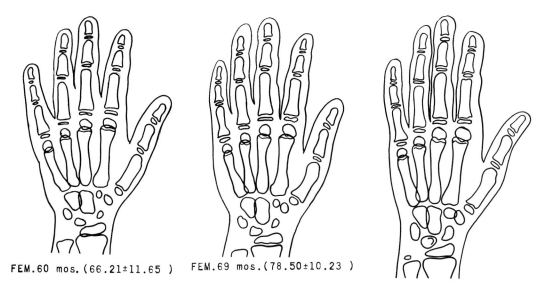

FEM.60 mos.(66.21±11.65)   FEM.69 mos.(78.50±10.23)

FEM.82 mos. (if 84 mos.:89.30±9.64

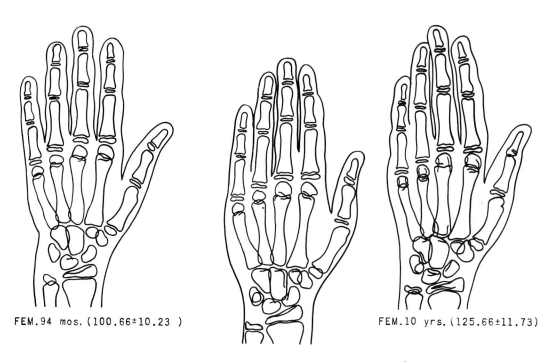

FEM.94 mos.(100.66±10.23)   FEM.10 yrs.(125.66±11.73)

FEM.106 mos.(if 9 yrs.:113.86±10.74)

Figure 4–15 *A* (*Continued*).

Figure 4–15 Osseous changes in the wrist and hand and foot in the male and female. (Modified from Greulich, W. W., and Pyle, S. I.: *Radiographic Atlas of Skeletal Development of the Hand and Wrist.* 2nd Ed. Stanford, Calif., Stanford University Press, 1959.) *A.* Female hand and wrist, birth to 18 years.

Figure 4–15 continued on following page.

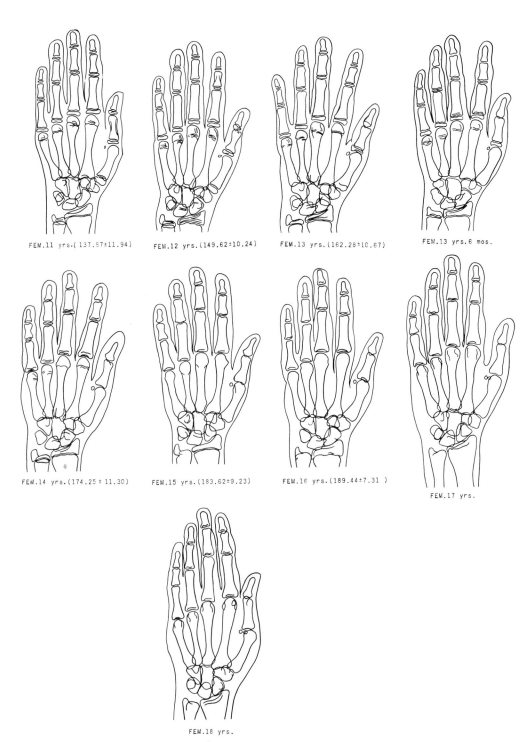

FEM.11 yrs.(137.87±11.94) FEM.12 yrs.(149.62±10.24) FEM.13 yrs.(162.28±10.67) FEM.13 yrs.6 mos.

FEM.14 yrs.(174.25±11.30) FEM.15 yrs.(183.62±9.23) FEM.16 yrs.(189.44±7.31) FEM.17 yrs.

FEM.18 yrs.

Figure 4–15 *A* (*Continued*).

Figure 4–15 continued on opposite page.

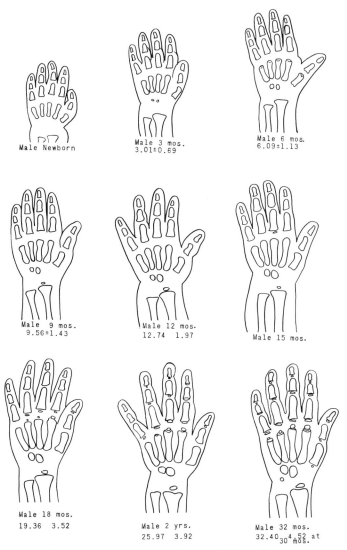

Figure 4–15 *B*. Male hand and wrist, birth to 17 years.

Figure 4–15 continued on following page.

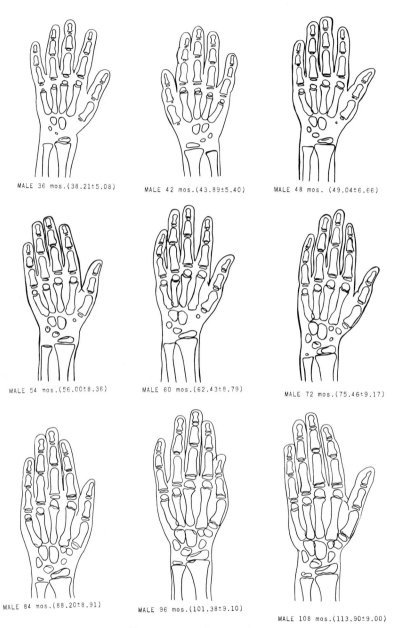

MALE 36 mos.(38.21±5.08)   MALE 42 mos.(43.89±5.40)   MALE 48 mos. (49.04±6.66)

MALE 54 mos.(56.00±8.36)   MALE 60 mos.(62.43±8.79)   MALE 72 mos.(75.46±9.17)

MALE 84 mos.(88.20±8.91)   MALE 96 mos.(101.38±9.10)   MALE 108 mos.(113.90±9.00)

Figure 4–15 *B* (*Continued*).

Figure 4–15 continued on opposite page.

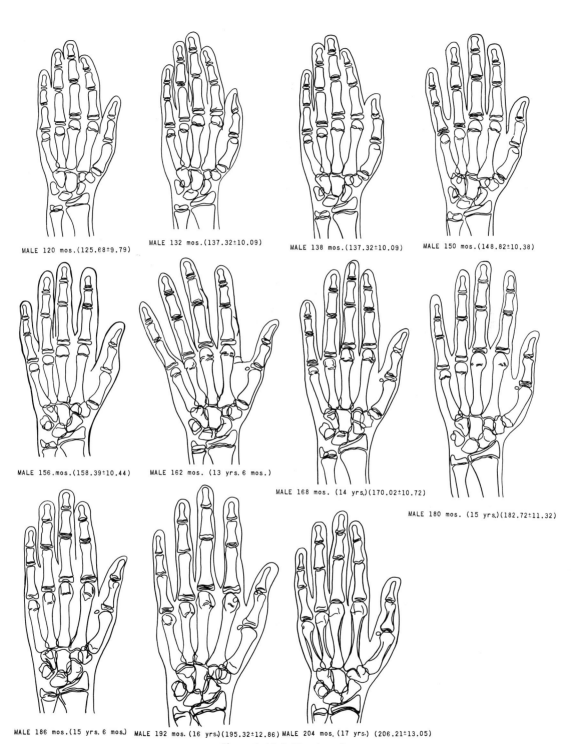

MALE 120 mos.(125.68±9.79)   MALE 132 mos.(137.32±10.09)   MALE 138 mos.(137.32±10.09)   MALE 150 mos.(148.82±10.38)

MALE 156.mos.(158.39±10.44)   MALE 162 mos. (13 yrs.6 mos.)

MALE 168 mos. (14 yrs.)(170.02±10.72)

MALE 180 mos. (15 yrs.)(182.72±11.32)

MALE 186 mos.(15 yrs. 6 mos.)   MALE 192 mos. (16 yrs.)(195.32±12.86) MALE 204 mos. (17 yrs.) (206.21±13.05)

Figure 4–15 *B* (*Continued*).

Figure 4–15 continued on following page.

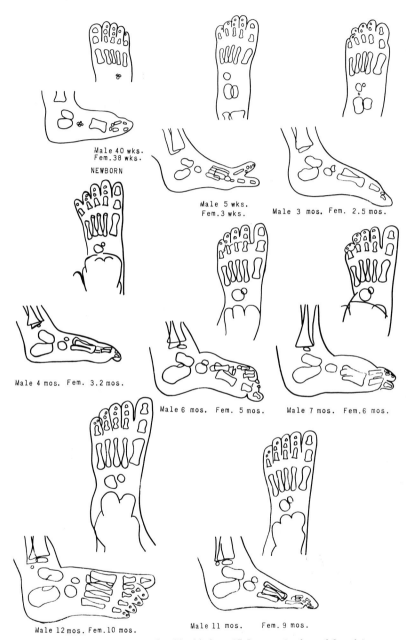

Male 40 wks.
Fem. 38 wks.

NEWBORN

Male 5 wks.
Fem. 3 wks.

Male 3 mos. Fem. 2.5 mos.

Male 4 mos. Fem. 3.2 mos.

Male 6 mos. Fem. 5 mos.

Male 7 mos. Fem. 6 mos.

Male 12 mos. Fem. 10 mos.

Male 11 mos. Fem. 9 mos.

Figure 4–15 *C.* Foot and ankle, birth to 17.5 years (male and female).

Figure 4–15 continued on opposite page.

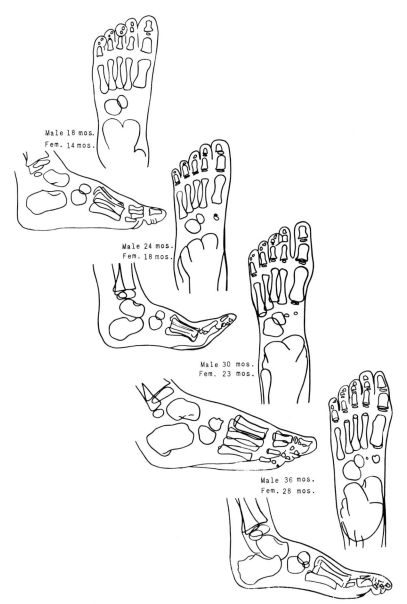

Figure 4–15   *C (Continued).*

Figure 4–15 continued on following page.

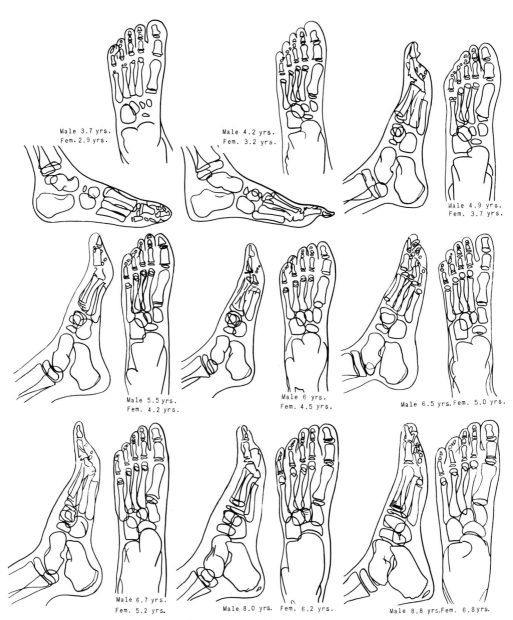

Male 3.7 yrs.
Fem. 2.9 yrs.

Male 4.2 yrs.
Fem. 3.2 yrs.

Male 4.9 yrs.
Fem. 3.7 yrs.

Male 5.5 yrs.
Fem. 4.2 yrs.

Male 6 yrs.
Fem. 4.5 yrs.

Male 6.5 yrs. Fem. 5.0 yrs.

Male 6.7 yrs.
Fem. 5.2 yrs.

Male 8.0 yrs. Fem. 6.2 yrs.

Male 8.8 yrs. Fem. 6.8 yrs.

Figure 4–15   *C   (Continued).*

Figure 4–15 continued on opposite page.

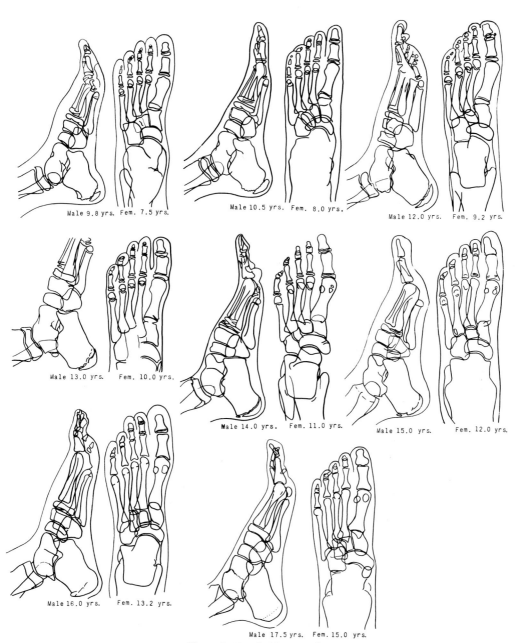

Male 9.8 yrs. Fem. 7.5 yrs.

Male 10.5 yrs. Fem. 8.0 yrs.

Male 12.0 yrs. Fem. 9.2 yrs.

Male 13.0 yrs. Fem. 10.0 yrs.

Male 14.0 yrs. Fem. 11.0 yrs.

Male 15.0 yrs. Fem. 12.0 yrs.

Male 16.0 yrs. Fem. 13.2 yrs.

Male 17.5 yrs. Fem. 15.0 yrs.

Figure 4–15   *C   (Continued).*

BONE AGE VERSUS CHRONOLOGICAL AGE: MATURATION OF THE SKELETON

Major Factors Studied in Skeletal Maturation:

1. *Ossification of the long and short bones* (usually complete *in utero*).
2. *Onset of ossification of the epiphyses* (Figures 4–13, 4–14).
3. *Completion of ossification* (Figures 4–13, 4–14) with fusion of the epiphyses and metaphyses (Todd; Rotch).
4. *Maturation indicators* in the wrist, hand, tarsus, foot, and knee (patella) (Figures 4–15, 4–16, 4–17).

Epiphyses begin to appear at birth and are ordinarily complete by puberty. Ossification is usually complete by the 20th year in the female and the 23rd year in the male.

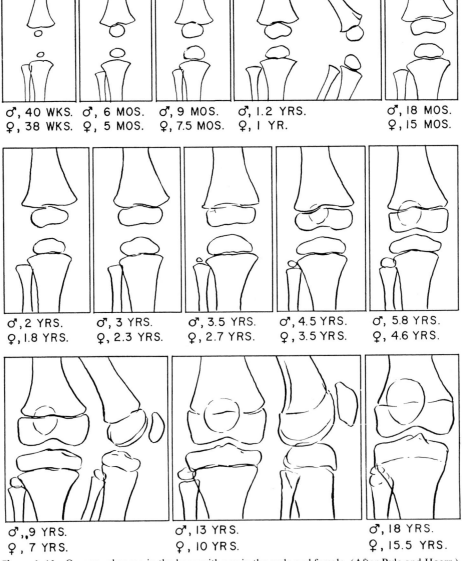

Figure 4–16 Osseous changes in the knee with age in the male and female. (After Pyle and Hoerr.)

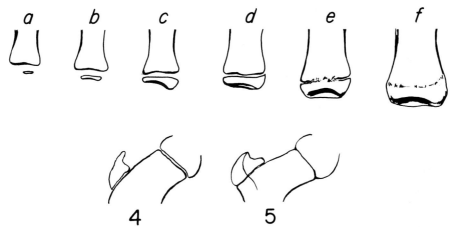

Figure 4–17   Six "universal" maturity indicators which can be applied to the growing end of any bone: *A*. First appearance; *B, C, D*. gradual maturation of the epiphyses; *E*. early fusion; *F*. complete fusion. (From Acheson, R. M.: Maturation of the Skeleton. *In* Falkner, Frank, ed., *Human Development*. Philadelphia, W. B. Saunders Co., 1966.)

Author's Recommended Method

1. Radiographs are obtained of the regions indicated in Figure 4–18, depending upon the chronological age of the child.

2. In these regions, onset of ossification and completion of ossification (fusion) are studied (Figures 4–13 and 4–14). The "age-at-appearance" percentiles for major postnatal ossification centers can be determined (Table 4–5).

3. Maturation indicators are studied in the hand, wrist, tarsus, foot, and knee as indicated by the age of the child. These are tabulated in relation to the mean age given plus the standard deviation (Figures 4–13, 4–14, 4–15).

4. All of these data are interrelated to give the most probable age. The 20 centers of ossification which are most valuable from the standpoint of evaluating postnatal ossification are shown in Figure 4–17B. Three radiographs can usually suffice. At puberty, however, more attention must be given to the centers of the hip, iliac bones, and the sesamoids of the thumb and other fingers.

Limitations of Skeletal Assessment

GENERAL RULES FOR USE OF BONE AGE DATA*

1. For children from birth to five years: registration of skeletal age by the time of appearance of centers of ossification.

2. For children five to 14 years of age: study maturation factors, and penetration of cartilaginous areas by reference to standards.

3. For children 14 to 25 years of age: register skeletal age by epiphyseal-diaphyseal union and reference to "Completion of Ossification" tables.

---

*Modified from Watson, E. H., and Lowrey, G. A.: Growth and Development of Children, 5th Ed. Chicago, Year Book Medical Publishers, 1967.

TABLE 4-5   AGE-AT-APPEARANCE (YEARS-MONTHS) PERCENTILES FOR SELECTED OSSIFICATION CENTERS*

Centers	Boys			Girls		
	5TH	50TH	95TH	5TH	50TH	95TH
1. Humerus, head	—	0- 0	0- 4	—	0- 0	0- 4
2. Tibia, proximal	—	0- 0	0- 1	—	0- 0	0- 0
3. Coracoid process of scapula	—	0- 0	0- 4	—	0- 0	0- 5
4. Cuboid	—	0- 1	0- 4	—	0- 1	0- 2
5. Capitate	—	0- 3	0- 7	—	0- 2	0- 7
6. Hamate	0- 0	0- 4	0-10	—	0- 2	0- 7
7. Capitellum of humerus	0- 1	0- 4	1- 1	0- 1	0- 3	0- 9
8. Femur, head	0- 1	0- 4	0- 8	0- 0	0- 4	0- 7
9. Cuneiform 3	0- 1	0- 6	1- 7	—	0- 3	1- 3
10. Humerus, greater tuberosity	0- 3	0-10	2- 4	0- 2	0- 6	1- 2
11. Toe phalanx 5M	—	1- 0	3-10	—	0- 9	2- 1
12. Radius, distal	0- 6	1- 1	2- 4	0- 5	0-10	1- 8
13. Toe phalanx 1D	0- 9	1- 3	2- 1	0- 5	0- 9	1- 8
14. Toe phalanx 4M	0- 5	1- 3	2-11	0- 5	0-11	3- 0
15. Finger phalanx 3P	0- 9	1- 4	2- 2	0- 5	0-10	1- 7
16. Toe phalanx 3M	0- 5	1- 5	4- 3	0- 3	1- 0	2- 6
17. Finger phalanx 2P	0- 9	1- 5	2- 2	0- 5	0-10	1- 8
18. Finger phalanx 4P	0-10	1- 6	2- 5	0- 5	0-11	1- 8
19. Finger phalanx 1D	0- 9	1- 6	2- 8	0- 5	1- 0	1- 9
20. Toe phalanx 3P	0-11	1- 7	2- 6	0- 6	1- 1	1-11
21. Metacarpal 2	0-11	1- 7	2-10	0- 8	1- 1	1- 8
22. Toe phalanx 4P	0-11	1- 8	2- 8	0- 7	1- 3	2- 1
23. Toe phalanx 2P	1- 0	1- 9	2- 8	0- 8	1- 2	2- 1
24. Metacarpal 3	0-11	1- 9	3- 0	0- 8	1- 2	1-11
25. Finger phalanx 5P	1- 0	1-10	2-10	0- 8	1- 2	2- 1
26. Finger phalanx 3M	1- 0	2- 0	3- 4	0- 8	1- 3	2- 4
27. Metacarpal 4	1- 1	2- 0	3- 7	0- 9	1- 3	2- 2
28. Toe phalanx 2M	0-11	2- 0	4- 1	0- 6	1- 2	2- 3
29. Finger phalanx 4M	1- 0	2- 1	3- 3	0- 8	1- 3	2- 5
30. Metacarpal 5	1- 3	2- 2	3-10	0-10	1- 4	2- 4
31. Cuneiform 1	0-11	2- 2	3- 9	0- 6	1- 5	2-10
32. Metatarsal 1	1- 5	2- 2	3- 1	1- 0	1- 7	2- 3
33. Finger phalanx 2M	1- 4	2- 2	3- 4	0- 8	1- 4	2- 6
34. Toe phalanx 1P	1- 5	2- 4	3- 4	0-11	1- 7	2- 6
35. Finger phalanx 3D	1- 4	2- 5	3- 9	0- 9	1- 6	2- 8
36. Triquetrum	0- 6	2- 5	5- 6	0- 3	1- 8	3- 9
37. Finger phalanx 4D	1- 4	2- 5	3- 9	0- 9	1- 6	2-10

(P = proximal, M = middle, D = distal)
*Modified by Graham from Garn et al.

Table 4-5 continued on opposite page.

1. Skeletal assessment has the greatest validity for normal children.
2. In some endocrinopathies, chromosomal aberrations, cases of Morquio's syndrome, and some dyschondroplasias, whole groups of ossification centers may fail to appear (Garn et al.).
3. Skeletal assessments have value in distinguishing between small size and retardation, in measuring the effects of thyroid therapy in hypothyroidism, and in steroid therapy in those requiring this form of treatment.
4. Assessment of one bone or joint is not necessarily a guide to the development of other bones or joints.
5. Irrespective of the "bone age assessment," the genetic pattern of the individual must be taken into consideration. For example, in populations where axillary and pubic hair are normally scarce, radiographic appraisal of the skeleton has particular value (Garn et al.).

TABLE 4–5 AGE-AT-APPEARANCE (YEARS-MONTHS) PERCENTILES
FOR SELECTED OSSIFICATION CENTERS* (*Continued*)

	Boys			Girls		
Centers	5TH	50TH	95TH	5TH	50TH	95TH
38. Toe phalanx 5P	1– 6	2– 5	3– 8	1– 0	1– 9	2– 8
39. Metacarpal 1	1– 5	2– 7	4– 4	0–11	1– 7	2– 8
40. Cuneiform 2	1– 2	2– 8	4– 3	0–10	1–10	3– 0
41. Metatarsal 2	1–11	2–10	4– 4	1– 3	2– 2	3– 5
42. Femur, greater trochanter	1–11	3– 0	4– 4	1– 0	1–10	3– 0
43. Finger phalanx 1P	1–10	3– 0	4– 7	0–11	1– 9	2–10
44. Navicular of foot	1– 1	3– 0	5– 5	0– 9	1–11	3– 7
45. Finger phalanx 2D	1–10	3– 2	5– 0	1– 1	2– 6	3– 3
46. Finger phalanx 5D	2– 1	3– 3	5– 0	1– 0	2– 0	3– 5
47. Finger phalanx 5M	1–11	3– 5	5–10	0–11	2– 0	3– 6
48. Fibula, proximal	1–10	3– 6	5– 3	1– 4	2– 7	3–11
49. Metatarsal 3	2– 4	3– 6	5– 0	1– 5	2– 6	3– 8
50. Toe phalanx 5D	2– 4	3–11	6– 4	1– 2	2– 4	4– 1
51. Patella	2– 7	4– 0	6– 0	1– 6	2– 6	4– 0
52. Metatarsal 4	2–11	4– 0	5– 9	1– 9	2–10	4– 1
53. Lunate	1– 6	4– 1	6– 9	1– 1	2– 7	5– 8
54. Toe phalanx 3D	3– 0	4– 4	6– 2	1– 4	2– 9	4– 1
55. Metatarsal 5	3– 1	4– 4	6– 4	2– 1	3– 3	4–11
56. Toe phalanx 4D	2–11	4– 5	6– 5	1– 4	2– 7	4– 1
57. Toe phalanx 2D	3– 3	4– 8	6– 9	1– 6	2–11	4– 6
58. Capitulum of radius	3– 0	5– 3	8– 0	2– 3	3–10	6– 3
59. Navicular of wrist	3– 7	5– 8	7–10	2– 4	4– 1	6– 0
60. Greater multangular	3– 6	5–10	9– 0	1–11	4– 1	6– 4
61. Lesser multangular	3– 1	6– 3	8– 6	2– 5	4– 2	6– 0
62. Medial epicondyle of humerus	4– 3	6– 3	8– 5	2– 1	3– 5	5– 1
63. Ulna, distal	5– 3	7– 1	9– 1	3– 3	5– 4	7– 8
64. Calcaneal apophysis	5– 2	7– 7	9– 7	3– 6	5– 4	7– 4
65. Olecranon of ulna	7– 9	9– 8	11–11	5– 7	8– 0	9–11
66. Lateral epicondyle of humerus	9– 3	11– 3	13– 8	7– 2	9– 3	11– 3
67. Tibial tubercle	9–11	11–10	13– 5	7–11	10– 3	11–10
68. Adductor sesamoid of thumb	11– 0	12– 9	14– 7	8– 8	10– 9	12– 8
69. Os acetabulum	11–11	13– 6	15– 4	9– 7	11– 6	13– 5
70. Acromion	12– 2	13– 9	15– 6	10– 4	11–11	13– 9
71. Iliac crest	12– 0	14– 0	15–11	10–10	12– 9	15– 4
72. Coracoid apophysis	12– 9	14– 4	16– 4	10– 4	12– 3	14– 4
73. Ischial tuberosity	13– 7	15– 3	17– 1	11– 9	13–11	16– 0

(P = proximal, M = middle, D = distal)
*Modified by Graham from Garn et al.

6. If the assessment is based upon developmental data compiled from a population which is not comparable to the individual being evaluated, allowances must be made for moderate deviations (Graham).
7. Caution must be exercised in "over-requesting" too many osseous centers (which will result in inordinate exposure to radiation) (Table 4–16), or in "overinterpreting" with a pictorial age-standard one specific body region, such as the hand and wrist, since the specific region may not reflect skeletal maturation as a whole. Moreover, there are long periods during which little bony change is occurring in the hand and wrist alone, or in the foot, and a single standard plate is virtually impossible (Graham).

Premature Fusion of Epiphyses (Currarino and Erlandson). Premature fusion of one or more epiphyses is uncommon but may occur under the following circumstances: (1) as a complication of infection or trauma involving the epiphyseal cartilage plate; (2) following scurvy, perhaps as a result of pathologic fracture of the epiphyseal plate; (3) as a complication of hypervitaminosis A; (4) as a developmental error of cartilage formation; (5) in Cooley's anemia; and (6) in the congenital adrenogenital syndrome with virilism (Kurlander).

Premature fusion is diagnosed on the basis of bony alteration of the epiphyseal line. There may be associated deformity and shortening of the affected bone.

In those patients over ten years old with Cooley's anemia, premature fusion is a relatively common finding if they also have homozygous thalassemia (23 per cent of patients). The sites of predilection are the proximal end of one or both humeri and the distal end of one or both femurs.

Disorders Which May Cause Small Stature*

Nutritional
  Malnutrition
  Hypervitaminosis D
Bone diseases
  Achondroplasia
  Hurler's syndrome
  Osteogenesis imperfecta
  Rickets
Central nervous system disorders
  Cerebral palsy
  Microcephaly
  Mongolism
  Porencephalia
  Postencephalitis
Chronic infections
  Bones, kidneys, or lungs
Congenital heart disease
Endocrine disorders
  Addison's disease
  Adrenogenital syndrome

Cretinism
Diabetes
Gonadal dysgenesis
Renal disorders
Hepatic disorders
  Atresia of bile ducts
  Cirrhosis
  Disorders of glycogen storage
  Galactosemia
Pulmonary disorders
  Asthma
  Cystic fibrosis
  Bronchiectasis
Blood diseases
  Severe anemia
Intestinal disorders
  Celiac syndrome
  Diaphragmatic hernia
  Fat or starch intolerance
  Gastrointestinal allergy

*From Watson, E. H., and Lowrey, G. A.: Growth and Development of Children, 5th Ed. Chicago, Year Book Medical Publishers, 1967.

Disorders Which May Cause Large Stature*

Pituitary hyperfunction
Testicular hypofunction
Adrenal cortex adenoma or carcinoma
Genital hyperfunction
Pineal tumors
Tumors of hypothalamus

*From Watson, E. H., and Lowrey, G. H.: Growth and Development of Children, 5th Ed. Chicago, Year Book Medical Publishers, 1967.

(*Text continued on page 98.*)

TABLE 4–6 ABNORMALITIES OF SKELETAL DEVELOPMENT*

Legend: N = normal   ↑ = advanced   ↓ = retarded
          (N) = probably normal (↑) = possibly advanced (↓) = possibly retarded

Condition	Skeletal Maturation	Growth and Stature	Comments
Central and General			
Hyperpituitarism (giantism)	N or (↓), may fuse late	↑ ↑	eosinophilic adenoma, acromegalic if late
Hypopituitarism (pan-, pituitary dwarfism)	↓ ↓, may never fuse	↓ ↓	? "normal" early
Primordial dwarfism (genetic, constitutional)	N or (↓)	↓	? bone maturation "scattered"
CNS disorders			(2° to neoplasm or other disease)
Pinealoma	↑	↑, adult? N	especially males
Fibrous dysplasia	↑	↑, adult? N	especially females
Craniopharyngioma	↓	↓	
Hypothalamic dysfunction	↑ or ↓	↑ or ↓	many associations, i.e., obesity
Exogenous obesity	N or (↑)	N or (↑), adult N	
Malnutrition and/or chronic disease	(↓)	(↓), adult may be N	
Chondro-osseous dysplasias and syndromes	↓ usually	↓ ↓ usually	rarely advanced, many die early
Gonads			
Hypergonadism (hyperplasia, neoplasm)	↑ ↑, fuse early	↑ ↑, adult ↓	(may be 2° to gonadotropin ↑ ↓)
Hypogonadism			
Eunuchoidism	N or (↓), fuse late	↑, long extremities	intrinsic, castration, 2° to disease
Pituitary	N	↓	not panhypopituitarism
Gonadal "dysplasias"			
Turner's syndrome	N or (↓), fuse late	↓	XO types, hypomineralization
Kleinfelter's syndrome	N or (↓), fuse late	↑, long extremities	XXY types
Abnormal sexual differentiation	(N)	(N)	pseudohermaphrodite types
Sexual developmental variations			
Delayed adolescence	(↓), then N	↓, adult N	
Premature pubarche	(↑), then N	↑, adult N	
Premature thelarche	N or (? ↑)	N	
Constitutional precocity	(↑), then N	↑, adult N	
Adrenals			
Cortical insufficiency (Addison's disease)	(↓)	(↓)	like a chronic disease (may be 2° to ACTH ↑ ↓)
Cortical hyperactivity (Cushing's disease)	(↓)	↓	cortisol ↑, hypomineralization
Adrenogenital syndrome (hyperplasia, neoplasm)	↑ ↑ ↑. fuse early	↑ ↑, adult ↓	usually masculinizing, rarely feminizing
Thyroid			
Hypothyroidism			(may be 2° to TSH ↑ ↓)
Congenital (cretinism)	↓ ↓ ↓ ↓	↓ ↓ ↓, infantile	epiphyseal dysgenesis hypermineralization
Acquired	↓	↓	
Hyperthyroidism	(↑)	(↑), adult N	? hypomineralization
Parathyroids			
Hyperparathyroidism (1° or 2°)	(N)	(N)	hypomineralization
Hypoparathyroidism	(N)	(N)	hypermineralization
(Pseudohypoparathyroidism)	(N)	↓	associated with XO types

*From Graham, C. B.: Personal communication, 1970.

TABLE 4–7   SOME ABERRATIONS IN OSSIFICATION IN BONE DISEASE

Probable Disturbance	Disease
The cartilaginous growth and the formation of the longitudinal calcified bars preparatory to their resorption and replacement by bone are normal. The ossification process is defective. The bone elongates by chondrogenesis, the limbs are fragile due to defective ossification. Multiple fractures ensue but the fractures heal with good osteoid, although inadequately calcified.	Osteogenesis imperfecta (hereditary fragility of bones with marked osteoporosis)
The cartilage cells retain their growth potential but the osteoblasts are in functional failure. Growth in length of the bones continues. The blood vessel walls are more permeable than normal and hemorrhages ensue. The osteoclastic activity proceeds also. Thus, the zone of preparatory calcification of the epiphyseal plate is widened but not replaced by new bone. There is a zone of rarefaction bordering upon this cartilaginous calcified area. There is friability and fragmentation of the calcified area. The bone is diffusely osteoporotic.	Scurvy (vitamin C deficiency)
The cartilaginous cells lack the power to grow at a normal rate whereas the osteoblasts continue to function. There is poor preparation for the longitudinal growth to long bones but the osteoblasts continue to function circumferentially. The bones tend to be broad, deformed, and stunted in size.	Achondroplasia
There is a proliferation of osteoid without calcification. There is also a deficiency of calcification in the cartilage zone and a failure of remodeling of the bone in the metaphysis. The blood vessels form brushlike structures penetrating the cartilage in all directions. There are bulbous enlargements of the ends of the bones and an increased bending of the bones with small stresses and strains due to poor calcification.	Rickets (vitamin D deficiency)
The damaged kidneys are unable to excrete the phosphates in adequate amounts. This stimulates the parathyroids to excrete increased quantities of parathormone which mobilizes calcium from the bones. The calcium deficiency in the bones produces the radiolucency and a lack of calcification seen in the zone of chondrocytic replacement of the metaphysis. This area appears frayed and broad.	Renal osteodystrophy and renal rickets
Both osteoblastic and chondroblastic activity are depressed in rate and the growth of the bone occurs more slowly than is normal. The secondary centers of ossification fail to ossify or are speckled in their appearance.	Hypothyroidism
Outright osteochondritis of the metaphyseal zone and a periostitis.	Congenital syphilis
Both osteoblastic and chondroblastic activity are depressed. Calcium is deposited in the "dead chondrocytic zone" or zone of provisional calcification. When the illness is overcome osteoblastic and chondroblastic activity are resumed but not all the calcium in the zone of provisional calcification is resorbed, and a "bypassed white line" remains in the metaphyses.	Severe systemic illness; acute leukemias

TABLE 4–8 ROENTGEN APPEARANCES OF BONE CORRELATED WITH BIOCHEMISTRY*

General Roentgen Appearances	Disease Suggested	Serum			Urine	
		Calcium	Inorganic Phosphorus	Alkaline Phosphatase	Calcium	Phosphorus
Diffuse hyperlucency of bone. Occasional "pseudocystic" lesions of bone (brown tumors). Cortical resorption—middle and distal phalanges. Resorption lamina dura around teeth. Soft tissue and renal calcifications. Peptic ulceration duodenum.	Hyperparathyroidism: Primary Early Advanced Terminal Secondary	↑ ↑ N-↓	N → ↑ ↑	S↑ ↑ R↑	↑ ↑ ↑	N → → →
Increased density of bones at times. Short metacarpals or metatarsals, especially fourth and fifth.	Hypoparathyroidism (Seabright Bantam) Pseudohypoparathyroidism Pseudo-pseudohypoparathyroidism	→ → N	↑ ↑ N	N-↓ N-↓ N	→ → N	→ → N
Hyperlucency of bone occasionally	Hyperthyroidism, marked	N	N	↑	↑	↑
Usually no change in adults. In *child* delayed ossification of epiphyses, retarded growth, and "stippled" epiphyses. Dwarfism. Vertebrae diminished in height.	Hypothyroidism	N	N	N	N	N
Severe radiolucency of bone generally. Aseptic necrosis of heads of femora and humeri. Vertebrae partially collapsed. In *child,* accelerated ossification and closure of epiphyses leading to dwarfism. Peptic ulceration duodenum.	Hypercortisonism (Cushing's disease or syndrome)	N	N	N	↑	↑
Diffuse hyperlucency of bones. Biconcave endplates of vertebrae ("fish-like") with collapse.	Senile osteoporosis	N	N-O↓	N	N	N

Table 4–8 continued on following page.

TABLE 4-8 ROENTGEN APPEARANCES OF BONE CORRELATED WITH BIOCHEMISTRY* (*Continued*)

General Roentgen Appearances	Disease Suggested	Serum			Urine	
		Calcium	Inorganic Phosphorus	Alkaline Phosphatase	Calcium	Phosphorus
Hyperlucency of bone distal to fracture (disuse atrophy).	Fracture healing (multiple and severe disuse atrophy).	↑	↑	↑	↑	N
Hyperlucency of bones. Expansion of metaphyses—"frayed" metaphyseal ossification, markedly diminished. Delayed ossification of epiphyses. Pathologic fractures and deformed bones under stress.	Hypovitaminosis D child rickets—active	↓	↓	↑	N	N
Marked hyperlucency of all bones—Biconcave appearances in vertebrae with partial collapse.	Adult—osteomalacia	N-↓	↓	↑	N	N
Hyperlucency of bones with some periosteal thickening. Soft tissue ectopic calcification.	Hypervitaminosis D	↑	N-↑	↑	↑	N
Hyperlucency of bone. In *child,* lucent strips in metaphyses with somewhat dense strip adjoining. Small spurs of bone at metaphyseal margins, which may be fractured. Epiphyses poorly ossified with white line around epiphyseal margins.	Hypovitaminosis C (untreated)	N	N	↓	N	N
Subperiosteal hemorrhages previously not manifest become calcified.	Healing scurvy	N	N	↑	N	N
Bizarre trabeculation of bones with thickened trabeculae interlaced with lucency—bones appear broadened, enlarged, and may be deformed.	Osteitis deformans (Paget's) mild—few bones Generalized and active	N R↑	N R↓	S-↑ ↑	N N	N N

Table 4–8 continued on opposite page.

Radiographic findings	Condition					
Early, there may be no changes. Circumscribed, indiscriminately scattered, lucent foci, or diffuse hyperlucency. Pathologic compressions and fracture.	Multiple myeloma Uncomplicated With renal involvement	↑ ↓	← ←	R↑ R↑	N-↑ ↑	← ←
Destroyed bone with reactive periosteal zone, and some bizarre calcification (in tumor osteoid).	Osteosarcoma	N	N	↑	N-↑	N
Circumscribed, indiscriminately scattered lucent or sclerotic foci, or both. Pathologic fractures. With some metastatic tumors, bones may be diffusely "white" (i.e., metastatic carcinoma of prostate).	Tumor, metastatic to bone	N	N	O↑	N	N-↑
Pseudocystic conglomerate foci with coarsened trabeculae and "shell of bone" appearance on margins of involved areas.	Polyostotic fibrous dysplasia	N	N	O↑	N	O↑

Code: N = Normal O = Occasionally
↑ = Increased S = Slight
↓ = Decreased R = Rarely

Sources:
  1. Bondy, P. K.: Duncan's Diseases of Metabolism. 6th Ed. Philadelphia. W. B. Saunders Company, 1969.
  2. Aegerter, E., and Kirkpatrick, J. A., Jr.: Orthopedic Diseases. 3rd Ed. Philadelphia, W. B. Saunders Company, 1968.
  3. Singleton, E. B., and Tseng, Ten, Ching: Pseudohypoparathyroidism with bone changes simulating hyperparathyroidism. Radiology, 78:388–393, 1962.

*Amalgamation of laboratory findings, courtesy of Dr. James L. Quinn, III.

TABLE 4–9 CHANGES IN CONTOUR OR SIZE OF THE BONE CHARACTERISTIC OF SOME DISEASE PROCESSES

Roentgen Appearances	Disease Suggested
Thickening of bone	Acromegaly
	Hypertrophic pulmonary osteoarthropathy
Increase in bony length	Arachnodactylia
	Englemann's disease
Diminution of diameter of bone	Osteogenesis imperfecta
	Osteopsathyrosis
Shortening in the length of bone	Achondroplasia
	Hypoplasia
	Phocomelia
	Peromelia
	Pituitary dwarfism
Irregular deformity of the bone grossly	Osteitis deformans (Paget's disease of bone)
	Chondrodysplasia (Ollier's disease)
Fracture	Traumatic fracture
	Pathologic fracture superimposed upon an underlying bone disease

Usefulness of Skeletal Maturation Studies

1. Diagnosis and management of certain endocrine disorders.
2. Evaluation of fetal maturity (Table 4–17).
3. Ability to anticipate onset of puberty.
4. Ability to predict growth potential.

However, the following factors must be taken into consideration:
1. Hereditary, individual, sexual, and population factors.
2. Anatomic variations.
3. Socioeconomic status.
4. Contemporary data, since there is a general trend toward earlier skeletal maturation (Graham).

METHODS OF ESTIMATING SKELETAL MATURATION

Rotch's method (1909), as modified by Bardeen (1921). This method was a description of clear-cut developmental stages in the hand, carpal bones, and distal radius and ulna. Thirteen stages or categories were originally described by Rotch and later amplified by Bardeen. The procedure did not allow for differences in genetic factors which have a part in determining the order of ossification of bony centers.

Direct measurements of the amount of relevant bony tissue on the radiograph. This method concentrated on the wrist, and used such expedients as planimetry and "bone area ratios" (Lowell and Woodrow, 1922; Carter, 1926; Flory, 1926).

Estimation of "bone age" from the epiphyses in which ossification has most recently begun (Sontag and Lipford).

Elgenmark's method (1946).   In this method the number of ossification centers were counted at different months of age, with a range of variations published for boys and girls indicating the mean and up to three standard deviations. Although accurate, this method required considerable radiation exposure to growing bones.

Description of "maturity indicators" by Todd (1937), and Greulich and Pyle (1959).   Maturity indicators were defined as the individual "features of bone" which mark the progress of the bone toward maturity and can be seen in the roentgenogram. These indicators usually concerned the appearance and gradual development of the epiphysis as well as the adjoining epiphyseal plate and metaphysis. This study by Todd, and later Greulich and Pyle, forms the basis of the Cleveland reference in Figure 4–15 for onset of ossification as well as completion. Children from "prosperous homes" in Cleveland were x-rayed "within three weeks of the birth date, and every six months, if the child was under five years; every twelve months if he was over five years." Standards were then developed so that every individual bone was precisely at the median stage of development for each sex separately. Atlases of the growing hand, wrist, foot, and knee were based upon this population study.

Unfortunately, the following determinants may alter the "average bone age concept" of Pyle: (1) genetic factors; (2) trauma; (3) systemic disease; and (4) skeletal maturation, which does not proceed at a constant rate throughout the developmental period. In the female there is a plateau in the development curve between ages six and ten, and in the male between ages seven and thirteen. In boys 13 to 18 years of age and in girls ten to 15 years of age there is a decelerating skeletal maturation.

Oxford method (Acheson).   This technique is a scoring system for the hand, wrist, and knee which permits maturation to be rated on a scale that does not require direct consideration of the size of the bone and is independent of the age of the child. A number is assigned to each maturity indicator and a total score is reached for each child.

The detractive factors in this method are: (1) considerable x-ray exposure is required for numerous epiphyses throughout the body, and (2) the scoring technique does not necessarily reflect as much actual information as the maturity indicators of Todd and Pyle.

Tanner Whitehouse method (Tanner and Whitehouse, 1959; Tanner, Whitehouse, and Healy, 1962).   This method is based on the definition of maturity indicators in each individual ossification center and has been worked out only for the hand and wrist. Eight maturity indicators are illustrated and described for all the centers of ossification except the radius, which has none, and the sesamoids, which are ignored. The unknown film is rated either in terms of a skeletal maturity score, which is in essence a percentage value, or by skeletal age. The scores are in proportion, totaling 1000 points in the fully developed adult, with arbitrary weights being given to certain individual bones.

The factors detracting from this method are: (1) there is no allowance for modification of indicators which may be distorted by disease; (2) the carpus is allowed to contribute half of the total maturity score of the hand and wrist and this is probably inordinate; (3) the order of ossification of long bones is to a considerable extent genetically determined and there is a wide variation (probably inherited) in size and the details of their shape.

Fels Research Institute technique (Sontag and Lipford, 1943; Garn and Rohmann, 1960; and Garn, Rohmann, and Davis, 1963).   This method confines itself to the "onset of ossification," and to secondary centers undergoing epiphyseal fusion, especially in the hand and foot. The researchers rated these centers according to

(Text continued on page 111.)

TABLE 4–10 RADIOGRAPHIC DIMINISHED BONE DENSITY HIGHLY SUGGESTIVE OF CERTAIN DISEASE ENTITIES

Roentgen Appearances	Disease Suggested

I. With systemic involvement (multiple extremities, skull possibly, vertebrae)
  A. Uniform radiolucency
	Osteogenesis imperfecta
	Hypovitaminosis D rickets
	Hypovitaminosis D osteomalacia
	Hypophosphatasia
	Hypophosphatemic and vitamin D refractory rickets
	Renal rickets
	Fanconi's syndrome
	Raynaud's disease or phenomenon
	Hyperparathyroidism (primary or secondary)
	Endocrine osteoporosis:
	1. Gonads:
	  a. Ovaries — postmenopausal osteoporosis due to inadequate estrogen stimulation.
	  b. Testes — osteoporosis of Fröhlich syndrome and possible acromegaly due to inadequate androgen stimulation.
	2. Adrenal cortex:
	  a. Cushing's syndrome — probably due to excessive sugar-active hormone, which is anti-anabolic.
	  b. Adrenal atrophy — senile osteoporosis due to adrenopause of Albright; a deficiency of the anabolic N hormone.
	3. Pituitary:
	  a. Cushing's syndrome — probably through the adrenal cortex.
	  b. Acromegaly — possibly through the gonads.
	4. Thyroid:
	Osteoporosis of long-standing hyperthyroidism — probably due to excessive use of proteins by the accelerated basal metabolic rate.
	5. Pancreas:
	Osteoporosis of diabetes mellitus — probably due to excessive utilization of protein.
	Disuse atrophy — osteoporosis due to loss of stress stimulus.
	Deficiency osteoporosis — inadequate intake, absorption, or utilization of proteins and vitamin C.

Table 4–10 continued on opposite page.

TABLE 4–10   RADIOGRAPHIC DIMINISHED BONE DENSITY HIGHLY SUGGESTIVE OF CERTAIN DISEASE ENTITIES (*Continued*)

B. Involvement primarily in multiple metaphyses	Scurvy Rickets Congenital syphilis Hypervitaminosis A
C. Multiple circumscribed radiolucencies	Inflammatory diseases of bone Neurofibromatosis Metastatic tumors Lipoid storage diseases and histiocytoses Hyperparathyroidism (primary and secondary) Polyostotic fibrous dysplasia Round cell tumors, such as Ewing's neuroblastoma, or reticulum cell sarcoma Multiple myeloma
D. Reticulolinear radiolucencies	Bone marrow disorders (anemias) Reticulum cell sarcoma
II. Involvement of a single extremity	
A. Affecting the epiphyses primarily	Focal aseptic necrosis Osteochondrosis Osteochondritis dissecans Epiphyseal chondroblastoma
B. Affecting the metaphyses primarily	Neurotrophic osteopathy Osteomyelitis; Brodie's abscess Osteosarcoma (prior to invasion of epiphysis) Giant cell tumors Bone cysts Giant osteoid osteoma (benign osteoblastoma)
C. Diaphyseal corticoperiosteal involvement primarily	Osteomyelitis Traumatic periostitis Round cell tumors (such as Ewing's and neuroblastoma) Neurofibromas of bone Hemangiomas of bone Fibrosarcomas
D. Adjoining articular surfaces	Pyogenic arthritis Rheumatoid arthritis Pigmented villonodular synovitis Tuberculosis Gout Hemorrhage in joints (as in hemophilia) Synovioma Sarcoid

TABLE 4–11 RADIOGRAPHIC INCREASED BONE DENSITY WIDELY
DISSEMINATED OR LOCALIZED IN ONE EXTREMITY

Roentgen Appearances	Diseases Suggested
I. Widely disseminated A. Diffuse 1. With dense sclerotic change	Osteopetrosis (marble bone disease) Englemann's disease Fluorine poisoning Juvenile and tertiary syphilis Urticaria pigmentosa (mastocytosis)
2. With moderate sclerotic change	Hypoparathyroidism Hypervitaminosis A Paget's disease Idiopathic hypercalcemia of infancy Anemias; lymphomas Myelofibrosis or sclerosis Metastatic carcinoma of prostate
B. Transverse bands in metaphyses	Heavy metal poisoning; phosphorus poisoning Cretinism Congenital syphilis Recovery following systemic debilitating illness Acute leukemia Scurvy Hypervitaminosis A and D
C. Longitudinal or corticoperiosteal sclerosis	Melorheostosis leri Juvenile and tertiary syphilis Infantile cortical hyperostosis of Caffey-Silverman Hypertrophic pulmonary osteoarthropathy Blood dyscrasias Osteomyelitis—chronic Neuroblastoma and Ewing's tumor occasionally Fibrous dysplasia In skull: meningioma, hyperostosis frontalis interna

Table 4–11 continued on opposite page.

TABLE 4–11   RADIOGRAPHIC INCREASED BONE DENSITY WIDELY DISSEMINATED
OR LOCALIZED IN ONE EXTREMITY (*Continued*)

Roentgen Appearances	Diseases Suggested
D. Irregular areas of indiscriminate distribution	Sclerotic bone islands Osteopoikilosis Osteitis deformans (Paget's disease) Osteosclerotic tumor metastases Occasional multiple myeloma Mastocytosis (urticaria pigmentosa) Osteosclerosis with parathyroid adenoma and renal failure
II. Localized or regional A. Epiphyseal	Epiphyseal dysplasia Hypothyroidism Congenital stippled epiphyses Osteochondrosis Bone infarction (epiphyseal type)
B. Metaphyseal	Bone infarcts (metaphyseal type) Osteitis condensans ilei Sclerotic bone islands Osteomyelitis of Garré

C. Diaphyseal corticoperiosteal	Osteoid osteoma
	Traumatic periostitis
	In skull:
	    Hyperostosis frontalis interna
	    Meningioma
	    Neuroblastoma
	    Osteoma
	    "Ossifying fibroma"
	In vertebrae:
	    Fibrous dysplasia
	    Idiopathic

D. Adjoining articular surfaces	Hypertrophic arthritis Peritendinitis calcarea Chondromatosis of joints Pseudogout

TABLE 4–12 DISEASES CHARACTERIZED BY MIXED INCREASED
RADIOLUCENCY OF BONE AND OSTEOSCLEROSIS

Roentgen Appearances	Disease Suggested
Sequestrum formation	Osteomyelitis Malignant bone neoplasms
Diffuse intermixed lucency and sclerosis	Chronic granulomatous infections (syphilis, blastomycosis) Lymphomas Malignant tumor metastases In the skull: meningioma
Zone of sclerosis around a zone of lucency	Very thin: cyst Very thick: fibrous dysplasia, or Brodie's abscess Intermediate: epidermoidoma, hemangioma, neurofibroma

TABLE 4–13 DISEASES CHARACTERIZED BY SOME DISORGANIZATION IN
THE ARCHITECTURAL TRABECULAR PATTERN OF THE BONE

Roentgen Appearances	Disease Suggested

"Mosaic" coarse trabecular pattern
  "Sheaves of grain" appearance
  "Picture frame" appearance in vertebral bodies
  "Maplike" appearance in the skull
  "Cotton-wool" pattern in skull
	Paget's disease of bone

Coarse, sclerotic irregular pattern	Chronic inflammation after repair
Coarse reticular, or linear medullary and cortical pattern.	Bone marrow disorders

TABLE 4–14 DISEASES CHARACTERIZED BY CHANGES IN THE
BONE RELATED TO ADJOINING PATHOLOGY

Roentgen Appearances	Pathology
Bones slender, cortex thin, adjoining soft tissues atrophic and thin; herring-bone pattern occasionally found in the muscles; calcification in plaques around joints.	Anterior poliomyelitis Amyotrophic lateral sclerosis
Bone sharply eroded by adjoining mass which contains numerous phlebolith-like calcific shadows.	Hemangioma
Bone sharply eroded by moderately dense soft tissue mass, sharply circumscribed, no calcification in mass.	Neurofibroma
Bone sharply eroded by adjoining mass which contains laminations of circumlinear calcification; or in vertebral bodies, anterior erosion sparing the intervertebral spaces.	Major artery (or in case of spine, the aorta) aneurysm
Bone invaded and destroyed by adjoining soft tissue mass; with or without amorphous calcification; with or without periosteal reaction; soft tissue mass larger than bone involvement.	Malignant soft tissue tumor such as fibrosarcoma or chondrosarcoma (with osteosarcoma, the bone destruction is usually of greater magnitude than the soft tissue mass accompanying; and the "calcium" in the mass may be recognized as calcified osteoid)
Bone destruction in a foot with extensive blood vessel (arterial) calcification, and soft tissue irregular swelling.	Secondary osteomyelitis, such as occurs in diabetes mellitus

TABLE 4–15   DISEASES SUGGESTED BY SITE OF INVOLVEMENT
WITHIN A LONG BONE

Roentgen Appearances	Disease Suggested
Circumscribed lytic lesion in epiphysis only	Epiphyseal chondroblastoma Osteochondrosis (early) Aseptic necrosis
Circumscribed lytic lesion involving epiphysis and metaphysis; no "white line" of margination (no "radiologic capsule")	Giant cell tumor Osteosarcoma Fibrosarcoma
Circumscribed lytic lesion which may involve epiphysis and metaphysis; intermittent "white line of margination"	Brodie's abscess
Partial lysis of epiphysis with "pointed" resorption of metaphysis	Neurotrophic disease of bone of atrophic type (such as leprosy)
Ill-defined lytic lesion involving metaphysis which stops at epiphyseal plate; often associated periosteal reaction	Osteomyelitis
Circumscribed and marginated lytic area in metaphysis (or diaphysis adjoining)	Bone cyst
Circumscribed and marginated lytic area of bone, with punctate foci of calcification	Enchondroma
Circumscribed lytic foci anywhere in bone, with "white lines of margination"	Hemangioma; lymphangioma
Circumscribed lytic foci in diaphysis; no "radiologic capsule" or incomplete faint white line around lesion	Reticuloendotheliosis or histiocytosis X Lipoid dyscrasias Eosinophilic granuloma
Circumscribed lytic foci anywhere in bone, with no "white lines of margination"	Metastatic tumors; multiple myeloma
Circumscribed lytic foci anywhere in bone with dense and thick "white lines of margination"	Fibrous dysplasia Brodie's abscess Sclerosing osteomyelitis of Garré

Table 4–15 continued on opposite page.

TABLE 4–15 DISEASES SUGGESTED BY SITE OF INVOLVEMENT
WITHIN A LONG BONE (*Continued*)

Roentgen Appearances	Disease Suggested
Sclerotic punctate foci in epiphysis only	Chondroangiopathia calcificans congenita (congenital stippled epiphyses) Cretinism Osteochondrosis (intermediate phase) Aseptic necrosis
Sclerotic foci in metaphysis only	Bone infarction (Caisson's disease)
Reticulolinear sclerosis in diaphysis	Reticulum cell sarcoma Hemangioma of vertebral bodies
Small foci of sclerosis indiscriminate	Sclerotic bone islands Osteopoikilosis Sclerotic types of metastatic tumor to bone
Diffuse sclerosis of diaphysis, but not of epiphyses or metaphyses	Engelmann's disease
Diffuse sclerosis of bone with Erlenmeyer flask shape of metaphysis	Osteopetrosis (marble bone disease)
Diffuse sclerosis of bone with no alteration in shape	Lymphoma of bone Metastatic carcinoma of bone, especially from prostatic carcinoma
Outgrowth from the bone metaphysis, sharply circumscribed like a mushroom	Osteochondroma (when multiple, and with malformed bone and enchondromas, Ollier's disease; when multiple purely of the exophytic type, diaphyseal aclasis, or multiple osteochondromatosis)
Ill-defined lytic lesion especially of diaphysis, with periosteal reaction, symmetrical expansion and destruction.	Ewing's disease of bone Neuroblastoma (Round cell tumors of bone generally)
Erlenmeyer flask shape of metaphyses	Osteopetrosis Gaucher's disease Metaphyseal dysplasia (Pyle's disease) Vitamin-D resistant rickets in an older child — partially treated

TABLE 4-16 NUMBER OF OSSIFICATION CENTERS AT DIFFERENT MONTHS OF AGE*

Boys

Age, Mo.	Av. No. Centers =M	Dev. =σ	Range of Variation					
			M−3σ	M−2½σ	M−σ	M+σ	M+2½σ	M+3σ
1	4.8	1.9	0	0	2.9	6.7	9.6	10.5
2	5.7	2.0	0	0.7	3.7	7.7	10.7	11.7
3	6.5	2.0	0.5	1.5	4.5	8.5	11.5	12.5
4	8.9	2.8	0.5	1.9	6.1	11.7	15.9	17.3
5	9.8	2.4	2.6	3.8	7.4	12.2	15.8	17.0
6	11.2	2.4	4.0	5.2	8.8	13.6	17.2	18.4
7	12.5	2.9	3.8	5.2	9.6	15.4	19.8	21.2
8	13.0	1.7	7.9	8.7	11.3	14.7	17.3	18.1
9	13.6	2.7	5.5	6.8	10.9	16.3	20.4	21.7
10	15.2	3.5	4.7	6.4	11.7	18.7	24.0	25.7
11	15.8	3.2	6.2	7.8	12.6	19.0	23.8	25.4
12	16.5	4.9	1.8	4.2	11.6	21.4	28.8	31.2
13–15	19.9	6.3	1.0	4.1	13.6	26.2	35.7	38.8
16–18	23.5	8.4	0	2.5	15.1	31.9	44.5	48.7
19–21	25.5	8.4	0.3	4.5	17.1	33.9	46.5	50.7
22–24	32.3	9.2	4.7	9.3	23.1	41.5	55.3	59.9
25–27	36.8	5.5	20.3	23.0	31.3	42.3	50.6	52.3
28–30	39.8	8.4	14.6	18.8	31.4	48.2	60.8	65.0
31–33	44.1	4.8	29.7	32.1	39.3	48.9	56.1	58.5
34–36	48.5	5.8	31.1	34.0	42.7	54.3	63.0	65.9
37–42	49.5	6.9	28.8	32.2	42.6	56.4	66.8	70.2
43–48	56.6	4.9	41.9	44.3	51.7	61.5	68.9	71.3
49–54	59.3	5.5	42.8	45.5	53.8	64.8	73.1	75.8
55–60	61.8	3.5	51.3	53.0	58.3	65.3	70.6	72.3

Girls

Age, Mo.	Av. No. Centers =M	Dev. =σ	Range of Variation					
			M−3σ	M−2½σ	M−σ	M+σ	M+2½σ	M+3σ
1	4.7	1.9	0	0	2.8	6.6	9.5	10.4
2	6.2	2.3	0	0.4	3.9	8.5	12.0	13.1
3	7.6	2.5	0.1	1.3	5.1	10.1	13.9	15.1
4	8.5	2.8	0.1	1.5	5.7	11.3	15.5	16.9
5	10.4	2.0	4.4	5.4	8.4	12.4	15.4	16.4
6	11.5	1.7	6.4	7.2	9.8	13.2	15.8	16.6
7	12.9	1.4	8.7	9.4	11.5	14.3	16.4	17.1
8	14.6	3.5	4.1	5.8	11.1	18.1	23.4	25.1
9	16.3	2.4	9.1	10.3	13.9	18.7	22.3	23.5
10	18.1	4.4	4.9	7.1	13.7	22.5	29.1	31.3
11	22.7	6.9	2.0	5.4	15.8	29.6	40.0	43.4
12	25.1	8.7	0	3.3	16.4	33.8	46.9	51.2
13–15	28.6	9.2	1.0	5.6	19.4	37.8	51.6	56.2
16–18	32.9	8.8	6.5	10.9	24.1	41.7	54.9	59.3
19–21	41.3	8.6	15.5	19.8	32.7	49.9	62.8	67.1
22–24	47.2	7.1	25.9	29.4	40.1	54.3	65.0	68.5
25–27	50.8	4.8	36.4	38.8	46.0	55.6	62.8	65.2
28–30	53.2	6.5	33.7	36.9	46.7	59.7	69.5	72.7
31–33	55.8	4.8	41.4	43.8	51.0	60.6	67.8	70.2
34–36	60.5	3.0	51.5	53.0	57.5	63.5	68.0	69.5
37–42	59.5	4.5	46.0	48.2	55.0	64.0	70.8	73.0
43–48	61.4	6.6	41.6	44.9	54.8	68.0	77.9	81.2
49–54	63.5	2.2	56.9	58.0	61.3	65.7	69.0	70.1
55–60	64.2	2.3	57.3	58.4	61.9	66.5	70.0	71.1

*From Elgenmark, O.: Acta Paediat., Vol. 33, Supp. 1, 1946.

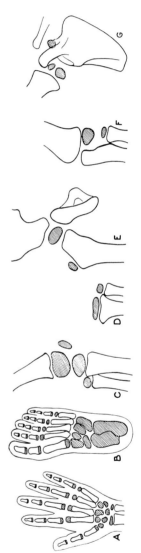

Secondary centers in one side of the skeleton which are counted in the Elgenmark method.
A, hand; B, foot; C, knee; D, wrist; E, hip; F, elbow; G, shoulder.

TABLE 4–17 PERCENTAGE OCCURRENCE OF NEWBORN OSSIFICATION CENTERS, DISTRIBUTED ACCORDING TO SEX, RACE (NEGRO/CAUCASIAN), AND BIRTHWEIGHT (GRAMS)*

Centers	<2,000	2,000–2,499	2,500–2,999	3,000–3,499	3,500–3,999	≥4,000
Calcaneus						
females N/C	100 / 100	100 / 100	100 / 100	100 / 100	100 / 100	100 / 100
males N/C	100 / 100	100 / 100	100 / 100	100 / 100	100 / 100	100 / 100
Talus						
females	100 / 83	100 / 100	100 / 100	100 / 100	100 / 100	100 / 100
males	91 / 73	100 / 100	100 / 100	100 / 99	100 / 100	100 / 100
Femur, distal						
females	50 / 50	94 / 92	99 / 98	100 / 100	100 / 100	100 / 100
males	18 / 9	89 / 75	91 / 85	94 / 100	100 / 100	100 / 100
Tibia, proximal						
females	14 / 0	41 / 54	77 / 76	88 / 86	86 / 91	100 / 91
males	0 / 0	39 / 19	63 / 53	76 / 79	80 / 84	93 / 97
Cuboid						
females	21 / 0	38 / 38	68 / 57	78 / 65	82 / 70	75 / 76
males	0 / 0	23 / 6	44 / 15	58 / 40	68 / 44	100 / 60
Humerus, proximal						
females	0 / 0	11 / 6	23 / 26	53 / 42	39 / 69	100 / 87
males	0 / 0	0 / 8	15 / 14	28 / 42	48 / 49	64 / 59
Capitate						
females	0 / 0	13 / 0	20 / 15	42 / 15	41 / 21	100 / 38
males	0 / 0	7 / 0	16 / 0	21 / 8	26 / 16	31 / 18
Hamate						
females	0 / 0	9 / 0	23 / 11	41 / 13	55 / 2/	67 / 33
males	0 / 0	16 / 7	16 / 6	18 / 6	44 / 10	28 / 11
Cuneiform, third						
females	0 / 0	6 / 0	14 / 0	17 / 0	18 / 6	25 / 10
males	0 / 0	4 / 0	8 / 0	15 / 3	14 / 2	14 / 3
Femur, proximal						
females	0 / 0	0 / 0	1 / 0	1 / 1	0 / 0	0 / 0
males	0 / 0	0 / 0	0 / 0	0 / 0	0 / 0	0 / 0

*Modified by Graham from Christie, A.: Prevalence and Distribution of Ossification Centers in the Newborn Infant. Amer. J. Dis. Child., 77:355–361, 1949. Basic data also in Caffey.

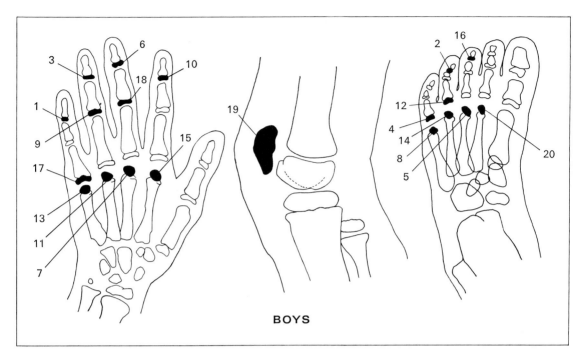

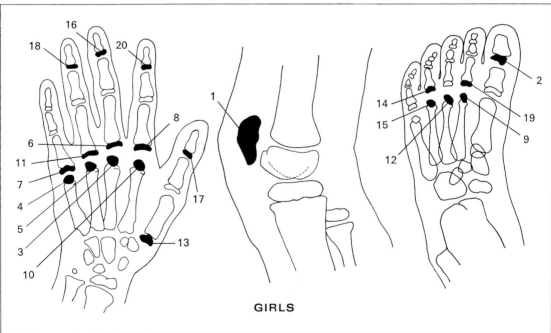

Figure 4–18 The 20 centers of maximum predictive value in boys and in girls. The postnatal ossification centers that have the highest statistical "communality" and hence the greatest predictive value in skeletal assessment are located in the hand, the foot, and the knee. Thus, three radiographs can actually provide more diagnostically useful information than the larger number often made. (From Garn, S. G., Rohmann, C. G., and Silverman, F. N.: Medical Radiography and Photography, *43*, Number 2, 1967.)

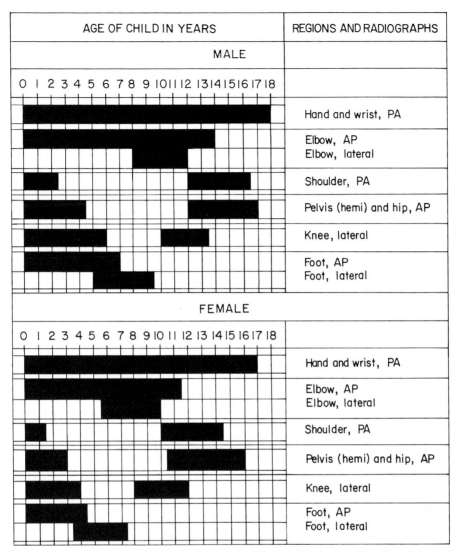

Figure 4-19   Bone age sampling method—suggested filming. (Fels Institute data from C. B. Graham, Instruction Course. Miami Beach, Amer. Roentgen. Ray Soc., 1970.)

their "maximum predictive value" (Figure 4-18). They felt that some of the short bones, as well as the radius, tibia, and fibula should also be excluded in order to allow a higher accuracy coefficient. The highest correlations for fusion apparently exist between the hand and foot, knee and elbow, and shoulder and hips. They are studying epiphyseal fusion in the knee, elbow, hip, and shoulder.

Unfortunately, any method of assessment which depends only on first appearances and epiphyseal closure must also include bony areas other than the hand and wrist.

Modification of the Fels Research Institute technique (Graham).   Figure 4-19 lists six body regions and the appropriate radiographs to be obtained for males and females at various ages. "The left side is examined by convention, but the right side may be substituted. When there is good correlation between the hand and wrist and other sampled regions, the assessment can be assumed to be reasonably accu-

TABLE 4–18 NORMAL RANGES OF AGE-AT-APPEARANCE OF PRINCIPAL CENTERS*

Age of Child		Range
MALE	FEMALE	**Range**
0– 1 year	0– 1 year	±3–6 months
3– 4 years	2– 3 years	±1–1.5 years
7–11 years	6–10 years	±2 years
13–14 years	12–13 years	±2 years plus

*Based on Fels Institute data in Graham, C. B.: Instruction course. Miami, American Roentgen Ray Society, 1970.

rate and is usually normal. Large discrepancies are more often associated with developmental abnormalities. . . . In these and in borderline situations, it is helpful to sample additional regions and at more frequent intervals on follow-up."*

The normal bone age range is unfortunately broad (Table 4–18). Thus, the normal bone age range for a three year old female is from 1.5 to 4.5 years. Moreover, females are considerably advanced over males (1 year at female ages two to three years; 2 years at female ages seven to eight years to the time of fusion).

Graham's table of "Age-at-Appearance (Years-Months) Percentiles for Selected Ossification Centers" is presented in Table 4–5 (modified from Garn et al., 1964).

Questions—Chapter 4

1. Describe the two main types of ossification.

2. What is the usual sequence of events in endochondral ossification?

3. Show diagrammatically the manner in which bone is deposited and resorbed to account for the remodeling that takes place at the ends of growing long bones that have flared extremities.

4. Draw a diagram of a high-power micrograph with a longitudinal section cut through the upper end of a long bone. The diagram should demonstrate the growing end of the epiphyseal plate as well as the adjoining metaphyses.

5. Describe the three main sources of blood supply of a long bone.

6. What three main groups of substances comprise the chemical constitution of bone?

7. List the various factors governing calcium metabolism and describe the interrelationship of these factors.

8. Where is phosphatase found and how does it act physiologically?

9. What is the principal function of parathyroid hormone (parathormone)?

10. What are the essential roles of vitamin D in respect to bone metabolism?

11. Indicate how the cortex and the medullary portions of the bone may be altered pathophysiologically, and give at least one example of a disease process where this occurs (there should be nine different alterations which may occur in respect to the cortex and medullary portions of bone in a general way).

12. Indicate an example of a disease process in which there are circumscribed foci of trabecular thickening or increase in number of trabeculae.

13. Indicate an example of a disease process in which there is reactive normal new bone formation with recognizable and well-defined margin.

*Graham, C. B.: Personal communication, 1970.

14. Indicate a disease process in which neoplastic new bone formation occurs characteristically.

15. Indicate a disease process in which a proliferative type of osteoid overlying the periosteum of the metaphyses occurs distally in the extremities.

16. Indicate a disease process in which local or regional changes of bone architecture result in a decreased density of bone.

17. Indicate at least six disease entities in which a study of the phalanges might help to determine the basic disease process. Describe the alterations which might occur.

18. Under what circumstances can ectopic calcification and/or ossification in soft tissues be observed?

19. Draw a diagram of a long bone and indicate a method of roentgenologic analysis which will ultimately allow a description of all the basic roentgenologic pathology.

20. Indicate where serum calcium and inorganic serum phosphorus are elevated or depressed in the following conditions: (a) primary hypoparathyroidism; (b) osteomalacia untreated; (c) menopausal osteoporosis; (d) multiple myeloma; (e) metastatic skeletal carcinosis; and (f) hyperthyroidism.

21. What is the main purpose in clinical medicine for the determination of bone age as compared with chronological age; and what is the system which was developed for radiographic determination of bone age?

22. Indicate the aberration of bone growth in the following conditions: (a) osteogenesis imperfecta; (b) scurvy; (c) achondroplasia; (d) rickets; (e) renal osteodystrophy; (f) hypothyroidism; and (g) congenital syphilis.

23. Define osteoporosis and differentiate this condition from osteomalacia.

24. Describe some of the changes in bone which may be related to adjoining structures, and indicate by it the importance of studying structures adjoining bone.

25. Summarize the areas of preferential localization in bone of such neoplasms as: (a) chondroblastoma; (b) giant cell tumors; (c) osteosarcoma; and (d) round cell tumors, such as Ewing's, reticulum cell sarcoma, and myeloma.

26. Summarize some of the causes of retarded or accelerated bone development.

27. Outline the system which the author has developed for consideration of bone radiology in the final synthesis of diagnosis.

References

Acheson, R. M.: A method of assessing skeletal maturity from radiographs. J. Anatomy (London), *88*:498–508, 1954.

Acheson, R. M.: The Oxford method of assessing skeletal maturity. Clin. Orthopedics, *10*:19–39, 1957.

Acheson, R. M.: Maturation of the Skeleton. Falkner, Frank, ed.: Human Development. Philadelphia, W. B. Saunders Co., 1966.

Acheson, R. M., Fowler, G. B., Fry, E. I., Janes, M., Koski, K., Urbano, O. P., and Vander-WerfftenBosch, J. J.: Studies in the reliability of assessing skeletal maturity from x-rays. Part I: Greulich-Pyle Atlas. Human Biology, *35*:317–349, 1963.

Acheson, R. M., Vicinus, J. H., and Fowler, G. B.: Studies in the reliability of assessing maturity from x-rays. Part II: The Bones: Specific Approach. Human Biology, *36*:211–228, 1964.

Acheson, R. M., Vicinus, J. H., and Fowler, G. B.: Studies in the reliability of assessing skeletal maturity from x-rays. Part III: The Methods Contrasted. Human Biology, *38*:204–218, 1966.

Adams, P. H., and Jowsey, J.: Sodium fluoride in the treatment of osteoporosis and other bone diseases. Ann. Intern. Med., *63*:1151–1155, 1965.

Aegerter, E., and Kirkpatrick, J. A., Jr.: Orthopedic Diseases. Second Edition. Philadelphia, W. B. Saunders Co., 1963.

Albright, F.: Osteoporosis. Ann. Intern. Med., *27*:861–882, 1947.

Aliapoulios, M. A., Berstein, D. S., and Balodimos, M. C.: Thyrocalcitonin, its role in calcium homeostasis. Arch. Intern. Med., *123*:88–94, 1969.

Bardeen, C. R.: The relation of ossification to physiological development. J. Radiology, *2*:1–8, 1921.

Barnhard, H. J., and Geyer, R. W.: Growth and development of bone, normal and abnormal. Radiology, *75*:942–947, 1960.

Caffey, J.: Pediatric X-ray Diagnosis. Fifth Edition. Chicago, Year Book Medical Publishers, 1967.

Carbone, P. P., Ziplin, I., Sokoloff, L., Frazier, P., Cook, P., and Mullins, F.: Fluoride effect on bone in plasma cell myeloma. Arch. Intern. Med., *121*:130–140, 1968.

Christie, A.: Prevalence and distribution of ossification centers in the newborn infant. Amer. J. Dis. Child., *77*:355–361, 1949.

Christie, A., Martin, M., Williams, E. L., Hudson, G., and Lanier, J. C., Jr.: Estimation of fetal maturity by roentgen studies of osseous development. Amer. J. Obstet. Gynec., *60*: 133–139, 1950.

Cohen, P.: Fluoride and calcium therapy for myeloma bone lesions. J.A.M.A., *198*:583–586, 1966.

Collins, D. H.: Pathology of Bone. London, Butterworths, 1966.

Copp, D. H.: Parathyroids, calcitonin, and control of plasma calcium. Recent Progress in Hormone Research, *20*:59–88, 1964.

Currarino, G., and Erlandson, M. E.: Premature fusion of epiphyses in Cooley's anemia. Radiology, *83*:656–664, 1964.

Dimich, A., Bedrossian, P. D., and Wallace, S.: Hypoparathyroidism. Arch. Intern. Med., *120*:449–458, 1967.

Edling, N. P. G.: Pathologic features of bone: Tentative classification of bone lesions. Acta Radiol. (Diagnosis), 7:449–456, 1968.

Elgenmark, O.: The normal development of the ossific centers during infancy and childhood; clinical, roentgenologic, and statistical study. Acta Paediat., *33*(Suppl. 1):1–79, 1946.

Engle, R. L., and Wallis, L. A.: Multiple myeloma and the adult Fanconi syndrome. Amer. J. Med., *22*:5–12, 1957.

Feist, J. H.: The biologic basis of radiologic findings in bone disease. Radiol. Clin. N. A., 8:182–206, 1970.

Flecker, H.: Time of appearance and fusion of ossification centers as observed by roentgenographic methods. Amer. J. Roentgenol., *47*: 97–159, 1942.

Foster, G. V.: Calcitonin (thyrocalcitonin). New Eng. J. Med., *279*:349–360, 1968.

Fraser, D.: Clinical manifestations of genetic aberrations of calcium and phosphorus metabolism. J.A.M.A., *176*:281–287, 1961.

Fraser, D.: Hypophosphatasia. Amer. J. Med., *22*:730–746, 1957.

Garn, S. M., and Rohmann, C. G.: Variability in the order of ossification of the bony centers of the hand and wrist. Amer. J. Phys. Anthropol., *18*:219–229, 1960.

Garn, S. M., Rohmann, C. G., and Davis, A. A.: Genetics of hand-wrist ossification. Amer. J. Phys. Anthropol., *21*:33–40, 1963.

Garn, S. M., Silverman, F. N., and Rohmann, C. G.: A rational approach to the assessment of skeletal maturation. Ann. Radiol. (Paris), 7:297–307, 1964.

Girdany, B. R., and Golden, R.: Centers of ossification of the skeleton. Amer. J. Roentgenol., *68*:922–924, 1952.

Goldbloom, R. B., Stein, P. B., Eisen, A., McSheffrey, J. B., Brown, B. St.J., and Wiglesworth, F. W.: Idiopathic periosteal hyperostosis with dysproteinemia. New Eng. J. Med., *274*:873–878, 1966.

Graham, C. B.: Assessment of bone maturation—methods and pitfalls. Radiol. Clin. N. Amer., *10*:185–202, 1972.

Graham, C. B.: Roentgenologic evaluation of skeletal development; Instruction course. Miami Beach, American Roentgen Ray Society, 1970.

Graham, C. B.: Skeletal development and assessment of bone age, in Brenneman-Kelly Practice of Pediatrics (Vol. IX), Hagerstown, Maryland, Harper & Row (in press).

Graham, C. B.: Skeletal maturation. Smith, D., and Marshall, R., eds.: Introduction to Clinical Pediatrics. Philadelphia, W. B. Saunders Co., 1972.

Greulich, W. W., and Pyle, S. I.: Radiographic Atlas of Skeletal Development of the Hand and Wrist. Stanford, Calif., Stanford University Press, 1950.

Greulich, W. W., and Pyle, S. I.: Radiographic Atlas of Skeletal Development of the Hand and Wrist. Second Edition. Stanford, Calif., Stanford University Press, 1959.

Ham, A. W.: Some histo-physiological problems peculiar to calcified tissues. J. Bone & Joint Surg., *34A*:701–728, 1952.

Hansman, C. F.: Appearance and fusion of ossification centers in the human skeleton. Amer. J. Roentgenol., *88*:476–482, 1962.

Hoerr, N. L., Pyle, S. I., and Francis, C. C.: Radiographic Atlas of Skeletal Development of the Foot and Ankle. Springfield, Ill., Charles C Thomas, 1962.

Hollander, J. L., ed.: Arthritis and allied conditions. Seventh Edition. Philadelphia, Lea & Febiger, 1966.

Johnston, F. E., and Jahina, S. B.: The contribution of carpal bones to the assessment of skeletal age. Amer. J. Phys. Anthropol., *23*:349–354, 1965.

Kleeman, C. R., ed.: Uremic osteodystrophy. Arch. Intern. Med., *124*:261–321 and 389–454, 1969.

Kurlander, G. J.: Roentgenology of the congenital adrenogenital syndrome. Amer. J. Roentgenol., *95*:189–199, 1965.

Luck, J. V.: Bone and Joint Disease. Springfield, Ill., Charles C Thomas, 1950.

McLean, F. C., and Urist, M. R.: Bone. Third Edition. Chicago, University of Chicago Press, 1968.

Meschan, I.: Atlas of Normal Radiographic Anatomy. Second Edition. Philadelphia, W. B. Saunders Co., 1959.

Munson, P. L.: Recent advances in parathyroid hormone research. Fed. Proc., *19*:593–601, 1960.

Park, E. A.: The imprinting of nutritional disturbances on the growing bone. Pediatrics, *33*:815–862, 1964.

Pryor, J. W.: The hereditary nature of variation in the ossification of bone. Anatomical Rec., *1*:84–88, 1907.

Pryor, J. W.: Differences in the time of development of centers of ossification in the male and female skeleton. Anatomical Rec., 25: 257–273, 1923.

Pyle, S. I., and Hoerr, N. I.: Radiographic Atlas

of Skeletal Development of the Knee. Spring-field, Ill., Charles C Thomas, 1955.

Pyle, S. I., Waterhouse, A. M., and Greulich, W. W.: A Radiographic Standard of Reference for the Growing Hand and Wrist. Chicago, Year Book Publishers, 1971.

Rich, C., Ensinck, J., and Ivanovich, P.: The effects of sodium fluoride on calcium metabolism of subjects with metabolic bone diseases. J. Clin. Invest., 43:545, 1964.

Rotch, T. M.: A study of the development of the bones in childhood by the roentgen method, with a view of establishing a developmental index for the grading and the protection of early life. Transactions Amer. Assoc. Physicians, 24:603–630, 1909.

Shapiro, L., and Stoller, N. M.: Erosion of phalanges by subungual warts. J.A.M.A., 176:379, 1961.

Shurtleff, D. B., Sparkes, R. S., Clawson, D. K., Guntheroth, W. G., and Mottet, N. K.: Hereditary osteolytis with hypertension and nephropathy. J.A.M.A., 188:363–368, 1964.

Sontag, L. W., and Lipford, J.: The effect of illness and other factors on appearance pattern of skeletal epiphyses. J. Pediat., 23:391–409, 1943.

Sontag, L. W., Snell, D., and Anderson, M.: Rate of appearance of ossification centers from birth to the age of five years. Amer. J. Dis. Child., 58:949–956, 1939.

Stein, I., Stein, R. O., and Beller, M. L.: Living Bone in Health and Disease. Philadelphia, J. B. Lippincott Co., 1955.

Stuart, H. C., Pyle, S. I., Cornoni, J., and Reed, R. B.: Onsets, completions and spans of ossification in the twenty-nine bone-growth centers of the hand and wrist. Pediatrics, 29:237–249, 1962.

Tanner, J. M., Whitehouse, R. H., and Healy, M. J. R.: A new system for estimating the maturity of the hand and wrist with standards derived from 2600 healthy British children. Part II. The Scoring System. Paris International Children's Center, 1962.

Todd, T. W.: Atlas of Skeletal Maturation: Part I. The Hand. St. Louis, C. V. Mosby Co., 1937.

Wallis, L. A., and Engle, R. L.: The adult Fanconi syndrome: Review of 19 cases. Amer. J. Med., 22:13–23, 1957.

Watson, E. H., and Lowery, G. A.: Growth and Development of Children. Fifth Edition. Chicago, Year Book Medical Publishers, 1967.

Weinman, J. P., and Sicher, H.: Bone and Bones: Fundamentals of Bone Biology. Second Edition. St. Louis, C. V. Mosby Co., 1955.

Wilkins, L.: Hormonal influences on skeletal growth. Ann. N. Y. Acad. Sci., 60:763–775, 1955.

Wilson, R. H., McCormick, W. E., Tatum, C. F., and Creech, J. L.: Occupational acroosteolysis. J.A.M.A., 201:577–581, 1967.

Worthen, H. G., and Good, R. A.: The deToni-Fanconi syndrome with cystinosis. Amer. J. Dis. Child., 95:653–688, 1958.

5

Fractures and Dislocations of the Extremities

Description of "Minimal" Study

The radiographs for a suspected fracture or dislocation must be made in a minimum of two planes at right angles to each other, and special views must at times be utilized.

The areas studied must be large enough to include at least one joint and preferably two joints if the bone in question lies between two joints.

The mechanism of trauma or injury must be understood so that the part being radiographed will include adjoining areas which may have undergone secondary injury. Thus, for example, in injuries involving a fall on the outstretched hand, the elbow or clavicle may also sustain a fracture in addition to the wrist.

An understanding of the routine radiographic examinations employed is fundamental. Although the routine radiographic studies for each anatomic part are summarized in greater detail in the author's other texts, a brief review will be rendered here because of its importance.

Major Items for Analysis on Radiographs of Extremities for Fractures. Assuming that appropriate radiographic views are in hand, *four major items require careful analysis:*

1. The degree of apposition of the fragments;
2. The alignment of the fragments with respect to the line of weight-bearing and movement of joints—diagrams in Chapter 11.
3. The degree of torsion of the fragments with respect to one another; and
4. The degree of shortening of the bone as a whole.

The radiographic method provides excellent data regarding the extent of the actual bone injury, the type of fracture (whether it is simple or comminuted, transverse, oblique, longitudinal, spiral, T-, V-, or Y-shaped), and whether there has been penetration by a pointed missile.

Some inferential information may also be gained: (1) Is there soft tissue caught between the fragments? (2) What is the associated soft tissue injury? (3) How much injury has been sustained in the periosteum? (4) How much cartilaginous or joint injury has been sustained?

The complete extent of associated soft tissue injury cannot be evaluated radiographically by simple radiographs and may sometimes require special arterial angiograms and neurological study.

> **Time Intervals Between Radiographic Studies.** Following the *initial diagnostic study,* films should be obtained as follows:
> 1. *Post-reduction and post-immobilization;*
> 2. *One or two weeks later, if position has changed;*
> 3. *After approximately six or eight weeks for primary callus;*
> 4. *After each plaster cast or traction change;* and
> 5. *Before final discharge of the patient.*

TYPES OF FRACTURES

The various types of fractures of the extremities are summarized in Figure 5–1. The following special comments are warranted regarding fracture types:

Avulsion- or Chip-type Fractures are often associated with forcible tearing of ligaments, tendons, or muscle attachments. This is the most serious aspect of this type of fracture.

The Most Important Consideration in the Oblique, Spiral, or Screwlike Fracture is the fact that soft tissue may be interposed between the fragments. Often these fractures are accompanied by contrecoup fractures in an adjoining bone, such as the fibula in respect to the tibia. The examination must be sufficiently inclusive to make such diagnoses whenever possible.

If interposition of soft tissues has occurred, impairment of the healing process may ensue.

Epiphysiolysis and Epiphyseal Injuries are classified into five types according to the Salter-Harris classification (Figure 5–2). Comparison films of the opposite uninvolved side should be obtained whenever possible. Significant disturbances in bone growth occur in only about 10 per cent of epiphyseal injuries because of the relationship of the usual fracture line to the epiphyseal plate and epiphyseal blood supply (DePalma; Rogers).

Types 4 and 5 in the Salter-Harris classification are most important to distinguish if at all possible. A minimum of two years is considered necessary before the possibility of shortening or deformity can be excluded. Radiographic evaluations should be performed at three to six month intervals, including comparison views with the opposite extremity.

Insufficiency, March, or Stress Fractures are also called "fatigue fractures," since they practically always occur at sites of maximal strain on bone, usually in connection with a type of unaccustomed activity. The second, third, or fourth metatarsals are frequent sites of occurrence, often without any demonstrable trauma. Another frequent localization is the upper third of the tibia. Sites affected with lesser

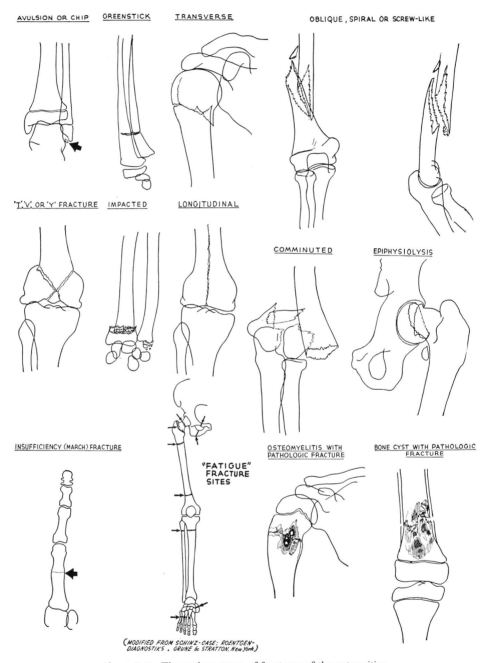

Figure 5–1 The various types of fractures of the extremities.

frequency are the lower third of the femur, the fibula, calcaneus, pelvis, first ribs, and neck of the femur.

Ordinarily with discontinued activity these fractures heal without incident.

When fatigue fractures are multiple and symmetrical, the condition is known as "Milkman's syndrome" and is characterized by so-called "multiple spontaneous idiopathic symmetrical fractures."

Related to insufficiency fractures is the condition known as "Looser's transformation zones" or "umbau zones." It is thought that actually these represent pseudofractures rather than true fractures. These lesions occur in a wide variety of pathological conditions of bone, such as osteomalacia, rickets, osteogenesis imperfecta, Paget's osteitis deformans, and starvation osteopathy, and it is thought that they represent pathological healing phases of fatigue fractures in these bone conditions.

Pathological Fractures are fractures superimposed upon an underlying pathological process in bone. Usually only minor trauma is associated. Metastatic disease, chronic osteomyelitis, aseptic osseous necrosis, malacic diseases, congenital defects of the skeleton, bone cysts, and bone tumors may all at times predispose a person to pathological fractures. It is important to recognize the underlying disease since the treatment of a fracture so sustained will depend to a great extent on the associated treatment of the underlying disease.

Bone Changes Following Electrical Injury (Brinn and Moseley).   The roentgenological findings associated with electrical accidents are usually due to associated mechanical trauma, including fracture and dislocation. Compression fractures of the vertebrae may also result from the convulsive contractions of the trunk muscles.

In addition to these injuries, there are changes within the bone proper which include rounded densities resembling "bone pearls" or "wax drippings"; these are probably related to foci of necrosis, secondary to the burn. Immobilization, soft tissue deformities, vascular injuries, and neurologic injuries are all involved in producing roentgenologic findings as well.

Other findings include mottled decalcification, thinning of the cortices and widening of the medullary cavities, and discrete areas of rarefaction, of which the cause is unknown.

Traumatic Cupping of the Metaphysis in Growing Bone (Caffey).   When growing bone is traumatized, there may be a shaftward depression of the metaphysis, a spreading and shortening of the shaft, a thinning of the cartilage plate in some cases, and a resulting deepening of the contiguous joint space. It is probable that a local oligemia is largely responsible for this occurrence.

SYSTEMATIC REVIEW OF FRACTURES OF THE APPENDICEAL SKELETON

Radiographic Technique of Study of the Extremities

The technique of radiographic study of the bones and joints of both the upper and lower extremities is illustrated in some detail in the author's companion text *Radiographic Positioning and Related Anatomy*. Antero-posterior and lateral views are invariably necessary, and in certain anatomic areas oblique views and special distorted views are employed for optimum detail.

The Most Common Sites of Fracture (and Dislocation) of the Upper Extremity (Figure 5–3).   The most common sites of fractures of the scapula, clavicle, and upper extremity are illustrated. The following special comment about specific regions is important.

TYPE I

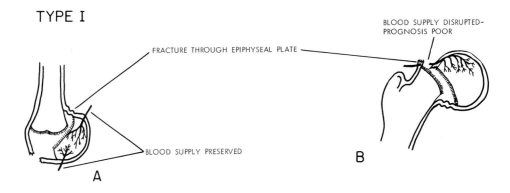

FRACTURE THROUGH EPIPHYSEAL PLATE

BLOOD SUPPLY DISRUPTED-
PROGNOSIS POOR

BLOOD SUPPLY PRESERVED

A

B

TYPE II

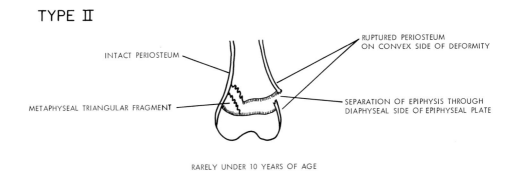

INTACT PERIOSTEUM

RUPTURED PERIOSTEUM
ON CONVEX SIDE OF DEFORMITY

METAPHYSEAL TRIANGULAR FRAGMENT

SEPARATION OF EPIPHYSIS THROUGH
DIAPHYSEAL SIDE OF EPIPHYSEAL PLATE

RARELY UNDER 10 YEARS OF AGE
PROGNOSIS GENERALLY GOOD

Figure 5–2   Salter-Harris classification of epiphyseal injuries. (Modified from DePalma, A. F.: *The Management of Fractures and Dislocations*. Philadelphia, W. B. Saunders Co., 1959.)

Figure 5–2 continued on opposite page.

TYPE III

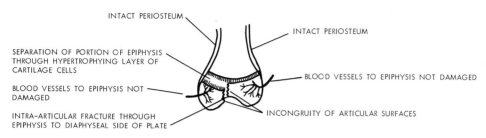

INTACT PERIOSTEUM

INTACT PERIOSTEUM

SEPARATION OF PORTION OF EPIPHYSIS THROUGH HYPERTROPHYING LAYER OF CARTILAGE CELLS

BLOOD VESSELS TO EPIPHYSIS NOT DAMAGED

BLOOD VESSELS TO EPIPHYSIS NOT DAMAGED

INCONGRUITY OF ARTICULAR SURFACES

INTRA-ARTICULAR FRACTURE THROUGH EPIPHYSIS TO DIAPHYSEAL SIDE OF PLATE

GENERALLY INVOLVES UPPER AND LOWER TIBIA.
PROGNOSIS GENERALLY FAVORABLE.

TYPE IV

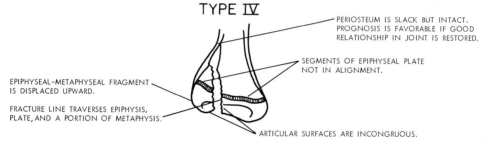

PERIOSTEUM IS SLACK BUT INTACT.
PROGNOSIS IS FAVORABLE IF GOOD
RELATIONSHIP IN JOINT IS RESTORED.

SEGMENTS OF EPIPHYSEAL PLATE
NOT IN ALIGNMENT.

EPIPHYSEAL-METAPHYSEAL FRAGMENT
IS DISPLACED UPWARD.

FRACTURE LINE TRAVERSES EPIPHYSIS,
PLATE, AND A PORTION OF METAPHYSIS.

ARTICULAR SURFACES ARE INCONGRUOUS.

MOST COMMON IN LATERAL CONDYLE
OF HUMERUS UNDER AGE 10.
INTERNAL FIXATION OFTEN NECESSARY.

TYPE V

INJURY TO EPIPHYSEAL PLATE.
NOTE: NO DISRUPTION OF
ARCHITECTURE OF EPIPHYSIS OR
METAPHYSIS OCCURS. SERIOUSNESS
OF LESION MANIFESTS ITSELF AFTER
A PERIOD OF GROWTH.

PORTION OF EPIPHYSEAL PLATE
HAS CLOSED PREMATURELY CAUSING
ANGULAR DEFORMITY.

KNEE AND ANKLE - 12 TO 16 YEARS.
ROENTGENOGRAMS ARE OFTEN NEGATIVE.
PROGNOSIS IS POOR - SHORTENING AND JOINT
DEFORMITY RESULT.

TYPES 4 AND 5 ARE, THEREFORE, MOST IMPORTANT TO DISTINGUISH IF AT
ALL POSSIBLE. A MINIMUM OF 2 YEARS IS CONSIDERED MINIMUM BEFORE ONE
CAN EXCLUDE THE POSSIBILITY OF SHORTENING OR DEFORMITY. RADIOGRAPHIC
RE-EVALUATION SHOULD BE PERFORMED AT 2 TO 6 MONTH INTERVALS, INCLUDING
COMPARISON VIEWS WITH THE OPPOSITE EXTREMITY.

Figure 5–2   *(Continued)*.

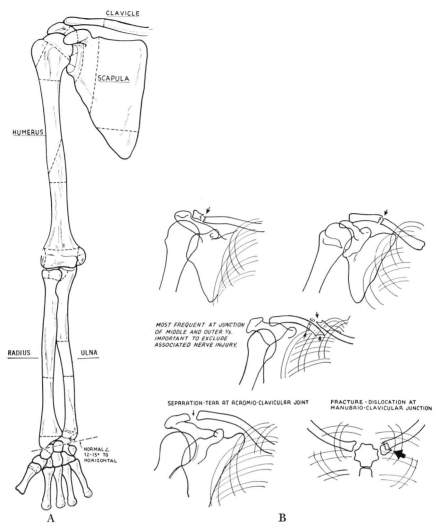

Figure 5–3 *A*. The most common sites of fractures of the scapula, clavicle, and upper extremity. *B*. Common injuries of the clavicle.

Fractures of the Clavicle (Figure 5–4).
Fractures or Dislocations of the Shoulder (Figure 5–5).
Dislocation of the shoulder complicated by a fracture of the greater tuberosity is relatively common and three types are encountered. These are shown in Figure 5–7.

ROENTGEN EVIDENCE OF POSTERIOR DISLOCATION OF THE SHOULDER (Figiel et al.; Arndt and Sears). In practically all posterior dislocations of the shoulder there is an associated fracture of the medial portion of the humeral head which is an important clue to the diagnosis of posterior dislocation. If this should go unrecognized, destruction of the humeral head and joint surface with functional impairment of the shoulder girdle will result.

Also, there is a widening between the anterior rim of the glenoid fossa and the medial margin of the humerus, which Arndt and Sears have called the "positive rim sign." In the normal shoulder, regardless of the rotation of the head of the humerus with respect to the glenoid fossa, the separation of the articular surfaces of the

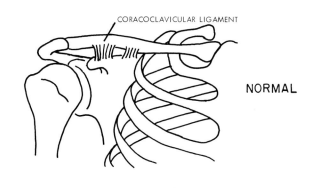

CORACOCLAVICULAR LIGAMENT

NORMAL

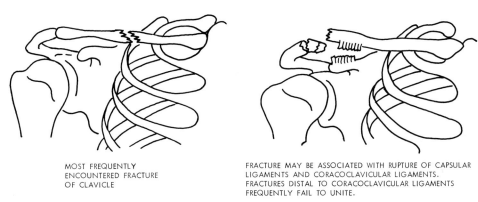

MOST FREQUENTLY
ENCOUNTERED FRACTURE
OF CLAVICLE

FRACTURE MAY BE ASSOCIATED WITH RUPTURE OF CAPSULAR
LIGAMENTS AND CORACOCLAVICULAR LIGAMENTS.
FRACTURES DISTAL TO CORACOCLAVICULAR LIGAMENTS
FREQUENTLY FAIL TO UNITE.

Figure 5–4 Fracture of the middle and outer third of the clavicle. Fracture distal to the coraco-clavicular ligaments with disruption of all ligaments usually requires surgical intervention.

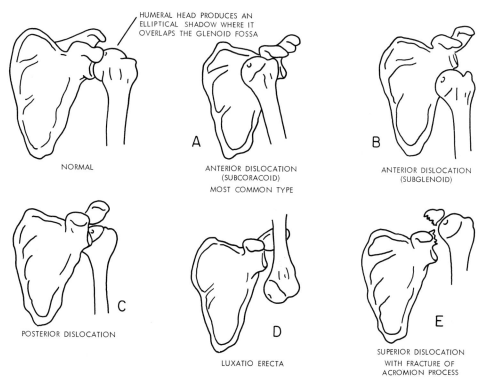

HUMERAL HEAD PRODUCES AN
ELLIPTICAL SHADOW WHERE IT
OVERLAPS THE GLENOID FOSSA

NORMAL

ANTERIOR DISLOCATION
(SUBCORACOID)
MOST COMMON TYPE

A

ANTERIOR DISLOCATION
(SUBGLENOID)

B

POSTERIOR DISLOCATION

C

LUXATIO ERECTA

D

SUPERIOR DISLOCATION
WITH FRACTURE OF
ACROMION PROCESS

E

Figure 5–5 Varieties of dislocations of the shoulder. (Modified from Zatzkin, H. R.: *Roentgen Diagnosis of Trauma.* Chicago, Year Book Medical Publishers, 1965, and DePalma.)

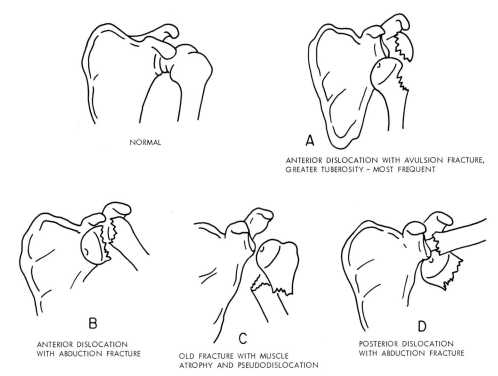

Figure 5–6   Varieties of fracture-dislocations of the shoulder. (After Zatzkin.)

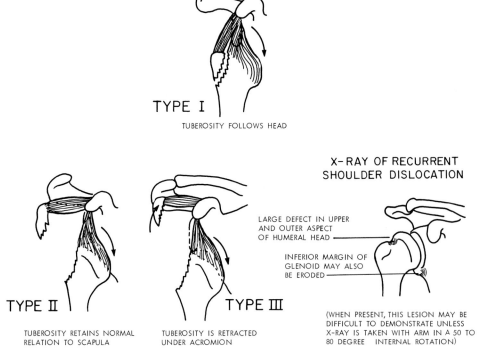

Figure 5–7   Dislocation complicated by fracture of the greater tuberosity of the humerus. (Modified from DePalma, p. 611.)

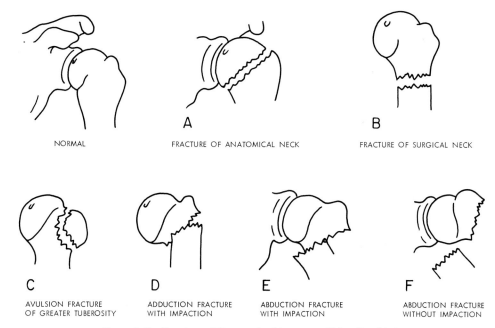

NORMAL   FRACTURE OF ANATOMICAL NECK   FRACTURE OF SURGICAL NECK

A   B

C   D   E   F

AVULSION FRACTURE   ADDUCTION FRACTURE   ABDUCTION FRACTURE   ABDUCTION FRACTURE
OF GREATER TUBEROSITY   WITH IMPACTION   WITH IMPACTION   WITHOUT IMPACTION

Figure 5–8   Fracture of the proximal humerus. (After Zatzkin.)

humerus and the glenoid never exceed 6 mm. With a "positive rim sign" the space between the medial margin of the humeral head and the anterior rim of the glenoid fossa is excessive—greater than 6 mm., regardless of the degree of rotation of the humerus (excluding children with incompletely ossified epiphyses).

Fractures of the Proximal Humerus (Figure 5–8).

Fractures of the Shaft of the Humerus.   Fractures of the shaft of the humerus are usually oblique or spiral in type but they may be transverse. *Radial nerve injury* most frequently occurs in fractures at the junction of the middle and lower thirds of the humerus, and in fractures of the middle third. At the lower end of the middle third, the radial nerve lies within the spiral groove and is therefore in a very vulnerable position.

For proper detection of the alignment of the major fragments of the humerus, a useful projection is *"through the body lateral view."* Although bony detail is lacking, a concept of alignment of fractures may be obtained by it.

Fractures of the lower third of the humerus offer considerably greater difficulty in reduction and are not infrequently sites of nonunion.

Fracture of the Supracondyloid Process.   The supracondyloid process is a bony prominence on the antero-medial aspect of the humerus approximately 5 to 7 cm. above the medial epicondyle. Although fracture of this process is a rare lesion, it is important because of the proximity of the brachial artery and the median nerve.

Fractures of the Lower End of the Humerus (Figure 5–9).

Epiphyseal Displacements of the Lower End of the Humerus.   Fracture of the medial epicondyle often occurs prior to fusion of the epiphysis of the medial epicondyle at about 18 years of age. In young boys it has been called "Little Leaguer's elbow" (Brogdon). The avulsed fragment is usually displaced into the fossa between the coronoid process and the trochlea. If not corrected, new bone formation in this

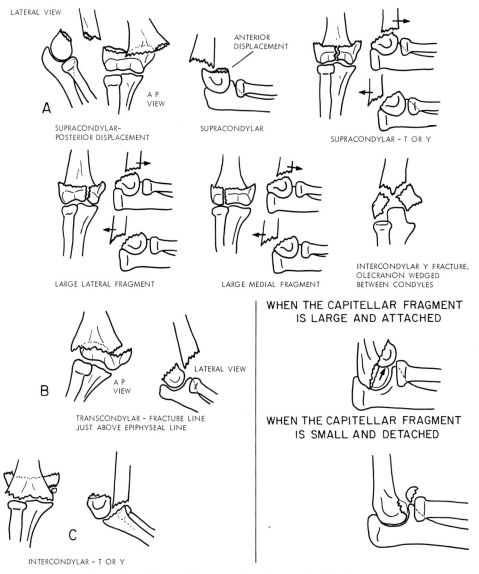

Figure 5-9   Types of fractures of the lower end of the humerus.

location will prevent complete flexion at the elbow joint. Open reduction is usually necessary.

Some variations of displacement of both medial and lateral condyle and epicondyle are illustrated in Figure 5–10. Note that the epiphyses in the lower humerus make an angle of approximately 25 degrees with the longitudinal axis of the shaft of the humerus. In treatment of fractures and displacements in this region, reconstitution of this angle is desirable as far as possible.

Supracondylar Fractures of the Humerus are a common cause of _Volkmann's ischemic contracture_ because of the vasospasm of the brachial artery. The muscles may undergo ischemic necrosis with later replacement by fibrosis, and considerable deformity of the wrist and hand may result. Apart from normal alignment of the

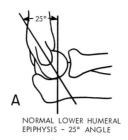

NORMAL LOWER HUMERAL
EPIPHYSIS - 25° ANGLE

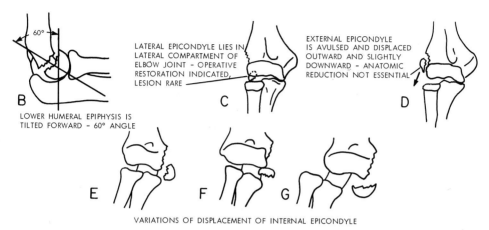

LOWER HUMERAL EPIPHYSIS IS
TILTED FORWARD - 60° ANGLE

LATERAL EPICONDYLE LIES IN
LATERAL COMPARTMENT OF
ELBOW JOINT - OPERATIVE
RESTORATION INDICATED,
LESION RARE

EXTERNAL EPICONDYLE
IS AVULSED AND DISPLACED
OUTWARD AND SLIGHTLY
DOWNWARD - ANATOMIC
REDUCTION NOT ESSENTIAL

VARIATIONS OF DISPLACEMENT OF INTERNAL EPICONDYLE

Figure 5–10   Epiphyseal fractures of the lower humerus. (After Watson-Jones, R.: *Fracture and Joint Injuries.* 4th Ed. Baltimore, Williams & Wilkins Co., 1955.)

condyles in the lateral projection, realignment in respect to the carrying angle is also important.

The variations of the normal carrying angle as derived from Smith are as follows: for girls, the range is from 0 to 12 degrees (average 6.1 degrees); for boys, the range is from 0 to 11 degrees (average 5.4 degrees). Forty-eight per cent of normal children have a carrying angle of 5 degrees or less.

Loss of the normal carrying angle may cause an increased stretching of the ulnar nerve with ultimate neuritis, palsy, and even paralysis.

Fractures and Dislocations of the Elbow

Varieties of Elbow Dislocations (Figure 5–11).   The posterior dislocation is the most frequent. In it, the brachialis anticus muscle may be torn from its attachment to the coronoid process, and the muscles of flexion may also be torn from their bony attachments. Rarely the brachial vessels and radial, ulnar, and median nerves are also injured.

Complicating fractures which may occur are (1) the coronoid process of the ulna; (2) the radius; (3) the condyles of the humerus; and (4) the epicondyles of the humerus.

If there is a fracture associated with the dislocation, the dislocation must be treated first (by reduction) and then the fracture.

Fractures of the Coronoid Process of the Ulna.   Chip fractures are small and are often associated with posterior dislocation. If the posterior dislocation has been

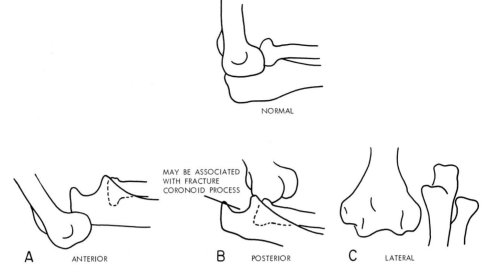

Figure 5–11   Varieties of dislocations of the elbow. (Modified from Zatzkin.)

corrected the fracture is of little significance unless it is displaced into the joint cavity.

Recognition of a chip fragment within the joint cavity is of considerable significance because the fragment must be excised (Figure 5–12A).

Fractures of the Olecranon of the Ulna (Figure 5–12B).   This group of fractures may be subdivided as follows: (1) fracture separations of the olecranon epiphysis; (2) simple fractures of the olecranon process; (3) comminuted fractures of the olecranon process; and (4) comminuted fractures of the olecranon process with dislocation.

The triceps tendon may or may not be intact.

With fracture-dislocations of the olecranon there is an anterior subluxation of both bones of the forearm, but usually the radius retains its normal relationship with the ulna. Since the ulnar nerve may be injured in the process, it is important to note any ulnar nerve deficit.

Fractures of the Head and Neck of the Radius.   The cause of this fracture is usually a fall, in which the shaft of the radius is driven against the capitellum of the humerus. In a child, the injury produces displacement of the radial epiphysis into the neck of the radius; involvement of the articular surface of the head of the radius is rare. There may, however, be an associated fracture of the medial epicondyle, and segments of the capitellum may be detached. *Care must be exercised to recognize loose bone fragments within the elbow joint.* Fractures of the radial head may conveniently be subdivided into (1) those which may be treated by conservative methods, and (2) those requiring excision of the radial head (DePalma) (Figure 5–13).

Generally, *those requiring excision of the radial head involve the articular surface with some displacement or tilt* of either a fragment of the head or the complete head of the radius. An impacted fracture of the neck of the radius can usually be treated conservatively.

POSTERIOR DISLOCATION OF THE ELBOW AND FRACTURE OF THE CORONOID PROCESS

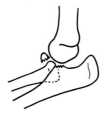

FRACTURE OF CORONOID FREQUENTLY COMPLICATES
POSTERIOR DISLOCATION OF ELBOW.
FRACTURE NEED NOT BE TREATED.
DISLOCATION IS REDUCED AND IMMOBILIZED.

A

VARIETIES OF FRACTURES OF THE OLECRANON PROCESS

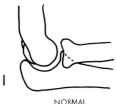

I

NORMAL

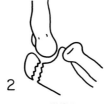

2

SIMPLE

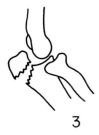

3

DISRUPTED TROCHLEAR NOTCH,
INTACT TRICEPS TENDON

4

COMMINUTED, WITH DISLOCATION

RADIUS AND ULNA HAVE MOVED
TOGETHER TO ANTERIOR POSITION.
ULNAR NERVE MAY BE INJURED.

5

COMMINUTED

B

Figure 5–12 *A*. Fractures of the coronoid process of the ulna. *B*. Fractures or dislocations of the olecranon process of the ulna.

TYPES OF FRACTURES TREATED BY CONSERVATIVE METHODS—NO DISPLACEMENT OF HEAD OR FRAGMENT

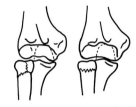

FISSURE FRACTURE   FRACTURE OF NECK

TYPES OF FRACTURES REQUIRING EXCISION OF THE RADIAL HEAD—DISPLACEMENT OF HEAD OR FRAGMENT

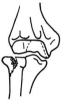 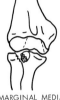 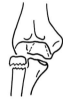 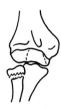 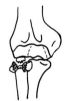

MARGINAL LATERAL   MARGINAL MEDIAL

DISLOCATION OF THE ELBOW WITH FRACTURE OF THE HEAD OF THE RADIUS

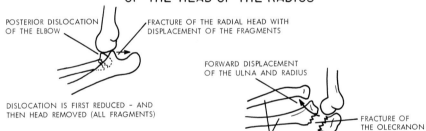

POSTERIOR DISLOCATION OF THE ELBOW

FRACTURE OF THE RADIAL HEAD WITH DISPLACEMENT OF THE FRAGMENTS

DISLOCATION IS FIRST REDUCED – AND THEN HEAD REMOVED (ALL FRAGMENTS)

FORWARD DISPLACEMENT OF THE ULNA AND RADIUS

FRACTURE OF THE OLECRANON

DISPLACEMENT OF THE RADIUS FROM THE ULNA INDICATIVE OF A TORN ORBICULAR LIGAMENT

Figure 5–13 Fracture-dislocations of the elbow with tears of the orbicular ligaments around the head of the radius.

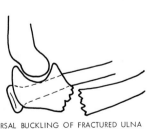

ANTERIOR

POSTERIOR

FRACTURE OF UPPER THIRD OF ULNA; FRAGMENTS ARE ANGULATED ANTERIORLY AND RADIALLY.
HEAD OF RADIUS IS DISLOCATED ANTERIORLY AND OUTWARD.

ANTEROPOSTERIOR

DORSAL BUCKLING OF FRACTURED ULNA SHAFT AND POSTERIOR DISPLACEMENT OF RADIAL HEAD

Figure 5–14 Varieties of Monteggia fractures or dislocations of the elbow.

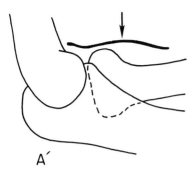

NORMAL ARM. SUPINATOR FAT PLANE ARISES FROM
ELBOW JOINT AND RUNS DISTALLY IN GENTLE VENTRAL
CURVE PARALLEL TO PROXIMAL THIRD OF THE RADIUS (ARROWS).

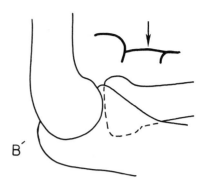

ARM WITH FRACTURE. FAT PLANE WIDENED,
BLURRED, AND VENTRALLY DISPLACED.

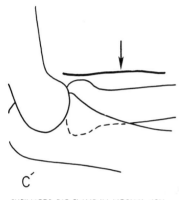

SUPINATOR FAT PLANE IN NORMAL ARM.

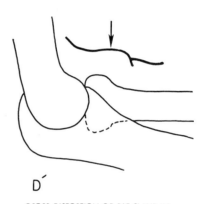

GROSS DISTORTION OF FAT PLANE IN
INFECTED ARM.

A

Figure 5–15 *A*. Change in the fat plane overlying the supinator muscle.

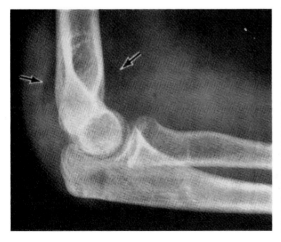
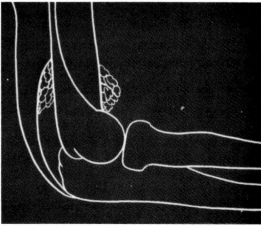

B

Figure 5–15 (*Continued*). *B*. Lateral radiograph of 13 year old girl who fell on her elbow, incurring a traumatic bursitis. No fracture was demonstrated. Arrows indicate anterior and posterior radiolucencies representing respectively displaced anterior and posterior fat pads. Note the concavity inferiorly in the posterior fat pad due to the impression of the distended synovial sac; also the rounded posterior contour of the triceps tendon. (From Bledsoe, R. C., and Izenstark, J. L.: Radiology, *73*:720, 1959.)

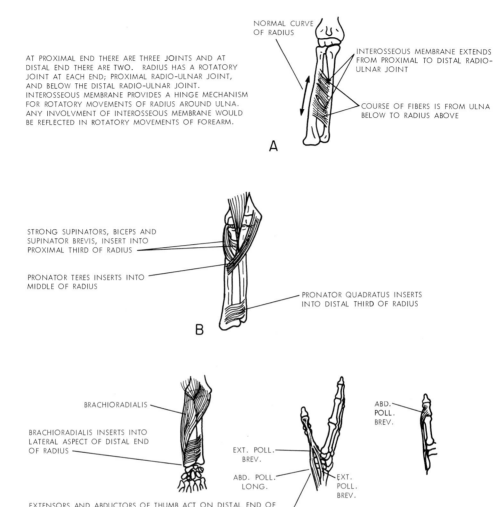

AT PROXIMAL END THERE ARE THREE JOINTS AND AT
DISTAL END THERE ARE TWO. RADIUS HAS A ROTATORY
JOINT AT EACH END; PROXIMAL RADIO-ULNAR JOINT,
AND BELOW THE DISTAL RADIO-ULNAR JOINT.
INTEROSSEOUS MEMBRANE PROVIDES A HINGE MECHANISM
FOR ROTATORY MOVEMENTS OF RADIUS AROUND ULNA.
ANY INVOLVMENT OF INTEROSSEOUS MEMBRANE WOULD
BE REFLECTED IN ROTATORY MOVEMENTS OF FOREARM.

NORMAL CURVE
OF RADIUS

INTEROSSEOUS MEMBRANE EXTENDS
FROM PROXIMAL TO DISTAL RADIO-
ULNAR JOINT

COURSE OF FIBERS IS FROM ULNA
BELOW TO RADIUS ABOVE

A

STRONG SUPINATORS, BICEPS AND
SUPINATOR BREVIS, INSERT INTO
PROXIMAL THIRD OF RADIUS

PRONATOR TERES INSERTS INTO
MIDDLE OF RADIUS

PRONATOR QUADRATUS INSERTS
INTO DISTAL THIRD OF RADIUS

B

BRACHIORADIALIS

BRACHIORADIALIS INSERTS INTO
LATERAL ASPECT OF DISTAL END
OF RADIUS

EXT. POLL.
BREV.

ABD. POLL.
LONG.

EXT.
POLL.
BREV.

ABD.
POLL.
BREV.

EXTENSORS AND ABDUCTORS OF THUMB ACT ON DISTAL END OF
RADIUS THROUGH THUMB IN FRACTURES OF DISTAL THIRD OF RADIUS

C

Figure 5–16 *A.* General anatomy of the interosseous membrane. *B.* Anatomy of the supinator and pronator muscles of the forearm. *C.* Anatomy of the brachioradialis and thumb muscles in respect to the bones of the forearm.

Figure 5–16 continued on opposite page.

Fracture-Dislocation of the Elbow with Tear of the Orbicular Ligament of the Radius.   In this lesion, apart from the recognition of fracture and dislocation, the displacement of the radius from the ulna, which indicates a torn orbicular ligament, can be noted (Figure 5–13).

Varieties of Monteggia Fracture-Dislocation.   The *anterior* Monteggia fracture is characterized by upward buckling and angulation of the fractured ulnar shaft, and an anterior dislocation of the radial head; in the *posterior* Monteggia fracture the angulation of the fractured ulna is posterior, and there is an associated posterior displacement of the radial head (Figure 5–14).

Changes in the Fat Plane Overlying the Supinator Muscle.   Normally there is a faintly visible fat plane just anterior to the proximal end of the humerus in the lateral view (Figure 5–15A). This fat plane can become widened, blurred, or ventrally displaced with trauma and inflammation, or it may be completely obliterated by severe swelling and edema (Rogers and MacEwen).

Similarly, there are radiolucent fat pads both anterior and posterior to the distal humerus. An effusion of 5 to 10 cc. or more will displace these fat zones, elevate

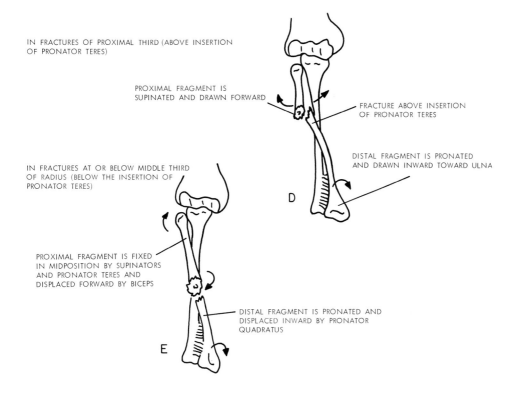

IN FRACTURES OF PROXIMAL THIRD (ABOVE INSERTION
OF PRONATOR TERES)

PROXIMAL FRAGMENT IS
SUPINATED AND DRAWN FORWARD

FRACTURE ABOVE INSERTION
OF PRONATOR TERES

DISTAL FRAGMENT IS PRONATED
AND DRAWN INWARD TOWARD ULNA

D

IN FRACTURES AT OR BELOW MIDDLE THIRD
OF RADIUS (BELOW THE INSERTION OF
PRONATOR TERES)

PROXIMAL FRAGMENT IS FIXED
IN MIDPOSITION BY SUPINATORS
AND PRONATOR TERES AND
DISPLACED FORWARD BY BICEPS

DISTAL FRAGMENT IS PRONATED AND
DISPLACED INWARD BY PRONATOR
QUADRATUS

E

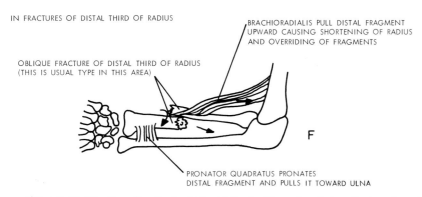

IN FRACTURES OF DISTAL THIRD OF RADIUS

BRACHIORADIALIS PULL DISTAL FRAGMENT
UPWARD CAUSING SHORTENING OF RADIUS
AND OVERRIDING OF FRAGMENTS

OBLIQUE FRACTURE OF DISTAL THIRD OF RADIUS
(THIS IS USUAL TYPE IN THIS AREA)

F

PRONATOR QUADRATUS PRONATES
DISTAL FRAGMENT AND PULLS IT TOWARD ULNA

Figure 5–16 (*Continued*).   *D.* Anatomy of the fractures at or below the insertion of the pronator teres muscle. *E.* Anatomy of the fractures at or below the insertion of the pronator teres muscle (at or below middle third of radius). (After DePalma.) *F.* Fractures of the distal third of the radius: important anatomic considerations.

the shadows, and become important roentgen signs (*displaced fat pad sign* of Norell; and Bledsoe and Izenstark) (Figure 5–15B). An additional useful finding is posterior bulging of the triceps brachii tendon in the presence of elbow-joint effusion.

Fractures of the Bones of the Forearm Distal to the Elbow (Proximal to the Wrist)

General Considerations.   The radius and ulna are attached to one another proximally and distally by joints and at the shaft level by an interosseous membrane which runs obliquely from below on the ulna to upward on the radius (Figure 5–16A). This membrane is intimately involved in the rotary movements of the forearm. Between the radius and ulna there are strong supinator and pronator muscles (Figure 5–16B). Also involved are the brachioradialis muscle and thumb muscles which attach to the distal end of the radius (Figure 5–16C).

Fractures of the proximal third of the radius usually lie above the insertion of the pronator teres muscle, whereas *fractures at or below the middle third of the radius lie below the insertion of this important muscle*. Difficult rotational deformities result in each of these lesions.

Similarly, fractures of the distal third of the radius present difficult management problems because of muscle pull.

Encroachment on the Interosseous Membrane.   Rotational deformities in fractures of the radius alone or combined fractures of the radius and ulna may cause encroachment on the interosseous membrane. Every effort must be made to "visualize" the approximate position of the interosseous membrane and to define its clarity and integrity, so that *when healing occurs, bridging of the interosseous membrane will not occur*, thus limiting pronation and supination functions.

ENCROACHMENT ON THE INTEROSSEOUS MEMBRANE

Rotational deformity produced by fractures of radius alone or by fractures of both radius and ulna causes encroachment of interosseous membrane.

Displacement of fragments is brought about by loss of muscle equilibrium and by gravity.

Fracture of radius alone above or below pronator teres causes marked rotational deformities as shown previously.

Fragments of unstable fractures of both bones may drift into positions of malalignment, producing angular and rotational deformities.

In fractures of both bones the radial curve may be flattened, causing distraction of ulnar fragments.

In the forearm the two bones are almost parallel, forming a parallelogram; it is impossible to shorten one arm of parallelogram without shortening the other.

A fracture of a single bone of forearm with shortening cannot remain as such. One of several concomitant lesions must occur:

Fracture of other forearm bone.

Dislocation or subluxation of proximal or distal radioulnar joints.

Generally when ulna is fractured and shortened the proximal radioulnar joint dislocates, as in a Monteggia fracture. When radius is fractured and shortened the distal radioulnar joint subluxates or dislocates, as in a Galeazzi fracture.

Fractures and Dislocations Involving the Radius in the Vicinity of the Distal Radioulnar Joint

Radius Types.   Varieties of fractures involving the lower end of the radius have been catalogued by eponyms and are illustrated in Figure 5–17 as follows:

1. *The reversed Colles' fracture or Smith fracture.*
2. *The Colles' fracture* (Figure 5–17C).
3. *Galeazzi's fracture in adults.* This is a fracture through the distal third of the radius with an associated dislocation of the distal radioulnar joints (Figure 5–17D).
4. *Barton's fracture.* This is an oblique fracture of the posterior lip of the distal end of the radius which usually is directed upward and backward (Figure 5–17E).
5. *Chauffeur's fracture.* This is a fracture of the radial styloid process involving the distal articular surface. There may be no displacement of the radial fragment. The fragment is usually directed upward and outward, and the carpus is generally shifted to the radial side along with the radial fragment (Figure 5–17F).

The system of lining shown in Figure 5–17G is very helpful in the determination of proper axial relationships of the wrist and the restoration of fragments to a good position.

Fractures and Dislocations of the Carpal Bones

Important Anatomic Considerations are (1) bony landmarks on antero-posterior and lateral views of the wrist (Figure 5–18), (2) joint surfaces in the wrist (Figure 5–19), (3) basic anatomy of the "carpal tunnel" (Figure 5–20), and (4) basic blood supply of the carpal navicular (scaphoid) bone.

Fractures of the Scaphoid (Figure 5–22) are most frequent among the carpal bones of the wrist. *Healing depends much on the integrity of the blood supply.* This may readily be interrupted by certain types of fractures. *The arteries enter the scaphoid on the dorsal surface in the region of the tubercle and in the waist of the bone or midposition.* When separated from this blood supply, avascular necrosis may result.

Scaphoid fractures may be associated with the following: (1) dislocations of the radiocarpal joint, (2) dislocation between the two rows of carpal bones, (3) fracture dislocations of the distal end of the radius, (4) an associated fracture at the base of the first metacarpal (Bennett's fracture), and (5) dislocations of the lunate and perilunate.

Lunate and Perilunate Dislocations. In *lunate dislocations* this carpal bone is virtually squeezed out of the wrist joint until it lies anterior to the wrist joint (Figure 5–23). Dorsal dislocation of the lunate is rare (Figure 5–25). In *perilunate dislocations* (Figure 5–24) the lunate-capitate articulation is disrupted and the *carpal bones, except for the lunate, are usually driven dorsally* and behind the lunate, whereas the radial-lunate relationship is preserved (Figure 5–24). Volar perilunate dislocations occur rarely (Figure 5–26). The perilunate dislocation may be associated with a fracture-dislocation of the scaphoid. Variations may also occur, in that portions of the scaphoid may remain with the lunate while a distal fragment of the scaphoid retains its normal relationship with the rest of the carpus and is displaced dorsally.

Dorsal perilunate dislocations may be complicated by a fracture of the capitate carpal bone as well.

When the lunate is dislocated, it has a triangular instead of a quadrilateral appearance in the antero-posterior projection (Figure 5–27).

Fractures of the Capitate. The capitate is an axial bone in respect to the anatomy of the wrist and is in a vulnerable position. Approximately 15 per cent of all fractures of the carpal bones involve the capitate. *Its blood supply is derived*

(Text continued on page 142)

FRACTURES OF THE LOWER END OF THE RADIUS

SMITH FRACTURE
(REVERSE OF COLLES' FRACTURE)

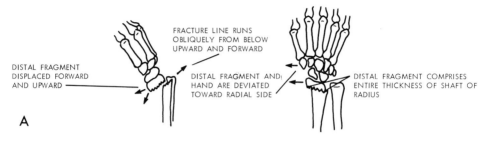

FRACTURE LINE RUNS OBLIQUELY FROM BELOW UPWARD AND FORWARD

DISTAL FRAGMENT DISPLACED FORWARD AND UPWARD

DISTAL FRAGMENT AND HAND ARE DEVIATED TOWARD RADIAL SIDE

DISTAL FRAGMENT COMPRISES ENTIRE THICKNESS OF SHAFT OF RADIUS

A

TYPICAL COLLES' FRACTURES

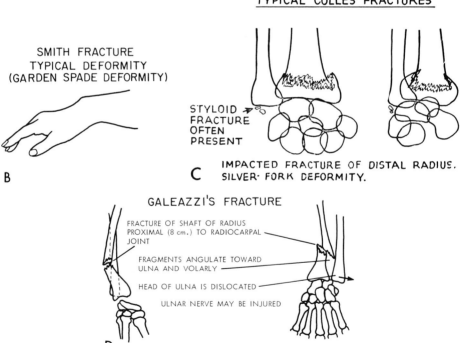

SMITH FRACTURE
TYPICAL DEFORMITY
(GARDEN SPADE DEFORMITY)

STYLOID FRACTURE OFTEN PRESENT

B

C IMPACTED FRACTURE OF DISTAL RADIUS. SILVER-FORK DEFORMITY.

GALEAZZI'S FRACTURE

FRACTURE OF SHAFT OF RADIUS PROXIMAL (8 cm.) TO RADIOCARPAL JOINT

FRAGMENTS ANGULATE TOWARD ULNA AND VOLARLY

HEAD OF ULNA IS DISLOCATED

ULNAR NERVE MAY BE INJURED

D

Figure 5–17 *A*. Reversed Colles' or Smith fracture. *B*. "Garden spade" deformity of the Smith fracture contrasted with "dinner fork" deformity of the Colles' fracture. *C*. Diagrams illustrating Colles' fracture. *D*. Galeazzi's fracture (distal third of radius and dislocation of the distal radioulnar joint).

Figure 5–17 continued on opposite page.

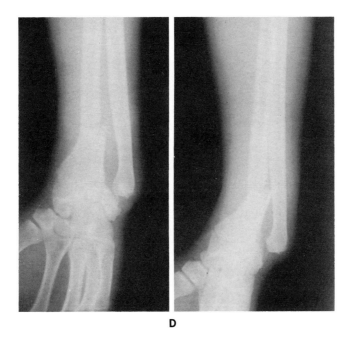

D

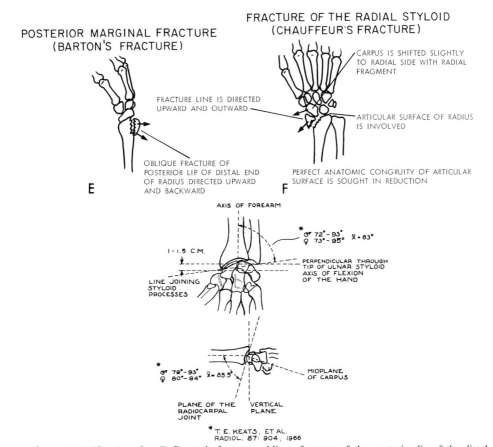

**POSTERIOR MARGINAL FRACTURE
(BARTON'S FRACTURE)**

FRACTURE LINE IS DIRECTED
UPWARD AND OUTWARD

OBLIQUE FRACTURE OF
POSTERIOR LIP OF DISTAL END
OF RADIUS DIRECTED UPWARD
AND BACKWARD

E

**FRACTURE OF THE RADIAL STYLOID
(CHAUFFEUR'S FRACTURE)**

CARPUS IS SHIFTED SLIGHTLY
TO RADIAL SIDE WITH RADIAL
FRAGMENT

ARTICULAR SURFACE OF RADIUS
IS INVOLVED

PERFECT ANATOMIC CONGRUITY OF ARTICULAR
SURFACE IS SOUGHT IN REDUCTION

F

AXIS OF FOREARM

♂ 72° - 93°   ♀ 73° - 95°   x̄ = 83°

1 - 1.5 C.M.

PERPENDICULAR THROUGH
TIP OF ULNAR STYLOID
AXIS OF FLEXION
OF THE HAND

LINE JOINING
STYLOID
PROCESSES

♂ 79° - 93°   ♀ 80° - 94°   x̄ = 85.5°

MIDPLANE
OF CARPUS

PLANE OF THE
RADIOCARPAL
JOINT

VERTICAL
PLANE

* T. E. KEATS, ET AL.
RADIOL. 87: 904, 1966

Figure 5–17 (*Continued*).   *E.* Barton's fracture: oblique fracture of the posterior lip of the distal end of the radius. *F.* Chauffeur's fracture (fracture of the radial styloid process). *G.* Lining system for determination of proper axial relationships of the wrist.

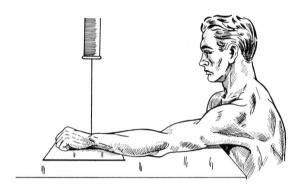

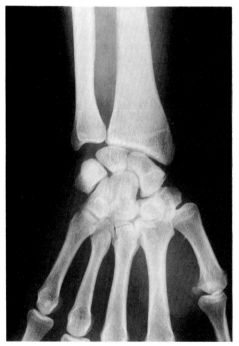

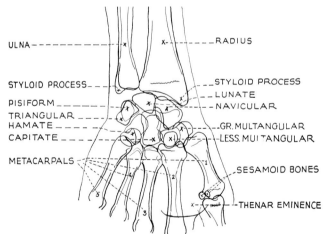

ULNA - - - - - - - - - - - - RADIUS

STYLOID PROCESS - - STYLOID PROCESS
PISIFORM - - - - - LUNATE
TRIANGULAR - - - - NAVICULAR
HAMATE - - - - GR. MULTANGULAR
CAPITATE - - - LESS. MULTANGULAR

METACARPALS - SESAMOID BONES

THENAR EMINENCE

Figure 5–18 *A*. Postero-anterior view of wrist.

Figure 5–18 continued on opposite page.

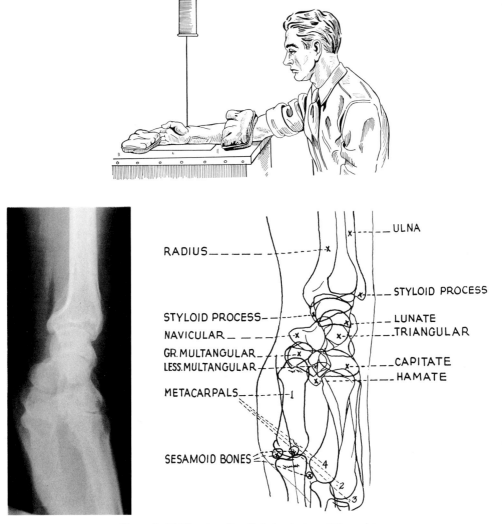

RADIUS

ULNA

STYLOID PROCESS

STYLOID PROCESS

LUNATE

NAVICULAR

TRIANGULAR

GR. MULTANGULAR

LESS. MULTANGULAR

CAPITATE

HAMATE

METACARPALS

SESAMOID BONES

Figure 5–18 (*Continued*).   *B*. Lateral view of the wrist.

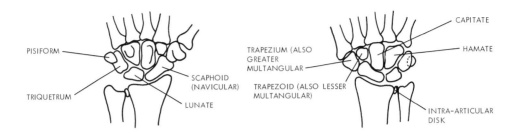

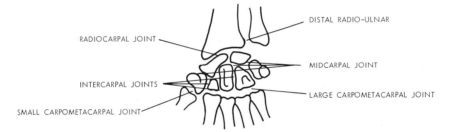

Figure 5-19   Joint cavities of the wrist.

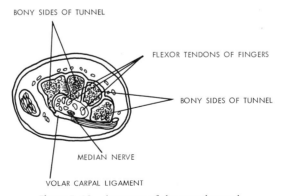

Figure 5-20   Anatomy of the carpal tunnel.

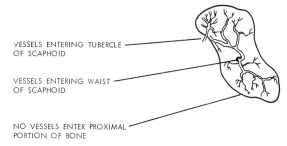

VESSELS ENTERING TUBERCLE
OF SCAPHOID

VESSELS ENTERING WAIST
OF SCAPHOID

NO VESSELS ENTER PROXIMAL
PORTION OF BONE

Figure 5–21 Blood supply of the scaphoid (navicular carpal) bone.

TYPES OF UNDISPLACED FRACTURES
USUALLY ENCOUNTERED

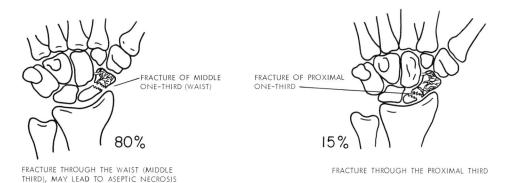

FRACTURE OF MIDDLE
ONE-THIRD (WAIST)

80%

FRACTURE THROUGH THE WAIST (MIDDLE
THIRD), MAY LEAD TO ASEPTIC NECROSIS
PROXIMAL FRAGMENT

FRACTURE OF PROXIMAL
ONE-THIRD

15%

FRACTURE THROUGH THE PROXIMAL THIRD

FRACTURE OF DISTAL
ONE-THIRD

5%

FRACTURE THROUGH THE DISTAL THIRD

FRACTURE OF TUBEROSITY

5%

FRACTURE THROUGH THE TUBERCLE

SOME OF THE ASSOCIATED INJURIES ARE:
DISLOCATION OF RADIOCARPAL JOINT.
DISLOCATION BETWEEN THE TWO ROWS OF CARPAL BONES.
FRACTURE-DISLOCATION OF DISTAL END OF RADIUS.
FRACTURE OF BASE OF THUMB METACARPAL (BENNETT'S FRACTURE).
DISLOCATION OF LUNATE.

NOTE: THERE MAY BE ANY COMBINATION
OF THESE AND OCCASIONALLY A
SEGMENTAL FRACTURE OF SCAPHOID
OCCURS

Figure 5–22 Classification of fractures of the scaphoid carpal bone.

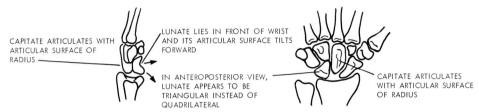

Figure 5–23 Volar dislocation of the lunate.

Figure 5–24 Dorsal perilunar dislocation.

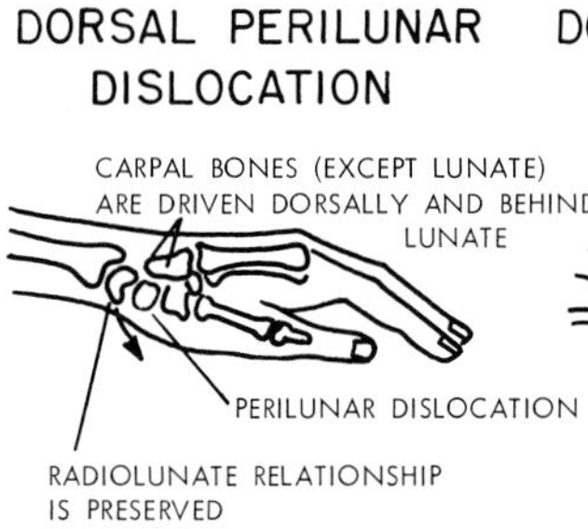

Figure 5–25 Dorsal dislocation of the lunate.

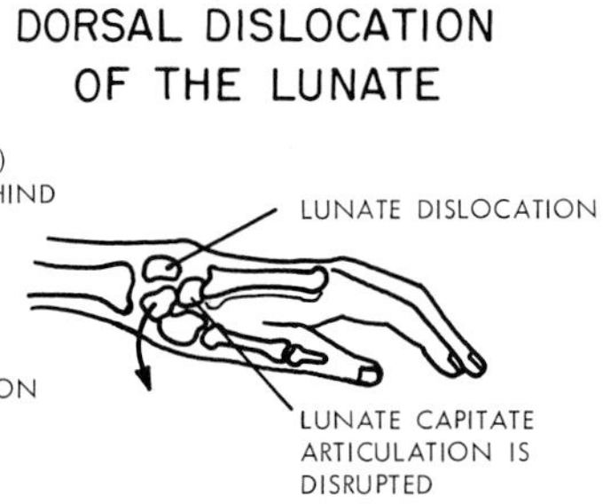

Figure 5–26 Volar perilunar dislocation.

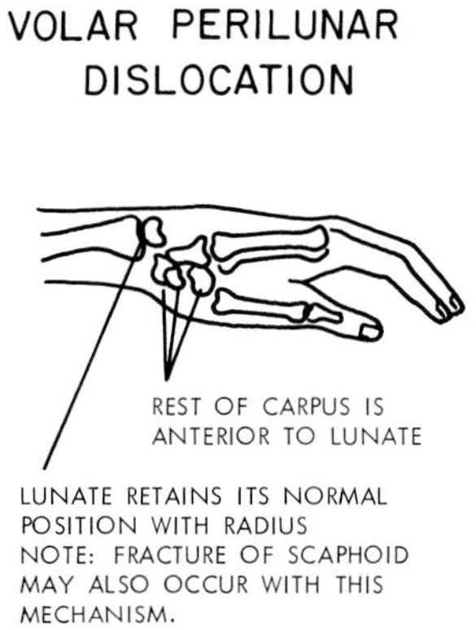

centrally in the neck and waist of the bone so that trauma may cause aseptic necrosis of a severed portion. Oblique views and body section radiographs are frequently required to establish the diagnosis. When the scaphoid and capitate bones alone are involved, the combination is referred to as the "scaphoid-capitate fracture syndrome."

Fractures of the Triquetrum. Oblique projections are essential to establish this diagnosis and fractures of this carpal bone rank second in frequency among fractures of the carpal bones.

Fracture of the Greater Multangular Carpal Bone (Trapezium). This carpal bone is essential to normal thumb motion. Fractures of this bone represent approximately 5 per cent of all carpal fractures.

Fat Plane Overlying the Pronator Quadratus Muscle in Trauma (MacEwan). Overlying the pronator quadratus muscle is a fat layer which, when seen in true lateral projections of the wrist, has a gentle convex curve just anterior to the lower sixth of the radius and ulna. The right and left sides are usually symmetrical. In fractures, the fat plane is displaced anteriorly and looks more bowed than normal. The fat appears blurred, irregular, and less well-defined.

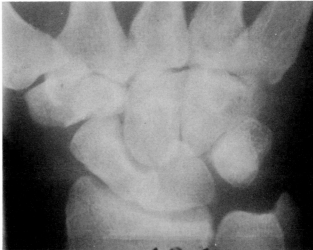
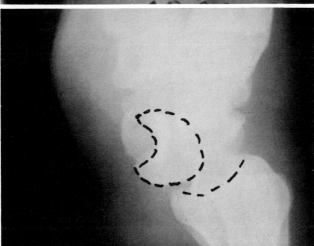

Figure 5–27   Antero-posterior and lateral radiographs showing the triangular appearance of the lunate in the antero-posterior projection when dislocated.

Fractures and Dislocations of the Hand

Dislocations of the Carpometacarpal Joint of the Thumb.

Fracture-Dislocation of the Carpometacarpal Joint of the Thumb (Bennett's Fracture).   In this injury there is a fracture through the base of the first metacarpal and dislocation of the radial portion of its articular surface, while its medial portion remains in normal relationship with the greater multangular (Figure 5–28).

Dislocations and Fracture-Dislocations of the Phalanges.   Dislocations of the interphalangeal joints are relatively common. These are often accompanied by fractures of the base of the distal phalanx.

Fractures of the Metacarpals.   These are common lesions of the hand and are second in frequency only to fractures of the phalanges. If not adequately corrected, severe deformities and disability of the hand may result. Usually fractures of the fourth and fifth metacarpals are accompanied by dorsal angulation, with the head being displaced toward the volar aspect of the hand. A shortening of the entire fourth or fifth digit may result.

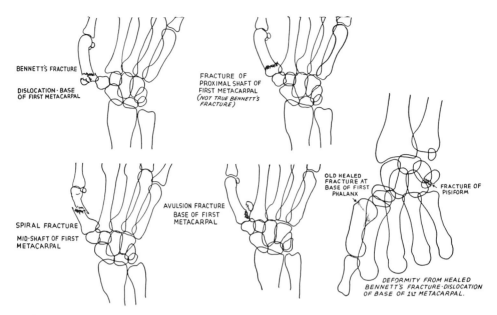

Figure 5–28 Bennett's fracture (fracture dislocation of the carpometacarpal joint of the thumb).

Fractures of the Phalanges. Usually fractures of the proximal phalanx are associated with a volar angulation of fragments.

In the case of the middle phalanx, if the fracture site is proximal to the insertion of the tendon, a dorsal angulation of fragments results. If the fracture site is distal to the insertion of the flexor sublimis tendon, a volar angulation of fragments results.

In the case of the distal phalanx, a comminuted fracture is the usual occurrence and very little displacement of fragments occurs. If the tufted end of the distal phalanx is severely traumatized, resorption may occur. Very often nonunion will result.

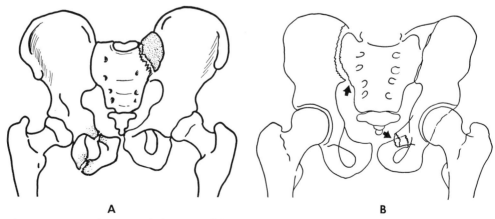

Figure 5–29 *A* and *B*. Example fractures of the pelvis and fracture-dislocation of the adjoining sacrum.

Figure 5–29 continued on opposite page.

Fractures of the Pelvis and Lower Extremities

The Pelvis.   Some of the more common fractures of the pelvis are illustrated in Figure 5–29.

Fractures of the Acetabulum.   The acetabulum has three anatomic portions: (1) a dome or superior portion; (2) a posterior portion; and (3) an anterior or inner wall.

Fractures of the acetabulum may be subdivided into the following categories:

1. *Linear fractures* without displacement.

2. *Rim fractures,* usually occurring through the posterior portion of the ace-

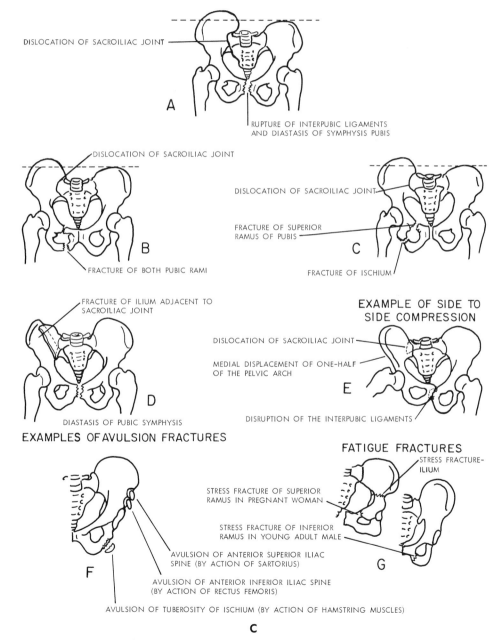

C

Figure 5–29 *(Continued).   C.* Fractures of the pelvis.

BLOOD SUPPLY OF THE FEMORAL CAPITAL EPIPHYSIS AND NECK OF THE FEMUR IN CHILDHOOD

BLOOD SUPPLY OF THE FEMORAL HEAD

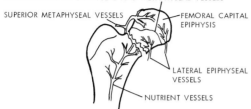

EPIPHYSEAL PLATE – THIS PLATE PRECLUDES ANASTOMOSIS OF EPIPHYSEAL AND METAPHYSEAL VESSELS

SUPERIOR METAPHYSEAL VESSELS

FEMORAL CAPITAL EPIPHYSIS

LATERAL EPIPHYSEAL VESSELS

NUTRIENT VESSELS

NOTE: BLOOD SUPPLY COMING THROUGH LIGAMENTUM TERES AT THIS AGE IS VERY INADEQUATE AND CONFINED TO A SMALL SEGMENT OF EPIPHYSIS

A

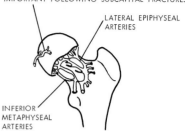

ARTERY OF LIGAMENTUM TERES, (NOT VERY SIGNIFICANT ORDINARILY, BUT MOST IMPORTANT FOLLOWING SUBCAPITAL FRACTURES)

LATERAL EPIPHYSEAL ARTERIES

INFERIOR METAPHYSEAL ARTERIES

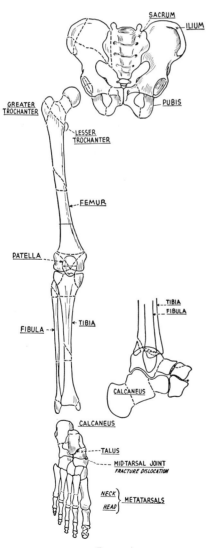

SACRUM

ILIUM

GREATER TROCHANTER

PUBIS

LESSER TROCHANTER

FEMUR

PATELLA

TIBIA
FIBULA

FIBULA

TIBIA

CALCANEUS

CALCANEUS

TALUS

MID-TARSAL JOINT
FRACTURE DISLOCATION

NECK
HEAD } METATARSALS

B

Figure 5–30 *A*. Blood supply of the head and neck of the femur. *B*. The most common sites of fractures of the pelvis and lower extremity.

tabulum. These may be *associated with a posterior dislocation of the hip.* Under these circumstances, aseptic necrosis or sciatic nerve involvement may be involved. Oblique views of the acetabulum may be necessary to demonstrate the posterior rim fractures (Berkebile et al.). In the lateral view of the pelvis, the posterior dislocation of the femoral head, plus the fracture fragments of the posterior rim of the acetabulum, form a double curved shadow which simulates the silhouette of a flying gull. This has been called the "gull-wing sign."

3. Superior or bursting fractures of the acetabulum, with possible total disruption of the acetabulum. In this group of disorders, the prognosis depends greatly on an intact superior acetabular dome. *Injury to the sciatic nerve in these lesions is relatively common* (20 to 25 per cent of cases). If there is an associated injury of the head of the femur, prognosis is usually poor.

The blood supply of the femoral capital epiphysis and neck is derived from the following: (1) ligamentum teres; (2) lateral epiphyseal and neck vessels; (3) nutrient vessels derived from the metaphysis and shaft of the femur; (4) superior metaphyseal vessels; and (5) vessels of the hip joint capsule proper.

Varieties of Dislocations of the Hip. These may be classified as shown in Figure 5–31:

1. *Posterior dislocation,* which may be either superior or inferior;

2. *Central dislocation,* usually accompanied by a bursting fracture of the acetabulum;

3. *Anterior dislocation,* which may be inferior or superior.

Congenital dislocation of the hip is thought by many to be due to defective ossification of the shelving portion of the acetabulum (*acetabular dysplasia*). This deficiency can be demonstrated by different lining techniques as illustrated in Figure 5–33 D.

Traumatic dislocations of the hip are rare and comprise only 2 to 5 per cent of

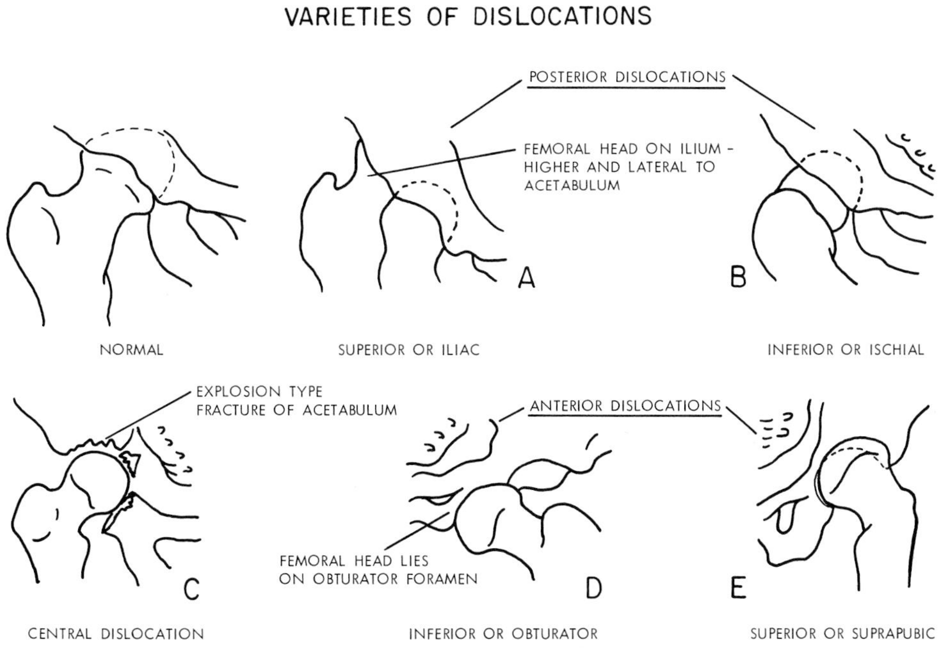

VARIETIES OF DISLOCATIONS

Figure 5–31 Dislocations of the hip.

VARIETIES OF HIP FRACTURES

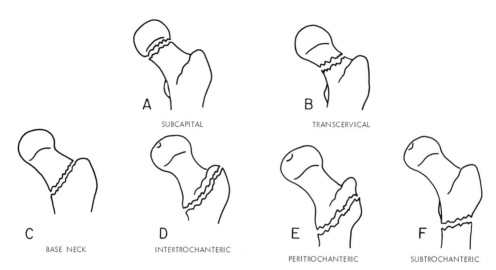

Figure 5–32   Fractures of the hip.

all dislocations, whereas traumatic dislocations of the shoulder make up about 50 per cent of all dislocations.

Varieties of Fractures of the Hip.   In obtaining antero-posterior films of the hip region it is important to rotate the thigh, leg, and foot *internally* if possible, so as not to foreshorten the neck of the femur. A fracture line may be overlooked if such foreshortening on the radiograph is permitted. The varieties of hip fractures are illustrated in Figure 5–32.

A slipped capital femoral epiphysis may also occur.

The integrity of the blood supply will to a great extent determine the result obtained. Here, as elsewhere, the *intracapsular fractures heal poorly* and frequently result in nonunion. The subcapital variety is universally intracapsular and the mid-cervical type fracture may or may not be completely contained within the capsular attachment. The intertrochanteric and subtrochanteric types are extracapsular and heal most readily.

Anterior angulation and a coxa vara deformity are most frequently obtained.

Usually the entire lower extremity appears shortened and externally rotated. *On the antero-posterior radiograph, Shenton's and Skinner's lines are disturbed* (Figure 5–33). It is most important to establish normal relationships in respect to these various lining techniques if at all possible.

When slippage of the capital femoral epiphysis occurs, it is important to determine *whether or not the slip is less than a third or greater than a third of the diameter of the femoral neck* from the standpoint of therapeutic management.

Fractures of the Upper End of the Femur

Classification.   These may be classified as:

1. Fractures of the greater trochanter;
2. Fractures of the lesser trochanter;

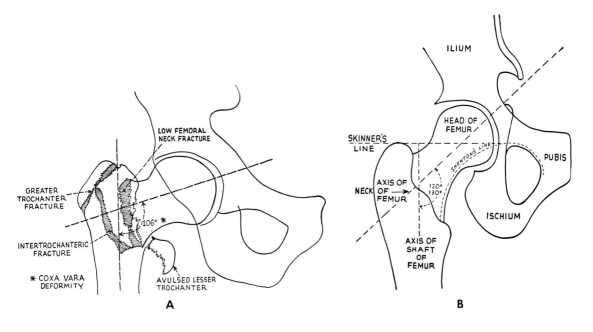

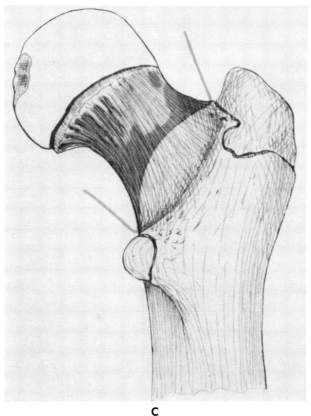

Figure 5–33 *A*, Tracing of an intertrochanteric fracture and an avulsion fracture of the neck of the femur. *B*, Lining techniques to demonstrate the proper axial relationships of the hip joint, for assistance in detection of fractures in the region of the hip. *C*. The line of attachment of the capsule of the hip joint. The posterior attachment is just distal to the midcervical portion of the neck of the femur. The anterior attachment is at the intertrochanteric ridge. (From Perry, in *Morris' Human Anatomy*. New York, Blakiston, 1953.)

3. Trochanteric fractures;

4. Fractures of the neck of the femur.

In trochanteric fractures and fractures of the neck of the femur an effort is made to determine whether the fracture is intracapsular or extracapsular.

The trochanteric fractures may be subdivided into the following types:

1. Intertrochanteric and extracapsular, but the greater and lesser trochanters are not involved.

2. Intertrochanteric and comminuted, with a varus deformity of the hip, and involvement of both the greater and lesser trochanter.

3. Involvement of both the greater and lesser trochanter with a conical sub-trochanteric fracture and a coxa vara deformity.

4. Intertrochanteric involvement, comminution of the greater trochanter, medial displacement of the lesser trochanter, and a spiral fracture involving the upper end of the femoral shaft.

Types 3 and 4 comprise about 30 per cent of all trochanteric fractures.

VARIETIES OF FRACTURES

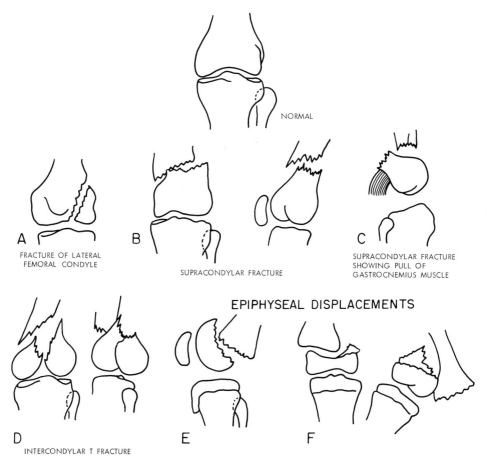

Figure 5–34 *A*. Types of fractures of the knee.

Figure 5–34 continued on opposite page.

Fractures of the Shaft of the Femur

Classification.   These may be transverse, oblique, spiral, or severely comminuted. In children occasionally they are greenstick.

Varieties of Fractures of the Lower End of the Femur.   These may be:
1. Lateral or medial condylar;
2. Supracondylar;
3. Intercondylar, T-, V-, or Y-fractures;
4. Supracondylar with marked posterior angulation as a result of the pull of the gastrocnemius muscle.

In children there may be various types of epiphyseal fractures or displacements in accordance with the previously described Salter-Harris classification (Figure 5–24).

Intercondylar fractures of the femur are always complicated by severe soft tissue damage and massive hemarthrosis.

Classification of Dislocations of the Knee Joint (Figure 5–34).
Most Common Varieties of Meniscal Tears (Figure 5–35).

Classification of Fractures of the Knee (Figures 5–36; 5–37; 5–38).
1. Anterior tibial tubercle;
2. Patella (with or without separation of fragments);
      a. With or without dislocation;
      b. With or without tear of adjoining ligaments.

In the interpretation of fractures of the patella, various anomalies of the patella must be borne in mind. Thus, the *bipartite* and *tripartite patella* contain incomplete

DISLOCATION OF THE KNEE JOINT

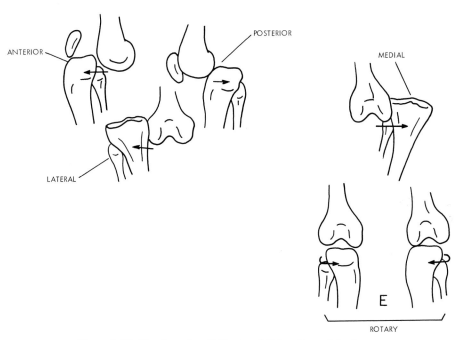

Figure 5–34 *(Continued).   B.* Types of dislocations of the knee.

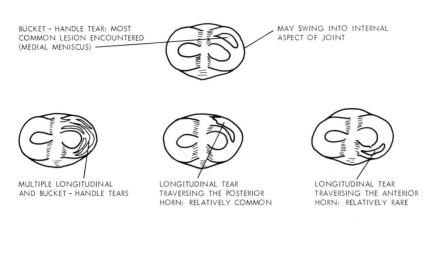

BUCKET - HANDLE TEAR: MOST COMMON LESION ENCOUNTERED (MEDIAL MENISCUS)

MAY SWING INTO INTERNAL ASPECT OF JOINT

MULTIPLE LONGITUDINAL AND BUCKET - HANDLE TEARS

LONGITUDINAL TEAR TRAVERSING THE POSTERIOR HORN: RELATIVELY COMMON

LONGITUDINAL TEAR TRAVERSING THE ANTERIOR HORN: RELATIVELY RARE

MULTIPLE SCORING OF INFERIOR SURFACE; ONE SMALL COMPLETE LONGITUDINAL TEAR

INCOMPLETE TEAR OF PERIPHERAL ATTACHMENTS OF POSTERIOR SEGMENT (MEDIAL MENISCUS)

INCOMPLETE TRANSVERSE TEAR (LATERAL MENISCUS): RARE LESION MORE FREQUENT IN LATERAL MENISCI

Figure 5–35 Types of meniscal tears.

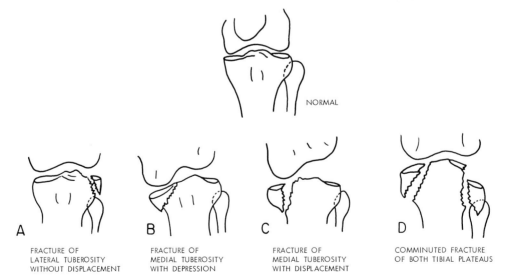

NORMAL

A
FRACTURE OF LATERAL TUBEROSITY WITHOUT DISPLACEMENT

B
FRACTURE OF MEDIAL TUBEROSITY WITH DEPRESSION

C
FRACTURE OF MEDIAL TUBEROSITY WITH DISPLACEMENT

D
COMMINUTED FRACTURE OF BOTH TIBIAL PLATEAUS

Figure 5–36 Types of fractures of the tibial condyle.

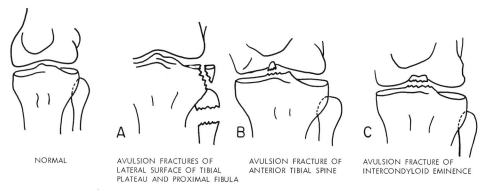

Figure 5–37   Types of condylar and plateau fractures of the tibia.

ossified segments of the patella. The unfused portions of the patella in these instances are in the *upper outer quadrant of the patella on its internal aspect in the lateral views* (Figure 5–39).

3. Fractures of the condyles of the tibia;
   a. Fractures of the medial condyle (rare);
   b. Depression of the central portion of the tibial plateau;
4. T- or Y-fractures of the upper end of the tibia, usually with downward depression of the tibial condyles.

Chip or avulsion fractures of the tibial eminence are often associated with and indicative of anterior or posterior cruciate ligament tears. The associated liga-

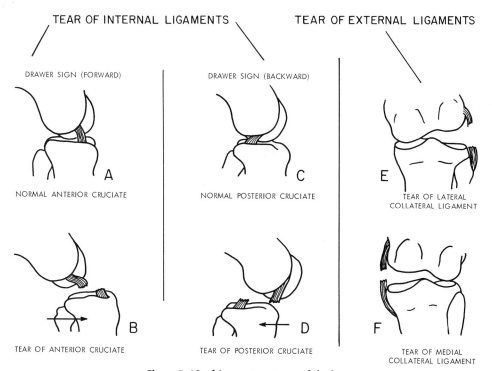

Figure 5–38   Ligamentous tears of the knee.

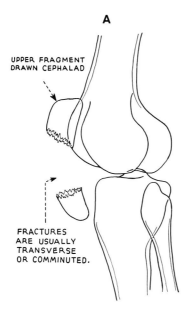

A

UPPER FRAGMENT
DRAWN CEPHALAD

FRACTURES
ARE USUALLY
TRANSVERSE
OR COMMINUTED.

Figure 5-39 *A*. Representative fracture of the patella. *B*. Bipartite patella.

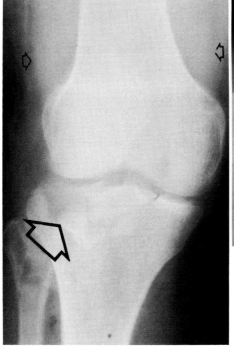

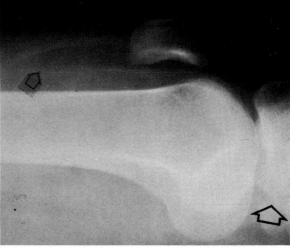

B

mentous injuries are by far the most serious consequences of this fracture. Internal derangement of the knee may also be associated, such as in meniscal tears and fractures. These can be diagnosed radiographically with the aid of special contrast studies (contrast arthrography).

Ligamentous Injuries of the Knee (Figure 5–38)

Fractures of the Shafts of the Tibia and Fibula

Union is notoriously slow and nonunion frequent. Ordinarily fractures of the upper shaft of the fibula can be disregarded, provided good alignment in the shaft of the tibia for weight bearing is obtained.

Fractures of the lower shaft of the fibula are often associated with fracture dislocations of the ankle.

A fracture in the lower shaft of the tibia is very often accompanied by a contrecoup upper shaft fracture in the fibula.

Dislocations (Fractures and Sprains) of the Ankle

Basic Anatomy.   The ankle is invested with a strong group of ligamentous structures which help to provide stability to the bony configuration. These ligaments bind the tibia and fibula firmly to one another and to the talus and calcaneus as well.

1. Anteriorly and posteriorly, extending between the distal ends of the tibia and fibula are the
   a. *Anterior tibiofibular ligaments,*
   b. The *posterior tibiofibular ligaments,* and
   c. The *interosseous membrane* (Figure 5–40).
2. The *medial collateral ligament* is attached to the navicular malleolus by a broad base and distally to the navicular and the talus tarsal bones. This is *also called the deltoid ligament.*
3. The *lateral collateral ligaments,* in addition to the previously indicated anterior and posterior talofibular component parts, also have a ligamentous structure extending between the calcaneus and the fibula.

Generally, injuries of the ankle are grouped into: (a) *inversion injuries* (Figure 5–41), and (b) *eversion injuries* (Figure 5–42). An effort is made, from the x-ray picture, to predict the ligamentous injury which has resulted. *At times, x-ray studies* (*Text continued on page 160*)

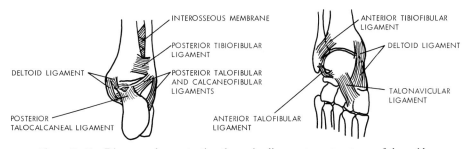

Figure 5–40   Diagrams demonstrating the major ligamentous structures of the ankle.

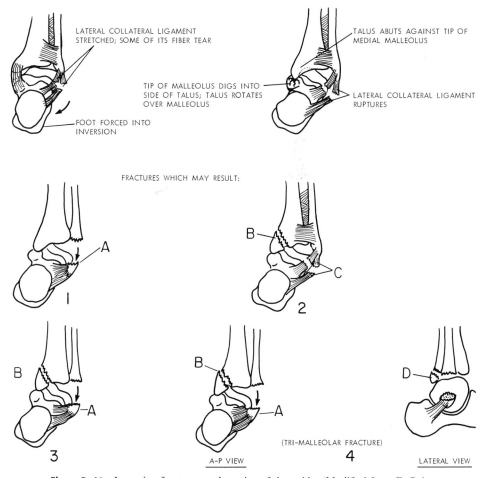

Figure 5–41   Inversion fractures and sprains of the ankle. (Modified from DePalma.)

Figure 5–41 continued on opposite page.

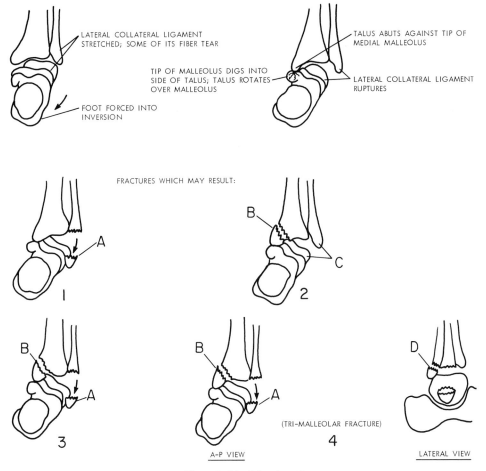

LATERAL COLLATERAL LIGAMENT
STRETCHED; SOME OF ITS FIBER TEAR

TIP OF MALLEOLUS DIGS INTO
SIDE OF TALUS; TALUS ROTATES
OVER MALLEOLUS

FOOT FORCED INTO
INVERSION

TALUS ABUTS AGAINST TIP OF
MEDIAL MALLEOLUS

LATERAL COLLATERAL LIGAMENT
RUPTURES

FRACTURES WHICH MAY RESULT:

1

2

3

4

(TRI-MALLEOLAR FRACTURE)

A-P VIEW

LATERAL VIEW

Figure 5–41 (*Continued*).

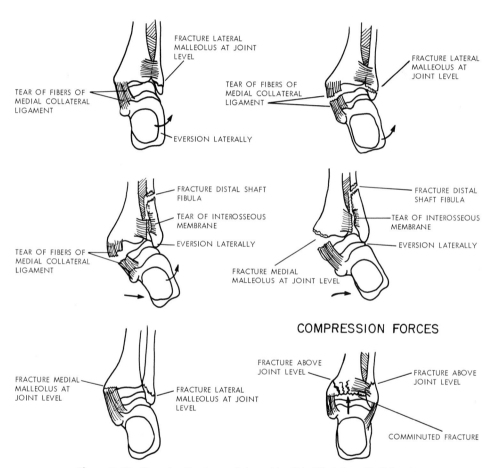

Figure 5–42   Eversion fractures of the ankle. (Modified from DePalma.)

Figure 5–42 continued on opposite page.

X-RAY TRACINGS

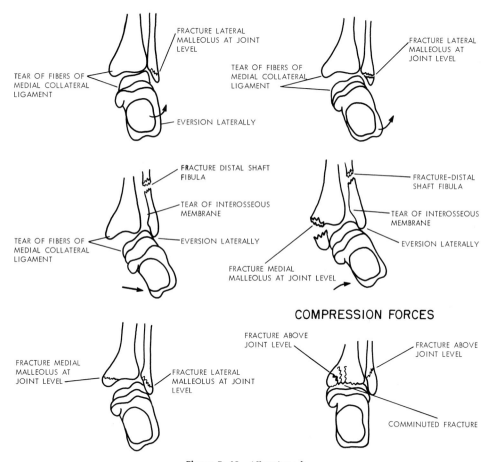

Figure 5–42 (*Continued*).

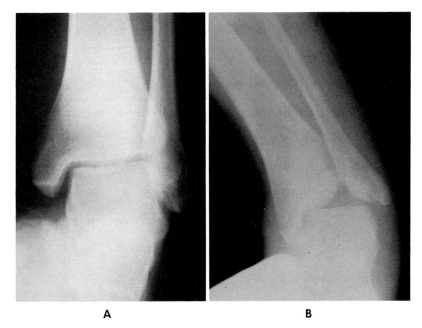

A   **B**

Figure 5–43   Stress films of the ankle demonstrating a tear in the lateral collateral ligament and fracture of the medial malleolus from an inversion injury of the ankle. *A.* Normal stress film demonstrating the preservation of the talotibial joint mortice with stress. *B.* Stress film demonstrating abnormal relaxation of the lateral collateral ligament of the ankle with stress.

of the ankle must be obtained under stress to establish ligamentous injuries beyond question (Figure 5–43).

With compression forces, such as a fall from a height, impaction of the distal articular surface of the tibia may result.

Dislocations of the ankle may occur either anteriorly or posteriorly with associated fractures of one or both malleoli. With the *posterior dislocation,* a posterior marginal fracture of the tibia may result; with *anterior dislocation,* an anterior marginal avulsion fracture of the tibia may occur.

In young persons in whom bony fusion of the distal epiphysis of the tibia has not yet occurred, it is important to diagnose correctly a crushing injury to the epiphyseal plate, since prognosis is poor in this case.

Soft Tissue Changes with Spontaneous Achilles Tendon Rupture (Reveno and Kittleson).   If spontaneous Achilles tendon rupture has occurred, the Achilles tendon, which on a straight lateral film of the ankle is ordinarily clearly outlined by fat, is obscured because of associated bleeding and edema. The tendon ends may be identified as a soft tissue mass after rupture and retraction. A posterior soft tissue defect may also be identified.

Fractures and Fracture-Dislocations of the Foot

Fractures of the Talus.   These may be classified as:
1. Fractures of the posterior process;
2. Fractures of the body of the talus;
3. Fractures of the neck of the talus without displacement;
4. Fractures of the neck of the talus with subluxation of the subtalar joint (Figure 5–44).

A

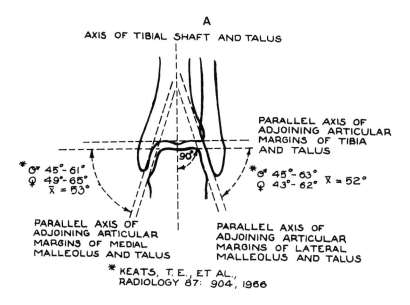

AXIS OF TIBIAL SHAFT AND TALUS

PARALLEL AXIS OF ADJOINING ARTICULAR MARGINS OF TIBIA AND TALUS

90°

* ♂ 45°- 61°
♀ 49°- 65°
X̄ = 53°

* ♂ 45°- 63°   X̄ = 52°
♀ 43°- 62°

PARALLEL AXIS OF ADJOINING ARTICULAR MARGINS OF MEDIAL MALLEOLUS AND TALUS

PARALLEL AXIS OF ADJOINING ARTICULAR MARGINS OF LATERAL MALLEOLUS AND TALUS

* KEATS, T. E., ET AL., RADIOLOGY 87: 904, 1966

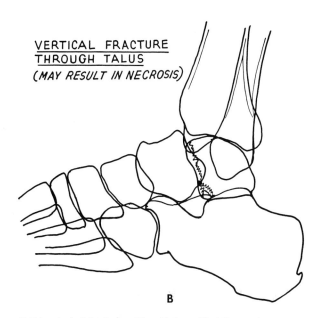

VERTICAL FRACTURE THROUGH TALUS (MAY RESULT IN NECROSIS)

B

Figure 5–44   *A.* Axial relationships of the ankle joint. *B.* Fracture of the talus.

Fractures through the neck of the talus are not infrequently associated with *avascular necrosis* of the body of the talus, which may lead ultimately to degenerative arthritis of the ankle and subtalar joints.

The Calcaneus.   Injuries to the spine are frequently associated with fractures of the calcaneus and should be carefully excluded.

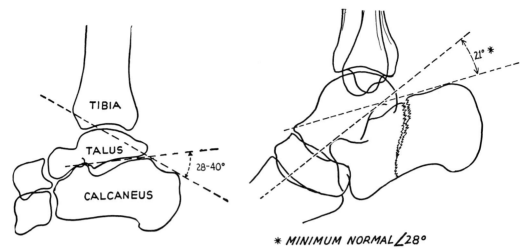

Figure 5–45 Tuber angle of the calcaneus. Normal: greater than 28 degrees and usually 35 to 40 degrees.

In addition to the usual lateral view of the calcaneus, an axial view should always be obtained.

Isolated fractures of a simple type may occur through the tuberosity or through the sustentaculum tali. If significant displacement is present, however, treatment becomes more complicated and assessment must therefore be accurate.

In all fractures of the calcaneus, assessment of the tuber angle (critical angle of Boehler) is essential (Figure 5–45).

In very severe injuries, disruption of the calcaneocuboid joint may also occur and must be assessed.

The Navicular Tarsal Bone. If a dorsal fragment of the navicular bone is displaced upward, aseptic necrosis and osteoarthritis are common sequels. Early recognition is essential, but even with the best treatment this complication may result and ultimate arthrodesis is necessitated.

Cuboid and Cuneiform Bone. Fractures of these bones are usually associated with dislocation at the midtarsal or tarsometatarsal joints. The midtarsal joints consist of the talonavicular and calcaneocuboid joints. Such dislocations must be recognized and reduced immediately.

In all injuries to this region as well as to the tarsometatarsal, thrombosis or spasm of the large arteries of the foot may occur.

Metatarsal Bones. Stress fractures of the metatarsals are frequent and are the so-called "march fractures."

At times a stress fracture will escape detection when it is first x-rayed and will become manifest only after callus has been deposited around the faint fracture line.

Fracture of the base of the fifth metatarsal bone requires some special consideration. This is an avulsion injury caused by inversion and plantar flexion of the foot. The base of the fifth metatarsal is pulled off by the tendon of the peroneus brevis muscle. *Careful differentiation from the peroneal sesamoid is essential.* Likewise, in young people, a normal epiphysis at the base of the fifth metatarsal must be differentiated.

Fractures of the Toes. The great toe is the most frequently involved. Usually displacement of fragments is minimal although at times the fractures can be comminuted.

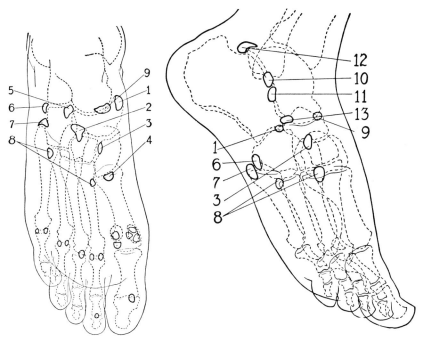

Figure 5–46   Schematic diagram to show sesamoid bones and supernumerary bones of the foot. (1) Os tibiale externum; (2) processus uncinatus; (3) intercuneiforme; (4) pars peronea metatarsalia I; (5) cuboides secundarium; (6) os peroneum; (7) os vesalianum; (8) intermetatarseum; (9) accessory navicular; (10) talus accessorius; (11) os sustentaculum; (12) os trigonum; (13) calcaneus secundarius. The most common of these are 1, 6, 7, 9 and 12. (From McNeill: *Roentgen Technique*. Springfield, Charles C Thomas, 1947.)

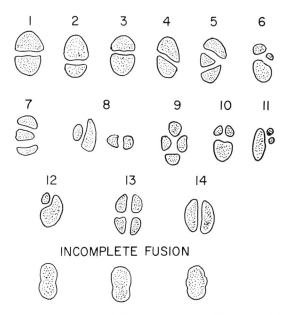

Figure 5–47   Developmental variations of hallux partite sesamoids arranged in descending order of frequency. (From Feldman et al., Radiology *96*:275–283, 1970.)

DISLOCATIONS OF THE ANKLE AND FOOT
VARIETIES OF DISLOCATIONS

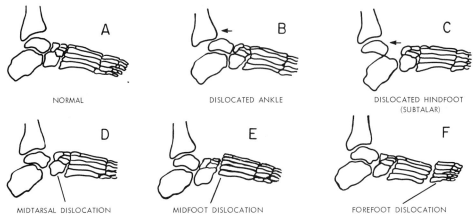

Figure 5–48   Dislocations of the foot. (Modified from DePalma and Zatzkin.)

Sesamoid Bones of the Foot and Ankle (Figure 5–46).   Sesamoid bones of the foot and ankle occasionally may be confused with avulsion-type fractures and they may not necessarily be symmetrical on both sides of the body. Nevertheless, comparison films of the opposite side are recommended. The most common sesamoids are os trigonum, os peroneum, and the accessory navicular.

Numerous variations in size and shape of the sesamoid bones have been described (Feldman, et al.) (Figure 5–47). The line of separation between two sesamoids is usually smooth, concavoconvex or transverse, oblique, or vertical with segments equal or unequal in size. Sesamoid fractures are very rare but they do occur and may be recognized radiographically.

The **roentgen criteria for sesamoid fractures** are: (1) irregular, serrated line of division; (2) interrupted peripheral cortex; (3) exaggerated separation of fragments; (4) unusual position; (5) multiplicity of fragments; (6) asymmetry with respect to the opposite foot; (7) callus formation after a suitable time interval; and (8) previous films showing a different appearance.

Questions – Chapter 5

1. What radiographic views are minimal requirements in suspected fracture or dislocation?

2. How large an area should be studied in any suspected fracture?

3. What are the four major items requiring careful analysis in respect to fractures of extremities?

4. What are the recommended time intervals between radiographic studies following a fracture?

5. Indicate the various types of fractures by classification.

   6. What is the importance of an avulsion- or chip-type fracture?

   7. Indicate the Salter-Harris classification of epiphyseal injuries.

   8. What is the significance of these five types and their relative incidence?

   9. Define the "insufficiency" or "stress fracture."

   10. What is "Milkman's syndrome"?

   11. Define "pathologic fracture."

   12. From the standpoint of potential complications, what is the most important site for fracture of the clavicle?

   13. What are the potential dangers in respect to vascular or radial injuries in fractures of the humerus and where are such fractures noted within the humerus?

   14. How may one obtain a good visualization of alignment of the fragments of the humerus when elevation of the humerus is not possible?

   15. What are the potential complications in respect to injured nerves and arteries of fracture of the supracondyloid process of the humerus?

   16. What is the importance of epiphyseal displacement of the lower end of the humerus in the growing adolescent if not corrected? When may open reduction be required?

   17. What is Volkmann's ischemic contracture and with what fracture is this frequently found?

   18. What is the importance of the carrying angle, especially in children?

   19. What is the importance of recognition of chip fragments around the elbow in association with the joints of the elbow?

   20. In fractures of the olecranon of the ulna, what possible complications must one anticipate in respect to nerves and major blood vessels?

   21. Why is it important to recognize loose bone fragments or altered configuration in fractures of the head and neck of the radius?

   22. What are the varieties of Monteggia's fracture-dislocation of the elbow?

   23. What is the importance of detection of the fat plane in the region of the elbow? What is the "displaced fat pad sign"?

   24. In fractures of the bones of the forearm, how may difficult rotational deformities result?

   25. Why is it important to attempt to visualize with clarity the position of the interosseous membrane?

   26. What are the various types of fractures involving the lower end of the radius? How have they been catalogued and described? Name five such fractures.

   27. Which are the most important fractures and dislocations of the carpal bones?

   28. What is the blood supply of the scaphoid carpal bone and how does this relate to potential complications? Wherein does frequent complication arise?

   29. What is the difference between lunate and perilunate dislocation? How many types of perilunate dislocations do we recognize?

   30. What is the importance of fractures of the capitate carpal bone in the wrist?

   31. What is the so-called "Bennett's fracture"?

   32. What are the various types of fractures of the acetabulum?

   33. Where may injury to the sciatic nerve result in fractures of the acetabulum? In approximately what percentage of cases?

   34. How is the blood supply of the femoral capital epiphysis and neck derived?

   35. What is the so-called "gull-wing sign"?

   36. Classify the dislocations of the hip.

   37. What is acetabular dysplasia and what is its importance?

   38. Why is it important to rotate the foot internally if possible in obtaining anteroposterior views for potential fracture of the neck of the femur?

   39. Where is the attachment of the hip joint capsule and what is its importance relative to fractures of the hip?

   40. What is the most frequent deformity in fracture of the neck of the femur?

   41. What is Shenton's line? Skinner's line? What is the importance of these lining techniques?

   42. In studying the capital femoral epiphysis for possible slippage, why is it important

to differentiate a slip of greater than a third or less than a third of the diameter of the femoral neck?

43. What is a useful classification for fractures of the upper end of the femur?

44. Classify the varieties of fractures of the lower end of the femur.

45. Why are intercondylar fractures of the femur especially important?

46. What are the most common varieties of meniscal tears within the knee?

47. Classify fractures of the knee.

48. Describe the basic ligamentous anatomy of the ankle and its importance in respect to fractures in this injury?

49. What injuries may result in inversion injury of the ankle?

50. What injuries of the ankle may result in eversion injuries?

51. Why is it important to bear in mind a particular classification of fractures of the talus in the tarsus?

52. What are the routine views for suspected injury to the calcaneus?

53. What is the tuber or critical angle of the calcaneus and what is its importance?

54. Why is it especially important to recognize fractures of the cuboid and cuneiform?

55. In all injuries to the tarsometatarsal region, what particular complication is especially prone to occur?

56. What are march fractures?

57. What are the most frequent sesamoid bones of the foot encountered?

58. How does one recognize sesamoid bone fractures?

References

Arndt, J. H., and Sears, A. D.: Posterior dislocation of the shoulder. Amer. J. Roentgenol., 94:639–645, 1965.

Berkebile, R. D., Fischer, D. L., and Albrecht, L. F.: Gull wing sign: value of lateral view of pelvis in fracture-dislocation of acetabular rim and posterior dislocation of the femoral head. Radiology, 84:937–939, 1965.

Bledsoe, R. C., and Izenstark, J. L.: Displacement of fat pads in disease and injury of elbow: New radiographic sign. Radiology, 73:717–724, 1959.

Brinn, L. B., and Moseley, J. E.: Bone changes following electrical injury: case report and review of literature. Amer. J. Roentgenol., 97:682–686, 1966.

Brogdon, B. G., and Crow, N. E.: Little Leaguer's elbow. Amer. J. Roentgenol., 83:671–675, 1960.

Caffey, J.: Pediatric X-ray Diagnosis. Fourth Edition. Chicago, Year Book Publishers, 1961.

Caffey, J.: Traumatic cupping of the metaphyses of growing bone. Amer. J. Roentgenol., 108:451–460, 1970.

DePalma, A. F.: The Management of Fractures and Dislocations. Philadelphia, W. B. Saunders Co., 1959.

Feldman, F., Pochaczevsky, R., and Hecht, H.: The case of the wandering sesamoid and other sesamoid afflictions. Radiology, 96:275–283, 1970.

Figiel, S. J., and Figiel, L. S.; Bardenstein, M. B., and Blodgett, W. H.: Posterior dislocation of the shoulder. Radiology, 87:737–740, 1966.

Friesen, S. R., Merendino, A., Baronofsky, I. D., Mears, F. B., and Wangensteen, O. H.: The relationship of bone trauma to the development of acute gastroduodenal lesions in ex-perimental animals and in man. Surgery, 24:134–159, 1948.

Kohn, A.: Soft tissue alterations in elbow trauma. Amer. J. Roentgenol., 82:867–874, 1959.

Kroenig, P. M., and Shelton, P. M.: Stress fractures. Amer. J. Roentgenol., 89:1281–1286, 1963.

MacEwan, D. W.: Changes due to trauma in the fat plane overlying the pronator quadratus muscle: A radiologic sign. Radiology, 82:879–886, 1964.

Meschan, I.: An Atlas of Normal Radiographic Anatomy. Second edition. Philadelphia, W. B. Saunders Co., 1959, pp. 178–182.

Meschan, I.: Synopsis of Roentgen Signs. Philadelphia, W. B. Saunders Co., 1962.

Monnet, P., and Beraud, C.: Osseous lesions in congenital insensitivity to pain in the infant. J. Radiol. et Electrol., 39:414–416, 1958.

Norell, G.: Roentgenologic visualization of the extracapsular fat. Its importance in diagnosis of traumatic injuries to the elbow. Acta Radiolog., 42:205–210, 1954.

Reveno, P. M., and Kittleson, A. C.: Spontaneous Achilles' tendon rupture. Radiology, 93:1341–1344, 1969.

Rogers, S. L., and MacEwan, D. W.: Changes due to trauma in the fat plane overlying the supinator muscle: A radiologic sign. Radiology, 92:954–958, 1969.

Rogers, Lee L. F.: The radiography of epiphyseal injuries. Radiology, 96:289–299, 1970.

Schinz et al. in J. T. Case, Ed.: Roentgen-Diagnostics, Volumes I and II. New York, Grune and Stratton, 1951–1952.

Zatzkin, H. R.: Roentgen Diagnosis of Trauma. Chicago, Year Book Medical Publishers, 1965.

6

Fracture Healing, Complications From Fractures, and Methods of Treatment from the Radiologic Standpoint

THE MAIN HISTOLOGIC STEPS IN FRACTURE HEALING AND CORRELATED RADIOGRAPHS

Main Steps in Fracture Healing (Figure 6–1). The main histologic steps in fracture healing may be summarized in the following outline:
1. Formation of hematoma.
2. Organization of hematoma.
3. Formation of fibrous callus.
4. Replacement of fibrous callus by primary bony callus.
5. Absorption of primary bony callus and transformation gradually to secondary bony callus.
6. Functional reconstruction of the bone in accordance with line of stress and adaptation by bone "modeling."

Every change in the position of fragments during the process of repair disturbs the formation of callus and therefore disturbs the repair process. If, in the course of healing, hyaline cartilage develops at the fracture margin, an actual false joint may in turn develop and nonunion ensue. The false joint is called a "neoarthrosis" and can be recognized by the formation of dense eburnated bone beneath the hyaline cartilage at the fracture margin (Figure 6–2).

Correlation of the Six Phases of Repair with Radiographic Appearances. The successive radiographic appearances in the process of fracture healing may be visualized as follows (Figures 6–3 through 6–7):

1. When the hematoma is formed there is considerable *soft tissue swelling* in the immediate vicinity of the fracture.

(Text continued on page 171)

STEPS IN THE HEALING OF FRACTURES

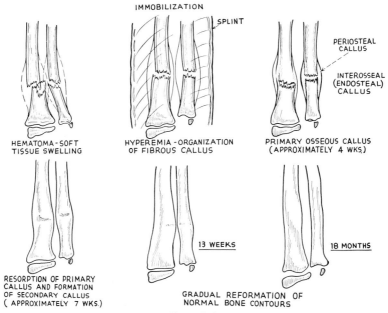

HEMATOMA-SOFT
TISSUE SWELLING

IMMOBILIZATION

SPLINT

HYPEREMIA-ORGANIZATION
OF FIBROUS CALLUS

PERIOSTEAL
CALLUS

INTEROSSEAL
(ENDOSTEAL)
CALLUS

PRIMARY OSSEOUS CALLUS
(APPROXIMATELY 4 WKS.)

RESORPTION OF PRIMARY
CALLUS AND FORMATION
OF SECONDARY CALLUS
(APPROXIMATELY 7 WKS.)

13 WEEKS

GRADUAL REFORMATION OF
NORMAL BONE CONTOURS

18 MONTHS

Figure 6–1

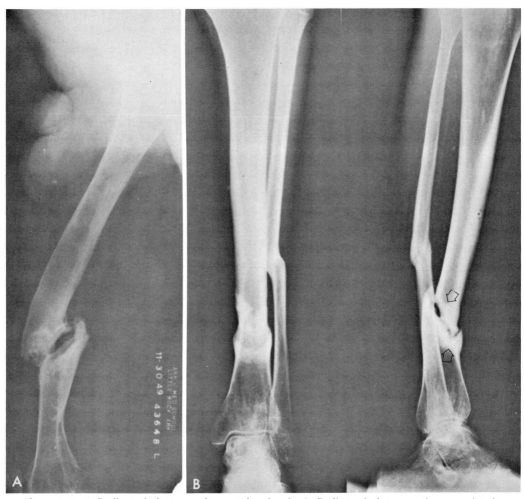

Figure 6–2 *A.* Radiograph demonstrating pseudoarthrosis. *B.* Radiograph demonstrating neoarthrosis. Note the eburnated smooth bone at the fracture margin.

168

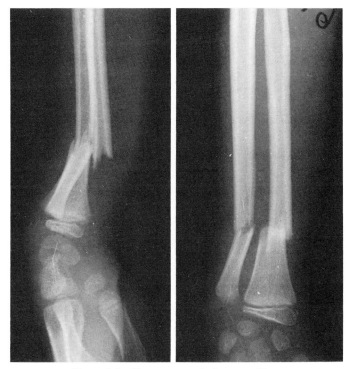

Figure 6–3   Hematoma, soft tissue swelling.

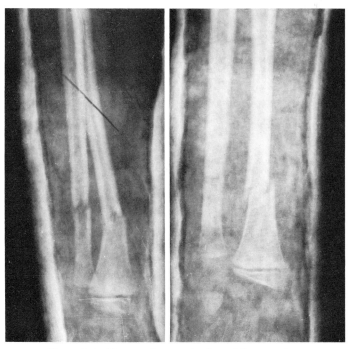

Figure 6–4   Hyperemia, organization of fibrous callus.

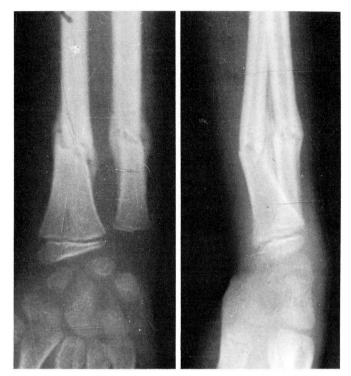

Figure 6–5   Primary osseous callus (approximately 4 weeks).

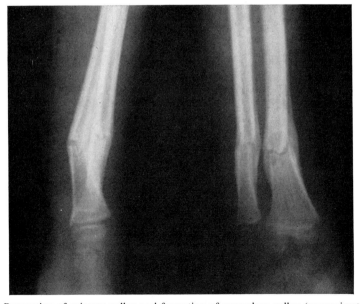

Figure 6–6   Resorption of primary callus and formation of secondary callus (approximately 7 weeks).

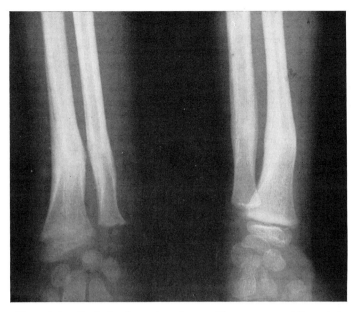

Figure 6–7   Gradual reformation of normal bone contours (13 weeks).

2. During the process of organization of the hematoma, there are a shrinkage of the swelling and the formation of fibrous callus with *progressive radiolucency of the bone surrounding the fragments.* There may be some resorption of bone along the fractured cleft, producing *the widened cleft.*

In the case of comminuted fractures, if there should be a devitalized fragment the surrounding bone will tend to become radiolucent, whereas the devitalized fragment will retain its original density and thus be readily identified as a *sequestrum.*

3. The *primary bone callus* is visualized as a faintly calcified area surrounding the fracture site. The time of appearance of bony callus is very variable and depends to a great extent upon the age of the patient and the fracture site. In young persons the bony callus is formed very rapidly, and in the newborn, massive bony callus may be visible by the end of one week.

4. The *primary bony callus becomes denser* and more sharply circumscribed and the bony cleft itself begins to be filled in by visible callus.

5. There is a *gradual and sharper delineation of the primary bony and periosteal callus* and actually a diminution in the size of the periosteal callus.

6. There is a gradual reformation of the normal appearing bony trabeculae and contour of the bone.

Pathogenesis of Delayed Union (with Pseudoarthrosis Formation) or Nonunion (Neoarthrosis). Normally primary bony callus consists of a metaplasia of fibrous granulation scar tissue to fibro- and hyaline cartilage with some calcification. The greater the development of hyaline cartilage (from motion of fragments or delay in repair), the more protracted is lamellated bone formation, and the more likely is *pseudoarthrosis.*

If an actual cleft forms in this pseudoarthrosis, and the hyaline cartilage fails to calcify, *neoarthrosis* is formed with calcification deposition adjoining the hyaline cartilage. This may be recognized radiographically by a dense line of compact bone adjoining the fracture line (Figure 6–2).

Major Items for Analysis on Radiographs of Extremities for Fractures

1. Degree of apposition of fragments.
2. Alignment with respect to:
    a. Adjoining joints.
    b. Line of weight bearing, or required action or movement of extremity as a whole.
3. Degree of torsion of fragments.
4. Degree of shortening of bone as a whole.

Inferential Information Possibly Gained

1. Is there soft tissue caught between fragments?
2. What is the associated soft tissue injury?
3. How much injury to periosteum?
4. How much cartilaginous or joint injury?

At What Time Intervals Should Fractured Extremities be Studied?

1. Initially.
2. Post-reduction and post-immobilization.
3. One or two weeks later to note if position has changed.
4. After approximately six or eight weeks for primary callus.
5. After each plaster cast or traction change.
6. Before final discharge of patient.

COMPLICATIONS FROM FRACTURES

The complications from fractures may be subdivided into the categories as illustrated in Figure 6–8.

When bony atrophy occurs with great rapidity, even though the initiating injury is trivial, and when it would appear that there is a reflex neurotrophic phenomenon occurring, the process is referred to as "Sudeck's atrophy." It is characterized by persistent pain, stiffness, and disability; after the injury, the extremity remains cold, tender, and cyanotic, and the joints are stiff and painful. This condition may persist over a period of months and may be very resistant to all forms of treatment.

Occasionally gastric hemorrhage and bleeding, erosions and ulcerations of the gastrointestinal tract have been encountered following severe trauma (Friesen).

Unrecognized Fractures of the Long Bones Suggesting Primary Bone Tumors. Occasionally, because of pain and disability, radiographs of an extremity are obtained which reveal an unsuspected healing fracture. The picture may suggest either primary bone tumor, osteomyelitis, or a healing fracture.

On other occasions, after a traumatic episode to bone, a radiograph will suggest the diagnosis of either a primary or metastatic bone tumor. *Biopsy may be necessary in order to make the correct diagnosis.* "Fatigue" or "stress" fractures as already described must also be considered.

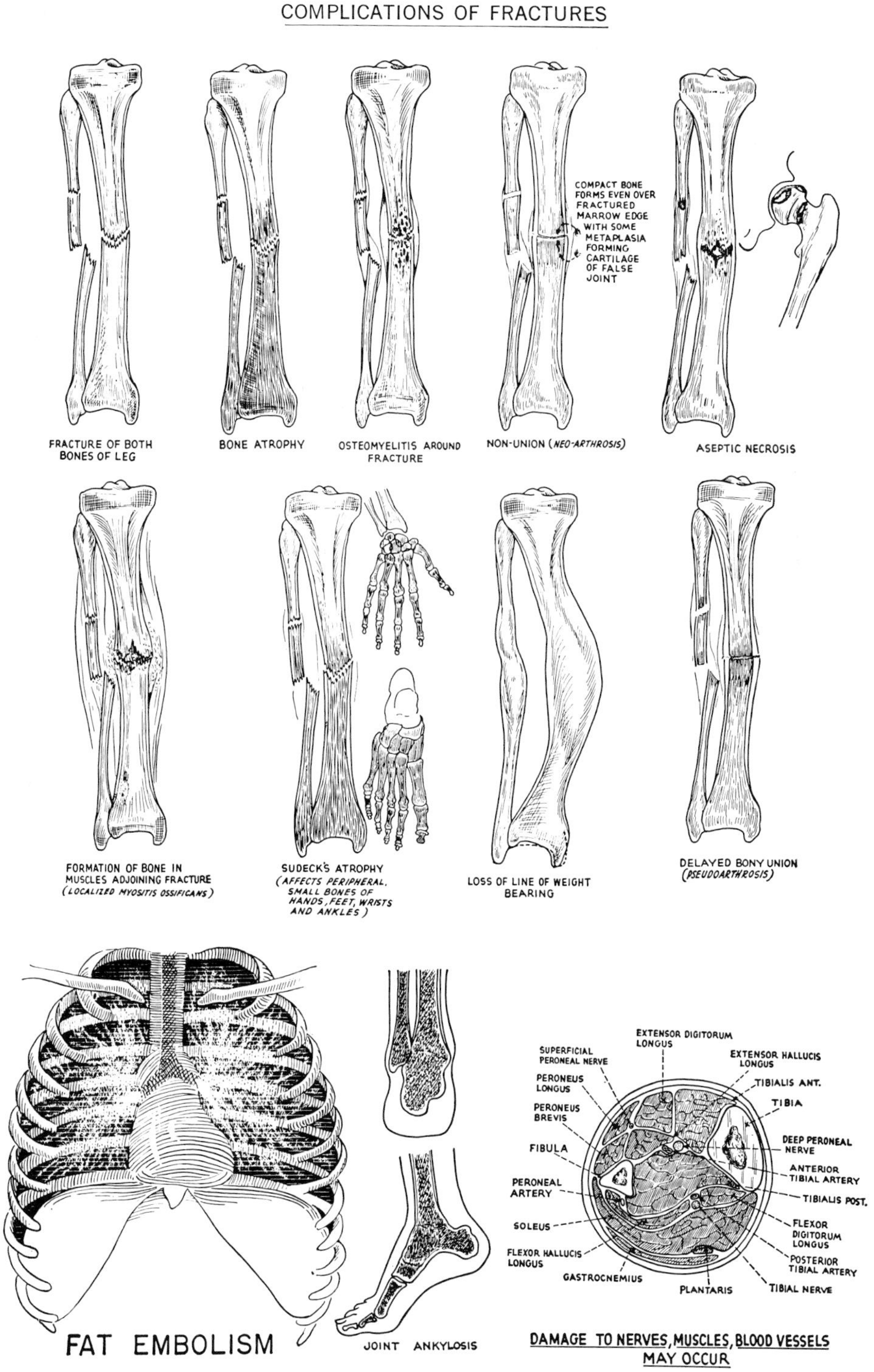

COMPLICATIONS OF FRACTURES

FRACTURE OF BOTH
BONES OF LEG

BONE ATROPHY

OSTEOMYELITIS AROUND
FRACTURE

COMPACT BONE
FORMS EVEN OVER
FRACTURED
MARROW EDGE
WITH SOME
METAPLASIA
FORMING
CARTILAGE
OF FALSE
JOINT

NON-UNION (*NEO-ARTHROSIS*)

ASEPTIC NECROSIS

FORMATION OF BONE IN
MUSCLES ADJOINING FRACTURE
(*LOCALIZED MYOSITIS OSSIFICANS*)

SUDECK'S ATROPHY
(*AFFECTS PERIPHERAL,
SMALL BONES OF
HANDS, FEET, WRISTS
AND ANKLES*)

LOSS OF LINE OF WEIGHT
BEARING

DELAYED BONY UNION
(*PSEUDOARTHROSIS*)

FAT EMBOLISM

JOINT ANKYLOSIS

EXTENSOR DIGITORUM
LONGUS

SUPERFICIAL
PERONEAL NERVE

EXTENSOR HALLUCIS
LONGUS

PERONEUS
LONGUS

TIBIALIS ANT.

PERONEUS
BREVIS

TIBIA

FIBULA

DEEP PERONEAL
NERVE

ANTERIOR
TIBIAL ARTERY

PERONEAL
ARTERY

TIBIALIS POST.

SOLEUS

FLEXOR
DIGITORUM
LONGUS

FLEXOR HALLUCIS
LONGUS

POSTERIOR
TIBIAL ARTERY

GASTROCNEMIUS

PLANTARIS

TIBIAL NERVE

DAMAGE TO NERVES, MUSCLES, BLOOD VESSELS
MAY OCCUR

Figure 6–8 Complications of fractures diagrammatically illustrated. It is implied that loss of line of weight bearing also indicates excessive deformity.

TRAUMATIC LESIONS OF THE SKELETON IN THE INFANT

("Battered Child" Syndrome)

Fractures or other manifestations of trauma are not infrequently discovered in infants incidental to some other examination. A history of trauma cannot always be obtained because of family concealment or because an older child may be responsible and the parents are unaware of the assault.

Infantile growth is rapid, and the periosteum is loosely applied and vascular. Radiographically the lesions tend to be multiple and superimposed on bones of normal density and architecture. Subperiosteal new bone beneath the elevated periosteum may involve an entire diaphysis (Figure 6–9). The metaphysis may be fragmented near the epiphyseal plate with or without gross epiphyseal displacement, especially around the elbows, knees, and ankles.

Subdural hematoma is often an associated abnormality.

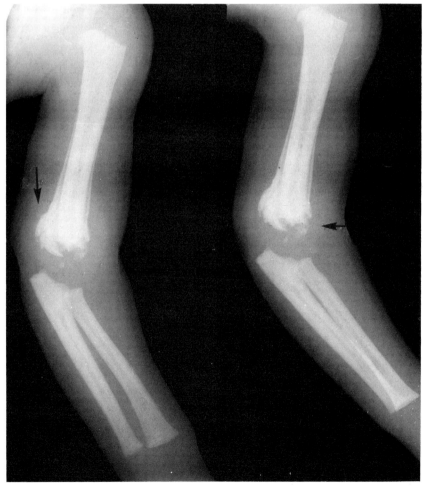

Figure 6–9 Radiographs of the arm and forearm of a child subjected to "battering" by an older sibling ("battered child syndrome"). (Courtesy of Dr. Joseph G. Gordon, Reynolds Memorial Hospital, Winston-Salem, N. C.)

The. *differential diagnosis* must include: scurvy, congenital syphilis, infantile cortical hyperostosis, and malignant neoplasia. Usually the presence of an outright fracture of the diaphysis, the absence of bone destruction, and the absence of a radiolucent zone adjoining the zone of provisional calcification make the diagnosis evident (Caffey).

BIZARRE SKELETAL LESIONS ASSOCIATED WITH CONGENITAL INSENSITIVITY TO PAIN (Figure 6–10)

Congenital insensitivity to pain is a poorly understood, probably hereditary condition which can be suspected on the basis of the radiographic appearances in bone (Silverman, et al.).

The fractures are usually in the lower extremities and are associated with extreme hypermobility of joints and questionable increased elasticity of the skin. The patients are sometimes thought to be afflicted with an *incomplete form of Ehlers-Danlos syndrome*. Local swellings and redness appear in the neighborhood of joints. It is difficult to know whether these are traumatic or infectious in origin. The x-ray examinations of these extremities frequently show fractures and epiphyseal separations in various stages of repair. Occasionally, focal metaphyseal radiolucencies with sclerotic borders are differentiated which represent foci of osteomyelitis. Except for the insensitivity to pain, no outstanding neurological signs or symptoms are present.

These lesions are perhaps the counterparts in children of Charcot joints in adults (Silverman, et al.; Monnet, et al.).

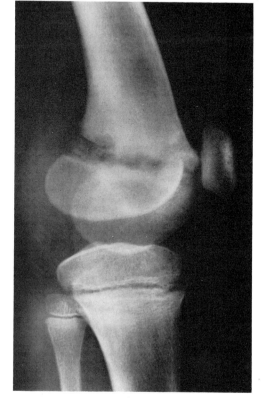

Figure 6–10 Congenital insensitivity to pain. "Aseptic necrosis-like lesion" near epiphyseal plate resembling epiphyseal separation. (From Silverman, F. N., and Gilden, J. J.: Radiology, *72*:183, 1959.)

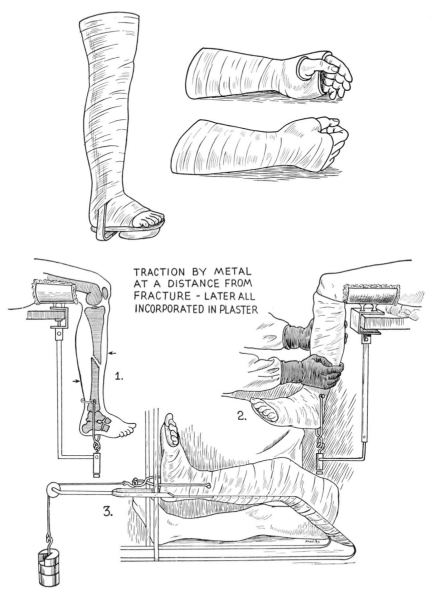

SIMPLE PLASTER IMMOBILIZATION

TRACTION BY METAL
AT A DISTANCE FROM
FRACTURE - LATER ALL
INCORPORATED IN PLASTER

1.

2.

3.

Figure 6–11   Diagrammatic summary of methods of treating fractures.

Figure 6–11 continued on opposite page.

APPLICATION OF METAL PLATES, SCREWS, WIRE, ETC.
ACROSS FRACTURE SITE

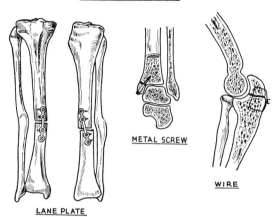

METAL SCREW

WIRE

LANE PLATE

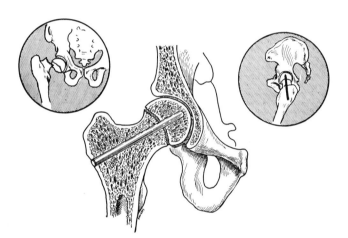

INTRAMEDULLARY FIXATION AT FRACTURE SITE BY OPEN REDUCTION
(BONE GRAFT)

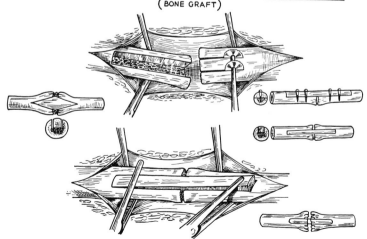

SOLID CORTICAL BONE GRAFTS

Figure 6–11   (*Continued*).

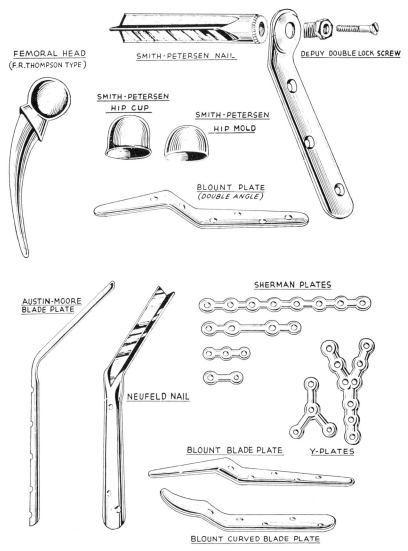

Figure 6–12 Representative metallic orthopedic fixation devices. More complete identification charts are available from surgical supply companies.

Immobilization of the Affected Part. This is achieved by:
1. Application of a plaster cast or splint.
2. Application of traction and countertraction to the bone itself by means of nails, clamps, or wire tension mechanisms.
3. Ultimately placing the whole arrangement in a plaster dressing.
4. Introduction of intramedullary nailing devices through the upper or lower metaphyses of a long bone, transfixing the fractured area without actual open operation over it.
5. Various open operative techniques in which the bone fragments are lined under direct vision and transfixed or immobilized by various special devices or bone grafts.

Figure 6–12 continued on opposite page.

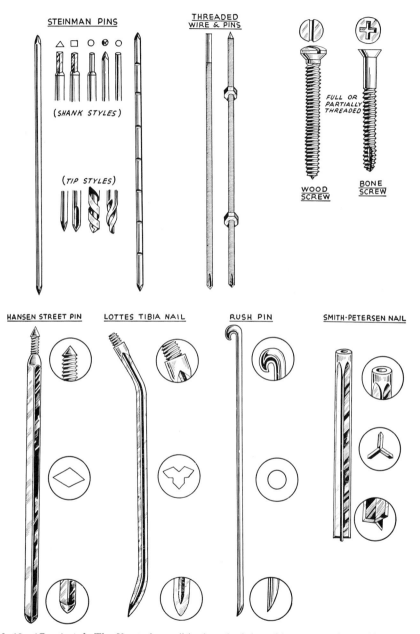

Figure 6–12 (*Continued*). The Kuntscher nail is cloverleaf shaped in cross section and is used similarly to the Hansen-Street.

METHODS OF TREATMENT OF FRACTURES FROM THE RADIOLOGIC STANDPOINT

Basic Principles

1. Treatment of the patient as a whole in respect to pain, shock, bleeding, care of open wounds, and anesthesia.
2. Correct immobilization.
3. Placement of the affected part in an optimal position.
4. Maintenance of this optimal position by any means possible.
5. Radiographs of the fractured extremity:
    (a) Initially.
    (b) Post-reduction.
    (c) Post-immobilization.
    (d) One or two weeks later to note if position has changed.
    (e) After each change of cast, or after each check for definitive consolidation in the fractured part.
    (f) After approximately six or eight weeks for primary callus.
    (g) Before final discharge of the patient.
6. Devise the earliest possible use of the injured part.

These various methods of immobilization and general mechanisms for fixation are illustrated in Figure 6–11.

Fixation Devices. These devices are highly variable and different in many institutions. Some of them are shown in the accompanying illustration (Figure 6–12).

It is important that the metal or alloy employed be relatively inert within the bone, since electrolysis within the bone must be avoided. This is recognized radiographically in the healing fracture by a lucent zone which surrounds the metallic function device.

In addition to those metallic devices illustrated, wire encircling methods may also be employed. In the adult, wires may be left in situ without concern. In the adolescent, their removal is indicated, since with the normal growth and the thickness of the bone, the wires will break or become embedded within the bone.

Bone Grafts. In the utilization of bone grafts, the following orthopedic principles have been demonstrated.

Osteogenesis occurs in bone grafts regardless of the integrity of the periosteum and endosteum, but is facilitated when the periosteum and endosteum are left intact.

There is an intimate fusion of the graft to the host bone even after 30 days.

Although vascularity within grafts can be demonstrated, they may have large areas of necrosis.

When stability at the site of a graft is needed through internal fixation, it is desirable to use a solid graft of compact bone, a metal plate, or both.

Since cancellous bone generally undergoes less necrosis than compact bone, the use of cancellous-chip grafts around a fracture site is desirable, even when a metal plate is used.

Necrotic areas in bone grafts are gradually replaced by "creeping substitution" made possible through the ingrowth of adjacent cellular and vascular elements.

After a fresh bone graft transplantation the first roentgenographic evidence detectable is usually a minimal bone callus surrounding the graft while the adjoining zone becomes atrophic. Later on, the transplant gradually becomes less dense because of the resorption of the dead bony tissues. The transplant itself does not become revascularized and remain alive. Ordinarily, the autoplastic transplant of calcific bony tissue dies along with the osteophytes contained therein. But meanwhile it still fills its mechanical function for a certain period of time. Only the osteoblasts and osteoclasts in the periosteum and endosteum of the graft remain alive; these proliferate and form new bony tissue, which replaces the original graft area by "creeping substitution."

Questions – Chapter 6

1. What are the six main steps in fracture healing?

2. What is meant by pseudoarthrosis and neoarthrosis and how may they be recognized radiographically?

3. What are the various phases of repair in bone healing following fractures, as recognized radiographically?

4. List the various complications from fractures.

5. What is meant by Sudeck's atrophy?

6. What are the major items for analysis on radiographs of extremities for fractures?

7. What is the inferential information which may possibly be gained by study of films for fractures?

8. At what time intervals should fractured extremities be studied following the initial x-rays?

9. What is the "battered child syndrome"?

10. What is the syndrome known as "congenital insensitivity to pain"?

11. Outline the general principles for definitive treatment of fractures.

12. What complications should be sought in the study of fractures treated by intramedullary fixation devices?

13. What are the six main orthopedic principles in the utilization of bone grafts?

14. What is the sequence of radiographic appearances following the application of bone graft transplantation in the treatment of fractures?

References

Aegerter, E., and Kirkpatrick, J. A., Jr.: Orthopedic Diseases. Second Edition. Philadelphia, W. B. Saunders Co., 1963, pp. 225–242.

Blount, W. P.: Fractures in Children. Baltimore, Williams and Wilkins Co., 1954.

Caffey, J.: Pediatric X-ray Diagnosis. Fourth Edition. Chicago, Year Book Publishers, 1961.

Campbell, W. S.: Operative Orthopedics. Second Edition. St. Louis, C. V. Mosby Co., 1949.

Christian, J. D., and Thompson, S. B.: Medullary fixation in fractures of long bones. J. Ark. Med. Soc., 49:126–129, 1953.

Friesen, S. R., Merendino, A., Baronofsky, I. D., Mears, F. B., and Wangensteen, O. H.: The relationship of bone trauma to the development of acute gastroduodenal lesions in experimental animals and in man. Surgery, 24:134–159, 1948.

Key, J. A., and Conwell, H. E.: Fractures, Dislocations and Sprains. Fifth Edition. St. Louis, C. V. Mosby Co., 1951.

Linscheid, R. L., and Coventry, M. B.: Staff meetings of Mayo Clinic, 37:599–606, 1962.

Monnet, P., and Beraud, C.: Osseous lesions in congenital insensitivity to pain in the infant. J. Radiol. et Electrol., 39:414–416, 1958.

Silverman, F. N., and Gilden, J. J.: Congenital insensitivity to pain: neurologic syndrome with bizarre skeletal lesions. Radiology, 72: 176–190, 1959.

Watson-Jones, R.: Fractures and Joint Injuries. Third Edition. Baltimore, Williams and Wilkins Co., 1943.

Weaver, J. B., and Francisco, C. B.: Pseudofractures: a manifestation of non-suppurative osteomyelitis. J. Bone & Joint Surg., 22:610–615, 1940.

Weinman, J. P., and Sicker, H.: Bone and Bones: Fundamentals of Bone Biology. Second Edition. St. Louis, C. V. Mosby Co., 1955.

7

Congenital and Hereditary Abnormalities of the Skeletal System

INTRODUCTION

The subject of congenital and hereditary abnormalities has become exceedingly complex and extends far beyond the scope of this text. Inborn errors of metabolism are more and more being identified as specific metabolic disorders which in turn may be related to genetic mutations or chromosomal aberrations.

This section is included so that the student may formulate a systematic approach to these problems from the radiologic standpoint, and so that he may utilize the outlined material as a framework around which he may build a concept of the complexity of the field and its detailed parts.

We may divide this group of disorders into *four major categories:*

1. *Underdevelopment of a bone or extremity.*
2. *Overdevelopment of single bones or an extremity or duplication of parts.*
3. *Maldevelopment of a skeletal part.*
   a. *Regional* — localized in one part of the skeleton.
   b. *General* (systemic in skeletal system — possibly associated with abnormalities in other systems).
      (1) Skeletal abnormalities in relation to known *chromosomal aberrations.*
4. *Diseases of bone* related to a *defect extrinsic* to the bone but involving the bone secondarily.

TABLE 7–1   CLASSIFICATION OF CONGENITAL AND HEREDITARY OSSEOUS MALFORMATIONS

Underdevelopment	Overdevelopment, Sclerosis, or Duplication	Maldevelopment				Primarily Extrinsic to Bone
		Regional	Epiphyseal	General		
				Metaphyseal	Bones or Tissues Diffusely	
Brachydactylia Oligodactylia Aplasias and phocomelias Cleidocranial dysostosis Idiopathic familial osteolysis Absent patella—fingernail syndrome (hereditary arthro-osteo-onycho-dysplasia)	Hyperphalangism Arachnodactylia (Marfan's syndrome) (Klinefelter's syndrome) Melorheostosis Partial gigantism Marble bone disease * Engelmann's disease or hereditary multiple diaphyseal sclerosis (Ribbing) * Osteopoikilosis * Osteopathia striata (Voorhoeve) Epiphyseal dysplasia † Congenital stippled † epiphyses (chondroangiopathia calcificans congenita)	Syndactylia Perodactylia Peromelia Madelung's deformity Vertical talus	Congenital stippled epiphyses Dysplasia epiphysialis multiplex	Ollier's disease Diaphyseal aclasis Metaphyseal dysplasia (Pyle's disease) Hypophosphatasia (hereditary) (see Chap. 8)	Achondroplasia Polytopic enchondral dysostosis (Morquio's; Pfaundler-Hurler; Leri) Osteogenesis imperfecta Acrocephalosyndactylia Mandibulofacial dystosis (Franceschetti's syndrome) (Treacher-Collins syndrome) Congenital dysplasia of face and extremities Craniometaphyseal dysplasia Chondroectodermal dysplasia (Ellis-van Creveld) Familial metaphyseal dysplasia (Pyle's syndrome) Mongolism (trisomy 21) Trisomy 16-18 (possibly trisomy 13-15 or triploid mosaicism) } Known chromosomal aberrations	Sprengel's deformity Myositis ossificans progressiva Neurofibromatosis Lipoid storage disease Hematopoietic disorders

*See Chapter 7 (sclerosis of bone).
†May also occur under *Epiphyseal.*

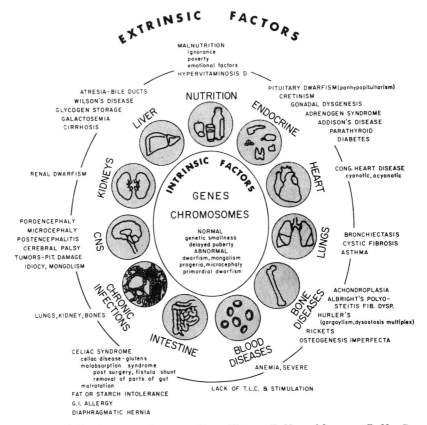

Conditions frequently leading to small stature. (From Watson, E. H., and Lowrey, G. H.: *Growth and Development of Children.* 5th Ed. Chicago, Year Book Medical Publishers, 1967.)

UNDERDEVELOPMENT OF A BONE OR EXTREMITY

This group of abnormalities comprises those in which:

1. An extremity or part of an extremity is absent (*aplastic*), or underdeveloped (*hypoplastic*), or too few in number.

2. There are associations of underdeveloped abnormalities which occur sufficiently frequently to be identified as a *syndrome*.

Three of these entities are described below, and a number of the others are included in a glossary of terms.

Cleidocranial Dysostosis (Scheuthauer-Marie-Sainton syndrome) (Soule) (Figure 7–1)

Radiographic Features. Aplasia of clavicles; delayed closure of the sutures of the skull; delayed and sometimes absent ossification in the bones of the pelvis, particularly in the pubes and ischia; curious shape of the phalanges; and moderately severe osteoporosis throughout.

The skull ordinarily contains numerous wormian bones in the vicinity of the lambdoid suture, deficient ossification of the bones of the cranial vault, large fontanelles, and a limited union of the frontal bone centrally. Usually there is also a deficient ossification in the symphysis of the mandible. The thorax often appears compressed from both sides.

PATHOLOGIC CONDITIONS ASSOCIATED WITH ABNORMALITIES OF OSSEOUS DEVELOPMENT*

Conditions associated with *advanced* osseous development
    Hyperthyroidism (acceleration is not a constant finding)
    Adrenogenital syndrome (tumor or hyperplasia of the adrenal cortex)
    Pubertas praecox (Fluhmann)
    Tumors of the ovary (granulosa cell, thecoma, teratoma)
    Interstitial cell tumor of the testes
    Pineal gland tumor (male only)
    Tumors of the third ventricle involving the hypothalamus
    Simple obesity associated with statural overgrowth
    McCune-Albright syndrome (polyostotic fibrous dysplasia)

Conditions associated with *delayed* osseous development
    Hypothyroidism
    Addison's disease
    Hypopituitarism (dwarfism)
    Pituitary cachexia (Simmonds' disease)
    Prolonged malnutrition
    Chronic illness
    Fröhlich's syndrome (adiposogenital dystrophy)
    Chondrodystrophy (achondroplasia)
    Hurler's syndrome (lipochondrodystrophy)
    Some cases of mental deficiency and mongolism
    Gonadal agenesis (Turner's syndrome)
    Hypogonadism

In addition to these classic findings, the following are sometimes noted (Keats):

(a) Deformity of the articular surfaces of the long bones.

(b) Scoliosis, with incomplete closure of the neural arches of the spine, and disturbances in growth of the vertebral bodies.

(c) The ossification of the base of the skull may also be disturbed and appear strikingly flat.

The Absent Patella-Fingernail Syndrome (Hereditary arthro-osteo-onychodysplasia) (Brixey et al.)

Clinical and Radiographic Features. Deficient development of the fingernails, absence of the patellae, subluxations of the radial head, iliac horns, and other anomalies. There may be associated cervical ribs, angiomatosis of the skin, pigeon chest, thoracic kyphosis, and congenital cataract.

The disorder is not sex-linked but a definite genetic linkage has been demonstrated.

Klippel Feil Syndrome (Brevicollis) (See Chapter 14, Figure 14–22)

Clinical and Radiographic Features. Extreme shortness of the neck with associated synostoses of vertebral segments as well as hemivertebrae. There

---

*From Watson, E. H., and Lowrey, G. H., Growth and Development of Children, 5th Ed. Chicago, Year Book Medical Publishers, 1967.

(Text continued on page 190)

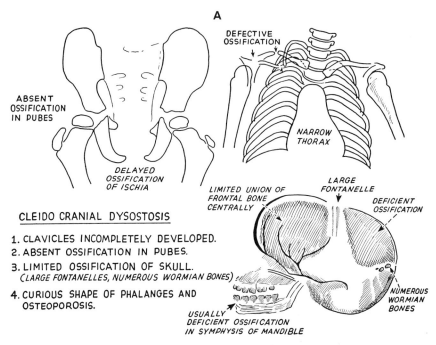

A

DEFECTIVE
OSSIFICATION

ABSENT
OSSIFICATION
IN PUBES

NARROW
THORAX

DELAYED
OSSIFICATION
OF ISCHIA

LARGE
FONTANELLE

LIMITED UNION OF
FRONTAL BONE
CENTRALLY

DEFICIENT
OSSIFICATION

CLEIDO CRANIAL DYSOSTOSIS

1. CLAVICLES INCOMPLETELY DEVELOPED.
2. ABSENT OSSIFICATION IN PUBES.
3. LIMITED OSSIFICATION OF SKULL.
   (LARGE FONTANELLES, NUMEROUS WORMIAN BONES)
4. CURIOUS SHAPE OF PHALANGES AND
   OSTEOPOROSIS.

NUMEROUS
WORMIAN
BONES

USUALLY
DEFICIENT OSSIFICATION
IN SYMPHYSIS OF MANDIBLE

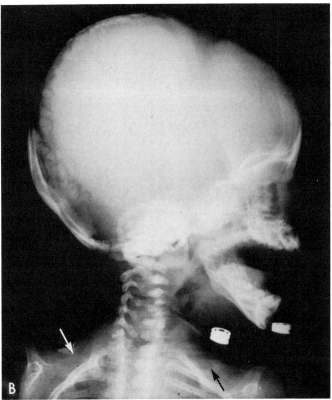

B

Figure 7–1   Cleidocranial dysostosis. *A*. Diagram. *B*. Radiograph.

Figure 7–1 continued on opposite page.

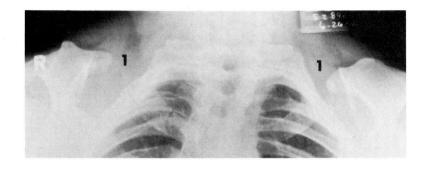

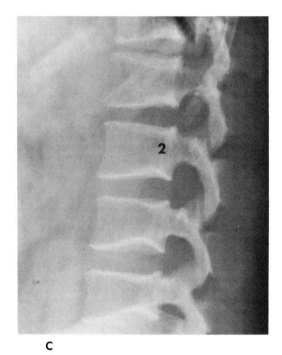

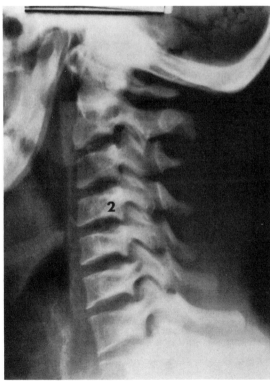

Figure 7–1 *(Continued).   C.* Radiographs of cleidocranial dysostosis in a 35 year old. (1) The absent clavicle and winged scapulae. (2) The deformed vertebral bodies with endplate indentations which are just proximal to the posterior aspects of the vertebral bodies in the cervical and lumbar region.

Figure 7–1 continued on following page.

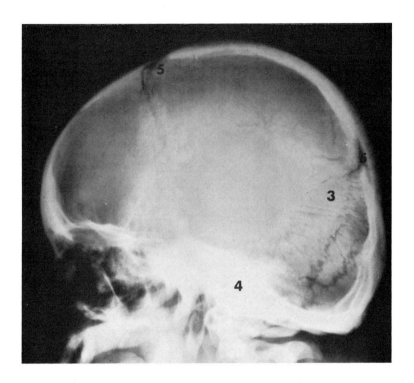

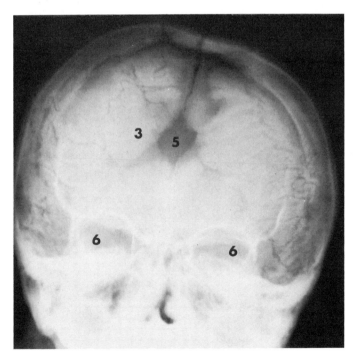

Figure 7–1 *C (Continued).* (3) The numerous wormian bones. (4) The flattened base of the skull (see platybasia, Chapter 12). (5) The large open fontanelles. (6) Reverse sloping of petrous ridges in association with the flattening of the skull.

Figure 7–1 continued on opposite page.

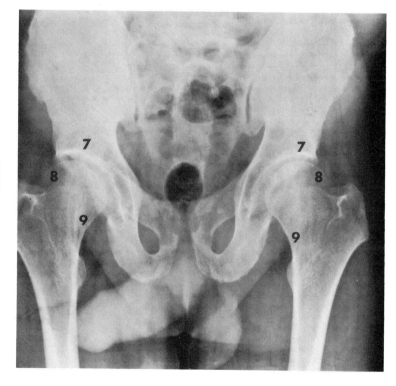

Figure 7–1 *C (Continued)*. (7) Shallow acetabulum. (8) The heads of the femora partially extruding beyond the shallow acetabulum. (9) Coxa valga deformities of both hips.

are often such associated anomalies as Sprengel's deformity and anomalies of the jaws, palate, skull, heart, and lung. This will be illustrated and discussed further in the chapter on the spine.

OVERDEVELOPMENT OF A PART OR SUPERNUMERARY PARTS, OR OVERPRODUCTION OF BONE-PRODUCING SCLEROSIS

This group of disorders includes those in which the bones are too numerous, too broad, or too long; or in which there are foci of sclerotic bone, suggesting overproduction. In this latter group the *sclerosis may be diffuse (marble bones), concentrated throughout the shaft (Engelmann's disease), or striated or spotted* in the bones.

A few of these entities are described below in greater detail, and the rest are appended in a glossary.

Arachnodactylia (Figure 7–2) merely refers to long slender fingers but is often associated with a systemic syndrome called *"Marfan's hereditary syndrome."*

Clinical Features. This is a rare, hereditary, congenital growth disturbance affecting the musculoskeletal, cardiovascular, and ocular systems. The individual is often tall and slender, and all the long bones may be elongated. The arch of the palate is usually high and there may be a double row of teeth. The head is apt to be dolichocephalic, the thorax funnel-shaped, and the muscles, tendons, and ligaments of poor tone and hypermobile.

A thumb protruding beyond the confines of the clenched fist appears to be a confirming sign of the Marfan syndrome (Steinberg); it has been proposed as a screening test for this syndrome.

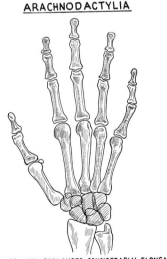

ARACHNODACTYLIA

1. PROXIMAL PHALANGES CONSIDERABLY ELONGATED WITH RESPECT TO METACARPALS.
2. FINGERS LONG AND TAPERED.
3. ? ASSOCIATION WITH PITUITARY DISORDER.

Figure 7–2 Arachnodactylia.

The most *common cardiovascular malformation is aneurysm formation,* usually of the dissecting type. However, *patent foramen ovale, mitral stenosis, or aortic insufficiency* may also be present.

Dislocation of the ocular lens is frequent and vision may be poor.

Radiographic Findings.   Markedly elongated metacarpals, metatarsals, and basal phalanges, with usually greater affection of the hands than of the feet. The skull deformity shows it to be large and the facial bones long and slender.

Homocystinuria (Morreels et al.).   There is a similarity between the predominant roentgenographic features of homocystinuria and Marfan's syndrome, although the roentgenographic features of homocystinuria are variable. Arachnodactyly and pectus excavatum or pectus carinatum are frequent in both syndromes.

General Comment.   Marfan's syndrome is included in the hereditary diseases of connective tissues along with others, such as chondrodystrophes, achondroplasia, osteogenesis imperfecta, osteopetrosis, the Ehlers–Danlos syndrome, and other less well-defined inherited disorders (the student is referred to the excellent monograph by McKusick for further elaboration). The cause of Marfan's syndrome may be an interference with normal chondroitin sulfate or zinc ion metabolism (Whittaker, et al.; McKusick).

Marble Bone Disease (Figure 7–3)

Clinical Features.   Pronounced thickening of the bones which, both microscopically and radiographically, give normal values for phosphorus and calcium, but the serum phosphatase may be markedly elevated. *Myelophthisic anemia* is apt to be the most troublesome complication and it is frequently the cause of death.

Radiographic Findings.   The long bones are Erlenmeyer-flask-shaped and broadened at both ends because the normal shaping processes brought about by osteoclastic activity do not occur. The bones are abnormally brittle with pathologic fractures frequently sustained, and children so affected are ordinarily retarded in physical development. The circumference of the head is abnormally large. The base of the skull is especially involved and there is often an associated hydrocephalus.

The teeth are small with severe caries and numerous enamel defects. Osteomyelitis and necrosis of the mandible are frequent.

At the level of the foramina of the skull and in the vertebrae, the openings are usually severely encroached upon, with impingement upon cranial and spinal nerves.

Engelmann's Disease (Progressive diaphyseal dysplasia) (Griffiths) (Figure 7–4)

Clinical Features.   Usually growth is disproportionate so that there is elongation of the extremities in comparison with the size of the trunk. Muscular atrophy, general wasting, and tenderness upon pressure are often associated. Ordinarily, the blood picture, sedimentation rate, and blood chemistry are normal.

Radiographic Features.   In this disease, there is usually a homogeneous fusiform enlargement of the cortical layers of the long bones in their diaphyseal portions particularly, and occasionally also of the short tubular bones as well. The marrow cavity is somewhat narrowed. In contrast to marble bone disease the epiphyses and metaphyses remain free from disease. Occasionally the mid-

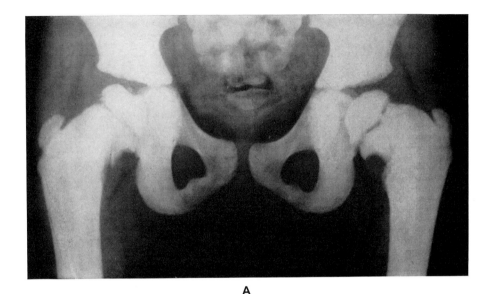

A

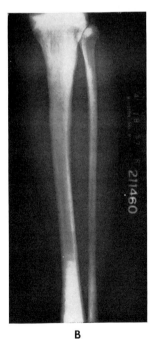

B

Figure 7–3 *A*. Osteopetrosis (marble bone disease). (Courtesy of L. R. Sante, M.D.) *B*. The healed fractured tibia in a patient with osteopetrosis. Note the "Erlenmeyer" flask deformity due to a failure of bone modeling.

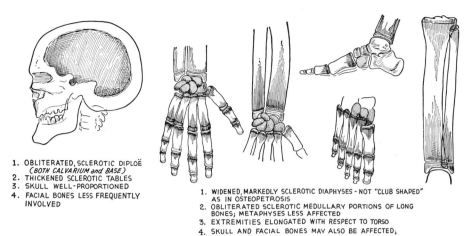

1. OBLITERATED, SCLEROTIC DIPLOË
   (BOTH CALVARIUM and BASE)
2. THICKENED SCLEROTIC TABLES
3. SKULL WELL-PROPORTIONED
4. FACIAL BONES LESS FREQUENTLY
   INVOLVED

1. WIDENED, MARKEDLY SCLEROTIC DIAPHYSES - NOT "CLUB SHAPED"
   AS IN OSTEOPETROSIS
2. OBLITERATED SCLEROTIC MEDULLARY PORTIONS OF LONG
   BONES; METAPHYSES LESS AFFECTED
3. EXTREMITIES ELONGATED WITH RESPECT TO TORSO
4. SKULL AND FACIAL BONES MAY ALSO BE AFFECTED;
   ALTHOUGH RARELY

Figure 7-4 Engelmann's disease.

dle part of the base of the skull and the frontal bones, the vertebral bodies, and the pelvis are also involved. There is a progressive increase in disease with the growth of the person.

Congenital Stippled Epiphyses (Chondrodysplasia punctata; chondroangiopathia calcificans congenita) (Figure 7–5)

Clinical and Pathologic Features. This disease represents a disturbance of vascularization of the epiphyseal cartilage associated with mottled, mucous degeneration. These changes favor considerable deformity of the epiphyses and bones of the wrist and ankle. Congenital cataract, dulled intellect, large head, and dwarfism are also present.

Radiographic Features. Punctate, sclerotic foci throughout many of the epiphyseal centers of ossification in the early growth period. As the child grows, there is a confluence of these punctate areas of calcification so that they appear to diminish in number or disappear completely if the child survives sufficiently long. There is dwarfism with a large head, bossing of the skull, blunt, short fingers, and flexion contractures of the joints (Allansmith and Senz).

Pathology. The diffuse stippling of the epiphyses is related most often to dystrophic calcification of the epiphyses and small hemangiomas within them.

Epiphyseal Dysplasia (Epiphyseal dysplasia puncticularis; dysplasia epiphysealis multiplex) (Figure 7–6) (Fairbank)

Clinical Features. Waddling gait; difficulty in walking; joint pain and stiffness or occasional laxity of joints; some shortening of stature occasionally.

Radiographic Findings. Irregularity and hypoplasia of the developing ossification centers of the epiphyses, usually bilateral. The appearance suggests a "mulberry" deformity, due to separate centers arising and blending together. Their density eventually becomes normal but the deformity is permanent and causes some restriction of motion. The hips, knees, and ankles are usually

(Text continued on page 197)

CHONDRO ANGIOPATHIA CALCIFICANS CONGENITA

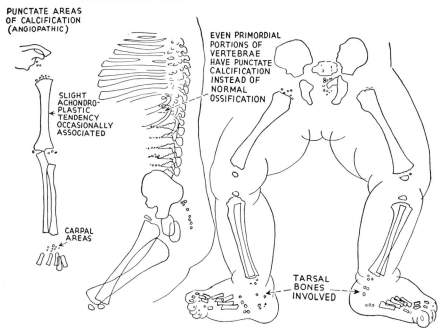

PUNCTATE AREAS
OF CALCIFICATION
(ANGIOPATHIC)

SLIGHT
ACHONDRO-
PLASTIC
TENDENCY
OCCASIONALLY
ASSOCIATED

CARPAL
AREAS

EVEN PRIMORDIAL
PORTIONS OF
VERTEBRAE
HAVE PUNCTATE
CALCIFICATION
INSTEAD OF
NORMAL
OSSIFICATION

TARSAL
BONES
INVOLVED

Figure 7–5 *A*. Chondroangiopathia calcificans congenita.

Figure 7–5 continued on following page.

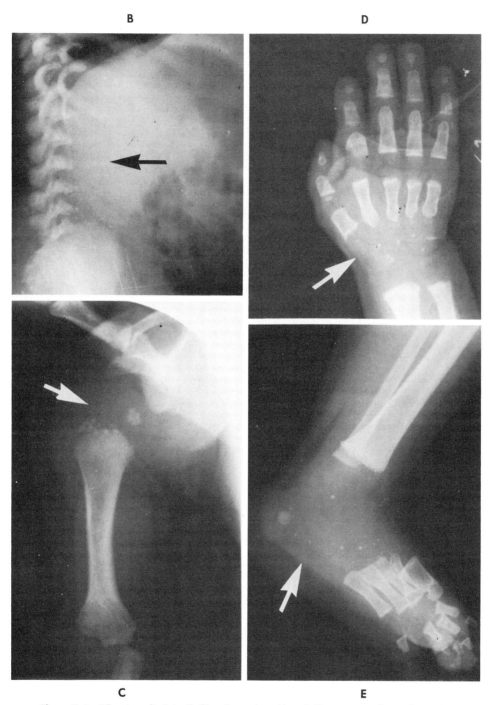

Figure 7–5   (*Continued*). *B* to *E*. Chondroangiopathia calcificans congenita: radiographs.

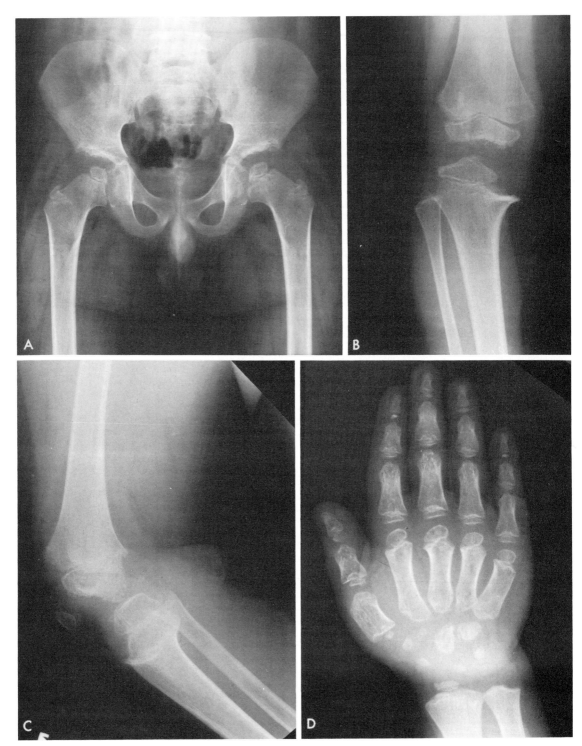

Figure 7–6   Epiphyseal dysplasia. *A*. Antero-posterior roentgenographic view of pelvis. Note small capital femoral epiphyses, wide joint space, and wide femoral necks. Acetabular margins are irregular. *B* and *C*. Antero-posterior and lateral views of the right knee showing fragmentation of the femoral and tibial epiphyses with lateral subluxation of the tibia. *D*. Antero-posterior view of right hand. Note short, broad metacarpals and phalanges. Ossification centers of capitate and hamate bones are irregular. (From Kaufman, E. E., and Coventry, M. B.: Proc. Mayo Clin., *38*:115, 1963.)

involved—shoulders, elbows, and wrists rarely. Subluxation may supervene if the deformity is severe, and degenerative arthritis is common because of stress. The adjoining joint space often appears widened and the metaphysis enlarged, although metaphyseal changes are rarely observed, and when present consist of fraying or irregular mineralization. The carpal and tarsal bones tend to appear late and look mottled and irregular. **The spine is usually normal.**

MALDEVELOPMENT OF AN ANATOMICAL PART—REGIONAL

The most important entities of this group are:

Syndactylia, or fusion of the fingers, in which the soft tissues or bones or both may be fused.

Perodactylia, in which the fingers appear to be amputated.

Peromelia, in which the extremities appear "flipperlike" and malformed.

Madelung's Deformity (Figure 7–7) (Paus), a hereditary overgrowth of the ulna, in which it extends distally and dorsally to the radius. There is also a bayonet-like projection of the distal end of the radius and the two bones tend to cross one another in lateral projection.

The Roentgenologic Criteria of Madelung's deformity may be summarized as follows:

A double lateral and dorsal bowing of the radius which involves the entire diaphysis but is most marked at the distal end.

A variable widening of the interosseous space due to the lateral curvature described above.

Shortening of the radius as compared with the normal standards for age and the relation to the size of the other bones of the upper extremity.

An alteration of the contour of the distal radius so that the articular surface of the epiphysis faces in an ulnar and palmar direction.

Premature fusion in the ulnar half of the epiphyseal line of the distal radius which contributes to accentuation of the deformity in early adolescence.

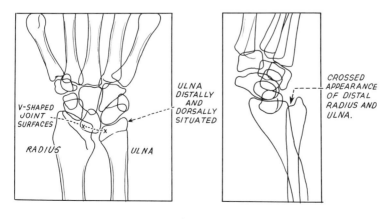

MADELUNG'S DEFORMITY

Figure 7–7

Dislocation or subluxation of inferior radial ulnar articulation with the distal ulna dorsal to the distal radius.

An area of decreased bone density on the ulnar border of the radius extending for a short distance proximal to the fused epiphyseal line.

Small bony excrescences, sometimes condensed into an exostosis along the inferior ulnar border of the radius.

Triangularization of the normally quadrangular outline of the distal radial epiphysis, with the apex of the triangle pointing medially.

Hypercondensation of trabeculations of the ulnar head.

A change in the inferior radial articular surface with modification of the relationship of the carpal bones wedging them between the deformed radius and protruding ulna and giving them a triangular configuration with the lunate at the apex.

An arched curvature of the carpal bone which is a continuation of the arch of the dorsal bowing of the radial diaphysis (Langer).

Vertical Talus (talonavicular dislocation with congenital flatfoot), in which the talus is vertically situated in the tarsus instead of at its usual oblique angle of 15 to 20 degrees with respect to the horizontal. This later results in an abnormal articulation of the navicular tarsal bone and an interposition of the talus between the calcaneus and the cuboid. Shortening of the Achilles tendon often occurs. Since ossification of the navicular tarsal occurs in the second or third year of life, this is usually when the disease becomes manifest.

Tarsal Coalition (Calcaneonavicular coalition) (Conway and Powell)

A rigid painful foot requires proper roentgenographic evaluation. Oblique views of the foot are necessary to exclude a calcaneonavicular coalition. The secondary signs include:

1. A "talor beak."
2. Broadening of the lateral process of the talus.
3. Narrowing of the posterior talocalcaneal facet.

Any of these signs requires an axial view of the calcaneus at the angle of the sustentacular joint for demonstration. Coalition between the talus and calcaneus may be located in the region of the anterior, middle, or posterior facets. Tomography may be necessary to exclude coalition, especially of the anterior facets (Conway and Powell).

MALDEVELOPMENT OF AN ANATOMICAL PART—GENERAL

Maldevelopments involving several extremities or the axial skeleton may be related to an inherited (genetic) disorder or to an intrauterine fetal affection. We shall briefly review these under four headings:

1. *Those involving the epiphyses primarily. Rubin, 1964, has also included a separate category related to the epiphyseal plate called "Physeal."*
2. *Those involving the metaphyses primarily.*
3. *Those affecting the bones and tissues generally,* often involving the axial skeleton as well.
4. *Those diseases related to a defect extrinsic* to the bone but involving the bone secondarily.

Involvement of the Epiphyses Primarily

The two most important entities of this group, *congenital stippled epiphyses* and *epiphyseal dysplasia,* have already been considered in our prior section.

Involvement of the Metaphyses Primarily

There are five major entities in this group:

1. *Chondrodysplasia* or *Ollier's disease.*
2. *Multiple cartilaginous exostoses* or *diaphyseal aclasis.*
3. *Metaphyseal dysplasia (Pyle's disease).*
4. *Hereditary hypophosphatasia (see Chapter 7).*
5. *Infantile familial or hereditary hypophosphatemia* (see Chapter 8).

Chondrodysplasia (Dyschondroplasia) or Ollier's disease is a disorder of the metaphyses primarily.

Radiographic Findings.   Cartilaginous enchondromata appear as irregular, vaguely delimited defects and radiolucencies within the metaphyses. These are due to masses of cartilage in these sites. The bone may develop tumor-like swellings and may be short, thick and angulated, and there may be an osteolysis of the bony cortex of the metaphyses (Figure 7–8). Exostoses may also occur. Apart from the four extremities, the other involved areas are the pelvis, ribs, and rarely, the base of the skull. These enchondromatous masses may ultimately become almost completely, or at least partially, calcified.

Prognosis.   The prognosis for life may be good, but there is usually pronounced invalidism produced by these tumor masses.

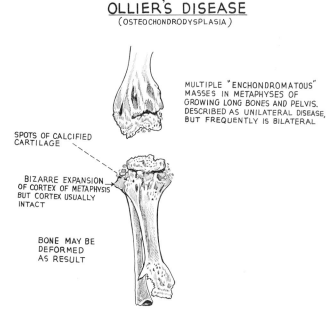

OLLIER'S DISEASE
(OSTEOCHONDRODYSPLASIA)

MULTIPLE "ENCHONDROMATOUS" MASSES IN METAPHYSES OF GROWING LONG BONES AND PELVIS. DESCRIBED AS UNILATERAL DISEASE, BUT FREQUENTLY IS BILATERAL

SPOTS OF CALCIFIED CARTILAGE

BIZARRE EXPANSION OF CORTEX OF METAPHYSIS BUT CORTEX USUALLY INTACT

BONE MAY BE DEFORMED AS RESULT

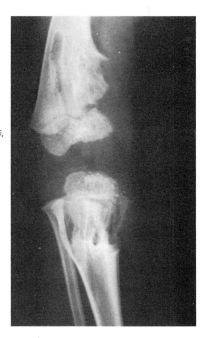

Figure 7–8

Differentiation from Diaphyseal Aclasis. These enchondromas differ from the multiple cartilaginous exostoses characteristic of diaphyseal aclasis since, in the latter condition, the osteochondromas grow externally from the metaphyses with only minimal internal extension. The osteochondromas in these instances are tumefactions, usually arising from metaphyses and producing a mushroomlike protrusion or tumefaction in one or more bones (Figure 7–9). Occasionally, these osteochondromas become malignant (osteochondrosarcoma). This is particularly true of the familial variety. Seventy per cent of cases of diaphyseal aclasis are in males (McKusick).

Enchondromas and ecchondromas associated with multiple hemangiomas of the skin, mucosae, and internal organs constitute a rare disorder called Maffucci's syndrome. Dwarfism, pathologic fractures, and sarcomas are frequent. The vascular lesions may occur anywhere in the subcutaneous tissues and may be recognized radiographically by the innumerable phleboliths in association with them.

Familial Metaphyseal Dysplasia (Pyle's disease) is a disturbance in the normal bone-modeling process of endochondral bone.

Radiographic Findings. The distal third of many long bones (femur, radius, and ulna especially) or of the proximal humerus assumes an Erlenmeyer-flask appearance. The tibia tends to be splayed at both ends. Unlike marble bone disease, in which this failure of modeling also occurs, the **cortex** of the bone is **thinner** than normal and readily subject to fracture on this basis. Stature is ordinarily increased (Kowins). The epiphyses appear normal. Any of the long bones may show the abnormality and the tubulation described.

Mori and Holt have noted cranial changes in Pyle's disease, principally symmetrical hyperostoses of the calvarium and mandible and ocular hypertelorism with retarded pneumatization of the paranasal sinuses.

Infantile Familial or Hereditary Hypophosphatemia is briefly mentioned in Chapter 8 (Williams, Winters, and Burnette).

Clinical Features. This condition is familial with four phenotypes, ranging be-

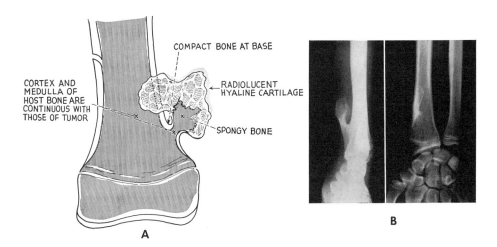

Figure 7–9 Osteochondroma (solitary). *A.* Diagrammatic illustration. *B.* Representative radiograph showing an osteochondroma of the distal radius.

tween: (1) an asymptomatic group; (2) adult with post-rachitic deformities; (3) adult with active osteomalacia; and (4) resistant rickets in childhood.

It is *due to a hereditary diminished renal tubular resorption of inorganic phosphate*. In children there may also be some diminished gastrointestinal calcium absorption. The diagnosis is made by: (1) radiographic evidence of rickets; (2) high serum phosphatase; (3) lower serum phosphate; and (4) periapical rarefaction around teeth without dental caries.

Affection of Bones or Tissues Diffusely

Only a few of the diseases in this category will be described, since so many groups and subgroups can be identified.

Achondroplasia or Chondrodystrophy (Maroteaux and Lamy) (Figure 7–10). This is a congenital growth disturbance of endochondral bone associated with dwarfism.

Radiographic Findings. All the bones of cartilaginous origin, such as the pelvis, spine, shoulder girdle, skull, and extremities, are usually affected. The bones tend to grow circumferentially, but ordinarily there are a marked shortening of bones of the extremities and the base of the skull and a **narrowness of the interpediculate dimension of the vertebral bodies.** The arms are well muscled but very short and usually terminate in a claw-like three-pronged hand. The excursion of the joints is restricted.

Because of the shortened base of the **skull,** the frontal bone appears to protrude, but the head is normal in size.

The pelvis usually shows a characteristic marked narrowness or flattening with a kidney-shaped pelvic inlet and a highly protuberant sacral promontory, and it has a wide pubic angle. The ilea are most affected (Caffey). The greater sciatic notch is flattened with a narrow and relatively deep cleft and the ileum appears rectangular. The acetabular angles are reduced to near zero.

The **spine is particularly characteristic** in that the individual vertebral bodies are small in width in relation to height and appear small in relation to the intervertebral disks, and there are a **progressive stenosis and narrowing** of the **spinal canal.** In adults dorso-lumbar kyphosis and hypertrophic arthritis may precipitate early neurological disturbances owing to the smallness of the spinal canal.

As growth proceeds, the epiphyseal plate presents an irregular undulating contour and the **epiphyseal ossification centers are incompletely developed and deformed.** Some of the epiphyseal plates close prematurely.

Many classifications of the bone dysplasias have been rendered but these are outside the scope of the present text (Table 7–2).

Diastrophic Dwarfism (Langer, 1965) resembles achondroplasia clinically in that the pelvic configuration is similar. In achondroplasia, however, there is an absence of the basal portion of the innominate bones so that these bones appear square on frontal view.

In addition, the **most characteristic changes of diastrophic dwarfism are in the hands and feet, where the first metacarpal is small and the other metacarpals are broad with the distal end wider than the proximal end.**

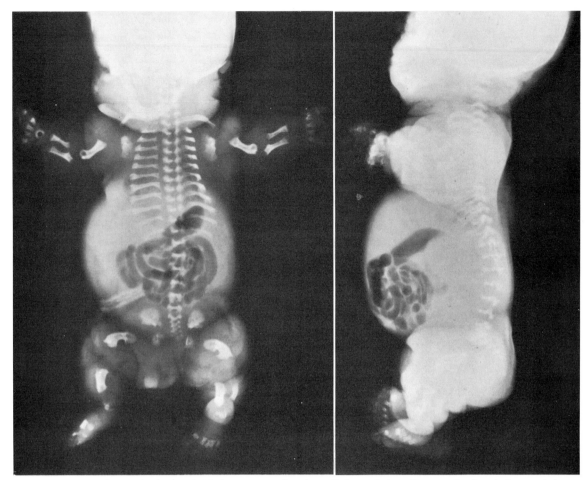

Figure 7–10 *A*. Thanatophoric dwarf. (1) Antero-posterior view. (2) Lateral view. See text for description. *B*. Achondroplasia. (1) Upper extremities. (2) Pelvis and lower extremities. See text for description.

Figure 7–10 continued on opposite page.

There is an equinovarus deformity present sometimes. The large tubular bones are short and have broad metaphyses. In the spine the *interpediculate distance increases from the level of L-1 to L-5 and is not narrowed as in the case of achondroplasia.* Also, *scoliosis is not present in early infancy.*

Thanatophoric Dwarfism (Keats et al.).   This type of dwarfism resembles a severe form of achondroplasia in respect to the following features: shortening of the base of the skull; prominence of the frontal bone with depression of the root of the nose; a long trunk with short limbs; narrow chest; and short ribs and reduction of the interpedicular distances of the last lumbar vertebrae. The iliac wings are small and square and have horizontal acetabular roofs and narrow sacrosciatic notches. The features distinguishing it from achondroplasia are the following:

1. Extreme flatness of the vertebral bodies, with excessive dimensions of the intervertebral spaces.
2. Tubular bones very short and bowed, particularly in the lower extremities.
3. Metaphyseal areas irregular in contour and frequently cupped.

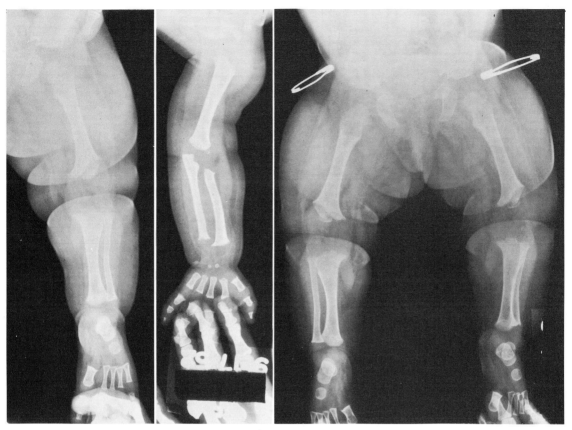

Figure 7–10 *B*

Whereas achondroplasia is transmitted as an autosomal dominant hereditary trait, with ominous genetic implications, this type of dwarfism is a dominant mutation apparently without a hereditary influence (Keats et al.).

In Morquio's Disease (Figure 7–11) there is a severe disorder of epiphyses and endochondral bone formation, and a severe kyphosis in the mid-dorsal or dorsolumbar region. An abnormality of mucopolysaccharide metabolism has also been demonstrated in the urine in a high percentage of patients (Robbins, Stevens, and Linker).

Radiographic Findings. The **arms are often very long** in contrast to those characteristic of achondroplasia, sometimes reaching to the knees, and in many cases they are held in valgus position. The knees are in genu valgum. The **skull is enlarged,** the frontal and parietal bones protrude, and saddle nose is frequently encountered.

The spine is composed of shallow vertebral bodies with a "beaking" of the vertebra immediately caudad to the kyphotic site. Morquio-Ullrich disease may be a variant of gargoylism (Hurler's disease) or Morquio's disease. The skeletal changes of Morquio's disease are present but only a few of the extraskeletal abnormalities are seen (Goidanich).

(Text continued on page 208)

TABLE 7–2 PRINCIPAL CHONDRODYSPLASIAS DETECTABLE AT BIRTH*

	Clinical Features in the Newborn	Extremities	Thorax	Vertebrae	Radiological Features in the Newborn		Misc.	Inheritance
					Pelvis	Skull		
Disorders incompatible with life.								
Thanatophoric dwarfism	Severe micromelia Narrowness of the thorax	Short, bowed (especially lower) Metaphyses irregular and cupped	Narrowness, but long trunk Ribs short	Platyspondyly Reduction of interpedicular distances of last lumbar	Iliac wings small and square Narrow sacro-sciatic notch	Shortened base Prominent frontal bone and depressed nose		Mutation
Achondrogenesis	Severe micromelic dwarfism	Micromelic		Severe dwarfism Defects in ossification, especially vertebrae				?
Disorders compatible with life.								
Achondroplasia	Micromelic dwarfism with characteristic craniofacial changes	Short, thick tubular bones—proximal bones worst Trident deformities—hands Epiphyses normal	Flat chested Ribs—club-shaped	Platyspondyly Reduction of lumbar interpediculate distances	Iliac wings square; sacro-sciatic notch acute	Short base, acute angle, hydrocephalus face small, prognathism		Dominant
Pseudoachondroplasia		Long bones short and thick Epiphyses irregular Brachydactyly Severe arthritis	Ribs normal with full round chest	Vertebra plana and platyspondyly	Iliac crests flared	Normal base and odontoid		
Chondrodysplasia punctata	Micromelic dwarfism, often asymmetrical cataract Ichthyosis	Micromelia; asymmetrical cataract often Small areas of calcification in joints Diaphyses normal	Stippling at anterior ribs and sternum	Small areas of calcification in vertebral bodies Vertical cleft in vertebrae	Stippling at iliac crests	Normal or head may be large		
Chondroectodermal dysplasia (Ellis-Van Creveld)	Polydactyly Ectodermal abnormalities Cardiac malformation	Polydactyly Metaphyseal notching Peripheral shortening of tubular bones Lateral defect in epiphysis of tibia leading to peaking	Narrow Clavicles horizontal		Horizontal acetabular roof with lateral spur projecting	Poorly developed	Ectodermal abnormalities Cardiac malformations in one-third of cases	Autosomal recessive

Table 7–2 continued on opposite page.

Asphyxiating thoracic dysplasia	Narrowness of the thorax Shortness of the limbs	Narrowness and asphyxiation Shortened ribs					Third cuneiforms often absent in feet	Autosomal recessive
Diastrophic dwarfism	Micromelic dwarfism Club foot Cleft palate Deformity of the external ear (at 1 or 2 months of age)	Micromelia Clubfoot (cuboid feet and hands) Changes in epiphyses and metaphyses Epiphyses appear late Joint luxations Short and massive tubular bones	Normal	Scoliosis but vertebrae normal		Cleft palate Deformed external ear Normal skull otherwise		Autosomal dominant
Metatrophic dwarfism	Micromelic dwarfism Kyphoscoliosis	Micromelia Widened metaphyses		Kyphoscoliosis Reduction in height of vertebral bodies				Autosomal recessive
Mesomelic dwarfism	Micromelia with selective involvement of the forearm and leg	Micromelia selectively involving forearm and leg Incurvation of radius Aplasia of fibula						Autosomal recessive
Spondylo-epiphyseal dysplasia (congenital)	Dwarfism with shortness of the trunk	Delay in ossification Epiphysis irregular Diaphyses narrow Brachydactyly	Ribs normal in length	Platyspondylia Hypoplasia of T_{12}, L_1 with an anterior tongue Odontoid process hypoplastic	Broadness of the base of the iliac wings Acetabuli protrusio	Normal or platybasia May be enlarged Saddle nose		Dominant
Gargoylism (Hurler's syndrome) May be a variant of Morquio's		Pinching of metaphyses and shortening with stunting Tapering of distal ulna and radius Tapered metacarpals with apex at wrist	Ribs narrow medially and broadened distally, resembling a "caveman's club"	Hypoplasia D_{12}, L_1 with stepping defect anteriorly	Stenosis of iliac base and proximal femoral necks	Scaphocephaly "Shoe-shaped" sella turcica		Progressive, leading to shortened life span Hereditary error in metabolism of mucopolysaccharides

*Maroteaux, 1969; P. Rubin, 1964; Langer, 1965; Keats et al., 1970.

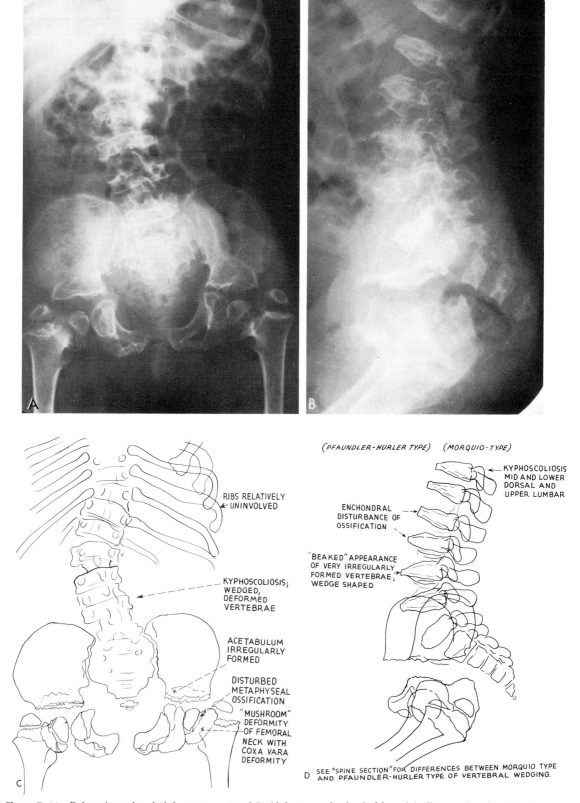

Figure 7–11 Polytopic enchondral dysostoses. *A* and *B*. Abdomen and spine in Morquio's disease. *C* and *D*. Tracings of *A* and *B* respectively.

Figure 7–11 continued on opposite page.

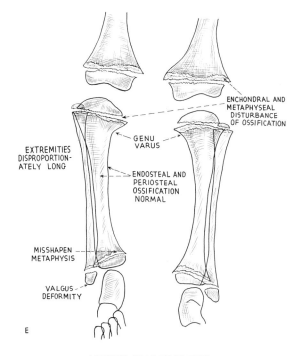

ENCHONDRAL AND METAPHYSEAL DISTURBANCE OF OSSIFICATION

GENU VARUS

EXTREMITIES DISPROPORTION- ATELY LONG

ENDOSTEAL AND PERIOSTEAL OSSIFICATION NORMAL

MISSHAPEN METAPHYSIS

VALGUS DEFORMITY

E

MORQUIO-BRAILSFORD TYPE

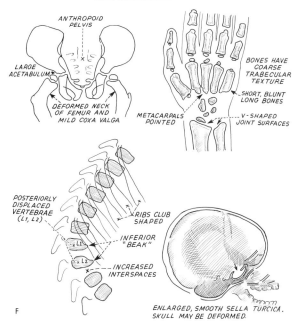

ANTHROPOID PELVIS

LARGE ACETABULUM

DEFORMED NECK OF FEMUR AND MILD COXA VALGA

BONES HAVE COARSE TRABECULAR TEXTURE

SHORT, BLUNT LONG BONES

METACARPALS POINTED

V-SHAPED JOINT SURFACES

POSTERIORLY DISPLACED VERTEBRAE (L1, L2)

RIBS CLUB SHAPED

INFERIOR "BEAK"

INCREASED INTERSPACES

x L1

x L2

F

ENLARGED, SMOOTH SELLA TURCICA. SKULL MAY BE DEFORMED.

Figure 7–11 (*Continued*). Polytopic enchondral dysostoses. *E.* Tracing with pertinent findings labeled in the Pfaundler-Hurler type. *F.* Tracing in the Morquio-Brailsford type.

Pfaundler-Hurler's Disease (Gargoylism; dysostosis multiplex) (Figure 7–12)

Clinical Features. Kyphosis, dwarfism, corneal clouding, impaired hearing, feeble-mindedness, dermatologic abnormalities with hirsutism, papular or nodular lesions, thick and firm skin distally on the fingers and toes. Small crateriform ulcers appear on the skin dorsal to the interphalangeal joints (Kambrick et al.; McKusick et al.; Berenson and Geer). The large head, thick lips and tongue, high palate, saddle nose, and widely separate eyes have given rise to the term "gargoylism."

As in Marfan's syndrome, there is a high incidence of heart disease—occurring probably in three-fourths of the patients. Septal defects, mitral valvular insufficiency, and aortic regurgitation are most frequent. Death prior to the age of 20 years usually results from heart failure.

Laboratory Findings. Blood cholesterol is usually abnormal. The disease represents a hereditary error in the metabolism of the mucopolysaccharides, which may be found in the urine (Berry and Spinanger).

Radiographic Findings. The upper extremities are short and the lower show the genu valgum deformity described for Morquio's disease. The spine findings are also similar, with kyphosis and "beaking" of the vertebral body in the vicinity of the kyphosis. Unlike Morquio's disease, there are usually a spleno-megaly, hepatomegaly, and enlargement of the sella turcica, with or without increased intracranial pressure.

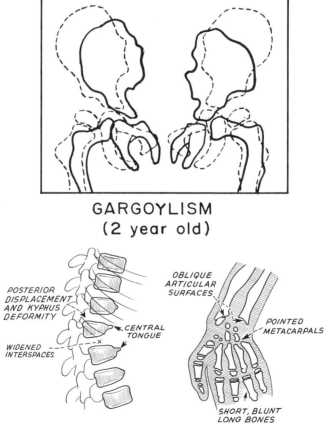

Figure 7–12 Polytopic enchondral dysostoses. Tracing with pertinent findings labeled in the Pfaundler-Hurler type.

Alterations in cardiac contour will depend upon whether the predominant lesions are septal or valvular in origin. Also, the findings of cardiac failure will later supervene.

Both Morquio's disease and Pfaundler-Hurler's disease have been referred to as "polytopic enchondral dysostosis" with many subgroups identified, or as the "mucopolysaccharide disorders."

Osteogenesis Imperfecta (Fragilitas ossium, Lobstein's disease, Van der Hoeve's syndrome)

Clinical Features.   Three clinical types are distinguished:
1. Osteogenesis imperfecta congenita.
2. Osteogenesis imperfecta tarda (osteopsathyrosis or Ekmann-Lobstein disease).
3. An additional form of the latter syndrome in which the fractures, which first appear at two to three years of age, seem to decline in frequency at about puberty.

Typically there is a high frequency of blue sclerae as a result of the abnormal thinness of the usually tough white supporting tunic of the eyeball and deafness from otosclerosis.

Hydrocephaly and congenital heart defects may coexist (McKusick; Elefant and Tosovsky; Caniggia et al.).

Pathology.   Osteoid is laid down relatively normally but the osseous development thereafter is deficient. When fractures occur, the cartilaginous callus develops, but ossification is defective so that considerable deformity of the fractured bone results.

Radiographic Findings.   The bone shafts are extremely thin, deficient in mineral structure, subject to frequent fractures, and highly deformed after healing of fracture has occurred.

In the skull there are multiple wormian bones that give a "jigsaw puzzle" pattern at sutural junctions. Hydrocephaly and congenital heart defect may also be found.

The roentgenographic features of osteogenesis imperfecta in the adult have been summarized by Levin as follows: (1) undermineralization of the bones; (2) biconcavity of the vertebral bodies; (3) multiple fractures which heal normally but with persistent deformity; (4) platybasia of the skull; (5) a tendency to a decrease in the trabecular pattern of most bones; (6) no dwarfism.

Chondroectodermal Dysplasia (Ellis-Van Creveld's disease) (Ellis and Andrew)

Clinical Features.   This disease consists of *ectodermal dysplasia, chondro-dysplasia, polydactylism,* and *congenital cardiac abnormalities.* The ectodermal dysplasia is characterized by defective nails and dentition and alopecia. The chondrodysplasia produces dwarfing and synostosis of the calvarium. The cardiac abnormalities are usually manifested by cyanosis, with patency of the interventricular or interatrial septa and transposition of the major blood vessels. Polydactyly is constant but fusion of the capitate and hamate bones is pathognomonic.

Radiographic Findings.   The long bones are generally thickened and coarse, with acceleration of maturation of the secondary centers of ossification, and retardation of the primary centers of ossification. In the distal tibiae and fibulae there may be areas of osteosclerosis intermingled with rarefaction, somewhat

DISORDERED OSSIFICATION *Generalized*

ACROCEPHALO-SYNDACTYIA

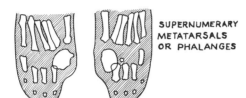

SUPERNUMERARY
METATARSALS
OR PHALANGES

Figure 7–13   Acrocephalosyndactylia.

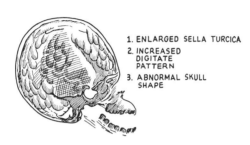

1. ENLARGED SELLA TURCICA
2. INCREASED
   DIGITATE
   PATTERN
3. ABNORMAL SKULL
   SHAPE

similar to chondrodysplasia. **Peaking of the proximal ends of the tibiae,** described by Caffey as pathognomonic, is often found. There is often a curvature of the humeri. The thorax is narrow with horizontal clavicles and the third cuneiforms are often absent in both feet.

Acrocephalosyndactylia (Apert's syndrome) (Figure 7–13) is a disease state consisting of *oxycephaly* (acrocephaly) and *syndactyly* of the fingers or toes. Often there are supernumerary metatarsals or phalanges. The *sella turcica tends to be enlarged* with an *accentuated digitate pattern* throughout the calvarium and premature fusion of the coronal or sagittal sutures. The skull tends to be "tower-shaped." The orbits are shallow, coexisting with hypertelorism and exophthalmos. The hard or soft palate is often malformed. *A single nail is common to the fused second, third, and fourth hand digits and is typical of Apert's syndrome* (Blank).

Arthrogryposis Multiplex Congenita.   This congenital disorder is characterized by *rigid joints* due to an infiltration of muscle fibers by fibrous and fatty tissue. The extremities become fusiform in shape and knees and elbows become fixed in flexion. The joints may be webbed, but their degree of involvement varies (Mead and Lithgow; Kanof et al.).

Contractures and decreased muscle tone are universally present. Poznanski and LaRowe have described a "carpal sign" in this condition as follows:

The "carpal angle" as described by Kosowicz in Turner's syndrome (Figure 7–20) is the angle between two lines tangent to the proximal aspect of the carpus. One line joins the scaphoid and lunate; the other, the lunate and triquetrum. In normal subjects this angle measures 131.5 degrees ±7.2. In Turner's syndrome there is a decrease in this angle; in arthrogryposis there is an increase in most patients who have hand abnormalities.

Ehlers-Danlos Syndrome (Hyperelastosis cutis).   This syndrome, in contrast to arthrogryposis, is characterized by *hyperlaxity and hyperextensibility of the joints and skin with increased fragility of the blood vessels.* There is an underlying defect, probably in the collagen. Hypertelorism, permanent epicanthic folds, and blue sclera are frequently associated. *Cardiovascular defects* include dissecting aneurysms of the aorta, aneurysms of the sinus of Valsalva, atrial septal defects, and anomalies of the pulmonary arteries. Other anomalies of lungs, kidneys, and bones are associated (Bruno and Narasimhan).

Mandibulofacial Dysostosis (Franceschetti's syndrome; Treacher-Collins syndrome). These are disturbances of the extremities such as *oligodactylia, radio-ulnar synostoses, vertebral synostoses, and facial mandibular maldevelopment.* The chin recedes, the palate is high, the mouth is large, and there is a complete absence of the nasofrontal angle, with the teeth in an abnormal position. These patients appear facially "fishlike" or "birdlike." There may be *associated deafness* and absence of the external auditory meati, with deformity of the pinnae.

In Craniometaphyseal Dysplasia there is a *failure of the metaphyseal modeling* of the long bones *associated with the skull changes.* There is a tendency toward genu valgus deformity and palpable expansions of the metaphyseal ends of the long bones. In this respect, the disease resembles metaphyseal dysplasia as well as marble bone disease. In the skull, the picture may resemble that of leontiasis ossea or fibrous dysplasia.

Craniofacial Dysostosis (Crouzon's disease). In the skull the main features of this syndrome are: (1) *premature cranial synostosis,* and (2) *hypoplasia of the maxilla,* resulting in a relative prominence of the mandible and a parrot-beaked nose. Exophthalmos may be severe. The skull radiographs show prominent digital markings with a large frontal protuberance and marked hypoplasia of the maxilla. *Syndactyly* is frequently associated, as are deafness, mental retardation, and dental abnormalities (Gorlin and Pindborg).

Mandibular Hypoplasia (Micrognathia). Micrognathia is often seen and associated with other syndromes such as Robin's syndrome, infantile hypercalcemia syndrome, Hanhart's syndrome, gonadal dysgenesis, renal agenesis, mandibulofacial dysostosis, Moebius syndrome, oculoauriculovertebral dysplasia, progeria, and hemifacial microsoma.

In Hanhart's Syndrome, in addition to micrognathia with low-set ears and congenitally missing teeth, there is usually a variable absence of digits or extremities below the knee or elbow (Waardenburg).

Robin's Syndrome (Cleft palate with micrognathia and glossoptosis). This syndrome is characterized by *hypoplasia of the mandible* and *displacement of the tongue backward* into the pharyngeal space, causing severe difficulty in respiration and feeding. *Heart defects, bone anomalies, and defects of the eye and ear* are often associated. Hydrocephalus and microcephaly are found occasionally.

THE PELVIS AS A GUIDE IN NEONATAL AND CONGENITAL DISEASES OF BONE

Some of the characteristic abnormalities of the pelvis in the neonatal and infantile period are illustrated in Figure 7–14 A which helps to characterize these various disease entities. In each instance the equivalent normal pelvis is shown in dotted lines superimposed upon the abnormal. In Figure 7–14 B, Rubin (1964) has represented the inner pelvic contour by different types of wine glasses. This concept, although not invariable, is helpful. In many of these entities, the so-called "acetabular angle" and "iliac angle" play an important role for identification (Figure 7–15). The range of normal values is indicated in Table 7–3.

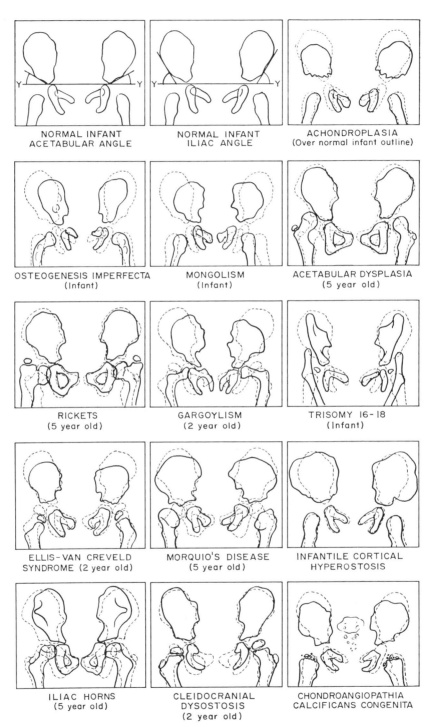

NORMAL INFANT
ACETABULAR ANGLE

NORMAL INFANT
ILIAC ANGLE

ACHONDROPLASIA
(Over normal infant outline)

OSTEOGENESIS IMPERFECTA
(Infant)

MONGOLISM
(Infant)

ACETABULAR DYSPLASIA
(5 year old)

RICKETS
(5 year old)

GARGOYLISM
(2 year old)

TRISOMY 16-18
(Infant)

ELLIS-VAN CREVELD
SYNDROME (2 year old)

MORQUIO'S DISEASE
(5 year old)

INFANTILE CORTICAL
HYPEROSTOSIS

ILIAC HORNS
(5 year old)

CLEIDOCRANIAL
DYSOSTOSIS
(2 year old)

CHONDROANGIOPATHIA
CALCIFICANS CONGENITA

Figure 7–14 *A*. The pelvis in normal, neonatal, and congenital diseases. In each instance the equivalent normal pelvis is shown in dotted lines superimposed upon the abnormal.

Figure 7–14 continued on opposite page.

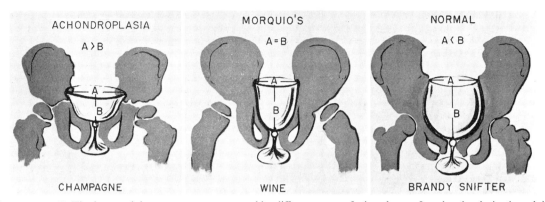

Figure 7–14   *B.* The inner pelvic contour as represented by different types of wine glasses. In achondroplasia, the pelvic width exceeds the depth due to decreased growth of the iliac base. The resulting appearance of the inner contour is that of a champagne glass. In spondyloepiphyseal dysplasia, the width and depth are equal and this results in a wine-glass shaped pelvis. The normal inner pelvic contour resembles a brandy snifter, the width of the pelvic inlet being less than its depth. The pelvis in multiple epiphyseal dysplasia corresponds to the normal. (From Rubin, P.: *Dynamic Classification of Bone Dysplasias.* Chicago, Year Book Medical Publishers, 1964.)

Garavaglia, by means of arthrography, has described an "arcuate line" in acetabular dysplasia and congenital dislocation of the hip. Initial roentgenologic signs of dysplasia begin at the upper end of the acetabular roof and consist of sclerosis and a shallow groove or fossa. An arcuate line on the outer aspect of the hip shows the nonosseous image of the epiphysis of the head of the femur and thus it assists in the diagnosis of this condition.

HEREDITARY OR CONGENITAL DISEASES OF BONE RELATED TO A DEFECT EXTRINSIC TO THE BONE BUT INVOLVING THE BONE SECONDARILY

For the most part this group of disorders has an inherited metabolic basis. Since the separate diseases are more readily discussed in conjunction with their objective roentgen appearances in Chapters 8, 9, and 10, discussions of the lipoid storage diseases, hematopoietic disorders, neurofibromatosis, and endocrine disorders will be deferred to these later chapters.

Sprengel's Deformity (Figure 7–16) is due to a *faulty descent of the scapula* from its fetal position adjoining the fourth cervical vertebra and to an *adjoining kyphoscoliosis* of the upper portion of the thoracic spine, so that the left shoulder girdle appears elevated. There may be *associated anomalies* such as synostoses of

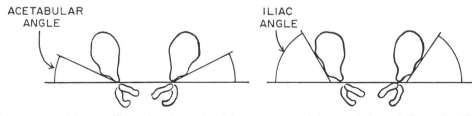

Figure 7–15   Diagrams illustrating the method of measurement of the acetabular and iliac angles. For range of normal values, see Table 7–3.

TABLE 7–3 RANGE OF NORMAL VALUES FOR ILIAC AND
ACETABULAR ANGLES (FROM CAFFEY, 1967)

Category	Mean Acetabular Angle	SD	± 2 SD	Actual Range
Young normal infants less than 3 months of age	28°	4.7	37–18	44–12
Normal infants 3–12 months of age	22°	4.2	30–14	34–8
	Mean Iliac Angle			
Less than 3 months	81°	8.0	97–65	97–68
3–12 months	79°	9.0	96–60	101–62

the vertebrae, cleft vertebrae, and wedge-shaped vertebrae. Occasionally an osseous band connects the scapula with the spine (*omovertebral bone*).

Myositis Ossificans Progressiva (Figure 7–17) is a progressive condition characterized by an *ossification of all of the voluntary muscles,* beginning before birth or in early childhood. Histologically, there is a proliferation of the connective tissue with secondary metaplasia into coarse fibrillar bone tissue and later into lamellar bone. The patient is ordinarily completely rigid by the age of 20 or 25, at which time there appears to be an arrest of the disease process. Usually the musculature of the face, eyes, tongue, larynx, abdomen, and sphincters escapes the ossifying process.

This disease entity should be differentiated from the following: interstitial calcinosis (calcinosis universalis), in which the deposits of calcium lie in the subcutaneous fatty tissues; localized ossifying myositis, which may be secondary to trauma and shows no evidence of systemic involvement; pseudohypoparathyroidism, in which hypoplasia of metacarpals and occasionally also basal ganglia calcification are apt to occur; and dermatomyositis, a "collagen disease."

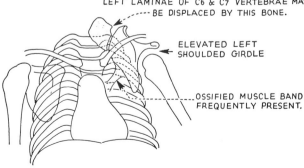

Figure 7–16 Sprengel's deformity. The defects are primarily external to bone.

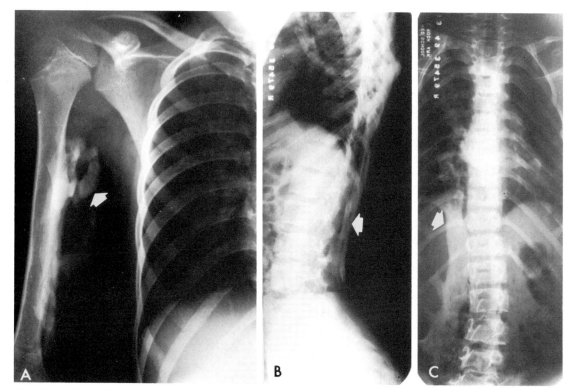

Figure 7–17 Myositis ossificans progressiva. *A*. Calcification of muscles of arm. *B*. Calcification of back muscles. *C*. Calcification of psoas muscle.

SKELETAL ABNORMALITIES IN RELATION TO KNOWN CHROMOSOMAL ABERRATIONS

The congenital disorders with known abnormal chromosomal constitution include the following:

1. *Mongolism* (trisomy 21 or Down's syndrome).
2. *Klinefelter's syndrome.*
3. *Turner's syndrome* (ovarian dysgenesis).
4. *Trisomy 13-15; 17-18; 19-20.*
5. *Monosomy 22.*
6. *Triploid mosaics.*
7. *Chromosomal satellites.*

There are, of course, many genetic inborn errors of metabolism, but karyotypic analysis ordinarily does not reveal grossly detectable aberration.

The **clinical disorders** in which chromosomal study is frequently rewarding include: **(1) mental deficiency; (2) congenital anomalies generally; (3) azoospermia in the male; and (4) primary amenorrhea and infertility in the female.**

Mongolism (Down's syndrome; trisomy 21) (Figure 7–18)

Clinical Features.   This is a variable congenital clinical syndrome characterized by a *mongoloid facial appearance, abnormal smallness of the hands and feet,* and variable degrees of *mental retardation*. The overall incidence is about 1.6 per 1000 births. There are three types differentiated: (1) regular mongols, defined as having 47 chromosomes and a trisomy of chromosome 21; (2) translocation mongols with only 46 chromosomes, in whose chromosome complement there is evidence that a translocation involving chromosome 21 has occurred; and (3) familial mongols in which there is sibship concentration, or the condition is found also on the maternal or paternal side. These latter may be either regular or translocation mongols and are important from the standpoint of the hereditary implications.

The eyes appear to be placed in small ovoid eye sockets with an internal strabismus, lateral nystagmus, and blepharitis.

There is an important *association between mongolism and acute leukemia in childhood* in that the chances for developing leukemia in mongols are about 15 times as great as for the population generally (Stewart et al.; and Tough et al.).

Radiographic Findings. No specific roentgen findings are present in all cases but the following findings are described in considerable numbers (Figure 7–18):

Skull: The nasal bones are usually hypoplastic; the jaws are hypoplastic; there is a persistence of the metopic suture; the frontal sinuses ordinarily fail to pneumatize; and dental abnormalities are frequent. The hard palate may appear shortened (Austin et al.).

The fingers and toes are hypoplastic, referred to as "acromicria," the converse of acromegaly.

The fifth fingers tend to be small and curved with alterations in the middle phalanges.

There is a gap between the first and second toe simulating the appearance of the thumb in its relationship to the index finger of the hand.

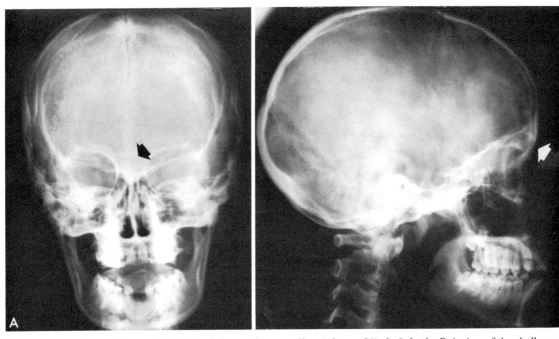

Figure 7–18 *A.* Some characteristic skeletal changes in mongolism (trisomy 21). *Left.* In the P-A view of the skull most patients have a persistent metopic suture and an absence of the frontal sinus. The absence of the frontal sinus is perhaps more clearly demonstrated at right.

Figure 7–18 continued on opposite page.

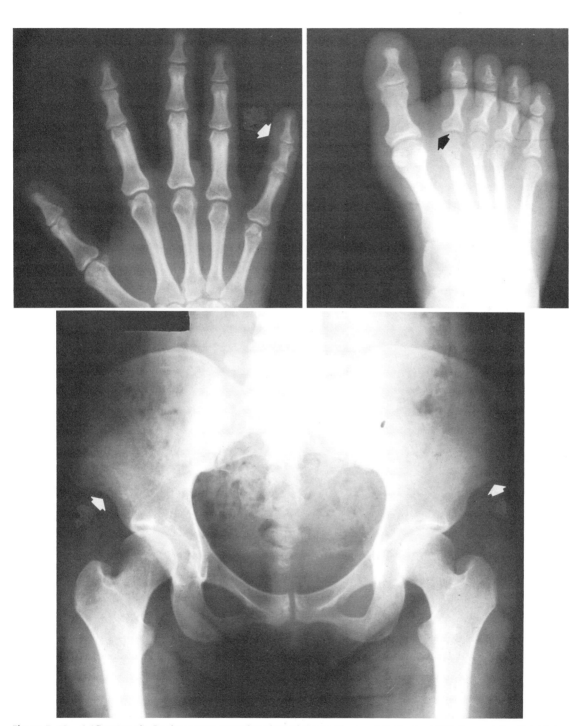

Figure 7–18   *A* (*Continued*). In the antero-posterior view of the hands, *top left*, the bent fifth finger at the distal inter-phalangeal joint is often characteristic. *Top right*. More readily demonstrated is the widened web space between the first and second toes of the feet. *Lower*. The marked flaring of the iliac crests of the innominate bones is also quite characteristic. (Courtesy of Dr. Leo Snow.)

Figure 7–18 continued on following page.

Pelvis: Both acetabular angles are flat and the iliac bones are widened bilaterally, so that the shape of the latter appears flared. The ischial rami appear slender on either side, and there is usually an associated bilateral coxa valga.

Atlanto-odontoid distance: This distance may be increased in mongolism (greater than 5 mm. in children and greater than 3 mm. in adults), but does not occur universally (Martel and Tishler).

Spine: The lumbar vertebrae may be increased in vertical diameter and decreased in antero-posterior diameter when viewed in the lateral projection. The anterior border of the vertebral bodies may appear straightened or concave posteriorly (Rabinowitz and Moseley).

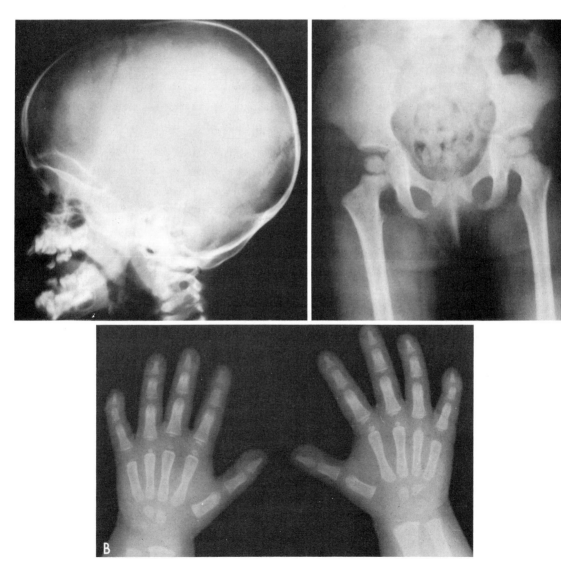

Figure 7–18 (*Continued*). *B. Top left.* The skull in a mongoloid patient. Note that the facial bones are hypoplastic and the roof of the mouth is highly arched. The paranasal sinuses are poorly developed. Closure of the sutures is delayed. The nasal bones particularly are hypoplastic or absent. The forehead appears large by contrast. A metopic suture is often present. The absence of the frontal sinuses and the poor development of the superciliary arches are prominent features in this disorder. *Top right.* The pelvis in infantile mongolism. The acetabular angles are flat and the iliac bones appear widened bilaterally. The ischial rami appear slender. This is usually a bilateral coxa valga. *Lower.* The hands in a mongoloid. These usually appear short and contain small curved fingers. In the feet there is often a gap between the first and second toes. Bone maturation may be normal, delayed, or accelerated.

Ribs: Eleven pairs of ribs instead of the normal 12 (Beber et al.).
Aberrant right subclavian artery (Goldstein).

Klinefelter's Syndrome.   Klinefelter's syndrome ordinarily does not declare itself until adolescence, at which time it consists of: (1) *small testes;* (2) *absence of evidence of spermatogenesis;* (3) *gynecomastia;* and (4) *high urinary excretion of gonadotropins* with low excretion of 17-ketosteroids. Most males with this syndrome are *chromatin-positive on nuclear sexing.* The majority of these patients have 47 chromosomes with an **XXY** constitution.

There is a positive association between Klinefelter's syndrome and mongolism and in these individuals a chromosome number of 48 can be differentiated.

The *long-limbed appearance* of these patients tends to raise the suspicion of Marfan's syndrome or arachnodactyly, but certain differences can be noted. *Congenital cardiac disease* is often present with Marfan's syndrome but *not in Klinefelter's syndrome,* and in addition, in Marfan's syndrome there is a hypotonic musculature and a diminished subcutaneous mass, with frequent bilateral dislocations of the ocular lenses and contracted pupils which do not respond to mydriatics.

Turner's Syndrome (Gonadal dysgenesis or agenesis) (Figures 7–19, 7–20) has 45 chromosomes with an XO constitution—where the O indicates absence of a chromosome.

Clinical Features.   Three basic clinical groups are differentiated in Turner's syndrome: (1) ovarian dysgenesis with webbing of the neck and usually other associated anomalies; (2) ovarian dysgenesis without webbing of the neck and with few other associated abnormalities and malformations except an invariable stunted stature; and (3) a third variant in which there is evidence of ovarian maldevelopment, but neither webbing of the neck nor stunting of stature is found.

In the *infant,* the presence of *unexplained peripheral edema* or a redundant skin fold at the back of the neck is highly suggestive of this diagnosis.

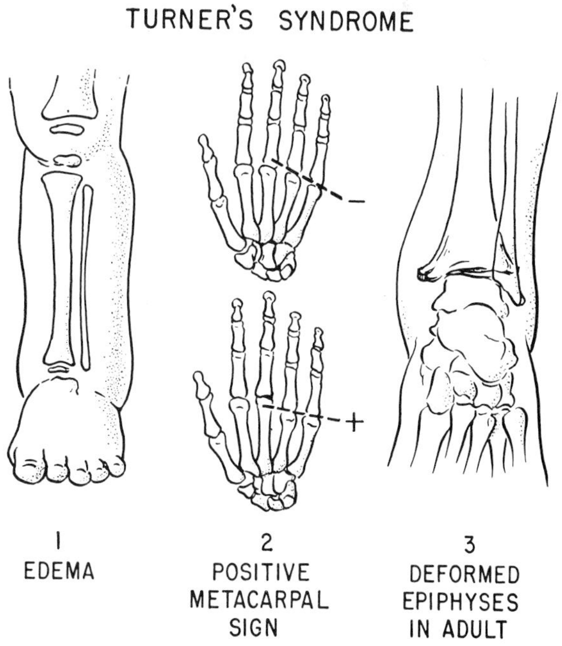

TURNER'S SYNDROME

Figure 7–19 Three of the common radiographic manifestations in Turner's syndrome. In the infant, peripheral edema as shown. In the adult, the positive metacarpal sign and deformed epiphyses.

I	2	3
EDEMA	POSITIVE METACARPAL SIGN	DEFORMED EPIPHYSES IN ADULT

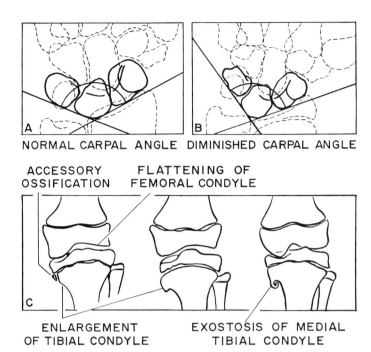

NORMAL CARPAL ANGLE   DIMINISHED CARPAL ANGLE

ACCESSORY   FLATTENING OF
OSSIFICATION   FEMORAL CONDYLE

ENLARGEMENT   EXOSTOSIS OF MEDIAL
OF TIBIAL CONDYLE   TIBIAL CONDYLE

Figure 7–20   *A* to *C*. Further radiographic manifestations with Turner's syndrome (according to Koso-wicz). Other radiologic manifestations are: (1) small and ridged sella turcica; (2) basilar impression of the skull; (3) increase in the carrying angle of the elbow (cubitus valgus); (4) changes in the spine resembling osteochondrosis; (5) hypoplasia of C-1 vertebral body; (6) male characteristics in the pelvis; and (7) thinness of lateral aspects of the clavicles and posterior aspect of the ribs.

The normal carpal angle is 131.5 ± 7.2°. (In arthrogryposis this angle is increased.)

During *childhood, dwarfing* is a very important finding and should be checked by cytogenetic analysis.

After puberty, primary *amenorrhea* and lack of secondary sex characteristics compose the diagnostic findings.

Radiographic Findings.   Despite the presence of webbing of the neck one does not ordinarily see fusion of the cervical vertebral segments. However, the **first cervical vertebra may be hypoplastic.** There is a **delayed fusion** of the epiphyseal centers and **osteoporosis** is frequent.

The characteristic changes in the skeleton otherwise are: (1) **edema** at the ends of the extremities on soft tissue study; and (2) shortness of the metacar-pals, which gives rise to the so-called **"positive metacarpal sign"** (Figure 7–19).

In addition to the above, a swelling over the medial tibial condyle bilaterally and symmetrically may be very pronounced as age advances, producing a vara-like deformity. Spurs tend to form after fusion of the centers with their shafts.

Irregularity and fragmentation of the epiphyseal plates of the vertebral bodies may occasionally be seen. However, there is usually no kyphosis in-volved in this deformity.

Kosowicz has reported that in roentgenograms of patients with gonadal dysgenesis, there is an **abnormal shape of the proximal carpal row of both hands.** These bones do not form an arch in normal fashion but rather an angle. The incidence of this "carpal sign" is ten times as frequent in gonadal dysgene-sis as might be expected in a normal population (Figure 7–20). Kosowicz has also reported **aseptic necrosis of the medial tibial condyle.**

Abnormalities of the urinary tract are found in high incidence in patients with gonadal dysgenesis. These abnormalities may include: horseshoe kidney, abnormal rotation, unilateral renal hypoplasia, hydronephrosis, and absence of a renal pelvis. Other abnormalities may also be seen, including partial uretero-pelvic obstruction and bilaterally incompletely rotated kidney (Hung and LoTresti).

The "pseudo-Turner" syndrome is characterized by normal chromosomal studies and normal buccal smears and yet these patients may have a webbed neck, short stature, and congenital heart disease. In contrast to Turner's syndrome, in which coarctation of the aorta is especially frequent, the congenital heart lesions here usually include atrial septal defect or pulmonic stenosis. No specific growth disturbances such as short metacarpals and deformities of the knee, or rotational renal anomalies are noted (Baker, Berdon et al.).

Other Chromosomal Aberrations with skeletal malformations might be described here but the student is referred to our larger text, *Roentgen Signs in Clinical Practice,* for more descriptions and for the bibliographic references which it contains for more extensive study.

Because of the very considerable confusion in respect to the nomenclature of constitutional or intrinsic diseases of bone, the European Society of Pediatric Radiology has tentatively proposed a standard nomenclature published in the Journal of Pediatrics, *78*:177–179, January 1971. The student is referred to this publication for further reference.

GLOSSARY OF SOME ADDITIONAL ENTITIES RELATING TO CONGENITAL AND HEREDITARY DISORDERS OF BONE:

Underdevelopment of a Bone or Extremity

Aplasia.   An extremity may be lacking in part or in its entirety. In recent times certain drugs (notably Thalidomide) administered early in the gestational period have been implicated in the causation of aplasia and phocomelia (congenital absence of the tibia) (Turek).

To the condition marked by total or partial absence of the phalanges and no reduction of other bony parts the term **ectrodactyly** has been applied (Frantz and O'Rahilly).

Brachydactyly: In this condition there is a hereditary abnormal shortness of the fingers or toes. Associated with it is Marchesani's syndrome (habitus opposite of Marfan's syndrome).

Dysgenesis of the Proximal Part of the Femur: Femoral shortening, bowing, and coxa vara, with the femur tapering proximally. The fibula may be either hypoplastic or absent (Amstutz and Wilson).

Hypoplasia of the Sacrum (Alexander et al.)

Oligodactylia: Too few fingers or toes.

Osteolysis, Familial: A rare entity in which complete resorption of phalanges, metatarsals, and sometimes tarsal bones may occur. It may be associated with hemophilia (Silber et al.), undifferentiated sarcoma (Fiore et al.), and many other diseases, and is perhaps related to angiomatosis (Johnson et al.).

Hemifacial Microsomia: Unilateral facial hypoplasia; malar or maxillary hypoplasia; microtia; deficiency of the external auditory meatus; hypoplasia or aplasia of the mandibular ramus or condyle; macrostomia; supernumerary skin tags; and malocclusion of the teeth.

Goldenhar's Syndrome (Oculoauriculovertebral dysplasia): Similar to hemifacial microsomia but in addition patients have epibulbar dermoids, colobomas of the eyelids, and vertebral anomalies (Darling et al.).

Overdevelopment

Diaphyseal Sclerosis, Hereditary Multiple: (Ribbing), probably same as Engelmann's disease.

Gigantism, Partial: Hypertrophy of a single bony part, such as a digit.

Hyperphalangism: Extra phalanges on either the hands or feet. (There may be other malformations associated.)

Melorheostosis (Flowing hyperostosis): Asymmetric overproduction of the cortex of a diaphysis, especially of the phalanges. This resembles a drop of wax flowing along the main shaft of a candle.

Osteopathia Striata (Voorhoeve's disease): Striation of the bones of the skeleton, especially the metaphyses of the long bones, running parallel to the bone axis (Fairbank).

Osteopoikilosis: Speckled appearance of the bones, widely disseminated.

Pyle's Disease: Symmetrical splaying of the long bones, due to a failure of bone modeling, imparting an Erlenmeyer-flask-shape to the long bones.

Maldevelopment

Aglossia-Adactylia Syndrome: Aplasia or hypoplasia of the tongue accompanied by failure of development of the digits. Hypoplasia of the mandible and salivary glands may be associated. (*Hanhart's syndrome* is the same, but there is no tongue defect. *Moebius syndrome* is also the same but there are anomalies of cranial nerves) (Gorlin and Pindborg).

Bird-Headed Dwarf of Seckel: Beaklike protrusion of the nose and premaxilla, with multiple skeletal anomalies such as shortness of stature, and microcephaly (Seckel).

Brachmann-DeLang Syndrome: A syndrome involving the skull, spine, extremities, chest, gastrointestinal tract, and in some cases, the genitourinary tract. For a summary of the roentgen findings see Kurlander and DeMeyer.

Craniocarpotarsal Dystrophy (Whistling face syndrome; Freeman-Sheldon syndrome): Long upper lip protrudes in whistling fashion. Flattened facial bones; microglossia; ulnar deviation of hands with contractures; equinovarus deformity of the feet; asymmetrical length and volume of the lower extremities; restricted mobility of the arms (Burian).

Farber's Disease (Disseminated lipogranulomatosis). The changes consist of nodular tumefaction around the joint; juxta-articular bone erosions; pulmonary parenchymal interstitial infiltration; and flaring of the costochondral junction (Schanche et al.).

Hand-Foot-Uterus Syndrome: Hereditary disorder with abnormalities involving the hands and feet; females with the disorder have a duplicated genital tract (Poznanski et al.).

Hemangiectatic Hypertrophy (Klippel-Trenaunay-Weber syndrome). Hypertrophy of the skeletal and soft tissues in a region which is involved with a "flame nevus." Predilection for involvement of the right side and lower extremities, and for maxillary division of the trigeminal nerve (Mullins).

Hemihypertrophy, Congenital (Hemigigantism): Total or partial hemihypertrophy of one side of the body. Frequently associated with it are: Wilm's tumor and adrenal cortical carcinoma (Miller et al.); Silver's syndrome which includes short stature and elevated gonadotropin levels; and hemangioma and compensatory scoliosis.

Holt-Oram Syndrome: Upper limb cardiovascular syndrome. It includes skeletal deformities involving the upper limbs with a wide spectrum of abnormalities such as hypoplasia, variations in carpal bones, synostoses, forward placement of the shoulders, and focal phocomelia. The most frequent cardiac defect is atrioseptal defect (Poznanski et al.; Rubin; Allen).

Hypertelorism: Increased distance between the eyes, due to an increase in size of the lesser wings of the sphenoids and diminution in size of the greater wings. Other congenital anomalies and syndromes are often associated (Rubin).

Hypercalcemia, Infantile Idiopathic: Increased density of all the skeletal structures, with underdevelopment of the mandible, low-set ears, supravalvular aortic stenosis (Black and Carter; Michael et al.; Joseph and Parrott).

Hypophosphatasia: Hereditary decrease in serum alkaline phosphatase which results in skeletal abnormalities closely resembling rickets. Oxycephaly, a "beaten-silver" skull, and notched ends of the long bones as in metaphyseal dysplasia are often associated (Bartter).

Larsen's Syndrome: Cleft palate, flattened facies, and multiple congenital dislocations.

Leri's Pleonosteosis: Marked thickening of the phalanges, metacarpals, and metatarsals with flexion contractures. Dwarfism and mongoloid facies (Watson-Jones).

Lipodystrophy, Total: Complete absence of body fat (Gwinn and Barnes).

Neurovisceral Storage Disease: Resembles Hurler's disease and is referred to as familial neurovisceral lipidosis and generalized gangliosidosis (Grossman and Danes).

Orodigitofacial Dysostosis (Gorlin-Psaume syndrome): Cleft mandible and maxilla with harelip and cleft tongue. Hydrocephalus and marked basal skull lordosis. Phalangeal synostosis or abnormality associated.

Oto-Palata-Digital Syndrome: Changes in the hands and feet involving multiple bones in combination with altered relationships between the clivus and cervical vertebrae. Usually appearing in patients over the age of five years. The skull may have prominent supraorbital ridges, thick frontal bones, and an absence of frontal sinuses with a thickened base of the anterior fossa. The posterior parietal and occipital regions may also be prominent with minimal pneumatization of the mastoid. The facial bones and maxillary sinuses appear small, as does the mandible, which has a more obtuse angle than normal. The posterior fossa may appear deep but the foramen magnum is usually small (Langer).

Progeria: Hutchinson-Gilford Syndrome (Margolin and Steinbach).

Definition. Premature aging characterized by alopecia, brown pigmented area on the trunk, atrophic skin, prominent veins, loss of subcutaneous fat, receding chin, beaked nose, exophthalmos, muscular atrophy, joint deformity, and accelerated premature degenerative processes with arteriosclerosis in coronary and other vessels.

Roentgen Findings include: hypoplastic facial bones, delay of cranial suture and fontanelle closure; thin, short clavicles; coxa valga. Views of the hand reveal striking resorption of the distal phalanges without loss of soft tissue. The shafts of long bones appear slender but the metaphyses of the proximal humeri may be widened.

Van der Woode's Syndrome: Cleft lip, cleft palate, and anomalies of the hands and feet.

Questions—Chapter 7

1. What are the major categories in the classification of congenital and hereditary abnormalities of the extremities?

2. Name some of the major categories in underdevelopment of a bone or extremity.

3. Name some of the examples of overdevelopment or duplication of extremities on a congenital and hereditary basis.

4. Describe some of the main roentgen findings in cleidocranial dysostosis.

5. What is meant by "arachnodactylia"?

6. What are some examples of maldevelopment of a regional portion of the body on a congenital and hereditary basis?

7. Describe perodactylia, peromelia, and Madelung's deformity.

8. Classify the congenital and hereditary abnormalities of extremities which represent a generalized maldevelopment of the skeleton. Indicate these by sub-groups as affecting the epiphyses primarily, the metaphyses primarily, or the bones rather diffusely.

9. Describe the radiographic findings in congenital stippled epiphyses.

10. Describe the radiographic findings in Ollier's disease (chondrodysplasia).

11. Describe the radiographic findings with diaphyseal aclasis and indicate another acceptable radiographic term for this disease. How does this disease differ from chondrodysplasia?

12. Describe the radiographic findings in familial, metaphyseal dysplasia (Pyle's disease).

13. Describe the clinical and radiographic findings in infantile familial or hereditary hypophosphatemia.

14. Describe the main radiographic findings in achondroplasia.

15. Describe the radiologic and clinical findings in Morquio's disease as well as in Pfaundler-Hurler's disease and indicate the differences between these two entities.

16. Describe the main radiographic findings in osteogenesis imperfecta.

17. Describe the clinical and radiographic findings in chondroectodermal dysplasia (Ellis-van Creveld's disease).

18. What are the main findings in acrocephalosyndactylia (Apert's syndrome)?

19. Describe the main radiographic and clinical findings in arthrogryposis multiplex congenita.

20. Describe the main clinical and radiographic findings in Ehlers-Danlos syndrome (hyperelastosis cutis).

21. Describe the main radiographic features in the following entities: mandibulofacial dysostosis; craniofacial dysostosis (Crouzon's disease); mandibular hypoplasia (micrognathia); Robin's syndrome (cleft palate with micrognathia and glossoptosis).

22. Indicate some of the more commonly considered congenital bone abnormalities that are actually primarily outside of bone.

23. What is meant by "Sprengel's deformity"?

24. What similarities exist between myositis ossificans progressiva and pseudohypoparathyroidism?

25. Describe the typical pelvic alterations in: achondroplasia; osteogenesis imperfecta; mongolism; acetabular dysplasia; Morquio's disease; iliac horns; cleidocranial dysostosis.

26. List at least four congenital disorders with known abnormal chromosomal aberrations which have been demonstrated.

27. Describe the roentgen findings often present in mongolism.

28. Describe the roentgen findings often present in Klinefelter's syndrome. How may one differentiate Klinefelter's syndrome from Marfan's syndrome?

29. Indicate positive or negative associations between mongolism, Klinefelter's syndrome, and acute leukemia in childhood.

30. Describe six radiographic changes in Turner's syndrome (gonadal dysgenesis). How does the spine in Turner's syndrome differ from that in juvenile kyphosis or Scheuermann's disease?

31. What is the most frequent manifestation of Turner's syndrome in the infant, during childhood, and after puberty?

References

Alexander, E., Jr., and Nashold, B. S., Jr.: Agenesis of the sacrococcygeal region. J. Neurosurg., 13:507–513, 1956.

Allansmith, M., and Senz, E.: Chondrodystrophia congenita punctata (Conradi's disease). Review of literature and report of case with unusual features. Amer. J. Dis. Child., 100:109–116, 1960.

Alvarez-Borja, A.: Ellis-van Creveld syndrome. Pediatrics, 26:301–309, 1960.

Amstutz, H. C., and Wilson, P. D., Jr.: Dysgenesis of proximal femur (coxa vara) and its surgical management. J. Bone Joint Surg., 44-A:1–24, 1962.

Andren, L., and Von Rosen, S.: The diagnosis of dislocations of the hip in the newborn. Acta Radiolog., 49:89–95, 1958.

Arkless, R., and Graham, C. B.: An unusual case of brachydactyly; peripheral dysostosis? pseudo-pseudohypoparathyroidism? cone epiphysis? Amer. J. Roentgenol., 99:724–735, 1967.

Austin, J. H. M., Preger, L., Siris, E., and Taybi, H.: Short, hard palate in newborn: roentgen sign of mongolism. Radiology, 92:775–776, 1969.

Baker, D. H., Berdon, W. E., Morishima, A., and Conte, F.: Turner's syndrome and pseudo-Turner's syndrome. Amer. J. Roentgenol., 100:40–47, 1967.

Barr, M. L., and Bertram, E. G.: A morphological distinction between neurones of the male and female, and the behaviours of the nucleolar satellite during accelerated nucleoprotein synthesis. Nature, 163:676–677, 1949.

Bartter, F. C.: Hypophosphatasia. In Stanbury, J. B., Wynegaarden, J. B., and Fredrickson, D. S. (editors), The Metabolic Basis of Inherited Disease. New York, McGraw-Hill, 1966.

Bean, W. B.: Dyschondroplasia and hemangiomata (Maffucci's syndrome). Arch. Intern. Med., 95:767–778, 1955.

Beber, B. A., Litt, R. E., and Altman, D. H.: A new radiographic finding in mongolism. Radiology, 86:332–333, 1966.

Berenson, G. S., and Geer, J. C.: Heart disease in the Hurler and Marfan syndromes. Arch. Intern. Med., 111:58–69, 1963.

Berg, P. K.: Dysplasia epiphysialis multiplex. A case report and review of the literature. Amer. J. Roentgenol., 97:31–38, 1966.

Berry, H. K., and Spinanger, J.: A paper spot test useful in study of Hurler's syndrome. J. Lab. Clin. Med., 55:136–138, 1960.

Birch-Jensen, A.: Congenital deformities of the upper extremities. Copenhagen, Munksgaard, 1949.

Black, J. A., and Carter, R. E.: Association between aortic stenosis and facies of severe infantile hypercalcemia. Lancet, 2:745–748, 1963.

Blank, C. E.: Apert's syndrome (a type of acrocephalosyndactyly). Observations on a British series of 39 cases. Ann. Human Genetics, 24:151–164, 1960.

Brixey, A. M., Jr., and Burke, R. M.: Arthroonycho dysplasia. Hereditary syndrome involving deformity of the head of the radius, absence of patellas, posterior iliac spurs, dystrophy of fingernails. Amer. J. Med. 8:738–744, 1950.

Bruno, M. S., and Narasimhan, P.: Ehlers-Danlos syndrome: A report of four cases in two generations of a Negro family. New Eng. J. Med., 264:274–277, 1961.

Burian, F.: The whistling face characteristic in a compound craniofacial corporal syndrome. Brit. J. Plastic Surg., 16:140–143, 1963.

Caffey, J.: Achondroplasia of the pelvis and lumbosacral spine: Some roentgenographic features. Amer. J. Roentgenol., 80:449–457, 1958.

Caffey, J.: Pediatric X-ray Diagnosis. Fifth Edition. Chicago, Year Book Medical Publishers, 1967.

Caffey, J., Ames, R., Silverman, W. A., Ryder, C. T., and Hough, G.: Contradiction of the congenital dysplasia-predislocation hypothesis and congenital dislocation of the hip through a study of the normal variation in acetabular angles at successive periods in infancy. Pediatrics, 17:632–651, 1956.

Caffey, J., and Ross, S.: Pelvic bones in infantile mongoloidism — roentgenographic features. Amer. J. Roentgenol., 80:458–467, 1958.

Caniggia, A., Stuart, C., Guideria, R.: Fragilitus ossium hereditaria tarda: Ekman-Lobstein disease. Acta Med. Scand. Supp. 340, 1958.

Carr, D. H.: Chromosomal abnormalities and

their relation to disease. Canad. Med. Assoc. J., *88*:456–461, 1963.

Carter, C., and MacCarthy, D.: Incidence of mongolism and its diagnosis in the newborn. Brit. J. Soc. Med., *5*:83–90, 1951.

Cockshott, W. P.: Carpal fusions. Amer. J. Roentgenol., *89*:1260–1271, 1963.

Conway, J. J., and Cowell, H. L.: Tarsal coalition: Clinical significance and roentgenographic demonstration. Radiology, *92*:799–811, 1969.

Coventry, M. B., and Johnson, E. W., Jr.: Congenital absence of fibula. J. Bone & Joint Surg., *34-A*:941–956, 1952.

Currarino, G., Neuhauser, E. B., Reyerspach, G. C., and Sobel, E. H.: Hypophosphatasia. Amer. J. Roentgenol., *78*:382–419, 1957.

Darling, D. B., Feingold, M., and Berkman, M.: Goldenhar's syndrome: Oculoauriculovertebral dysplasia. Radiology, *91*:254–260, 1968.

Edwards, J. H., Harnden, D. G., Cameron, A. H., Crosse, V. M., and Wolff, O. H.: New trisomy syndrome. Lancet, *1*:787–789, 1960.

Elefant, E., and Tosovsky, V.: Osteogenesis imperfecta congenita. Ann. Paediat., *202*:285–292, 1964.

Elliot, K. R., Elliot, G. B., and Kindrachuk, W. H.: The "radial subluxation-fingernail defect-absent patella" syndrome: Observations on its nature. Amer. J. Roentgenol., *87*:1067–1074, 1962.

Ellis, R. W. B., and Andrew, J. D.: Chondroectodermal dysplasia. J. Bone & Joint Surg., *44-B*:626–636, 1962.

Ellis, R. W. B., and van Creveld, S.: Syndrome characterized by ectodermal dysplasia, polydactyly, chondrodysplasia, and congenital morbis cordis; report of 3 cases. Arch. Dis. Child., *15*:65–84, 1940.

Evans, R., and Caffey, J.: Metaphyseal dysostosis resembling vitamin D-refractory rickets. Amer. J. Dis. Child., *95*:640–648, 1958.

Fairbank, T.: Dysplasia epiphysialis multiplex. Brit. J. Surg., *34*:225–232, 1947.

Fairbank, T.: Generalized diseases of the skeleton. Proc. Royal Soc. Med., *28*:1611–1619, 1935.

Fairbank, T.: An Atlas of General Affections of the Skeleton. Edinburgh, E. & S. Livingstone, Ltd., 1951, pp. 111–119.

Fairbank, T.: An Atlas of General Affections of the Skeleton. Baltimore, Williams and Wilkins Co., 1951.

Feinberg, S. B., and Fisch, R. O.: Roentgenologic findings in growing long bones in phenylketonuria: Preliminary study. Radiology, *78*:394–398, 1962.

Felman, A. H.: Multiple epiphyseal dysplasia. Radiology, *93*:119–125, 1969.

Felman, A. H., and Kirkpatrick, J. A.: Madelung's deformity: Observations in 17 patients. Radiology, *93*:1037–1042, 1969.

Finby, N., and Archibald, R. M.: Skeletal abnormalities associated with gonadal dysgenesis. Amer. J. Roentgenol., *89*:1222–1235, 1963.

Fiore, J. M., and Smyth, W. T.: Massive osteolysis of bone: Report of a fatal case with temporary reconstitution of the affected bone following irradiation. Ann. Intern. Med., *53*:807–816, 1960.

Ford, C. E., Jacobs, P. A., and Lajtha, L. G.: Human somatic chromosomes. Nature, *181*:1565–1568, 1958.

Frantz, C. H., and O'Rahilly, R.: Congenital skeletal limb deficiencies. J. Bone & Joint Surg., *43-A*:1202–1224, 1961.

Fraser, D.: Clinical manifestations of genetic aberrations of calcium and phosphorus metabolism. J.A.M.A., *176*:281–287, 1961.

Friedenberg, Z. B.: Protrusio acetabuli in childhood. J. Bone & Joint Surg., *45-A*:373, 1963.

Garavaglia, C.: Early diagnosis of congenital dysplasia of the hip; new roentgenologic signs. Amer. J. Roentgenol., *110*:587–590, 1970.

Goidanich, I. F., and Lenzi, L.: Morquio-Ullrich disease. J. Bone & Joint Surg., *46-A*:734–746, 1954.

Goldstein, H.: Congenital acromicria syndrome. Arch. Pediat., *73*:115–124, 1956.

Goldstein, W. B.: Aberrant right subclavian artery in mongolism. Amer. J. Roentgenol., *95*:131–134, 1965.

Gorlin, R. J., and Pindborg, J. J.: Syndromes of the Head and Neck, New York, McGraw-Hill, 1964.

Gorlin, R. J., and Psaume, J.: Orodigitofacial dysostosis: A new syndrome. A study of 22 cases. J. Pediat., *61*:520–530, 1962.

Gram, P. B., Fleming, J. L., and Fine, G.: Metaphyseal dysostosis. J. Bone & Joint Surg., *41-A*:951–959, 1959.

Griffiths, D. L.: Engelmann's disease. J. Bone & Joint Surg., *38-B*:312–326, 1956.

Grossman, H., and Danes, B. S.: Neurovisceral storage disease: roentgenographic features and mode of inheritance. Amer. J. Roentgenol., *103*:149–153, 1968.

Hambrick, G. W., and Scheie, H. G.: Studies of the skin in Hurler's syndrome: mucopolysaccharidosis. Arch. Derm., *85*:455–471, 1962.

Hamerton, J. L.: Chromosomes in medicine. Little Clubs Clin. in Developmental Med., *5*:1–231, 1962.

Haveson, S. B.: Congenital flat foot due to talonavicular dislocation (vertical talus). Radiology, *72*:19–25, 1959.

Holman, G. H.: Infantile cortical hyperostosis: A review. Quart. Rev. Pediat., *17*:24–31, 1962.

Hung, W., and LoPresti, J. M.: Urinary tract anomalies in gonadal dysgenesis. Amer. J. Roentgenol., *95*:439–441, 1965.

Jackson, W. P. U., Hanelin, J., and Albright, F.: Metaphyseal dysplasia, epiphyseal dysplasia, diaphyseal dysplasia and related conditions: familial metaphyseal dysplasia and craniometaphyseal dysplasia; their relation to leontiasis ossea and osteopetrosis; disorders of "bone remodeling." Arch. Intern. Med., *94*:871–885, 1954.

James, A. E., Jr., Belcourt, C. L., Atkins, L., and Janower, M. L.: Trisomy 13-15. Radiology, *92*:44–49, 1969.

James, A. E., Jr., Belcourt, C. L., Atkins, L., and Janower, M. L.: Trisomy 18. Radiology, *92*:37–43, 1969.

Johnson, P. M., and McClure, J. G.: Observations on massive osteolysis. Review of literature and report of a case. Radiology, 71:28–42, 1958.

Joseph, M. C., and Parrott, D.: Severe infantile hypercalcemia with special reference to the facies. Arch. Dis. Child., 33:385–395, 1958.

Kalayjian, B. S., Herbut, P. A., and Erf, L. A.: The bone changes of leukemia in children. Radiology, 47:223–233, 1946.

Kanof, A., Aronson, S. M., and Volk, B. W.: Arthrogryposis: A clinical and pathologic study of three cases. Pediatrics, 17:532–540, 1956.

Karpinski, F. E., and Martin, J. F.: The skeletal lesions of leukemic children treated with Aminopterin. J. Pediat., 37:208–223, 1950.

Kaufman, E. E., and Coventry, M. B.: Multiple epiphyseal dysplasia in a mother and son. Proc. Mayo Clin., 38:115–124, 1963.

Keats, T. E.: Cleidocranial dysostosis: some atypical roentgen manifestations. Amer. J. Roentgenol., 100:71–74, 1967.

Keats, T. E., Rivervold, H. O., and Michaelis, L. L.: Thanatophoric dwarfism. Amer. J. Roentgenol., 108:473–480, 1970.

Kosowicz, J.: Changes in medial tibial condyle – common findings in Turner's syndrome. Acta Endocrin., 31:321–323, 1959.

Kosowicz, J.: The carpal sign in gonadal dysgenesis. J. Clin. Endocrin., 22:949–952, 1962.

Kowins, C.: Familial metaphyseal dysplasia (Pyle's disease). Brit. J. Radiol., 27:670–675, 1954.

Kozlowski, K., and Budzinska, A.: Metaphyseal and epiphyseal dysostosis. Amer. J. Roentgenol., 97:21–30, 1966.

Kurlander, G. J., and DeMeyer, W.: Roentgenology of the Brachmann-DeLang syndrome. Radiology, 88:101–110, 1967.

Kurlander, G. J., Lavy, N. W., and Campbell, J. A.: Roentgen differentiation of the oculodentodigital syndrome and the Hallermann-Streiff syndrome in infancy. Radiology, 86:77–85, 1966.

Langer, L. O. Jr.: Dyschondro-osteosis, a heritable bone dysplasia with characteristic roentgenographic features. Amer. J. Roentgenol., 95:178–188, 1965.

Langer, L. O., Jr.: Spondyloepiphyseal dysplasia tarda. Radiology, 82:833–839, 1964.

Langer, L. O. Jr.: Diastrophic dwarfism in early infancy. Amer. J. Roentgenol., 93:399–404, 1965.

Langer, L. O. Jr., and Carey, L. S.: The roentgenographic features of KS mucopolysaccharidosis (Morquio-Brailsford's disease). Amer. J. Roentgenol., 97:1–20, 1966.

Langer, L. O., Jr., Peterson, D., and Spranger, J. W.: An unusual bone dysplasia: parastremmatic dwarfism. Amer. J. Roentgenol., 110:550–560, 1969.

Langer, L. O. Jr., Spranger, J. W., Greinacher, I., and Herdman, R. C.: Thanatrophoric dwarfism. Radiology, 92:285–294, 1969.

Langer, L. O. Jr.: The roentgenographic features of the oto-palato-digital (OPD) syndrome. Amer. J. Roentgenol. 100:63–70, 1967.

Larose, J. H., and Gay, B. B., Jr.: Metatrophic dwarfism. Amer. J. Roentgenol., 106:156–161, 1969.

Larsen, L. J., Schottstaedt, E. R., and Bost, F.: Multiple congenital dislocations associated with characteristic facial abnormality. J. Pediat., 37:574–581, 1950.

Ledeboer, R., and VanMeel, P. J.: Dysplasia epiphysialis multiplex. Nederl. Tydschr. Geneesk., 102:2257, 1958.

Lee, F. A., and Kenny, F. M.: Skeletal changes in the Cornelia DeLang syndrome. Amer. J. Roentgenol., 100:27–39, 1967.

Leeds, N. E.: Epiphyseal dysplasia multiplex. Amer. J. Roentgenol., 84:506–510, 1960.

Leucutia, T.: Autosomal trisomy syndromes (editorial). Amer. J. Roentgenol., 89:1092–1094, 1963.

Levin, E. J.: Osteogenesis imperfecta in the adult. Amer. J. Roentgenol., 91:973–978, 1964.

Lile, H. A., Rogers, J. F., and Gerald, B.: The basal cell nevus syndrome. Amer. J. Roentgenol., 103:214–217, 1968.

Margolin, F. R., and Steinbach, H. L.: Progeria: Hutchinson-Gilford syndrome. Amer. J. Roentgenol., 103:173–178, 1968.

Maroteaux, P.: The chondrodystrophies detectable at birth. In Fraser, F. C., McKusick, V. A., and Robinson, R. (editors): Congenital Malformations. Proceedings of the Third International Conference. The Hague, The Netherlands, 1969. Excerpta Medica, Amsterdam – New York, 1969.

Maroteaux, P., and Lamy, M.: Metaphyseal dysostosis. Semaine Lop, Paris, 34:402–408, 1958.

Maroteaux, P., and Lamy, M.: Achondroplasia in man and animals. Clin. Orthop., 33:91–103, 1964.

Martel, W., and Tishler, J. M.: Observations on the spine in mongoloidism. Amer. J. Roentgenol., 97:630–638, 1966.

McKusick, V. A.: Heritable Disorders of Connective Tissue. Second Edition. St. Louis, C. V. Mosby Co., 1960.

McKusick, V. A.: Medical Genetics. St. Louis, C. V. Mosby Co., 1961.

McNeill, K. A., and Wynter-Wedderburn, L.: Choanal atresia – A manifestation of Treacher-Collins syndrome. J. Laryng. & Otol., 67:365–369, 1953.

Mead, N. G., Lithgow, W. C., and Sweeny, H. J.: Arthrogryposis multiplex congenita. J. Bone & Joint Surg., 40-A:1285–1309, 1958.

Michael, A. F., Jr., Hong, R., and West, C. D.: Hypercalcemia in infancy. Amer. J. Dis. Child., 104:235–244, 1962.

Miller, R. W., Fraumeni, J. F., and Manning, M. D.: Association of Wilms' tumor with aniridiahemi-hypertrophy and other congenital malformations. New Eng. J. Med., 270:922–927, 1964.

Mori, P. A., and Holt, J. F.: Cranial manifestations of familial metaphyseal dysplasia. Radiology, 66:335–343, 1956.

Morreels, C. L. Jr., Fletcher, B. D., Weilboecher, R. G., and Dorst, J. P.: Roentgenographic features of hemocystinuria. Radiology, 90:1150–1158, 1968.

Moseley, J. E., Moloshok, R. E., and Freiberger,

R. H.: The silver syndrome: congenital asymmetry, short stature and variations in sexual development; roentgen features. Amer. J. Roentgenol., 97:74–81, 1966.

Moseley, J., Wolf, B. S., and Gottlieb, M. I.: The trisomy 17-18 syndrome: Roentgen features. Amer. J. Roentgenol., 89:905–913, 1963.

Mullins, J. F., Naylor, D., and Redetski, J.: The Klippel-Trenaunay-Weber syndrome. Arch. Dermatol., 86:202–206, 1962.

A nomenclature of constitutional (intrinsic) diseases of bone. J. Pediat., 78:177–179, 1971.

Ozonoff, M. B., and Clemett, A. R.: Progressive osteolysis in progeria. Amer. J. Roentgenol., 100:75–79, 1969.

Palacios, E., and Schimke, R. N.: Craniosynostosis-syndactylism. Amer. J. Roentgenol., 106:144–155, 1969.

Papadimitriou, D. G.: Hereditary arthro-osteo-onychodysplasia. South. Med. J., 53:186–193, 1960.

Papavasiliou, C. G., Gargano, F. P., and Walls, W. I.: Idiopathic nonfamilial acro-osteolysis associated with other bone abnormalities. Amer. J. Roentgenol., 83:687–691, 1960.

Patau, K., Smith, D. W., Therman, E., Inhorn, S. L., and Wagner, H. P.: Multiple congenital anomalies caused by extra autosomes. Lancet, 1:790–793, 1960.

Paus, B.: Madelung's deformity: Its etiology and pathogenesis. Acta Orth. Scand., 21:249–258, 1951.

Penrose, L. S.: The relative aetiological importance of birth order and maternal age in mongolism. Proc. Royal Soc. (Biol.), 115:431–450, 1934.

Poznanski, A. K., Gall, J. C. Jr., and Stern, A. M.: Skeletal manifestations of the Holt-Oram syndrome. Radiology, 94:45–53, 1970.

Poznanski, A. K., and LaRowe, P. C.: Radiographic manifestations of the arthrogryposis syndrome. Radiology, 95:353–358, 1970.

Poznanski, A. K., Stern, A. M., and Gall, J. C., Jr.: Radiographic findings in the hand-foot-uterus syndrome (HFUS). Radiology, 95:129–134, 1970.

Rabinowitz, J. G., and Moseley, J. E.: The lateral lumbar spine in Down's syndrome: a new roentgen feature. Radiology, 83:74–79, 1964.

Ribbing, S.: Hereditary multiple diaphyseal sclerosis. Acta Radiol., 31:522–536, 1949.

Ringrose, R. E., Jabbour, J. T., and Keele, D. K.: Hemihypertrophy. Pediatrics, 36:434–448, 1965.

Riordan, D. C.: Congenital absence of radius. J. Bone & Joint Surg., 37-A:1129–1140, 1955.

Robbins, M. M., Stevens, H. F., and Linker, A.: Morquio's disease: an abnormality of mucopolysaccharide metabolism. J. Pediatrics, 62:881–889, 1963.

Rubin, A.: Handbook of Congenital Malformations. Philadelphia, W. B. Saunders Co., 1967.

Rubin, P.: Dynamic Classification of Bone Dysplasias. Chicago, Year Book Medical Publishers, 1964.

Schauerte, E. W., and St.-Aubin, P. M.: Progressive synosteosis in Apert's syndrome (acrocephalosyndactyly); with a description of

roentgenographic changes in the feet. Amer. J. Roentgenol., 97:67–73, 1966.

Schanche, A. F., Bierman, S. M., Sopher, R. L., and O'Loughlin, B. J.: Disseminated lipogranulomatosis: Early roentgenographic changes. Radiology, 82:675–678, 1964.

Schinz, H. R., Baensch, W. E., Friedl, E., and Vehlinger, E.: Roentgen-Diagnostics. J. T. Case, editor and translator. Volume I. New York, Grune and Stratton, 1951.

Schwarz, E.: Craniometaphyseal dysplasia. Amer. J. Roentgenol., 84:461–466, 1960.

Schwarz, E., and Fish, A.: Roentgenographic features of a new congenital dysplasia. Amer. J. Roentgenol., 84:511–517, 1960.

Schwarz, E., and Rivellini, G.: Symphalangism. Amer. J. Roentgenol., 89:1256–1259, 1963.

Sear, H. R.: Englemann's disease. Brit. J. Radiol., 21:236, 1948.

Seckel, H. P. G.: Bird Headed Dwarfs. Springfield, Ill., Charles C Thomas, Publishers, 1960.

Seward, F. S., Roche, A. G., and Sunderland, S.: The lateral cranial silhouette in mongolism. Amer. J. Roentgenol., 85:653–658, 1961.

Silber, R., and Christenson, W. R.: Pseudotumor of hemophilia in a patient with PTC deficiency. Blood, 14:584–590, 1959.

Silverman, F. N.: Epiphyseal dysplasias: Protean entity. Ann. Radiology, 4:833–967, 1961.

Smith, H. L., and Hand, A. M.: Chondro-ectodermal dysplasia (Ellis-van Creveld syndrome): Report of two cases. Pediatrics, 21:298–307, 1958.

Soule, A. B. Jr.: Mutational dysostosis (cleidocranial dysostosis). J. Bone & Joint Surg., 28:81–102, 1946.

Spitzer, R., Rabinowitch, J. Y., and Wybar, K. C.: A study of the abnormalities of the skull, teeth and lenses in mongolism. Canad. Med. Assoc. J., 84:567–572, 1961.

Spranger, J. W., and Langer, L. O. Jr.: Spondyloepiphyseal dysplasia congenita. Radiology, 94:313–322, 1970.

Stanbury, J. B., Wyngaarden, J. B., and Frederickson, D. I.: The Metabolic Basis for Inherited Disease. New York, McGraw-Hill, 1960.

Steinbach, H. L., and Brown, R. A.: Epiphyseal dysostosis. Amer. J. Roentgenol., 105:860–869, 1969.

Steinberg, I.: Screening test for the Marfan syndrome. Amer. J. Roentgenol., 97:118–124, 1966.

Stewart, A., Webb, J., and Hewitt, D.: A survey of childhood malignancies. Brit. Med. J., 1:1495–1508, 1958.

Stover, C. N., Hayes, J. T., and Holt, J. F.: Diastrophic dwarfism. Amer. J. Roentgenol., 89:914–922, 1963.

Taussig, H. B.: Thalidomide and focomelia. Pediatrics, 30:654–659, 1962.

Taybi, H.: Diastrophic dwarfism. Radiology, 80:1010, 1963.

Taybi, H.: Generalized skeletal dysplasia with multiple anomalies: A note on Pyle's disease. Amer. J. Roentgenol., 88:450–457, 1962.

Taybi, H., and Rubinstein, J. H.: Broad thumbs and toes, and unusual facial features: a probable mental retardation syndrome. Amer. J. Roentgenol., *93*:362–366, 1965.

Thieffry, S., and Sorrell-Dejerine, J.: Forme spéciale d'ostéolyse essentielle heréditaire familiale à stabilisation spontanée, survenant dans l'enfance. Presse méd., *66*:1858–1861, 1958.

Tough, I. M., Court Brown, W. M., Baikie, A. G., Buckton, K. E., Harnden, D. G., Jacobs, P. A., King, M. J., and McBride, J. A.: Cytogenetic studies in chronic myeloid leukemia and acute leukemia associated with mongolism. Lancet, *1*:411–417, 1961.

Turek, S. L.: Orthopaedics. Second Edition. Philadelphia, J. B. Lippincott, 1967.

Van der Woude, A.: Fistula labii inferioris congenita and its association with cleft lip and palate. Amer. J. Human Genetics, *6*: 244–256, 1954.

Waardenburg, P. J., Franceschetti, A., and Klein, D.: Genetics and Ophthalmology, Springfield, Ill., Charles C Thomas, 1961.

Walls, W. L., Altman, D. H., and Winslow, O. P.: Chondroectodermal dysplasia (Ellis-van Creveld syndrome). Amer. J. Dis. Child., *98*: 242–248, 1959.

Watson, E. H., and Lowery, G. H.: Growth and Development of Children. Fifth Edition. Chicago, Year Book Publishers, 1967.

Watson, R. J., and Lichtman, H. C.: Symposium on basic sciences in medical practice. The anemias. Med. Clin. N. Amer., *39*:735–749, 1955.

Watson-Jones, R.: Leri's pleonosteosis. J. Bone & Joint Surg., *31-B*:560–571, 1949.

Wesenberg, R. L., Gwinn, J. L., and Barnes, G. R. Jr.: The roentgenographic findings in total lipodystrophy. Amer. J. Roentgenol., *103*:154–164, 1968.

White, J. E., Binford, C. C., Robinson, R. R., and Blackard, W. G.: Familial hypophosphatemia. Arch. Intern. Med., *111*:460–464, 1963.

Whittaker, S. R., and Seehan, J. D.: Dissecting aortic aneurysm in Marfan's syndrome. Lancet, 2:791–792, 1954.

Williams, T. F., Winters, R. W., and Burnette, C. H.: Familial (hereditary) vitamin D-resistant rickets with hypophosphatemia. *In* Stanbury, J. B., Wyngaarden, J. B., and Fredrickson, D. S. (editors), Metabolic Basis of Inherited Disease. Second Edition, New York, McGraw-Hill, 1966.

Willson, J. K. V.: The bone lesions of childhood leukemia; a survey of 140 cases. Radiology, *72*:672–681, 1959.

Winchester, P., Grossman, H., Lim, W. N., and Danes, B. S.: Acid mucopolysaccharidosis with skeletal deformities simulating rheumatoid arthritis. Amer. J. Roentgenol., *106*: 121–128, 1969.

Yunis, J. J.: Human Chromosomes in Disease. *In* Yunis, J. J., (editor), Human Chromosome Methodology. New York, Academic Press, 1965.

8

Radiolucent Bone Diseases of Multiple Extremities or Regions

INTRODUCTION

Radiolucent Bone Diseases involving extremities or regions may be categorized as follows (Figure 8–1):

MULTIPLE OSTEOLYTIC LESIONS
OF MULTIPLE EXTREMITIES

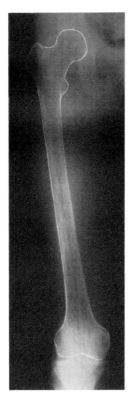 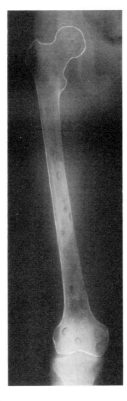 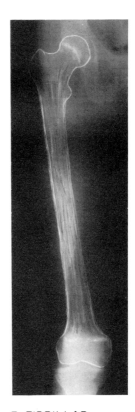 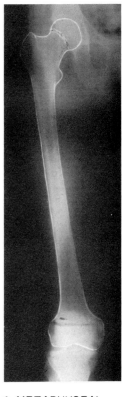

I. UNIFORM
   RADIOLUCENCY

2. CIRCUMSCRIBED
   MULTIPLE AREAS
   OF RADIOLUCENCY

3. FIBRILLAR
   OSTEOPOROSIS
   WITH COARSENING
   OF TRABECULAE

4. METAPHYSEAL
   TRANSVERSE
   OSTEOPOROSIS

Figure 8–1   Classification of radiolucent bone diseases of multiple extremities.

Figure 8–1 *continued on opposite page.*

1. *Uniform radiolucency.*
2. *Sharply circumscribed areas of radiolucency.*
3. *Longitudinally fibrillar or reticular areas of radiolucency.*
4. *Transverse radiolucencies, particularly of the metaphyses,* especially occurring in young growing bones.

This spectrum fades almost imperceptibly into the *sclerotic diseases* involving many bones, so that these will be categorized in the following chapter:

5. *Transverse sclerotic foci, especially of the metaphyses.*
6. *Horizontally fibrillar or reticular areas of sclerosis.*
7. *Sharply circumscribed areas of osteosclerosis or increased density.*
8. *Uniform increased bone density.*
9. *Cortico-periosteal, asymmetrical sclerosis.*

DIAGRAMMATIC REPRESENTATION OF RADIOGRAPHIC CATEGORIZATION OF BONE DISEASES

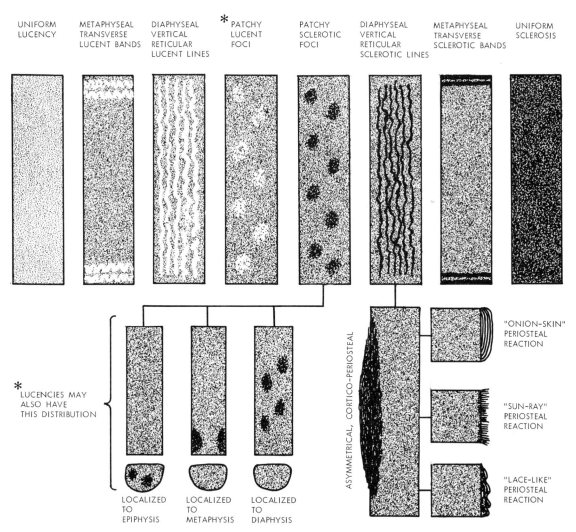

Figure 8–1 *(Continued).*

There is considerable overlap between the fourth and fifth "bands" in this spectrum, as well as the third and sixth. Indeed, the same diseases will be found in these categories in many instances.

Sharp lines of distinction cannot be drawn, and the student must recognize that these categories have been artificially created to facilitate the learning process.

A tenth category may be added called:

10. *"Hypertrophic" disease of bone.*

RADIOLUCENT BONE DISEASES OF MULTIPLE EXTREMITIES INVOLVING BONE DIFFUSELY

Polyostotic Diseases Characterized by Uniform Radiolucency (Figure 8–2).

The entities in this group may be classified as follows:

1. **Osteomalacia**

2. **Calcium Deposition Deficiency** related to the gastrointestinal diseases such as disturbances of the fat and carbohydrate metabolism

3. **Renal Rickets** (renal osteodystrophy; secondary hyperparathyroidism; renal osteitis fibrosis cystica)

4. **Fanconi's Syndrome**

5. **Protein Deficiency Osteopathy**

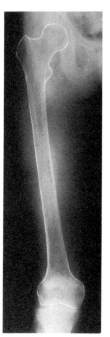

UNIFORM RADIOLUCENCY

1. OSTEOMALACIA

2. CALCIUM DEFICIENCY DUE TO INTESTINAL DISTURBANCES

3. RENAL RICKETS (RENAL OSTEODYSTROPHY) (SECONDARY HYPERPARATHYROIDISM)

4. FANCONI'S SYNDROME

5. PROTEIN DEFICIENCY OSTEOPATHY

6. ENDOCRINE OSTEOPATHY

7. RAYNAUD'S DISEASE

8. HYPOPHOSPHATEMIC-VITAMIN D REFRACTORY RICKETS

9. HYPERPARATHYROIDISM

Figure 8–2 Diseases characterized by uniform radiolucency.

6. **Endocrinosteopathies** producing generalized radiolucency:

   a. Pituitary dwarfism
   b. Hyperthyroidism
   c. Cretinism
   d. Primary and secondary hyperparathyroidism
   e. Cushing's syndrome and bone appearances following steroid therapy

7. **Raynaud's Disease**

8. **Hypophosphatemic and Vitamin D Refractory Rickets**

9. **Primary Hyperparathyroidism** (plus or minus adenoma)

The radiolucency in these disease entities may be due to:

1. *Insufficient osteoid matrix,* upon which the calcium salts may be laid;
2. *Insufficient calcium salts;*
3. *Active osteoclastic activity* which has removed both the mineral as well as the osteoid component of bone, transforming much of the compact bone to a cancellous variety. New osteoid may be deposited around the old cannibalized trabeculae, but these may remain unossified due to a deficiency of any of the following: vitamin D; calcium; phosphorus in the diet; disturbances of absorption of calcium or vitamin D; or excessive serum phosphorus loss from the kidneys.

Because of loss of substance, the *bones become very waxlike* and subject to grotesque deformities, with occasional infractions or fractures. When fractures occur, the callus is present without calcification, and the process may be extremely painful.

In the *spine* there is a *tendency toward concave indentation* of the superior and inferior end-plates, producing what are called fishlike vertebrae and kyphoscoliotic deformities.

At times translucent transverse zones (called *Looser's or umbau zones*) occur which actually represent pathologic healing of small infractions in the bones throughout the weight-bearing portion of the body. When these are widely distributed the condition is referred to as *Milkman's syndrome.*

Renal Rickets (Figure 8–3)

Clinical Features. In the presence of markedly damaged kidneys, which are unable to excrete phosphate, there is also thought to be a deficient formation of ammonia-base in the renal tubules. The calcium ions are used as alkali and a depletion of calcium results, bringing about acidosis, hyperphosphatemia, stimulation of the parathyroid glands, and a *secondary hyperparathyroidism.* The bones are called upon to supply calcium as a base, and *growing bone is deprived of its calcium at the epiphyseal plate.* Available dietary calcium is utilized to combine with excess phosphate excreted in the gastrointestinal tract.

Radiographic Findings (Figure 8–3)

A **frayed appearance of the metaphysis** adjoining the epiphyseal plate, in the child or adolescent.

Increased radiolucency of the bones, generally with thinness of the cortex, and some bending or fracturing in the bone.

Subcortical erosion of the phalanges and pointing of the tufted ends of the distal phalanges.

Ectopic calcium deposition in all tissues where chloride or carbon dioxide ions are found in relative abundance, such as the lung alveoli, renal tubules,

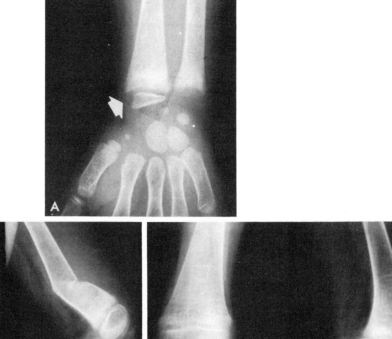

Figure 8–3   Renal rickets. *A*. P-A view of the wrist and hand demonstrating the great similarity of this process to avitaminosis D. *B*. A-P and lateral views of the right knee showing a diffuse osteoporosis as well as a pathologic fracture in the distal shaft of the femur. Note the typical frayed appearance in the distal metaphysis of the femur. *C*. Somewhat similar appearance of the left knee, although a pathologic fracture is not present. Note the marked anterior bowing, however, of the distal shaft of the femur (called "renal osteitis fibrosa cystica" by Albright and Reifenstein).

gastric mucosa, media of the medium-sized arteries throughout the body, and interstitially everywhere. In the kidney there is a characteristic **nephrocalcinosis** with calcium deposit in the renal pyramids (see section on primary hyperparathyroidism).

In some bones there are **circumscribed areas of lucency** suggesting "cystic" or "pseudocystic" appearances in the bone. (Osteitis fibrosa cystica with its so-called "brown tumors.")

Endocrine Osteopathies Producing Generalized Radiolucency.   The hormones, in general, exert the following influences on the skeletal system: (1) determination of the rate of growth of the long bones; (2) the maturation of bones; (3) the time of closure of the epiphyseal plate. This establishes the absolute overall length of the bone, growth and thickness of the bone, and mobilization of the calcium salts from the bones to the blood and vice versa.

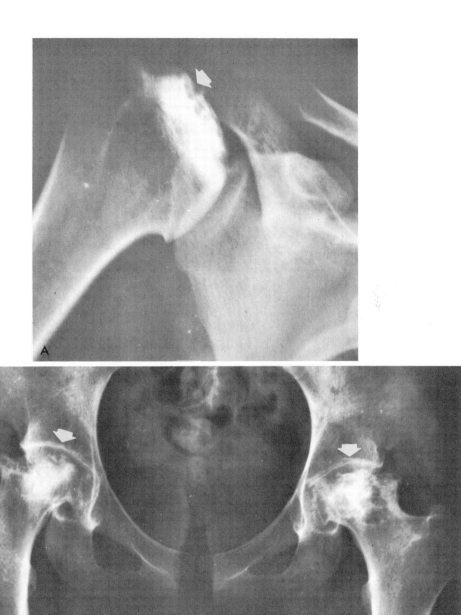

Figure 8–4   Aseptic necrosis resulting from steroid therapy, along with severe osteoporosis. *A*. Head of humerus. *B*. Head of femora.

THE ROENTGENOGRAPHIC MANIFESTATION OF CUSHING'S SYNDROME IN INFANCY (Darling et al.)

1. Atrophy of thymus.
2. Excessive deposits of fat.
3. Atrophy of muscles in the extremities.
4. Osteoporosis.
5. Retarded bone maturation.
6. Possible changes in the adrenal gland as revealed by: excretory urography; selective angiography; retroperitoneal air insufflation.

The radiolucent skeletal diseases which have their origin in disturbances in various endocrine glands are:

1. *Pituitary dwarfism;*
2. *Hypothyroidism (cretinism);*
3. *Primary hyperparathyroidism;*
4. *Secondary hyperparathyroidism;*
5. *Adult hypogonadism;*
6. *Pancreatic osteoporosis* in association with diabetes mellitus;
7. *Diabetic dwarfism;*
8. *Steroid therapy* may result in severe *skeletal osteoporosis, pathological fracture* and abnormal callus formation. The skull, ribs, pelvis, and vertebrae may be particularly affected. Pathological fracture, however, with the appearance of *aseptic necrosis* occurs especially in the heads of the femora and humeri (Figure 8–4).

Hyperparathyroidism (Figure 8–5).   In hyperparathyroidism arising from either parathyroid adenoma or hyperplasia, there is an excessive excretion of calcium and phosphate in the urine associated with high calcium and low phosphate levels in the blood. The increased calcium requirements of the blood may or may not call upon the bones for satiation; thus, *not all cases of hyperparathyroidism are associated with changes in the bones.* If the exogenous supply of calcium is deficient, the bones of the body may show any degree of change, from osteoporosis to marked osteitis fibrosis cystica, and the appearances are those already described under secondary hyperparathyroidism and illustrated in Figure 8–5.

Hypophosphatemic-Vitamin D Refractory Rickets.   There are six types of this disorder identified:

1. Vitamin D resistant rickets;
2. Aminoaciduria;
3. Rickets with aminoaciduria and acidosis (Fanconi's syndrome);
4. Rickets with cystine storage disease;
5. Rickets with hyperglycinuria;
6. Lowe's diseases (oculocerebrorenal syndrome); rickets with mental retardation and glaucoma.

The cause of the reabsorption defect varies. In some patients it may be due to a congenital enzymatic deficiency. In others it may be due to a congenital malforma-

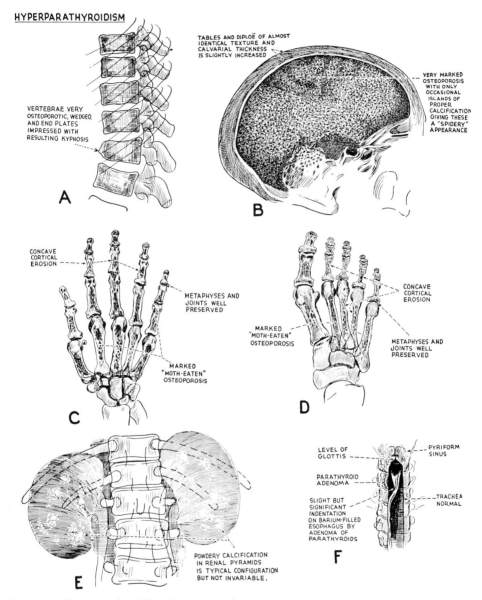

HYPERPARATHYROIDISM

TABLES AND DIPLOË OF ALMOST
IDENTICAL TEXTURE AND
CALVARIAL THICKNESS
IS SLIGHTLY INCREASED

VERY MARKED
OSTEOPOROSIS
WITH ONLY
OCCASIONAL
ISLANDS OF
PROPER
CALCIFICATION
GIVING THESE
A "SPIDERY"
APPEARANCE

VERTEBRAE VERY
OSTEOPOROTIC, WEDGED,
AND END PLATES
IMPRESSED WITH
RESULTING KYPHOSIS

A

B

CONCAVE
CORTICAL
EROSION

METAPHYSES AND
JOINTS WELL
PRESERVED

MARKED
"MOTH-EATEN"
OSTEOPOROSIS

C

CONCAVE
CORTICAL
EROSION

MARKED
"MOTH-EATEN"
OSTEOPOROSIS

METAPHYSES AND
JOINTS WELL
PRESERVED

D

LEVEL OF
GLOTTIS

PYRIFORM
SINUS

PARATHYROID
ADENOMA

SLIGHT BUT
SIGNIFICANT
INDENTATION
ON BARIUM-FILLED
ESOPHAGUS BY
ADENOMA OF
PARATHYROIDS

TRACHEA
NORMAL

F

POWDERY CALCIFICATION
IN RENAL PYRAMIDS
IS TYPICAL CONFIGURATION
BUT NOT INVARIABLE.

E

Figure 8–5 Hyperparathyroidism due to a parathyroid adenoma. *A* to *F*. Labeled tracings of the spine, skull, hand, foot, kidney areas, and neck region respectively in patient with a parathyroid adenoma. Note the extremely slight displacement of the esophagus by the adenoma. Note also the powdery calcification in the renal pyramids rather typical of the type of nephrocalcinosis which occurs in this condition.

Figure 8–5 *continued on following page.*

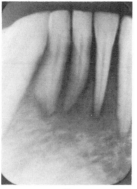

G

Figure 8–5 *(Continued).* *G.* Loss of lamina dura in the alveolar ridges adjoining the teeth. *H* and *I.* Cortico-periosteal erosion of middle phalanges especially with diffuse hyperlucency of bones. *J.* Esophagram prior to removal of parathyroid adenoma, demonstrating indentation by the adenoma—absent after removal of the tumor in *K.*

Figure 8–5 *continued on opposite page.*

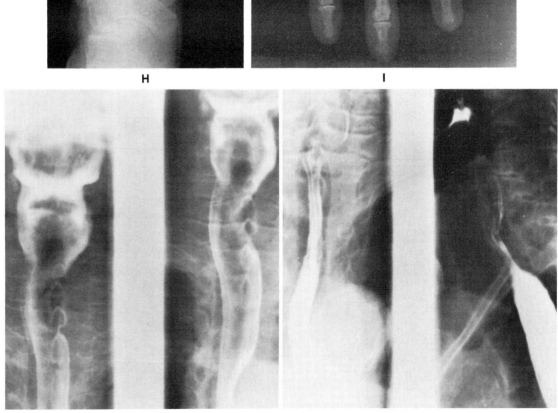

H

I

J

K

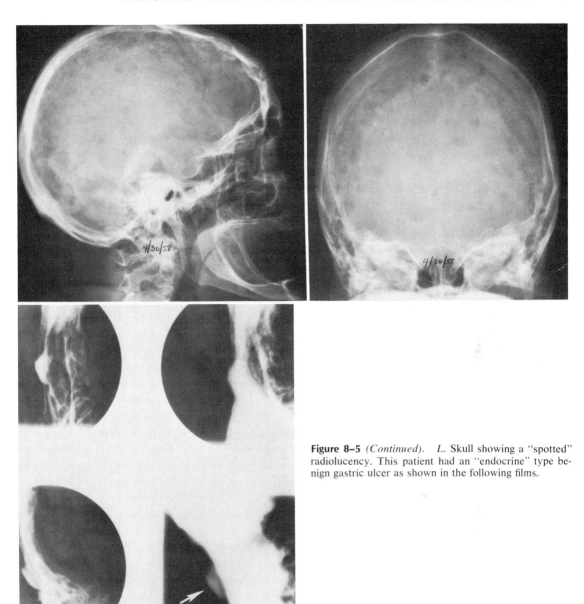

L

Figure 8–5 *(Continued). L.* Skull showing a "spotted" radiolucency. This patient had an "endocrine" type benign gastric ulcer as shown in the following films.

Figure 8–5 *continued on following page.*

tion of the proximal tubules. In still others it may be related to toxic agents acting upon the tubule lining cell.

The **radiographic manifestations** are those of rickets of any cause since the underlying bony disturbance is that of poor mineralization of osteoid. These patients, however, are usually older and the deformity of bones is a prominent feature. It includes: (1) generalized radiolucency; (2) coarsening of the trabecular pattern; (3) the formation of transverse Looser's zones; and (4) widening of the bulbous ends of some of the bones, particularly the femur.

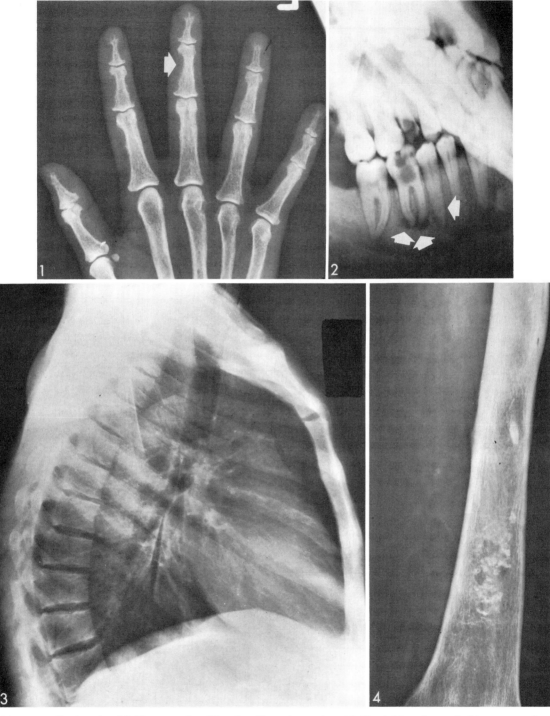

Figure 8–5 *(Continued).*   *M.* Hyperparathyroidism in still another patient. (1) Hand. Note the cortical bony resorption, particularly of the middle phalanges of the fingers. In this instance, there is also advanced resorption of the cortices of other phalanges as well. (2) Mandible. The single arrow indicates the area of resorption of the lamina dura. The double arrow may represent periapical abscess formation rather than a focus of osteitis fibrosa cystica. Note the marked crown decay in this tooth also. (3) Thoracic spine and (4) femur demonstrate the occasional sclerotic appearance in bone in association with hyperparathyroidism. Here the trabeculae appear coarsened. The clavicle is an area where such coarsening is very apt to appear.

DISEASES CAUSING MULTIPLE AREAS OF CIRCUMSCRIBED, PATCHY RADIOLUCENCY, WITH NO SCLEROTIC MARGIN

Some diseases included in this group are listed and partially illustrated in Figure 8–6. We shall limit our discussion to just a few of these entities.

Of the entities mentioned, the most frequent in this category are:

1. Metastatic bone tumors, including multiple myeloma;
2. The histiocytoses or reticuloendothelioses, including the lipoid storage diseases even though the latter are not related;

CIRCUMSCRIBED MULTIPLE AREAS OF RADIOLUCENCY

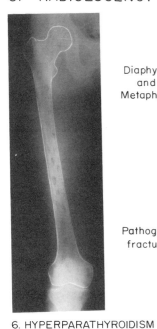

Diaphysis
and
Metaphysis

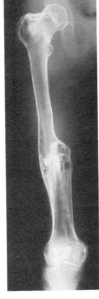

Pathogenic
fracture

6. HYPERPARATHYROIDISM
   (may be confined to
   "moth eaten" appearance
   of epiphysis)

7. POLYOSTOTIC
   FIBROUS
   DYSPLASIA

I. ACUTE DISSEMINATED INFECTIONS OF BONE—OSTEOMYELITIS
2. YEAST AND FUNGUS INFECTIONS OF BONE LESS NUMEROUS THAN ACTINOMYCOSIS. AFFECTS JAWS AND RIBS. BLASTO-MYCOSIS GENERALIZED
3. NEUROFIBROMATOSIS WITH BONY INVOLVE-MENT. BONE IS INVADED FROM WITHOUT IN RIB CAGE PARTICULARLY
4. METASTATIC BONE TUMORS—INTERMEDIATE NUMERICALLY BETWEEN I AND 2
5. LIPOID GRANULOMATOSES AND HISTIO-CYTOSES, OR RETICULOSES
8. OXALOSIS
9. "ROUND CELL" TUMORS
   A—MULTIPLE MYELOMA
   B—EWING'S TUMOR
   C—NEUROBLASTOMA
   D—RETICULUM CELL SARCOMA

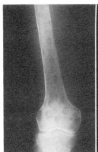

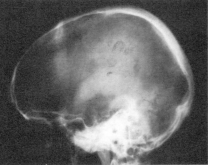

9. MULTIPLE MYELOMA—DISCRETE PUNCHED OUT AREAS—NO REACTIVE SCLEROSIS

Figure 8–6 Diseases causing multiple areas of circumscribed radiolucency. (Intensified.)

3. Hyperparathyroidism with osteitis fibrosa cystica;
4. Widely disseminated inflammatory diseases of bone, both acute and chronic.

Metastatic Bone Tumors

Radiographic Findings. Metastatic osteolytic bone tumors have a variable appearance radiographically, ranging from only a **fine granularity** of the bones **to well-defined areas of osteolysis** in many bones of the body.

General Comment. The greater proportion of bone tumors after the third decade of life are metastatic carcinomas. The most common metastatic lesions come from the breast, lung, prostate, thyroid, and kidney. (Prostatic carcinoma usually produces sclerotic metastases—see Chapter 10.) In an adult male, carcinoma of the lung, and in an adult female, carcinoma of the breast (in at least one-half of the cases) stand high on the list. Carcinoma of the kidneys is responsible for metastases in about 20 to 30 per cent of the cases of metastatic tumors to bone; and the thyroid is responsible for about 25 per cent of cases.

Extraintestinal malignancies are responsible for the majority of metastases to bone (Edeiken and Hodes); of all metastases from extraintestinal malignancies, about 25 per cent are metastases to bone.

In a child, the most probable cause of osteolytic metastases is neuroblastoma.

About two-thirds of all patients with malignancies show metastases when first seen clinically. Of these the distribution of metastases is as follows: lymph nodes, one-half; liver, one-third; lungs, one-fifth; bone, one-tenth.

The lytic metastases from carcinoma of the kidney and thyroid often produce a somewhat "bubbly" appearance roentgenographically (Greenfield).

Distribution of Metastases in the Skeleton, considering multiple foci of involvement, is as follows: (1) spine, 80 per cent; (2) femur, 40 per cent; (3) ribs and sternum, 25 per cent; (4) skull and pelvis, 20 per cent; (5) upper shoulder girdles, 7 per cent; and (6) other extremity bones, 1 to 2 per cent.

Metastases distal to the elbows and knees are rare but do occur (Figure 8–7) (Mulvey).

Metastatic Bone Tumors Which May Evoke a Periosteal Response (Norman and Ulin). Approximately 37 per cent of metastatic solitary bone lesions evoke a periosteal reaction, whereas 78 per cent of primary bone tumors elicit this response.

The metastatic bone tumors which are most apt to react in this manner include neuroblastoma and tumors that arise in the colon and prostate. Only about one-third of the metastases from lung carcinoma and 20 per cent from kidney carcinoma produce a periosteal reaction. Metastases from prostatic carcinoma are usually osteoblastic (Chapter 10), with dense periosteal new bone formation.

By comparison, some primary osseous tumors which elicit a periosteal response are: Ewing's sarcoma, 100 per cent; fibrosarcoma, 100 per cent; osteogenic sarcoma, 91 per cent; reticulum cell sarcoma, 85 per cent; chondrosarcoma, 50 per cent; and the malignant lymphomas, only 20 per cent.

Multiple Myeloma (Plasma Cell Myeloma, Myelocytoma, Erythroblastoma, Lymphocytoma) (Figure 8–8)

Clinical Features. Multiple myeloma, or plasma cell myeloma, accounts for about one-third of all primary bone malignancies. It is thus the most common of all malignant primary bone tumors, and may appear as an isolated entity, but usually there are multiple foci. Predominant affection occurs in the skull, spine, pelvis,

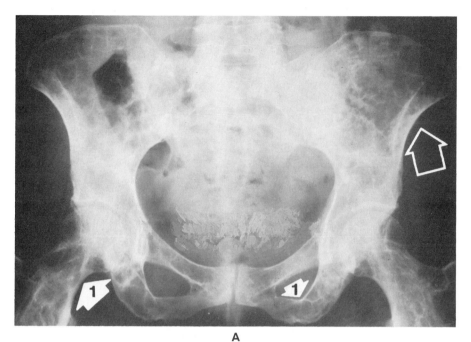

A

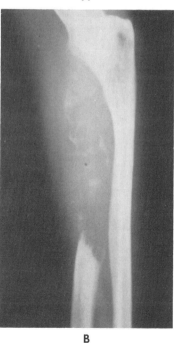

B

Figure 8–7   *A*. Pelvis in a patient with metastases from a carcinoma of the breast. The open arrow points to a lytic lesion in the left iliac bone. The large arrow (1) points to large lytic lesions extending into the neck and upper shaft of the right femur, and the small arrow (1) points to lytic metastases in the left pubis and ischium. *B*. Hodgkin's disease affecting the shafts of the radius.

MULTIPLE MYELOMA

(PLASMA CELL, MYELOCYTOMA, ERYTHROBLASTOMA, and LYMPHOCYTOMA)

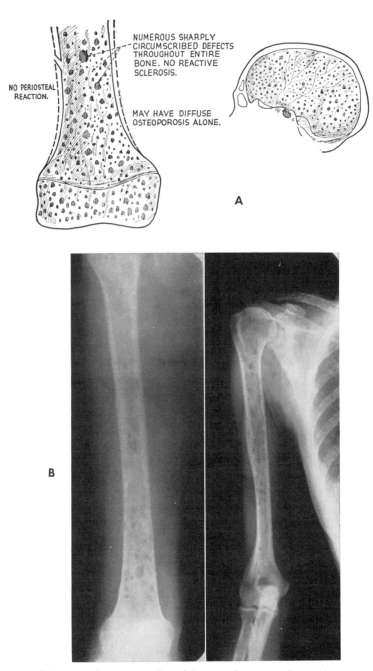

Figure 8–8 *A*. Diagrammatic representation of the most frequent radiographic appearances in the long bones and the skull. *B*. Antero-posterior view of the arm showing the "punched out" lesions in the humerus.

Figure 8–8 *continued on opposite page.*

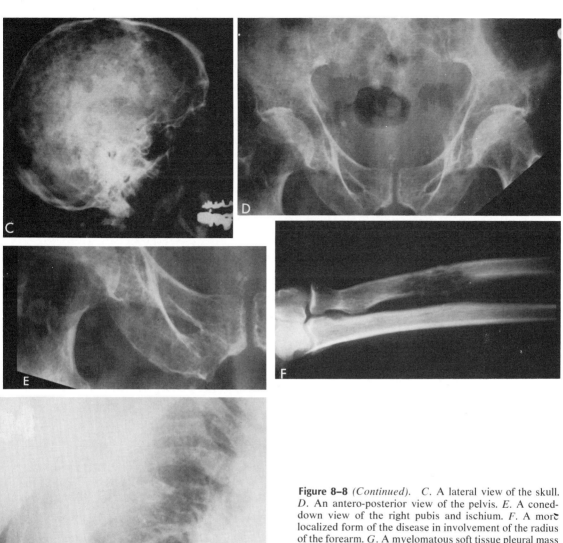

Figure 8–8 *(Continued). C.* A lateral view of the skull. *D.* An antero-posterior view of the pelvis. *E.* A coned-down view of the right pubis and ischium. *F.* A more localized form of the disease in involvement of the radius of the forearm. *G.* A myelomatous soft tissue pleural mass contiguous with involvement of the ribs in the chest wall.

femora, humeri, ribs, and sternum. Myelomatous foci seldom occur beyond the elbow or knee. Pathological fractures at the sites of involvement are frequent.

Radiographic Findings

Numerous sharply circumscribed defects throughout the bone with no reactive marginal sclerosis.

There may also be a diffuse osteoporosis with no particular punched-out area. Usually there is no periosteal reaction.

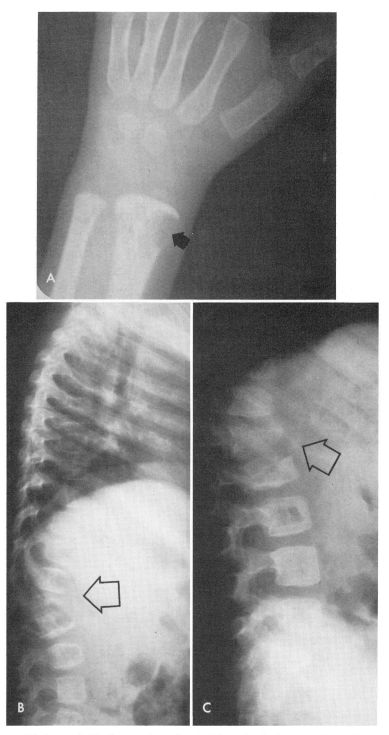

Figure 8–9 *A*. Histiocytosis X affecting the radius. *B*. The spine in Letterer-Siwe's disease. *C*. Same patient with magnified view of the upper lumbar vertebrae demonstrating the circumscribed lytic process coupled with irregular collapse of involved vertebrae. There is a tendency to diffuse flattening of vertebral bodies so involved.

Figure 8–9 *continued on opposite page.*

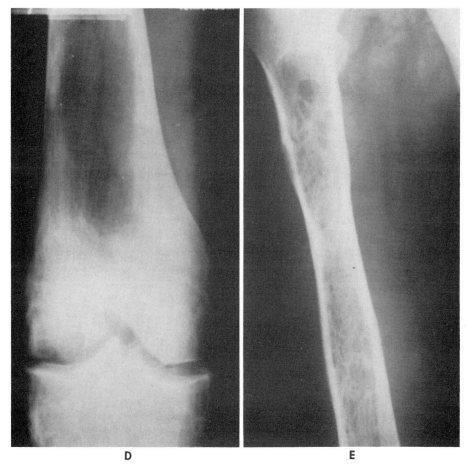

D   **E**

Figure 8–9 *(Continued).*   *D* and *E*. Views of long bones in a patient with Gaucher's disease.

Some cases show no radiographic changes.

In the flat bones of the pelvis and occasionally in the ribs or sternum, the plasmocytoma may appear as an expanding radiolucent lesion with a thin coating of compact bone surrounding the lesion. Incomplete trabeculae may traverse the lesion.

The radiographic differential diagnosis must always include metastatic carcinosis and hyperparathyroidism, and often these entities are indistinguishable.

Reticuloendothelioses, Reticuloses, or Histiocytosis (the Lipid Granulomatoses) (Figure 8–9)

General Clinical Considerations.   This group of diseases is basically due to histiocytic proliferation with lipid deposits in the sites of histiocytosis. The Hand-Schüller-Christian complex is probably an inflammatory histiocytic proliferation, with the *secondary* accumulation of cholesterol in many instances, whereas Niemann-Pick disease is due to a true metabolic defect in sphingomyelin, and Gaucher's disease to a defect in kerasin.

The Hand-Schüller-Christian complex consists of: Letterer-Siwe disease, Hand-

Schüller-Christian disease, and eosinophilic granuloma (Robbins), perhaps all part of a continuous spectrum, with rapid proliferation in the very young (Letterer-Siwe disease), and slower and focal proliferation in older persons (eosinophilic granuloma).

Any organ containing reticuloendothelial tissue may be affected. *Letterer-Siwe disease* affects the skin, lymph nodes, liver, and spleen especially, but the bones may be affected early. In *Hand-Schüller-Christian disease,* there is a much more chronic affection of the soft tissues and bones in infants or adults. When the skull is affected (as it is in about half the cases, especially at the base of the skull and orbit) diabetes insipidus and exophthalmos are also present. *Bone lesions are present in about 80 per cent of the cases.* With *eosinophilic granuloma,* the bones of the skull are often first affected, but any bone may become involved. Lymph node involvement, skin infiltration, and splenohepatomegaly are rare.

Niemann-Pick disease is a rare, familial disease, with a usual (although not invariable) onset in infancy, and it is characterized by early involvement of the central nervous system, spleen, and liver. Since any organ may be affected, the bones are almost invariably involved, usually in a diffuse fashion rather than focally as in the other diseases in this group.

Gaucher's disease is also characterized by splenohepatomegaly, pigmentations of the skin, thickening of the sclerae of the eye, and pulmonary and bone involvement. The abnormal histiocytic cells are rich in acid phosphatase, producing elevated serum levels of this enzyme (similar to carcinoma of the prostate).

Radiographic Findings

IN THE HAND-SCHÜLLER-CHRISTIAN COMPLEX—consisting of histiocytosis X, Letterer-Siwe disease, Hand-Schüller-Christian disease, and eosinophilic granuloma—radiographic findings are similar where osseous changes occur.

In Letterer-Siwe disease bone lesions are absent when the disease is first recognized, but may appear in the course of several months.

The roentgenologic features of the Hand-Schüller-Christian complex may be summarized as follows:

1. The bone defects are sharply demarcated, large, and "map-like" (Figure 8–9), especially in the skull. Both the inner and outer tables of the cranial vault seem to be equally affected, with no evidence of periosteal reaction, repair, or a sclerotic margin.

2. In particular, the mandible (in the infant) is frequently involved, producing the "floating tooth" appearance (Figure 8–9).

3. Pathologic fractures are frequent. Collapsed vertebrae (vertebra plana) may assume a sclerotic pattern.

4. Bone lesions may be absent from about 20 per cent of cases of Hand-Schüller-Christian disease. The exophthalmos and diabetes insipidus, when they occur in about half of these cases, are associated with bony lesions in the skull and orbit (forming the "classic triad" of this disease).

NIEMANN-PICK DISEASE differs from Hand-Schüller-Christian disease in that it is a constitutional metabolic defect in the metabolism of sphingomyelin (complex lipid). In it, the bones are involved in a diffuse fashion, unlike the focal characteristics of the Hand-Schüller-Christian complex or Gaucher's disease. The marrow may be virtually completely replaced by the lipophages characteristic of this disease. The dominant changes occur in all of the reticuloendothelial organs of the body.

GAUCHER'S DISEASE

In the infant, this condition may be indistinguishable from Letterer-Siwe disease, although it differs from the latter by its constitutional metabolic defect in kerasin compounds.

When the long bones are affected (Figure 8–9) there is often a metaphyseal expansion of the bone, giving it an Erlenmeyer-flask contour, around a large lytic focus.

These lytic foci may have a thin sclerotic margin, or even a periosteal reaction.

The trabecular texture of the pelvis may be altered, with a tendency to sclerotic change in the vicinity of the pubis and sacroiliac joints.

With ischemic necrosis of the femoral heads, a mixed lysis and sclerosis may ensue.

The most frequent sites of bone involvement are: femora; spine; hips; shoulders; tubular bones generally; and pelvis. The bones of the thoracic cage and skull are also often involved (Greenfield).

Widely Disseminated Osteomyelitis, Acute or Chronic (Figure 8–10).

Ordinarily acute hematogenous osteomyelitis occurs at one site, but occasionally there are multiple foci of involvement, especially when there is a deficient immune mechanism. The usual location is in the metaphysis of a long bone. The lower femur and upper tibia are involved most frequently.

Radiographic Findings. **The radiographic appearance may not become manifest for as long as two to three weeks.** The usual sequence is as follows (Figure 8–10, B, C, and D):

1. Soft tissue swelling;
2. Periosteal reaction;
3. Bone destruction in a small nidus near the metaphysis that progresses to involve the diaphysis diffusely but does not cross the epiphyseal plate prior to closure of the plate. (In adults this may not be true.)
4. Sequestration; accompanied usually by
5. Involucrum formation.

Since the advent of antibiotic therapy, sequestration may not occur, particularly if therapy is instituted early in the course of the disease.

Usually the destructive process does not cross the epiphyseal line into the epiphysis prior to closure of the epiphyseal plate, and any extension to a joint is usually secondary to soft tissue involvement and perforation of the joint capsule. However, if a destructive process does involve a joint, it is most apt to be infectious in origin. It is very exceptional for a bone sequestrum to develop in an epiphyseal focus. **Indeed, this failure to cross the epiphyseal plate prior to its closure is an important differential feature, differentiating osteomyelitis from malignant neoplasia of bone.** Extension of osteomyelitis into an adjoining joint is more likely in young infants and adults.

When sequestration occurs, the dead bone gradually becomes separated from the surrounding vitalized bone and is therefore surrounded by a pool of exudate. The dead bone is called a **sequestrum** and can be **recognized radiographically** by its retention of a **relatively normal or even increased density,** whereas all the surrounding bone has become markedly osteoporotic. The exudate produces a lucency surrounding the sequestrum.

At the same time that the dead bone is forming a sequestrum through demarcation, there is a simultaneous effort on the part of the bone for **regranu-**

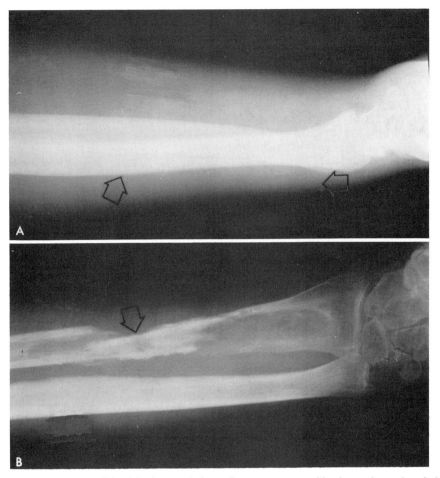

Figure 8–10   *A*. Osteomyelitis of the forearm in its earliest roentgenographic phase when only soft tissue swelling and periosteal elevation are noted. *B*. Osteomyelitis in a late phase demonstrating marked destruction and sequestration formation (arrow).

Figure 8–10 *continued on opposite page.*

lation of the diseased area, which in turn gives rise to the so-called **"involucrum" formation.**

With the removal or resorption of the sequestrum, healing may proceed slowly but very often a disturbance of the trabecular pattern remains as permanent evidence of the prior existence of this disorder.

GENERAL COMMENT.   Certain mycotic infections also would appear to have a predilection for bone, producing chronic granulomatous infections. For example, actinomycosis is particularly apt to occur either in the mandible or in the ribs. Blastomycosis may occur anywhere, even peripherally in the bones of the tarsus or the ankle (Figure 8–11). Usually the lesions involve the cortex but they demonstrate a sharply demarcated contour and, *unlike the metastatic malignancies and reticuloendothelioses, a zone of sclerosis surrounding the inflammatory process can usually be differentiated.* Usually associated with it is evidence of fungus disease elsewhere in the body, swelling of the adjoining soft tissues, draining sinuses, and parenchymal involvement of the lungs.

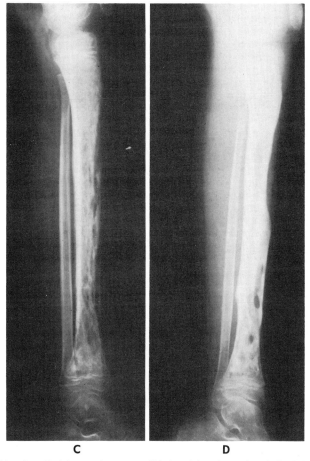

Figure 8–10 *(Continued)*. *C*. Advanced osteomyelitis involving the entire shaft of the tibia before treatment with Chloromycetin. *D*. Same leg in this patient approximately three months after Chloromycetin therapy showing spontaneous reossification with removal of sequestrae.

Fibrous Dysplasia of Jaffe-Lichtenstein and Albright Syndrome (Figure 8–12)

General Comment. This is an intramedullary replacement process of bone, with a proliferation of abnormal fibrous tissue. The disease may be monostotic or polyostotic.

Histopathologically, the main feature is a fibro-osseous metaplasia.

Pigmented nonelevated skin patches occur in about one-third of the cases, on the trunk, scalp, neck, or thigh on the same side as the bone lesion. They have a geographic outline varying from a few millimeters in diameter to ten or more centimeters. They have a chestnut color (Gorlin et al.).

Endocrine disturbances or skin manifestations rarely accompany solitary lesions; the endocrine dysfunction, when it occurs, almost invariably occurs in females. There is a precocious menstruation in about 20 per cent of cases, and the menarche appears early. The menses are irregular in amount and periodicity until puberty. Precocious skeletal growth is also reported, with premature closure of the epiphyseal centers. Although serum phosphatase may be elevated, the serum values for calcium and phosphorus are normal, as are the urinary 17-ketosteroid values.

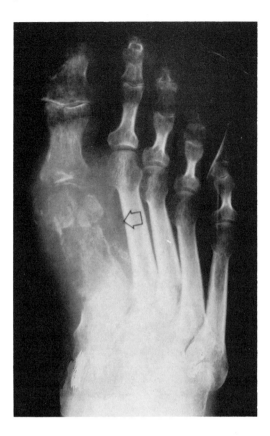

Figure 8–11   Blastomycosis involving the first metatarsal and great toe of the right foot. Note the calcification of the blood vessels of this foot as well.

POLYOSTOTIC FIBROUS DYSPLASIA
(JAFFE -LICHTENSTEIN-ALBRIGHT)

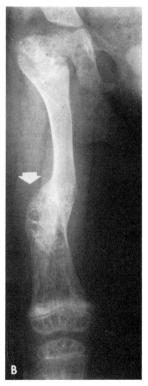

DIAPHYSIS AND METAPHYSIS OCCUPIED BY LARGE FIBROUS AREAS SIMULATING FIBROCYSTIC DISEASE. -USUALLY UNILATERAL. -MAY BE MONOSTOTIC.

A

B

Figure 8–12   *A*. Salient radiographic findings in polyostotic fibrous dysplasia. *B*. Representative radiograph of a femur affected by polyostotic fibrous dysplasia, showing an area of healed pathologic fracture in the midshaft of the femur.

Roentgenologic Features

Sites of predilection: none usually; there is a slight predilection for long bones of extremities in the cases with endocrine involvement.

The lesions are lucent and covered by a thin shell of bone, or irregularly radiopaque.

The cortex appears to be eroded from within, while the periosteum **appears to lay down a new shell of normal bone on the outer surface** as the process expands the bone from within.

Protrusions from the normal contours of the bone are common. When the orbit is involved, exophthalmos results.

In serial roentgenograms, there is a tendency toward distal progress of the lesions.

The process within the shaft of the bone appears "pseudocystic" with multilocular "cavities" surrounded by thin sclerotic margins. The lytic foci do not re-ossify (Schlumberger, Albright, et al.; Lichtenstein and Jaffe; McIntosh et al.).

DISEASES CAUSING MULTIPLE "RETICULAR" OR "FIBRILLAR" AREAS OF OSTEOPOROSIS WITH COARSENING OF THE TRABECULAE (Figure 8–13).
(For irregular mosaic admixture of lucency and sclerosis as found in osteitis deformans or Paget's disease of bone, see Chapter 10.)

The *hemolytic anemias*, anemias due to marrow hypofunction, and the bone changes resulting from leukemic and lymphomatous infiltration of bone all have certain changes in common in their radiographic appearances (Figure 8–13).

The *hemolytic anemias* may be classified as follows (modified from Robbins):
1. Anemia due to a defect inherent in the red cells.
    a. Hereditary spherocytosis (Congenital hemolytic anemia).
    b. Thalassemia (Mediterranean anemia; Cooley's anemia).
    c. Sickle cell anemia, hemoglobin S disease.
    d. Other hemoglobinopathies.
    e. Paroxysmal nocturnal hemoglobinuria.
2. Anemia due to a defect extrinsic to the red cells.
    a. Erythroblastosis fetalis.
    b. Autoimmune hemolytic disease.
    c. Acquired hemolytic anemia due to toxic, bacterial, and physical agents.
3. Anemias due to defects both intrinsic and extrinsic to red cells.
    a. Lead poisoning.
    b. Vitamin B deficiency.
    c. Glucose-6-phosphate dehydrogenase deficiency.

Hereditary Spherocytosis is characterized especially by a markedly enlarged spleen. Expansion of the erythropoietic marrow may cause *resorption of the inner layers of cortical bone* with *new appositional growth on the outer layers,* and an irregular outer layer may form subperiosteally. In the skull perpendicular rays of increased density form, giving the "hair-on-end" appearance. Cholelithiasis occurs in 50 to 85 per cent of the cases.

MULTIPLE "RETICULAR" OR "FIBRILLAR"
AREAS OF OSTEOPOROSIS WITH
COARSENING OF TRABECULAE

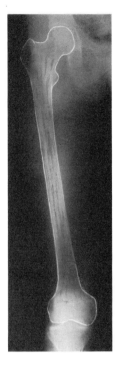

I. HEMOLYTIC ANEMIAS
    A—THALASSEMIA
    B—SPHEROCYTIC ANEMIA
    C—SICKLE CELL ANEMIA

2. LEUKEMIAS, LYMPHOMAS

3. CHRONIC POISONING, OR
    HORMONAL EFFECT

Figure 8–13 (Intensified diagrammatic radiograph.)

Sickle Cell Anemia is characterized by packing of sickle-shaped red cells into vessels, causing *vascular stasis* and tissue anoxia. Although 8 to 11 per cent of Negroes in the United States carry the sickle cell trait, only two and a half per cent of these are homozygous for hemoglobin S and have sickle cell anemia (Robbins). *Radiographically* the manifestations in bone resemble those of hereditary spherocytosis due to expansion of the red marrow. In the early phase of the disease the spleen is enlarged, but in older individuals erythroblastosis leads to thrombosis and infarction with progressive shrinkage of the spleen, ultimately resulting in an autosplenectomy. *Infarctions* may also occur in the liver, brain, kidney, bone marrow, and lungs. *Pigment gallstones* may form in some patients. Leg ulcers are especially frequent in adults.

SICKLE CELL ANEMIA IN CHILDHOOD

1. Coarse osseous trabeculations and demineralization, 48 per cent. Increases with age.

2. Vertebral end-plate deformity ("fish" vertebra), 18 per cent. The indented nucleus pulposus has a rectangular appearance in many cases. Increases with age in older children.

3. Splenomegaly, 32 per cent. Decreases with age in childhood.

4. Hepatomegaly, most marked in three to six year old group in children, 25 per cent.

5. Cardiomegaly, 77 per cent, same in all age groups in children.

6. Pneumonia, 42 per cent. No significant difference in ages.

7. Pleural reaction, 13 per cent. Increases with age in childhood.

8. Hilar congestion, 55 per cent. Slightly increases in children three to 12 years of age.

9. Anterior vertebral vascular notches, increased in all age groups.

10. Caliectasis and poor renal function frequent in younger individuals and adults (Margulies and Minkin).

Thalassemia Major is a homozygous genetic defect characterized by marked anemia in infants and children. There is a decreased synthesis of hemoglobin A. The major morphologic alterations occur in the bone marrow and spleen. The expansion of the bone marrow results in much the *same appearance previously described for the other hemolytic anemias*—not only in the skull but in the long bones and face. *Splenomegaly* is usually very marked. Thalassemia minor is a heterozygous form of the disease and is usually asymptomatic.

Iron Deficiency Anemias are usually accompanied by hyperplastic marrow. In the skull, there is a widening of the diploic space and atrophy of the outer table. There may be radial striations running perpendicular to the outer table, resembling Cooley's anemia in infants and children (Chapter 12).

In 164 cases (147 fully verified) studied by Agarwal et al., the **roentgenologic changes** were described as follows:

In all cases mild to moderate osteoporosis was observed;

In 8 per cent there were findings of rickets;

In the skull the changes consisted of atrophy, osteoporosis, and thinning of the cortex;

In 90 per cent of the cases there was an osteoporosis and thinning of the cortex of the bones of the hand. Atrophy of the spongiosa of the small bones of the hands was noted in at least 50 per cent of the patients.

Two additional features of the iron deficiency anemias are atrophic glossitis and esophageal webs (a shelflike anterior partition or ridge in the upper esophagus: see Chapter 27).

Aplastic Anemias are attributed to bone marrow failure with a pancytopenia. Although usually the marrow is acellular with an increase in the amount of fat, the marrow may be hypercellular or even normocellular. The marrow may become diffusely infiltrated with lymphocytes and plasma cells. Thrombocytopenia with bleeding tendencies and granulocytopenia with superimposed infections may ensue.

Myelophthisic Anemias result from destruction or depression of marrow by metastatic cancer, especially from primary lesions of the breast, lung, prostate, thyroid, or adrenals. Multiple myeloma, leukemia, the lymphomas, and reticuloendothelioses may also be implicated. Myelofibrosis may result, and with it a tendency to *increased density of the bones*. Similar increased density of some bones (*especially clavicles*) may result from anemias secondary to renal disease as well.

Erythroblastosis Fetalis Is Not Related to Thalassemia and is a hemolytic disease of the newborn due to iso-immunization of an Rh-negative pregnant woman by Rh-positive fetal erythrocytes. The maternal antiagglutinins cross the placenta to the fetal circulation and hemolyze the vulnerable fetal red blood cells.

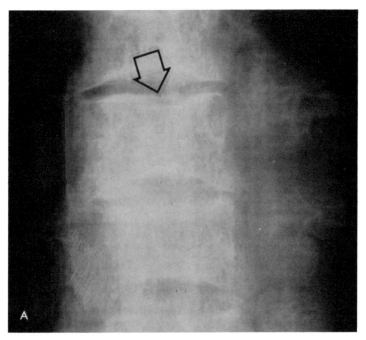

Figure 8–14   Sickle cell anemia. *A*. The vertebral body shows the squared-off appearance of the indented endplate thought to be due to infarction immediately beneath the nucleus pulposus involving the endplate and immediately adjoining the vertebral body.

Figure 8–14 *continued on opposite page.*

In most cases there are **no roentgen changes in the skeleton.** In some instances, however, endochondral bone formation is interfered with and transverse bands of increased and diminished density develop in the ends of the shaft. Other findings described are (1) diffuse sclerosis of the shaft; (2) an absence of the normal fetal kyphosis due to **enlargement of the liver and the spleen, ascites, and anasarca;** and (3) extension of the thighs and flexion of the knees, likewise due to the abdominal distention called the **"Buddha" attitude.**

Radiographic Findings in the Anemias with an Intrinsic Red Cell Defect.   Tracings of roentgenograms of fibulae in sickle cell anemia showing the spectrum of changes found in this disorder are well illustrated in Figure 8–14. Skull changes with the widened diploë, thin outer table and the "hair-on-end" appearance are illustrated in Chapter 12.

In the vertebral column there is a coarsening of the trabecular pattern of the vertebral body with progression to "fish" vertebrae, which is a sequel of disk invagination into the cancellous bone of the body. **In sickle cell anemia, (Figure 8–14) the indentation may be rectangular.**

Reynolds proposed that the spinal changes in sickle cell anemia were those of a growth disturbance, with a central depression in the vertebral endplate probably due to a relative ischemia of this area (Figure 8–14B). A similar change, however, has also been found in thalassemia major (Cassady et al.).

Absent, Hypoplastic or Supernumerary Thumb in the Hypoplastic Anemias of Childhood, Especially Fanconi's Anemia.   Minagi and Steinbach have called attention to the high order of frequency of absent hypoplastic or supernumerary thumb in patients with Fanconi's anemia (34 of 44 patients). They also noted a fairly high order of hypoplastic or absent radius (nine of 44 patients). Other less frequent

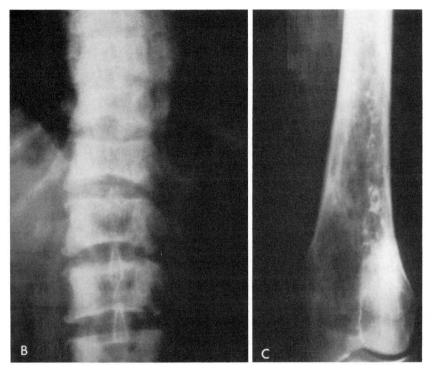

Figure 8–14 *(Continued).   B.* Antero-posterior view of the lower thoracic and lumbar spine showing the coarsened, fibrillar sclerosis of the bony texture. *C.* Infarction of the distal shaft of the femur in sickle cell anemia.

skeletal deformities included congenital hip dislocation, webbing of the second and third toes, Klippel-Feil deformity, clubfoot, extraterminal phalanges of third and fourth toes, and Sprengel's deformity in one case.

Especially frequent are renal anomalies, which occur in a fourth of the patients, and cardiovascular anomalies, which occur in about 11 to 12 per cent of the patients.

"Acute" (-Blastic) Leukemias

Pathologic Considerations and Radiographic Findings. Bone changes are frequently seen in individuals younger than ten years old. An incidence of over 80 per cent of bone lesions has been reported in this group. Bone changes with acute leukemias in children are related to (1) the **destruction of the marrow** by the proliferating reticulocytic elements; (2) a **tendency for the marrow to proliferate** (Figure 8–14A) in an effort to overcome cellular deficiencies; and (3) the **invasion of the periosteum** by the neoplastic elements, causing a periosteal elevation, proliferation, and so-called **"sun-ray striations"** of the periosteum or "hair-on-end" appearance. (4) Commonly there is a **transverse line of radiolucency** at the ends of the long bones beneath the metaphysis (Figure 8–15B). This occurs in over one-half the cases (Willson). Osteolytic lesions occur in 38 per cent, and periosteal reactions have been noted in 19 per cent (Karpinski and Martin; Kalayjian et al.).

The changes described show a predilection for the areas of most rapid bone growth, such as the knees, wrists, ankles, and shoulders. Because of this transverse appearance in the metaphyses, this entity must be mentioned in the next category for discussion.

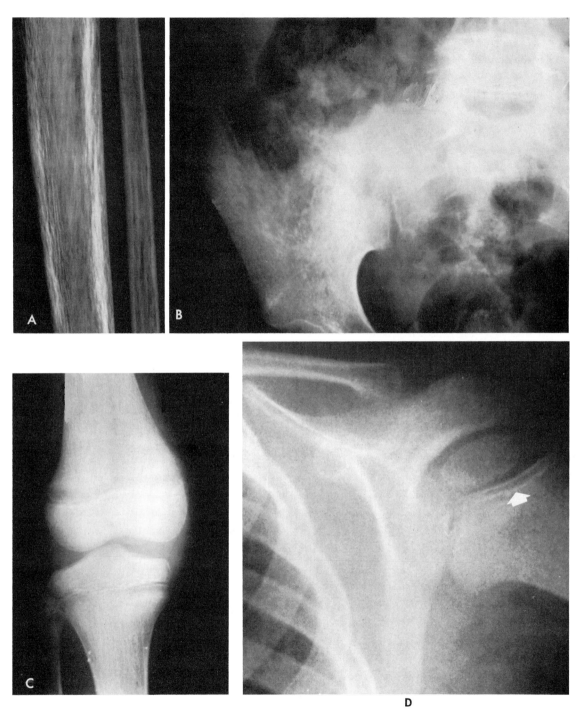

Figure 8–15   Bones in monocytic leukemia. *A.* Note the coarse linear trabeculation of the shafts of the tibia and fibula. *B.* Coarse trabeculation of the right innominate bone. *C.* The adjoining metaphyses of the femur and tibia around the knee show the broad lucent zone in a young individual with acute leukemia. *D.* Antero-posterior view of the shoulder in an infant with acute leukemia; this was actually discovered by inclusion of this region on a routine film of the chest.

Figure 8–15 *continued on opposite page.*

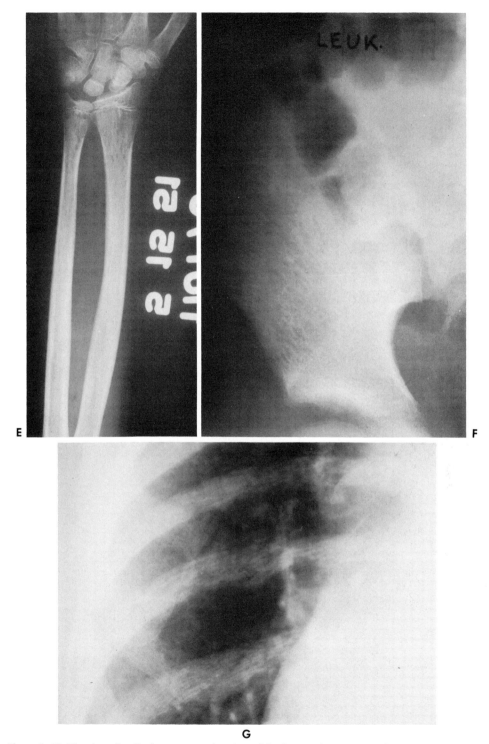

Figure 8–15 *(Continued). E.* Antero-posterior view of the forearm in a young patient with an acute leukemia showing the lucency of the metaphyses of the radius and ulna. *F.* The right innominate bone in this patient showing the coarsened trabecular pattern and lucency. *G.* The coarsened trabecular pattern of the ribs.

Lymphangiomatosis of Bone.   The bone lesions of angiomatosis consist of scattered lucent foci finely etched by a very thin sclerotic margin. Both the cortex and the spongiosa of the medullary cavity of bone are affected. The medullary lesions may be quite large, with mild expansion of the bone and thinning of the cortex. The skull and flat bones are also involved, but the small bones of the extremities are usually spared.

In differential diagnosis one may exclude marrow abnormalities since the marrow is relatively spared in comparison with such diseases as fibrous dysplasia and Gaucher's disease. In histiocytosis X and metastatic disease, there are no sclerotic thin borders as in this instance (Nixon).

Tuberous Sclerosis of Bone (Teplick).   The bones undergo a cystlike change, especially in the phalanges, where the walls of the cysts suggest local bulges of periosteal new bone formation and some thickening of the trabeculae. The trabeculae of the shaft of the metacarpals, tibia, and fibula may also be somewhat thickened. These cystlike changes and thickened trabeculae with periosteal new bone formation occur in about two-thirds of the patients and are highly suggestive. There is some resemblance to sarcoidosis and hyperparathyroidism but the periosteal new bone and the complete absence of subperiosteal resorption are against these latter two diagnoses. In the spine there is a tendency to sclerosis of the pedicles of vertebrae, especially lumbar vertebrae, and the posterior elements of the spine appear to be especially affected.

Pulmonary changes, while characteristic of tuberous sclerosis, are the least frequent finding. These consist of large cyst-like areas in any portion of the lung, indistinguishable from the honey-comb lung of histiocytosis, sarcoidosis, advanced collagen disease, pneumoconiosis, and Hamman-Rich disease.

Thus, there is a close resemblance to sarcoid in its many manifestations.

There may also be intracranial calcifications, especially paraventricular, basal ganglia, and in the cerebellum. The basal ganglia calcification occurs in about 50 per cent of the cases and the cerebellar calcification in 7 to 15 per cent.

RADIOLUCENCIES OCCURRING PRIMARILY TRANSVERSELY IN MULTIPLE METAPHYSES

The diseases which fall readily into this category are illustrated in Figure 8–16.

In general, these are disturbances occurring in childhood causing an *interruption of the normal bone growth sequences at the epiphyseal plate and metaphyseal junction.* As noted, they include the following disorders:
1. *Hypervitaminosis A (excessive osteoclastic activity in metaphysis, with active proliferation of new bone in diaphysis).*
2. *Hypovitaminosis C (scurvy).*
3. *Hypovitaminosis D (rickets).*
4. *Chronic renal osteodystrophy or renal rickets.*
5. *Hypophosphatasia.*
6. *Phenylketonuria.*
7. *Congenital syphilis.*
8. *Congenital rubella syndrome.*
9. *Acute leukemia of infants.*

The Osteomalacic Disorders.   These include vitamin D deficiency in the adult or child, renal tubular acidosis (renal tubular defect), the chronic renal insufficiency

METAPHYSEAL TRANSVERSE OSTEOPOROSIS

1. ACUTE LEUKEMIA
   (CHILDHOOD)

2. HYPERVITAMINOSIS A

3. HYPERVITAMINOSIS D

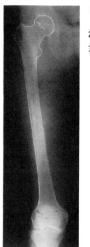

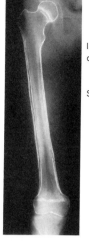

Increased zone
of rarefaction

Subperiosteal
    new bone
    formation

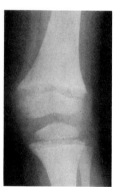

Cartilage zone
increased and
no calcifi‐
  cation of
  epiphysis

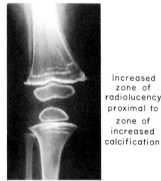

Increased
  zone of
radiolucency
proximal to
   zone of
  increased
 calcification

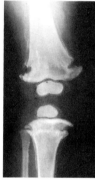

Transverse zone
    of no
  calcification

Slipped epiphysis

Poorly ossified
   spongiosa

4. RENAL RICKETS
7. HYPOPHOSPHATASIA
8. PHENYLKETONURIA

5. SCURVY

6. SYPHILIS

Figure 8–16   Radiolucent diseases characterized by osteoporosis arranged transversely, predominantly in the region of the metaphysis.

diseases, and the hereditary disorders predisposing to osteomalacia—familial vitamin D resistance; Fanconi syndrome; and hypophosphatasia, an abnormal reduction in the activity of alkaline phosphatase in serum, many tissues, and bone. In all these disorders, there is a defective mineralization of the osteoid matrix and a slowing down of matrix formation. The bones are fragile and subject to fracture, bending forces, and stress.

ROENTGEN APPEARANCES OF THE SKELETON IN OSTEOMALACIA AND RICKETS (Steinbach and Noetzli)

There are three distinct roentgenologic patterns:

a. A decreased density of the skeleton with pseudofractures—usually indicating malabsorption and dietary deficiencies;

b. An increase in the density of the skeleton rather than a decrease—

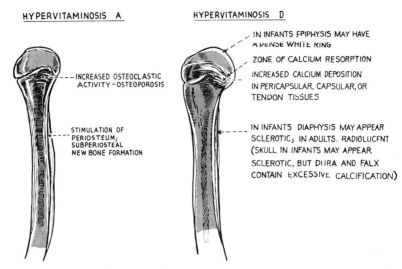

Figure 8–17   Diagram illustrating radiographic changes with hypervitaminosis A and hypervitaminosis D.

usually a manifestation of renal tubular insufficiency (vitamin D resistant osteomalacia or rickets);

c. A variable density in the bones with irregular mineralization presenting occasional horizontal bands of increased density. This third type is especially characteristic of chronic renal glomerular failure.

Radiographic Findings

In the child, since most rapid change is occurring at the metaphyseal-epiphyseal junction, the lack of mineralization imparts a lucent striped appear-

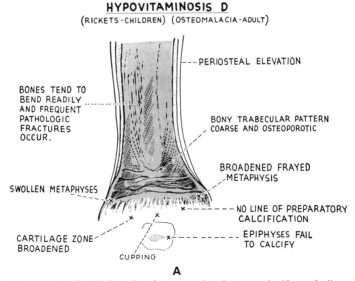

Figure 8–18   A. Labeled tracing demonstrating the most significant findings.

Figure 8–18 continued on opposite page.

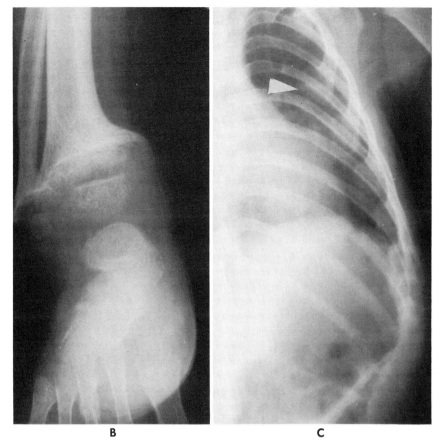

B   **C**

Figure 8–18 *(Continued).*   *B.* Antero-posterior view of an ankle. *C.* Views of the ribs showing the flared appearance at the costochondral junctions corresponding with a rachitic rosary.

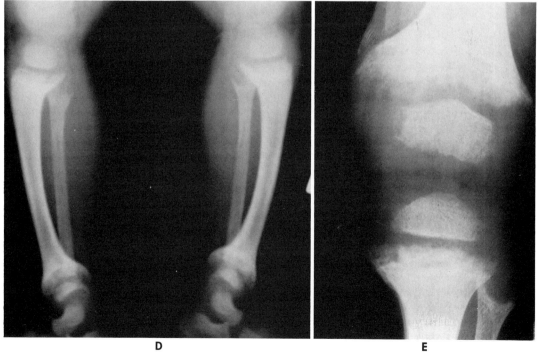

D   **E**

Figure 8–18 *(Continued).*   *D.* Lateral views of both legs in rickets, demonstrating the marked fraying and cupping at the metaphyses of the tibia and fibula and the deformity of the tarsal bones. *E.* Closeup view of the knee showing the frayed expanded appearance of the metaphyses of the femur and tibia and the irregular poorly ossified epiphyses of the femur and tibia.

ance to the radiographs of long bones in this zone. In older children a "hair brush" pattern results.

Some of the differences among these entities are detailed in the accompanying illustrations (Figures 8–17, 8–18, 8–19, 8–20 and 8–21).

In this group of disorders the striped appearance of the metaphysis at times includes transverse zones of whiteness (mineral deposition) alternating with the zones of lucency.

Scurvy

Clinical Considerations

Vitamin C deficiency in infants causes a drop in the alkaline phosphatase activity as well as osteoid formation by the osteoblast. Cement substance necessary to maintain the integrity of capillary walls is also deficient, and underlies the hemorrhagic diathesis characteristic of this condition. The chondroblastic activity at the metaphyseal-epiphyseal junction proceeds well and the zone of provisional calcification can be identified, but the osteoblasts are incapable of forming osteoid. Resorption of the cartilage fails or slows down and at times the cartilage "overgrows," giving rise to bulbous enlargements at the costochondral junctions.

Radiographic Findings

The formation of new osteoid matrix on the degenerating cartilage and zone of provisional calcification is lacking, but when this zone persists somewhat, a **striped appearance** results.

The poorly "cemented" capillaries rupture and hemorrhage takes place alongside small fractures in the deficient bone. Because the periosteum is loosely attached (owing to the lack of cement substance), extensive **subperiosteal hemorrhages** are common. Following the administration of vitamin C,

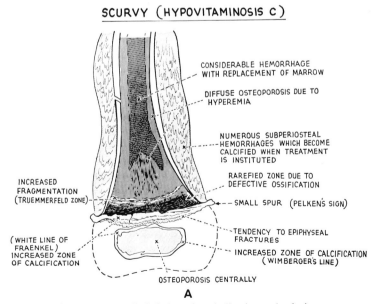

SCURVY (HYPOVITAMINOSIS C)

CONSIDERABLE HEMORRHAGE WITH REPLACEMENT OF MARROW

DIFFUSE OSTEOPOROSIS DUE TO HYPEREMIA

NUMEROUS SUBPERIOSTEAL HEMORRHAGES WHICH BECOME CALCIFIED WHEN TREATMENT IS INSTITUTED

RAREFIED ZONE DUE TO DEFECTIVE OSSIFICATION

SMALL SPUR (PELKEN'S SIGN)

TENDENCY TO EPIPHYSEAL FRACTURES

INCREASED ZONE OF CALCIFICATION (WIMBERGER'S LINE)

INCREASED FRAGMENTATION (TRUEMMERFELD ZONE)

(WHITE LINE OF FRAENKEL) INCREASED ZONE OF CALCIFICATION

OSTEOPOROSIS CENTRALLY

A

Figure 8–19 *A.* Labeled tracings indicating major lesions.

Figure 8–19 *continued on opposite page.*

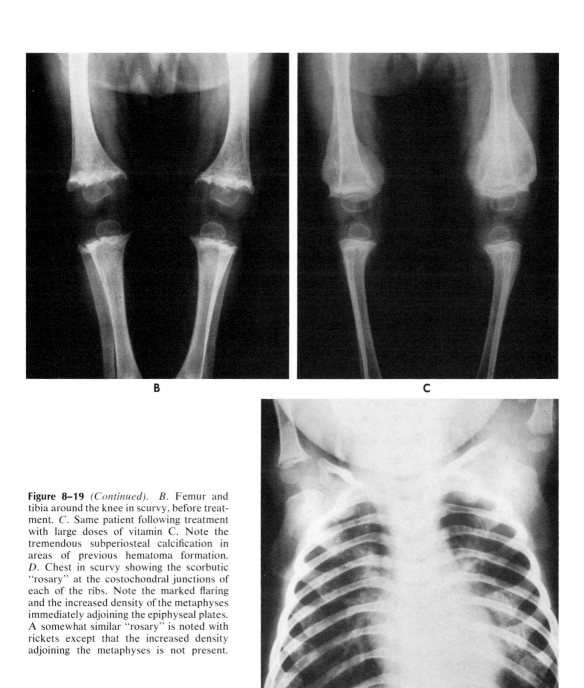

Figure 8–19 *(Continued).* *B.* Femur and tibia around the knee in scurvy, before treatment. *C.* Same patient following treatment with large doses of vitamin C. Note the tremendous subperiosteal calcification in areas of previous hematoma formation. *D.* Chest in scurvy showing the scorbutic "rosary" at the costochondral junctions of each of the ribs. Note the marked flaring and the increased density of the metaphyses immediately adjoining the epiphyseal plates. A somewhat similar "rosary" is noted with rickets except that the increased density adjoining the metaphyses is not present.

B

C

D

CONGENITAL SYPHILIS

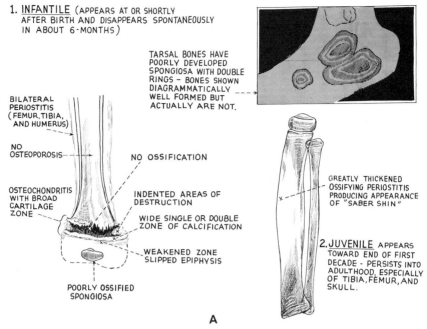

1. <u>INFANTILE</u> (APPEARS AT OR SHORTLY AFTER BIRTH AND DISAPPEARS SPONTANEOUSLY IN ABOUT 6-MONTHS)

TARSAL BONES HAVE POORLY DEVELOPED SPONGIOSA WITH DOUBLE RINGS – BONES SHOWN DIAGRAMMATICALLY WELL FORMED BUT ACTUALLY ARE NOT.

BILATERAL PERIOSTITIS (FEMUR, TIBIA, AND HUMERUS)

NO OSTEOPOROSIS

NO OSSIFICATION

OSTEOCHONDRITIS WITH BROAD CARTILAGE ZONE

INDENTED AREAS OF DESTRUCTION

WIDE SINGLE OR DOUBLE ZONE OF CALCIFICATION

WEAKENED ZONE SLIPPED EPIPHYSIS

POORLY OSSIFIED SPONGIOSA

GREATLY THICKENED OSSIFYING PERIOSTITIS PRODUCING APPEARANCE OF "SABER SHIN"

2. <u>JUVENILE</u> APPEARS TOWARD END OF FIRST DECADE - PERSISTS INTO ADULTHOOD, ESPECIALLY OF TIBIA, FEMUR, AND SKULL.

A

Figure 8–20   Congenital syphilis. *A*. Diagram.

Figure 8–20 *continued on opposite page.*

these subperiosteal hemorrhages undergo calcification and then reveal marked elevation and distribution of the entire periosteal envelope of a long bone.

There is a **bulbous enlargement at the costochondral junction.** The bulbous enlargement of the ends of the long bones and ribs in "renal rickets" is not nearly as great as with hypovitaminosis C and D, since affected children are older and the bones are growing in length more than circumference in these age groups.

Hypophosphatasia (Currarino et al.; Fraser; White et al.).   Unlike rickets, hypophosphatasia may become apparent in the immediate post-natal period. The metaphyseal ossification is streaked and ragged with frequent infractions. The epiphyseal "lines" are wide and irregular, with irregularity also of the diaphyseal margins. In the skull the cranial sutures, which at first are widened, are often subject to premature closure by the 20th month, thus producing the pattern of a craniostenosis.

Wilson's Disease (Cavallino and Grossman; Mindelzun et al.).   This disease is an inherited disorder of copper metabolism; it may produce bone roentgen manifestations which are indistinguishable from those of classical rickets or secondary hyperparathyroidism because of the kidney damage which accompanies the disease.

Apart from these changes the following have also been described: (1) small bone cysts with marginal sclerosis in the vicinity of the small joints of the hands, wrists, ankles, and feet; and (2) an appearance which suggests osteochondritis in the heads of the femurs.

Phenylketonuria.   In this condition there is considerable metaphyseal cupping but no dissolution or fraying of the metaphyseal margins, and no widening of the

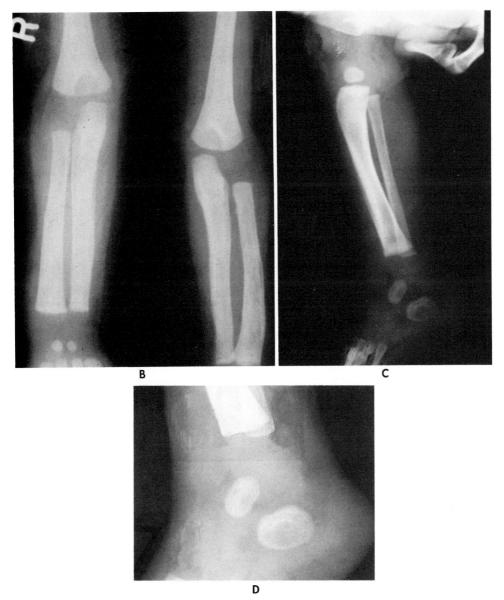

Figure 8–20 *(Continued).* *B.* Forearm and distal humerus demonstrating the thickening of the cortical periosteum. *C.* The leg in congenital syphilis showing the periosteal elevation and concentric lamination of the tarsal bone. *D.* Closeup view of the concentric ossification and/or lamination of the ossification of the os calcis.

metaphyses of the long bones, such as occurs in hypovitaminosis D. Also, there is an irregular hairlike spiculation of the zone of calcification extending into the metaphyseal side of the epiphyseal plate into the proliferating cartilage zone. After the cupping disappears the zone of provisional calcification appears inordinately dense, almost like that in heavy metal poisoning (which is included with the osteosclerotic diseases of the metaphyses) (Feinberg et al.).

Congenital Rubella Syndrome (Figure 8–21)

Clinical Considerations. Changes fall into the following categories: (1) retardation of growth, thrombocytopenia, hepatosplenomegaly, and central nervous system disease; (2) skeletal abnormalities; (3) eye abnormalities such as cataract and

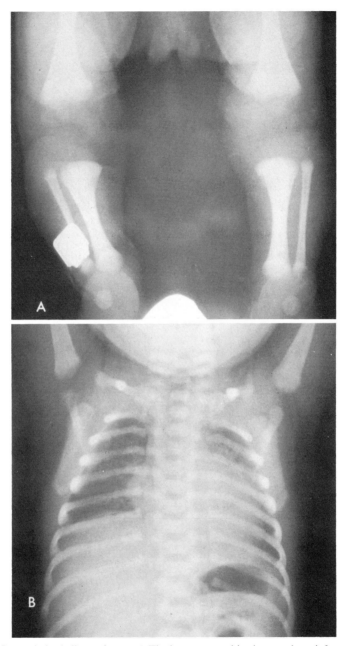

Figure 8–21 Congenital rubella syndrome. *A.* The lower extremities in a newborn infant with congenital rubella syndrome. *B.* The chest in this patient with congenital rubella syndrome, demonstrating the markedly enlarged heart. Note also the frayed appearance of the proximal metaphyses of the humeri.

glaucoma; (4) congenital heart disease, especially patent ductus arteriosus and pulmonary stenosis.

The degree of damage to the fetus depends primarily on the time of infection of the mother in relation to the pregnancy. When infection occurs early in gestation, more than 50 per cent of pregnancies end in abortion, stillbirth, or fetal malformation (Rubin). If infection occurs at the end of the first trimester, the probability of malformation is only slightly higher than for an uncomplicated pregnancy.

Radiographic Findings

The most striking manifestations are in the long bones, and the **bones at the knee are most frequently involved.** There are alternating transverse zones of lucency and sclerosis in the metaphyses, with an irregular density and contour of the zone of provisional calcification. At times there is only the broad band of lucency in the metaphysis.

There are linear and ovoid areas of radiolucency alternating with coarse trabeculae. The zone of provisional calcification is absent, thus creating a demineralized ragged appearance or splaying at the margins of the metaphysis, an appearance which to some extent resembles rickets or hypophosphatasia.

The lesions tend to disappear over a period of two to three months, or the zone of provisional calcification may remain inordinately dense. These changes are apparently due to a defect in the deposition and mineralization of the osteoid, and to defective calcification (in the zone of provisional calcification) of the cartilage prior to engulfment. (Aegerter and Kirkpatrick; Singleton et al.; Rabinowitz et al.).

Congenital Syphilis also begins *in utero,* and is in a secondary stage at birth, subsiding spontaneously at about six months of age.

Radiographic Findings

The primary manifestations in the bones are:
Diffuse periostitis of the long bones;
Retardation of growth, with a broad zone of unossified osteoid;
Frayed and excessive zone of provisional calcification;
"Chewed-out" appearance of the metaphysis marginal to the epiphyseal plate;
Concentric rings of calcification in the tarsal bones;
Slipped epiphyses frequently;
Some resorption of the nasal bones at the bridge of the nose.

"Acute" or -Blastic Leukemia (Figure 8–15).   The bone changes in individuals younger than ten years of age are characterized not only by destruction of marrow by the proliferating marrow elements and invasion (with elevation) of the periosteum, but also by transverse lines of radiolucency at the ends of the long bones beneath the metaphysis. As previously indicated, this latter change occurs in 53 per cent of the cases, according to Willson.

The radiolucent metaphyseal zones are most frequently seen in the knees, wrists, ankles, and shoulders.

Milkman's Syndrome refers to *bilateral, frequently symmetrical, incomplete fractures,* tending to occur especially in the scapulae. Albright (1946) classified the syndrome as caused by a calcium deficiency due to renal tubular dysfunction which resulted in osteomalacia. Engle and Wallis (1957) also related it to a disorder of renal tubular function, but from a wider variety of disorders (such as poisoning, multiple myeloma, and Wilson's disease). Steinbach noted similar fractures in the inferior ramus of the pubis. These incomplete fractures impart to the bone involved a "striped" appearance due to the superimposition of callus upon the incompletely united fracture.

Questions—Chapter 8

1. What four main categories of radiolucent bone diseases of multiple extremities do we distinguish in our method of classification?

2. What are the main radiolucent diseases occurring in the epiphyseal-metaphyseal junction area?

3. What are the main nutritional disorders of growing children and how may they be differentiated radiographically?

4. What are the main radiographic features of acute leukemia in children?

5. What are the main radiographic features of renal osteodystrophy in children?

6. What are the main radiographic features of congenital syphilis?

7. What main disease categories are characterized by generalized radiolucency that is not sharply demarcated?

8. What is the basic defect in osteomalacia and what are the various types of osteomalacia?

9. What are some of the main endocrine osteopathies which produce generalized radiolucency?

10. What is meant by hypophosphatasia and what are some of its radiographic and clinical features?

11. What are the main roentgen characteristics of the generalized radiolucency which is not sharply demarcated?

12. Name the main categories of disease that are characterized by generalized radiolucency in scattered circumscribed defects throughout the bony skeleton.

13. What malignancies are mainly believed to cause metastatic bone tumor?

14. Are all metastatic bone tumors osteolytic in appearance? If not, which ones are predominantly radiolucent?

15. Classify the lipoid storage diseases and the reticuloendothelioses and indicate their predominant radiographic features.

16. What are the main clinical and radiographic features of primary hyperparathyroidism?

17. What are the main radiographic features of the mycotic and fungus infections of bone?

18. What are the main clinical and radiographic features of the nonspecific widespread inflammatory diseases of bone?

19. What are the main bone entities characterized by generalized radiolucency with a linear coarsening of the trabecular pattern of bone?

20. Indicate at least two and, if possible, three diseases of the systemic group which are characterized by lucency of epiphyses.

21. Indicate at least four diseases characterized by radiolucency of metaphyses in this systemic category.

22. Indicate several diseases which are characterized by widespread radiolucency involving epiphyses and metaphyses to a great extent.

23. Indicate several diseases characterized by elevation of the periosteum where the elevation is also combined with radiolucency of the bones. Indicate whether the elevation of the periosteum is more likely to appear "layered," "lacelike," or "spiculated."

24. Indicate those systemic radiolucent diseases which are accompanied by one or another form of metaphyseal expansion.

25. How would you characterize the skeletal findings in the so-called "reticuloendothelial marrow disorders"?

26. What is the "congenital rubella syndrome" and how does it affect the fetal skeleton?

27. What is "Milkman's syndrome"?

References

Adams, F. D.: Reversible uremia with hypercalcemia due to vitamin-D intoxication. New Eng. J. Med., *244*:590–592, 1951.

Aegerter, E., and Kirkpatrick, J. A.: Orthopedic Diseases. Third Edition. Philadelphia, W. B. Saunders Co., 1968.

Agarwal, K. N., Dhar, N., Shah, M. M., and Bhardwaj, O. P.: Roentgenologic changes in iron deficiency anemia. Amer. J. Roentgenol., *110*:635–637, 1970.

Agerty, H. A.: The pediatric aspects of cancer. CA, *8*:97–100, 1958.

Albright, F., and Reifenstein, E. C., Jr.: Parathyroid Glands and Metabolic Bone Disease. Baltimore, Williams and Wilkins Co., 1948.

Albright, F., Burnett, C. H., Parson, W., Reifenstein, E. C., and Roos, A.: Osteomalacia and late rickets; various etiologies met in the United States with emphasis on that resulting from a specific form of renal acidosis, therapeutic indications for each etiological subgroup, and relationship between osteomalacia and Milkman's syndrome. Medicine, *25*: 399–479, 1946.

Albright, F., Butler, A. M., Hampton, A. O., and Smith, P.: Syndrome characterized by osteitis fibrosis disseminata, areas of pigmentation and endocrine dysfunction, with precocious puberty in females; report of 5 cases. New Eng. J. Med., *216*:727–746, 1937.

Arcomano, J. P., Barnett, J. C., and Wunderlich, H. O.: Histiocytosis X. Amer. J. Roentgenol., *85*:663–679, 1961.

Barton, C. J., and Cockshott, W. P.: Bone changes in hemoglobin SC disease. Amer. J. Roentgenol., *88*:523–532, 1962.

Becker, J. A.: Hemoglobin SC disease. Amer. J. Roentgenol., *88*:503–511, 1962.

Blount, A. W., Jr., and Cohen, M.: Tissue lipid patterns in a case of xanthoma disseminatum. Arch. Intern. Med., *111*:511–517, 1963.

Burko, H., Watson, J., and Robinson, M.: Unusual bone changes in sickle-cell disease in childhood. Radiology, *80*:957–962, 1963.

Caffey, J.: Chronic poisoning due to excess of vitamin A; description of clinical and roentgen manifestations in 7 infants and young children. Amer. J. Roentgenol., *65*:12–26, 1951.

Caffey, J.: Pediatric X-ray Diagnosis. Fourth Edition. Chicago, Year Book Publishers, 1961, pp. 1116–1118.

Calenoff, L., and Friederici, H. H.: Unilateral angiomatosis: roentgen and pathologic features. Amer. J. Roentgenol., *89*:1305–1313, 1963.

Cassady, J. R., Berdon, W. E., and Baker, D. H.:

"Typical" spine changes of sickle cell anemia in patient with thalassemia major (Cooley's anemia). Radiology, *89*:1065–1068, 1967.

Cavallino, R., and Grossman, H.: Wilson's disease presenting with rickets, Radiology, *90*: 493–494, 1968.

Currarino, G., Neuhauser, E. B., Reyerspach, G. C., and Sobel, E. H.: Hypophosphatasia. Amer. J. Roentgenol., *78*:392–419, 1957.

Darling, D. B., Loridan, L., and Senior, B.: Roentgenographic manifestations of Cushing's syndrome in infancy. Radiology, *96*:503–508, 1970.

Diggs, L. W., Pulliam, H. N., and King, J. C.: The bone changes in sickle-cell anemia. South. Med. J., *30*:249–259, 1937.

Dodds, W. J., and Steinbach, H. L.: Primary hyperparathyroidism and articular cartilage calcification. Amer. J. Roentgenol., *104*:884–892, 1968.

Dolan, P. A.: Reticulum cell sarcoma of bone. Amer. J. Roentgenol., *87*:121–127, 1962.

Edeiken, J., and Hodes, P. J.: Roentgen Diagnosis of Diseases of Bone. Baltimore, Williams and Wilkins Co., 1967.

Ellis, K., and Hochstin, R. J.: The skull and hyperparathyroid bone disease. Amer. J. Roentgenol., *83*:732–742, 1960.

Engle, R. L., Jr., and Wallis, L. A.: Multiple myeloma and the adult Fanconi syndrome. I. Report of a case with crystal-like deposits in the tumor cells and in the epithelial cells of the kidney. Amer. J. Med., *22*:5–23, 1957.

Fanconi, G.: Non-diabetic glycosuria and hyperglycemia in older children. Jahrb. f. Kinderheit, *133*:57, 1931.

Feinberg, S. B., and Fisch, R. O.: Roentgenologic findings in growing long bones in phenylketonuria. Preliminary study. Radiology, *78*: 394–398, 1962.

Finby, N., and Bearn, A. G.: Roentgenographic abnormalities of skeletal system in Wilson's disease (hepatolenticular degeneration). Amer. J. Roentgenol., *79*:603–611, 1958.

Fraser, D.: Clinical manifestations of genetic aberrations of calcium and phosphorus metabolism. J.A.M.A., *176*:281–287, 1961.

Fraser, D.: Hypophosphatasia. Amer. J. Med., *22*:730–746, 1957.

Fucilla, I. S., and Hamann, A.: Hodgkin's disease in bone. Radiology, *77*:53–60, 1961.

Gehweiler, J. A., Capp, M. P., and Chick, E. W.: Observations on the roentgen pattern in blastomycosis of bone. Amer. J. Roentgenol., *108*:497–510, 1970.

Gerber, A., Raab, A. P., and Sobel, A. E.:

Vitamin A poisoning in adults with description of case. Amer. J. Med., *16*:729–745, 1954.

Gorlin, R., and Chaudhry, A. P.: Oral melanotic pigmentation in polyostotic fibrous dysplasia, Albright's syndrome. Oral Surgery, *10*:857–862, 1957.

Greenfield, G. B.: Bone changes in chronic adult Gaucher's disease. Amer. J. Roentgenol., *110*:800–807, 1970.

Greenfield, G. B.: Radiology of Bone Diseases. Philadelphia, J. B. Lippincott Co., 1969.

Grossman, R. E., and Hensley, G. T.: Bone lesions in primary amyloidosis. Amer. J. Roentgenol., *101*:872–875, 1967.

Hibbs, R. E., and Rush, H. P.: Albright's syndrome. Ann. Intern. Med., *37*:587–593, 1952.

Hodges, P. C., Phemister, D. B., and Brunschwig, A.: The roentgen-ray diagnosis of diseases of bone. In Golden, R. (Ed.): Diagnostic Roentgenology, Volume I. New York, Thomas Nelson and Sons, 1950.

Holt, J. F., and Wright, E. M.: Radiologic features of neurofibromatosis. Radiology, *51*:647–663, 1948.

Hunt, J. C., and Pugh, D. G.: Skeletal lesions in neurofibromatosis. Radiology, *76*:1–20, 1961.

Jacobson, H. G., Rifkin, H., and Zucker-Franklin, D.: Werner's syndrome; a clinical roentgen entity. Radiology, *74*:373–385, 1960.

Kalayjian, B. S., Herbut, P. A., and Erf, L. A.: The bone changes of leukemia in children. Radiology, *47*:223–233, 1946.

Karpinski, F. E., and Martin, J. F.: The skeletal lesions of leukemic children treated with Aminopterin. J. Pediatrics, *37*:208–223, 1950.

Kolb, F. O., and Steinbach, H. L.: The syndrome of pseudo-hypohyperparathyroidism. Periodica Copenhagen, First International Congress of Endocrinology, "Advanced Abstract of Short Communications," 1960.

Levin, B.: Gaucher's disease: clinical and roentgenologic manifestations. Amer. J. Roentgenol., *85*:685–696, 1961.

Lichtenstein, L.: Polyostotic fibrous dysplasia. Arch. Surg., *36*:874–898, 1938.

Lichtenstein, L., and Jaffe, H. L.: Fibrous dysplasia of bones; condition affecting one, several or many bones, grave cases of which may present abnormal pigmentation of skin, premature sexual development, hyperthyroidism or still other extraskeletal abnormalities. Arch. Path., *33*:777–816, 1942.

Lowe, C. U., Terrey, M., and MacLachlan, E. A.: Organic-aciduria, decreased renal ammonia production, hydrophthalmos and mental retardation; clinical entity. Amer. J. Dis. Child., *83*:164–184, 1952.

McIntosh, H. P., Miller, D. E., Gleason, W. L., and Goldner, J. L.: The circulatory dynamics of polyostotic fibrous dysplasia. Amer. J. Med., *32*:393–403, 1962.

Margulies, S. I., and Minkin, S. D.: Sickle cell disease: The roentgenologic manifestations of urinary tract abnormalities in adults. Amer. J. Roentgenol., *107*:702–710, 1969.

Meema, H. E., and Schatz, D. L.: Simple radiologic demonstration of cortical bone loss in thyrotoxicosis. Radiology, *97*:9–15, 1970.

Milkman, L. M.: Multiple spontaneous; idiopathic symmetrical fractures. Amer. J. Roentgenol., *32*:622–634, 1934.

Minagi, H., and Steinbach, H. L.: Roentgen appearance of anomalies associated with hypoplastic anemias of childhood: Fanconi's anemia and congenital hypoplastic anemia. Amer. J. Roentgenol., *97*:100–109, 1966.

Mindelzun, R., Elkin, M., Scheinberg, I. H., and Sternlieb, I.: Skeletal changes in Wilson's disease. Radiology, *94*:127–132, 1970.

Moseley, J. E., and Starobin, S. G.: Cystic angiomatosis of bone: Manifestation of hamartomatous disease entity. Amer. J. Roentgenol., *91*:1114–1120, 1964.

Mulvey, R. B.: Peripheral bone metastases. Amer. J. Roentgenol., *91*:155–160, 1964.

Murray, R. O.: Steroids and the skeleton. Radiology, *77*:729–743, 1961.

Nixon, G. W.: Lymphangiomatosis of bone demonstrated by lymphangiography. Amer. J. Roentgenol., *110*:582–586, 1970.

Norman, A., and Ulin, R.: A comparative study of periosteal new bone response and metastatic bone tumors (solitary) and primary bone sarcoma. Radiology, *92*:705–708, 1969.

Papavasiliou, C. G., Gargano, F. P., and Walls, W. L.: Idiopathic non-familial acro-osteolysis associated with other bone abnormalities. Amer. J. Roentgenol., *83*:687–691, 1960.

Pedersen, H. E., and McCarroll, H. R.: Vitamin-resistant rickets. J. Bone & Joint Surg., *33A*:203–223, 1951.

Pugh, D. G.: The roentgenologic diagnosis of diseases of bone. In Golden, R. (Ed.): Diagnostic Roentgenology, Volume I. New York, Thomas Nelson and Sons, 1950.

Rabinowitz, J. G., Wolf, B. S., Greenberg, E. I., and Rausen, A. R.: Osseous changes in rubella embryopathy. Radiology, *85*:494–499, 1965.

Reynolds, J.: A re-evaluation of the "fish vertebra" sign in sickle cell hemoglobinopathy. Amer. J. Roentgenol., *97*:693–707, 1966.

Reynolds, J.: Roentgenographic and clinical appraisal of sickle cell hemoglobin C disease. Amer. J. Roentgenol., *88*:512–522, 1962.

Riggs, W. Jr., and Rockett, J. F.: Roentgen chest findings in childhood sickle cell anemia. Amer. J. Roentgenol., *104*:838–845, 1968.

Robbins, L. L.: Roentgenologic demonstration of spinal metastases from leiomyosarcoma of the uterus. Arch. Surg., *47*:462–467, 1943.

Rourke, J. A., and Heslin, D. J.: Gaucher's disease: Roentgenologic bone changes over a 20 year interval. Amer. J. Roentgenol., *94*:621–630, 1965.

Rubin, A.: Handbook of Congenital Malformations. Philadelphia, W. B. Saunders Co., 1967.

Schlumberger, H. G.: Fibrous dysplasia of single bones (monostotic fibrous dysplasia). Mil. Surg., *99*:504–527, 1946.

Singleton, E. N., and Teng, C.: Pseudohypoparathyroidism with bone changes simulating hyperparathyroidism. Report of a case. Radiology, *78*:388–393, 1962.

Singleton, E. B., Rudolph, A. J., Rosenberg, H. S., and Singer, D. B.: Roentgenographic manifestations of rubella syndrome in newborn infants. Amer. J. Roentgenol., *97*:82–91, 1966.

Steinbach, H. L., and Noetzli, M.: The roentgen appearance of the skeleton in osteomalacia and rickets. Amer. J. Roentgenol., *91*:955–972, 1964.

Steinbach, H. L., Gordon, G. S., Eisenberg, E., Crane, J. J., Silverman, S., and Goldman, L.: Primary hyperparathyroidism: A correlation of roentgen, clinical, and pathologic features. Amer. J. Roentgenol., *86*:329–343, 1961.

Steiner, G. M., Farmar, J., and Lawson, J. P.: Lymphangiomatosis of bone. Radiology, *93*:1093–1098, 1969.

Teng, C., and Nathan, M. H.: Primary hyperparathyroidism. Amer. J. Roentgenol., *83*:716–731, 1960.

Teplick, J. G.: Tuberous sclerosis. Radiology, *93*:53–55, 1969.

Tori, G.: Clinical and radiological observations on 102 cases of sickle cell anemia. Radiol. Clin., *23*:87–108, 1954.

Wallis, L. A., and Engle, R. L., Jr.: The adult Fanconi syndrome. II. Review of eighteen cases. Amer. J. Med., *22*:13–23, 1957.

Watson, R. J., and Lichtman, H. C.: Symposium on basic sciences in medical practice. The anemias. Med. Clin. N. Amer., *39*:735–749, 1955.

White, J. E., Binford, C. C., Robinson, R. R., and Blackard, W. G.: Familial hypophosphatemia. Arch. Intern. Med., *111*:460–464, 1963.

Williams, H. J., and Carey, L. S.: Rubella embryopathy: Roentgenologic features. Amer. J. Roentgenol., *97*:92–99, 1966.

Williams, T. F., Winters, R. W., and Burnette, C. H.: Familial (hereditary) vitamin-D resistant rickets with hypophosphatemia. In Stanbury, J. B., Wyngaarden, J. B., and Fredrickson, D. S. (Eds.): Metabolic Basis of Inherited Disease. Second Edition. New York, McGraw Hill Book Co., 1966.

Willson, J. K. V.: The bone lesions of childhood leukemia: a survey of 140 cases. Radiology, *72*:672–681, 1959.

Wolbach, S. B.: Vitamin-A deficiency and excess in relation to skeletal growth. J. Bone Joint Surg., *29*:171, 1947.

9

Radiolucent Bone Diseases of a Single Extremity

INTRODUCTION

Many of the diseases which have been described in the preceding chapter as widespread begin by initial involvement of single bones or single regions. Nevertheless, by the time these diseases are seen clinically, their manifestations are often widespread. It will be our purpose in this chapter to describe those diseases which tend to remain localized to a single region or to a single bone.

The following classification will be followed (Figure 9–1):
1. *Diseases affecting the epiphyses* primarily.
2. Radiolucent bone diseases affecting both the *metaphyses and epiphyses.*
3. Radiolucent bone diseases affecting the *metaphyses primarily with thick or thin marginal sclerosis.*
4. Radiolucent diseases affecting the *metaphyses primarily without marginal sclerosis.*
5. *Diaphyseal corticoperiosteal radiolucent* lesions.

DISEASES AFFECTING THE EPIPHYSES
PRIMARILY (Figure 9–2)

The most important entities in this category are illustrated in Figure 9–2.

The Osteochondroses (Focal Aseptic Necrosis of Bone). Osteochondrosis is a focal aseptic necrosis of centers of ossification of unknown etiology but not of inflammatory origin.

The Sites of Occurrence are illustrated in Figure 9–3. Actually, there is no reason to believe that any epiphysis is immune from an osteochondrosis. Sometimes there are multiple foci of involvement.

RADIOLUCENT DISEASE OF SINGLE EXTREMITY

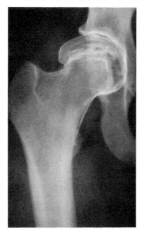

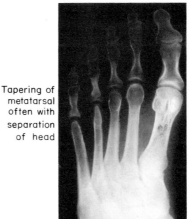

Tapering of
metatarsal
often with
separation
of head

Punctate
"honey
combing"

AFFECTING
EPIPHYSIS
PRIMARILY

AFFECTING
EPIPHYSIS AND
METAPHYSIS

Elevation of
periosteum
by exudate

Area of
absorption
in shaft

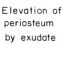

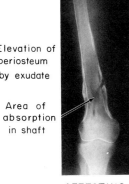

Infection
enters via
nutrient
shaft

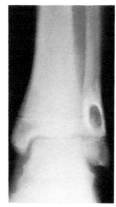

Marginal
sclerosis

Sharply
demarcated
area of
reabsorption

No sequestrae

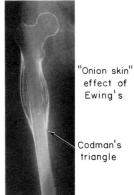

"Onion skin"
effect of
Ewing's

Codman's
triangle

AFFECTING
METAPHYSIS
PRIMARILY

NO MARGINAL
SCLEROSIS

AFFECTING
METAPHYSIS
WITH MARGINAL
SCLEROSIS

CORTICO-PERIOSTEAL
LESIONS

Figure 9–1 Classification of radiolucent bone diseases tending to remain localized to a single extremity or region. (Radiographs intensified.)

AFFECTING EPIPHYSIS PRIMARILY

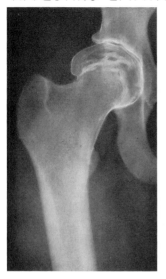

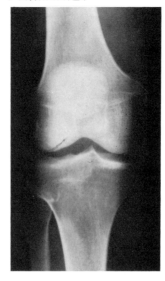

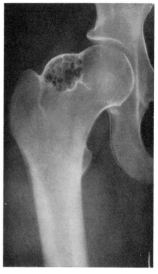

I. FOCAL ASEPTIC NECROSES
OR THE OSTEOCHONDROSES
DEFORMED FEMORAL HEAD
OF LATE PERTHES' DISEASE

2. OSTEOCHONDRITIS
DISSECANS OF KNEE

3. EPIPHYSEAL
CHONDROBLASTOMA
NUMEROUS CALCIFIC
FOCI IN EPIPHYSIS AND
ADJOINING METAPHYSIS

Figure 9–2 Diseases affecting the epiphyses primarily. (Radiograph intensified.)

The Pathogenesis of the disease and its three radiographic stages are illustrated in Figure 9–4. It is thought that the underlying pathology is a local ischemia of bone resulting in aseptic necrosis.

Three stages of the disease are identified:

Stage 1, *the necrotic stage:* Histologically, at the junction of the epiphysis and diaphysis there is a periosteal connective tissue proliferation and some bony resorption. Later a hyperemia develops around small foci of necrotic bone and marrow. The cartilage remains viable, since it derives its nutrition from the adjoining synovial membrane. A subchondral fissure develops and gradually becomes larger.

Radiologically, at this stage there may be no alterations in size or shape of the epiphysis. Soon, however, the necrotic bone becomes demarcated from the surrounding bone by its "whiteness." Later a depression and deformity of the necrotic elements become radiographically manifest.

Stage 2, *the regenerative stage:* Tongues of granulation tissue accompanied by capillaries project themselves into the marrow spaces of the necrotic elements. Phagocytes absorb the necrotic bony trabeculae. Osteoclasts and osteoblasts function simultaneously. Complete regeneration may require months or even years.

Radiologically, there is an increasing fragmentation of the involved area owing to the tonguelike inroads of granulation and fibrous tissue projecting themselves into a larger necrotic element. The deformity may increase.

Stage 3, *the healed stage:* There is complete bony replacement of the necrotic cortex and marrow. The microscopic appearance of the bone reverts to normal.

Radiologically, the bony appearance takes on a normal trabecular architecture, but the deformity persists. If the changes are juxta-articular, a degenerative secondary arthritis usually ensues. Alterations also often occur in the metaphysis adjoining the involved foci. In the case of the femoral neck, the structure becomes broad and short and the acetabulum also becomes deformed in order to adapt itself to the deformed femoral head.

Prognosis may be predicted by careful analysis of the radiographic appearances (Figure 9–4C).

In the **healed** stage any deformity present will persist, and in a juxta-articular situation degenerative arthritis may be superimposed after several years.

Alterations often occur in the metaphysis adjoining the epiphysis involved. The case of the femoral neck mentioned earlier is an example.

Osteochondrosis in Certain Areas

THE CAPITAL FEMORAL EPIPHYSIS (LEGG-CALVÉ-PERTHES DISEASE). This appears in childhood between the ages of 3 and 12, and more frequently in boys than in girls. It is bilateral in about 10 per cent of the cases. The recovery stage lasts for about two to four years.

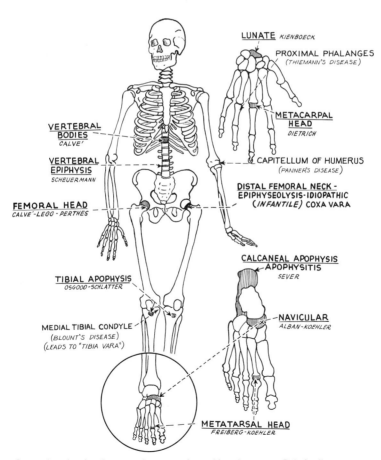

Figure 9–3 Osteochondrosis: the most frequent sites of involvement. Calvés disease, or vertebra plana, may more frequently, if not always, be due to involvement by eosinophilic granuloma, hyperparathyroidism, lipoid dyscrasia, Hodgkin's disease, or other, unidentified malignant disease (Weston and Goodson).

OSTEOCHONDROSIS

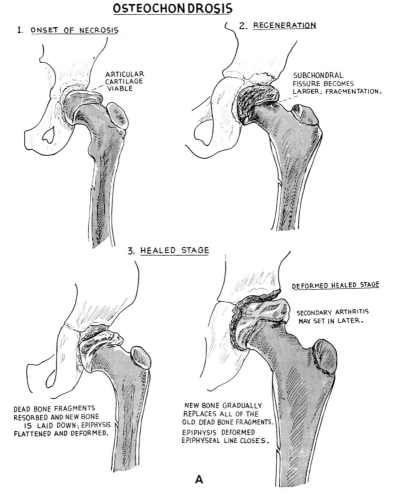

Figure 9–4   *A.* The pathogenesis of osteochondrosis as presented in the femoral head.

Figure 9–4 continued on opposite page.

One of the earliest signs of osteochondrosis of the hip is a widening of the distance as seen on the antero-posterior roentgenograms, from the lateral margin of the so-called pelvic teardrop to the medial border of the proximal femoral metaphysis. This has been widely referred to as the teardrop distance (Figure 9–4B). Eyring et al. have measured this distance in early cases of osteochondrosis as well as in a large normal population and have found that in patients with no known hip joint disease the mean measurement of the teardrop distance is 8.8 mm., with a standard deviation of 1.3 mm. Ninety-five per cent of all measurements were between 6 mm. and 11 mm. They also found that no normal hip had a teardrop distance greater than 10 mm. or greater than the teardrop distance of the affected hip. If the difference between the two sides was at least 2 mm., the disease was invariably present in the hip with the greater teardrop distance. Worded another way, the teardrop distance when greater than 11 mm., or more than 2 mm. greater than that of the opposite hip, was found to be a sensitive indicator of hip joint disease. Admittedly the disease present is not specifically osteochondrosis.

THE TIBIAL TUBERCLE (OSGOOD-SCHLATTER DISEASE).   The epiphysis of the tibial tubercle becomes fragmented, often following a history of trauma, and it occurs in boys more frequently than in girls during the age period of ten to 15 years. Since

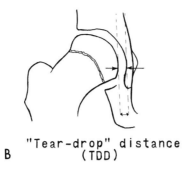

"Tear-drop" distance
B   (TDD)

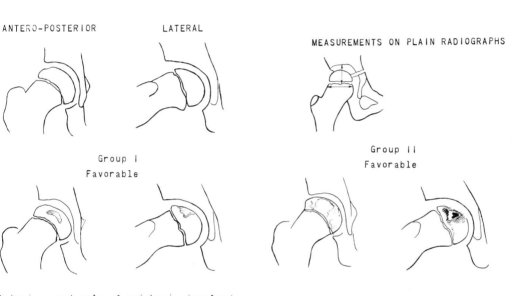

NORMAL

ANTERO-POSTERIOR   LATERAL

MEASUREMENTS ON PLAIN RADIOGRAPHS

Group I
Favorable

Group II
Favorable

Anterior part only of epiphysis involved
No collapse
No sequestrum
Cystic appearance on A-P
Height maintained
Minimal metaphyseal change

C

More of anterior part of epiphysis involved
Collapse of involved area
Sequestrum present
Height maintained
"V" separation of sequestrum on lateral view
Cystic appearance on A-P view disappears
with healing

Figure 9–4 *(Continued). B.* From Eyring, Bjornson, and Peterson: Am. J. Roentgenol., *93:*382–387, 1966. *C.* Modified from Catterall, A.: J. Bone Joint Surg. (Brit.), *53–B:*37–53, 1971.

Figure 9–4 continued on following page.

fusion of this epiphysis with the tibia does not occur until approximately 20 years of age, this process may occur at any time prior to this age. The deformity and discomfort at the site of the tibial tubercle—at the insertion of the quadriceps tendon—may require surgical intervention.

VERTEBRAL END-PLATES (SCHEUERMANN'S DISEASE). Both sexes are equally affected and the peak incidence is at about 16 years of age. The most commonly affected zone is the lower one-third of the thoracic spine, but so-called "vertebral epiphysitis" may occur in the lumbar vertebrae as well. The vertebral end-plates become fragmented, and a steplike deformity and wedging results. The vertebral body is narrowed anteriorly and there is a kyphotic deformity of the spine. The kyphosis—called juvenile kyphosis—persists and secondary degenerative changes develop in the part of the spine involved.

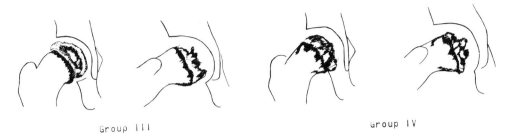

Group III

Only small part of epiphysis not sequestrated
"Head within head" appearance on A-P early
Collapsed sequestrum centrally later
Broadened neck (with regeneration)
Sequestrum resorbed before regeneration begins
at periphery
More generalized metaphyseal changes with broad neck

Group IV

Entire epiphysis sequestrated
Dense line on A-P
Loss of height
Mushroom head
No posterior viable portion
        (on lateral view)
Metaphyseal changes are extensive

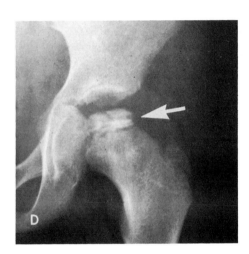

Figure 9–4 *(Continued).*

SECOND METATARSAL HEAD. This affects girls ten to 18 years of age especially, and is associated with a painful metatarsal head. The head of the involved metatarsal becomes flattened, and the adjoining joint becomes narrowed and atrophic.

NAVICULAR TARSAL BONE. This usually develops in children prior to the age of six years. The lesion is more frequent in boys than in girls—often following a history of trauma. The navicular tarsal bone becomes sclerotic and compressed to one-half or even one-fourth of its normal width. After two to three years the bone may be completely restored to a normal appearance.

CARPAL LUNATE BONE. This is usually seen in adults following a history of trauma. The bone appears wedged and sclerotic. A secondary degenerative arthritis may ensue.

SECONDARY EPIPHYSIS OF THE OS CALCIS (SEVER'S DISEASE). Fragmentation of this epiphysis must be interpreted with caution, since its normal appearance is fragmented. Comparison views with the normal side are helpful. Apart from the fragmentation of this secondary ossification center, there is often soft tissue swelling, broadening of the base, deformity, and asymmetrical increased density of necrotic fragments. Regeneration usually proceeds without ultimate deformity, although the course of the disease may be long and protracted.

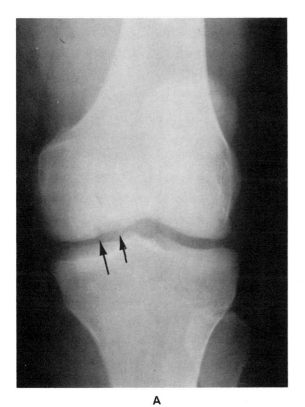

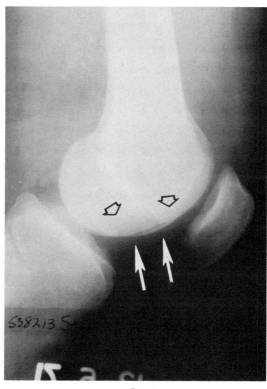

A   B

Figure 9–5 *A* and *B*. Osteochondritis dissecans of the knee, involving the medial femoral condyle. This is a well-circumscribed osteolysis or sequestration of subchondral bone and overlying cartilage of a portion of an epiphysis. The dissected fragment may become totally separated from the rest of the bone, drop into the joint as a loose body, or retain a small particle of connection from which it derives its blood supply. A degenerative arthritis may supervene.

Osteochondritis Dissecans and Benign Chondroblastoma (epiphyseal chondroblastoma) are illustrated in Figures 9–5 and 9–6 respectively.

Transitory Demineralization of the Femoral Head (Rosen).   Transitory demineralization of the femoral head may occur with accompanying pain and disability.

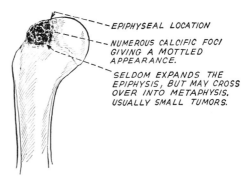

EPIPHYSEAL LOCATION

NUMEROUS CALCIFIC FOCI GIVING A MOTTLED APPEARANCE.

SELDOM EXPANDS THE EPIPHYSIS, BUT MAY CROSS OVER INTO METAPHYSIS. USUALLY SMALL TUMORS.

Figure 9–6   Benign epiphyseal chondroblastoma.

PATHOLOGY: BENIGN TUMOR ORIGINATING IN EPIPHYSES OF UPPER HUMERUS, UPPER TIBIA, AND LOWER FEMUR ESPECIALLY, 1 to 6cm. DIAMETER. CONTAINS NUMEROUS GIANT CELLS AND CALCIFIED CARTILAGE MASSES.

CLINICALLY: 1. PREDOMINANTLY IN MALES AND IN 'TEENS.
2. SLOWLY INCREASING PAIN, AND RESTRICTED MOBILITY LOCAL HEAT.

There may be joint effusion and diffuse osteoporosis of the hips with a loss of the subarticular zone of sclerosis. The medullary bones may appear mottled. These findings persist for approximately one month after the onset of symptoms and resolve themselves without evidence of complication over an interval of two to four months, regardless of therapy.

DIABETIC OSTEOPATHY
(Pogonowska et al.)

1. Osteoporosis.
2. Juxta-articular cortical bone defect.
3. Localized loss of cortex of the metaphysis.
4. Some lysis of the ends of bone with fragmentation but preservation of the articular surface until late.
5. "Pencil-like" or "candlestick" deformity.
6. Loss of adjacent ends of two bones with telescoping of the remainder of these bones.
7. Loss of tips of distal phalanges.
8. Destruction of an entire bone at times.
9. Slight periosteal reaction along the shaft.
10. Occasional sclerosis of the shafts of bones.
11. Reconstruction of phalanges which appear to have been destroyed previously.
12. Occurs predominantly in the distal foot and is probably caused by a vasculotrophic and/or neuropathic disorder with superimposed trauma and infection.

RADIOLUCENT BONE DISEASES OF METAPHYSIS AND EPIPHYSIS, THE "GROWING END"

Neurotrophic or Neurovasculotrophic Osteopathy (Figure 9–7)

Idiopathic Nonfamilial Acro-osteolysis (Figure 9–8).   This lesion may be caused by the direct influence of the nerves on local bone metabolism or by indirect effects of the nerves on blood vessels (vasa nervorum). The conditions which are most prominently associated with such disturbances are leprosy, Raynaud's disease, sclerodactylia, syringomyelia, certain tumors, and injuries of the spinal cord. The *neurogenic arthropathies,* which may accompany the neurotrophic osteopathies, are discussed with joints in Chapter 11.

Massive Osteolysis and Angiomatosis (Halliday et al.; Johnson and McClure). Apart from the other appearances of angiomatosis, the main roentgenographic change in this variety is the tapering of the bone to a conelike spicule at the edges of the lesion. This is apparently due to intraosseous involvement, which removes the medullary support, and to extraosseous involvement, which impresses itself on the bone to the point of complete resorption.

Roentgenologic Features of Ainhum (Fetterman et al.).   The soft tissue changes consist of (1) eversion of the fifth toe; (2) swelling of the soft tissues distally until

A

NEUROTROPHIC OSTEOPATHY

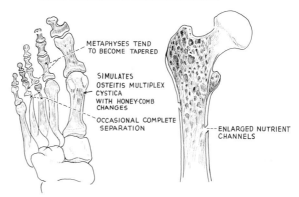

METAPHYSES TEND
TO BECOME TAPERED

SIMULATES
OSTEITIS MULTIPLEX
CYSTICA
WITH HONEY-COMB
CHANGES

OCCASIONAL COMPLETE
SEPARATION

ENLARGED NUTRIENT
CHANNELS

Figure 9–7 *A.* Line tracings of various types of neurotrophic osteopathy. *B.* Radiograph representing neurotrophic lesions of both feet. Note that the toes have not as yet completely sloughed away despite the very considerable osteolysis of the distal metaphysis of the metatarsals.

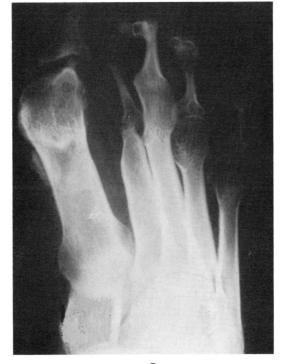

B

the end of the digits assumes a bulbous, spherical character; (3) the presence of a soft tissue groove or sulcus, which gives rise to a ringlike narrowness around the toe.

The bone changes consist largely of dissolution or resorption, which is sharply demarcated. There is no periosteal reaction.

Typically, this condition occurs in the fifth toe of a Negro patient.

Hereditary Sensory Radicular Neuropathy (Pallis and Schneeweins) is also a familial severe relapsing ulceration of the feet, and is of neurotrophic origin. In it, there is progressive destruction of the tarsus, metatarsals, and phalanges in a distal sensory syndrome usually confined to the legs.

(*Text continued on page 288*)

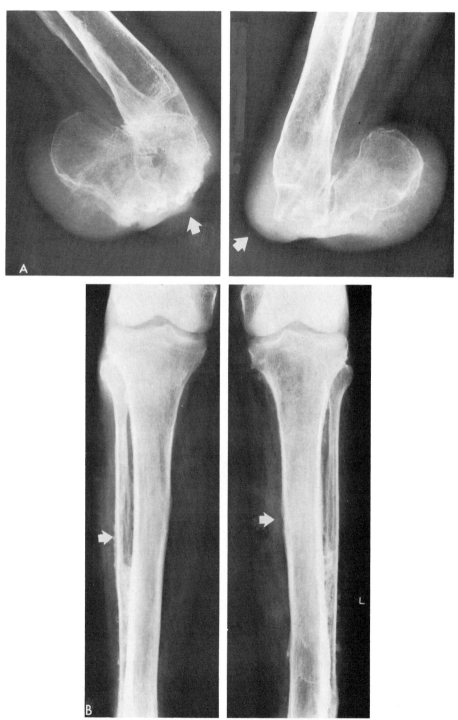

Figure 9–8 *A* and *B*. Idiopathic familial acro-osteolysis. There may be a lysis of the shafts of the distal phalanges, with preservation of the tufts and bases of the phalanges. Skin ulcerations may occur with secondary osteomyelitis, which may involve the metatarsals as well. The nonfamilial variety of this disease is apt to be more generalized, and there may be resorption of the upper and lower alveolar processes of both jaws. There may be multiple wormian bones of the skull and lack of tubulation of the long bones (Papavaisiliou et al.).

AFFECTING METAPHYSIS WITH
MARGINAL SCLEROSIS

Marginal
Sclerosis

Sharply
demarcated
area of
resorption

No sequestrae

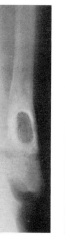

Distortion of
host bone

Bone wall
well defined

Punctate
calcification

I. BRODIE'S ABSCESS   2. ENCHONDROMATA

3. CHONDROMYXOID FIBROMA

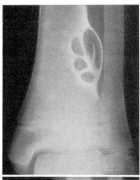

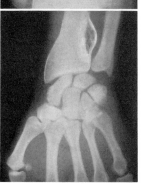

SITES: LONG TUBULAR BONES
        SMALL TUBULAR BONES
        FLAT BONES
SIZE: 3 x 2 x 2 cm.
RADIOGRAPHIC APPEARANCE:
A– OVERLYING CORTEX EXPANDED AND
    THIN DUE TO PRESSURE
B– SMOOTH BORDER WITH LOBULATION
C– WELL DEFINED MEDULLARY BORDER
D– OCCASIONAL RIM OF SCLEROSIS
E– ABSENT PERIOSTEAL REACTION
F– PUNCTATE CALCIFICATION.
    LIMITED BY PERIOSTEUM
G– PSEUDO–SEPTAE

Figure 9–9 *A.* Radiolucent lesions affecting metaphyses primarily with marginal sclerosis. (Radiographs intensified.)

Figure 9–9 continued on following page.

Sharp outer
margin

Few thin
trabeculae

Slight
expansion
cortex

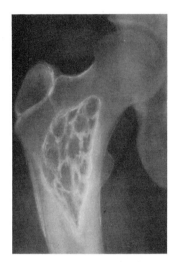

4. SOLITARY BONE CYST

6. FIBROXANTHOMA (NON–OSTEOGENIC
   FIBROMA)

7. "CHONDROMYXOSARCOMA"

8. ANEURYSMAL BONE CYST

Irregular
circumscribed
destruction of
bone with
thick sclerotic
margin

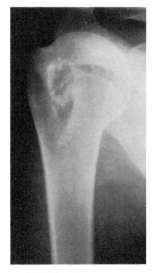

5. FIBROUS DYSPLASIA

Figure 9–9 *A (Continued).*

Figure 9–9 continued on opposite page.

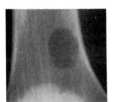
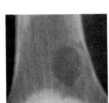
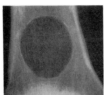

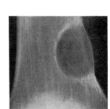

NO "RADIOLOGIC" CAPSULE

MALIGNANT TUMOR METASTASES

MULTIPLE MYELOMA

EOSINOPHILIC GRANULOMA

LIPOID DYSCRASIA

GIANT CELL
TUMOR   USUALLY
                           SOAP-
ANEURYSMAL BONE   BUBBLE
CYST   INTERIOR

DISCONTINUOUS THIN
"RADIOLOGIC" CAPSULE

OSTEITIS FIBROSA CYSTICA
("BROWN TUMOR")

GAUCHER'S DISEASE

BRODIE'S ABSCESS

CONTINUOUS THIN
"RADIOLOGIC" CAPSULE

BRODIE'S ABSCESS

THICK "RADIOLOGIC" CAPSULE

CHRONIC GRANULOMA
OR ABSCESS

FIBROUS DYSPLASIA

BRODIE'S ABSCESS

THICK "RADIOLOGIC" CAPSULE
CORTICAL

FIBROUS CORTICAL DEFECT

FIBROMAS (CHONDROMYXOID)

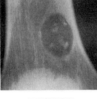
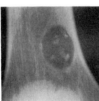

BONE CYST

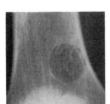

ENCHONDROMA

HEMANGIOMA

Figure 9–9 *(Continued).*   *B*. Analysis of solitary radiolucent lesions of bone by their marginal ("radio-logic capsule") and inner architecture.

RADIOLUCENT OSSEOUS LESIONS AFFECTING METAPHYSES PRIMARILY WITH MARGINAL SCLEROSIS (Figure 9–9)

As indicated in Figure 9–9, these lesions include:
1. Brodie's abscess (Figure 9–10);
2. Enchondromata (Figure 9–11);
3. Chondromyxoid fibroma (Figure 9–12);
4. Solitary bone cyst (Figure 9–13);
5. Fibrous dysplasia (Figure 9–9);
6. Fibroxanthoma (nonosteogenic fibroma) (Figure 9–15);
7. Aneurysmal bone cyst (Figure 9–16);
8. Benign osteoblastoma (giant osteoid osteoma) (Figure 9–17);
9. "Chondromyxosarcoma."

Brodie's Abscess (Figure 9–10).   This entity is a focal abscess of bone surrounded by a thick wall of granulation. The pus is usually sterile.

Radiographic Findings

Well-defined zone of lucency, surrounded by a thick reactive zone of sclerosis.

No sequestrum, no periosteal reaction and no sinus tract formation.

The tibia is probably the most frequently affected bone.

Enchondromas (Figure 9–11).   Solitary enchondromas are found mainly in persons over 20 years of age, in contrast to enchondromatosis, which occurs in younger people in a congenital pattern (Aegerter and Kirkpatrick). These are slow-growing cartilage masses which gradually replace the metaphyses of cylindrical bones, especially the short bones of the hands and feet. The humerus and femur may also be sites of involvement.

Radiographic Findings

There is a lucent replacement of the medullary trabeculae of the short bones so involved and a thin shell of cortex can be identified.

When the cortex becomes very thin, pathologic fracture may ensue. No periosteal reaction can be identified until a fracture induces callus formation.

Osteoblastoma (giant osteoid osteoma), although more frequently affecting

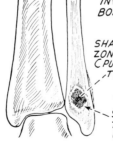

INVOLVES MEDULLARY BONE PARTICULARLY

SHARPLY CIRCUMSCRIBED ZONE OF BONE ABSORPTION (PUS OR GRANULATION TISSUE)

NO SEQUESTRA

SCLEROTIC ZONE UP TO 1 CM. IN WIDTH (NEW BONE FORMATION)

PATHOGENESIS:
RELATIVELY AVIRULENT INFECTION AFFECTING MEDULLARY BONE WITH ONLY MODERATE LOCAL SYMPTOMS AND SIGNS OF INFLAMMATION

CLINICALLY: MAY OR MAY NOT HAVE SYSTEMIC SYMPTOMS

A   **Figure 9–10**   Brodie's abscess. A. Diagram.

Figure 9–10 continued on opposite page.

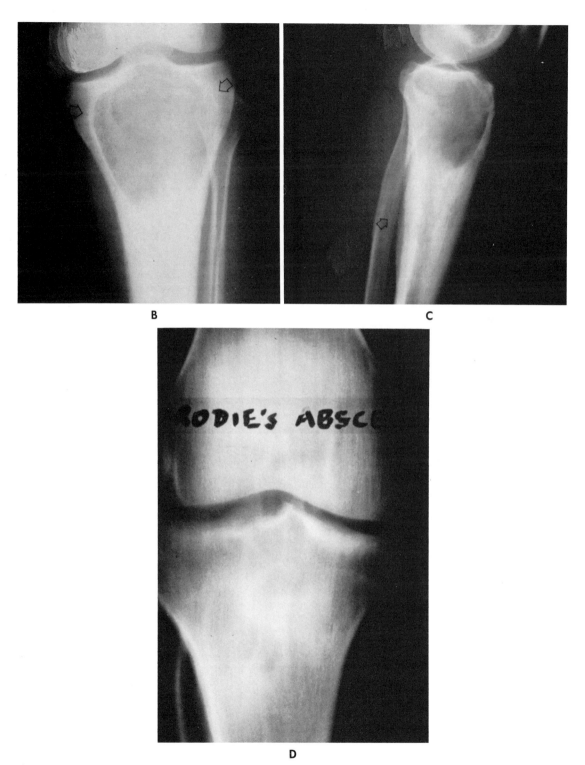

Figure 9-10 (*Continued*).   *B*. Large abscess involving the upper shaft of the tibia in antero-posterior projection. *C*. Lateral view. *D*. Brodie's abscess in a different patient demonstrating the irregular osteolysis with minimal sclerosis surrounding the bone destruction and no sequestration.

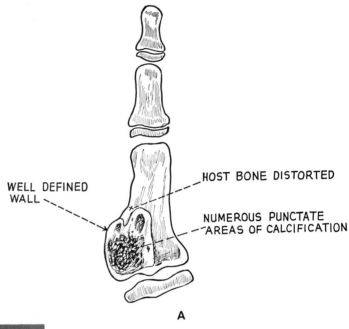

WELL DEFINED
WALL

HOST BONE DISTORTED

NUMEROUS PUNCTATE
AREAS OF CALCIFICATION

A

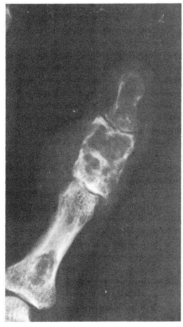

B

Figure 9–11   Benign enchondroma. *A*. Line tracing. *B*. Enchondroma of the middle phalanx of the fifth finger.

Figure 9–11 continued on opposite page.

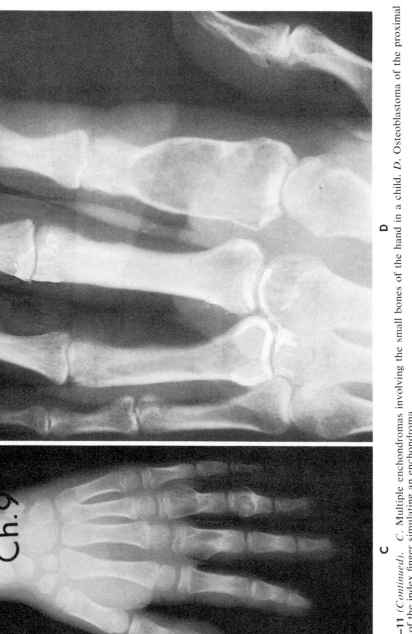

Figure 9–11 *(Continued).* *C.* Multiple enchondromas involving the small bones of the hand in a child. *D.* Osteoblastoma of the proximal phalanx of the index finger simulating an enchondroma.

Figure 9–11 continued on following page.

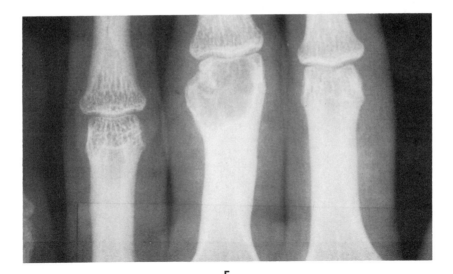

E

Figure 9–11 *(Continued).*   *E.* Fibrous dysplasia of the third proximal phalanx, simulating an enchondroma.

the neural arch and processes of the spine, may also affect the small bones of the hand and foot in an identical fashion (Figure 9–17).

The Chondromyxoid Fibroma (Figure 9–12) (Jaffe and Lichtenstein) is usually small and slow-growing, averaging 2 to 3 cm. in diameter, but lesions as large as 8 cm. in diameter have been described.

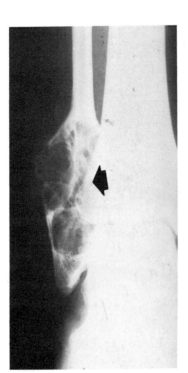

Figure 9–12   Chondromyxoid fibroma of the distal shaft and adjoining epiphysis of the fibula. (Courtesy of the Armed Forces Institute of Pathology, Washington 25, D.C.)

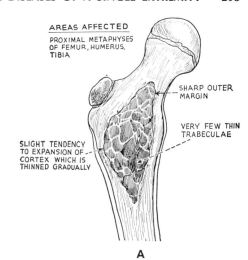

Figure 9–13   *A.* Line tracings of solitary bone cyst. *B.* A-P view demonstrating solitary bone cyst of left femur. *C.* Lateral view. *D.* Lipomatous cyst of the os calcis. This is a fairly common lesion of the os calcis. *E.* Lipoma of the forearm distal to the elbow. The radiolucency, sharp circumscription, trabeculation of the lesion, and lack of adjoining bone involvement suggest this diagnosis strongly.

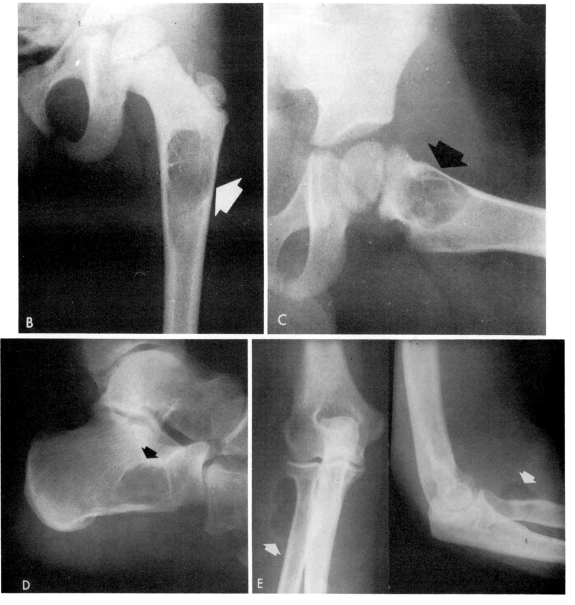

Radiographic Findings

This circumscribed elongated radiolucent lesion is usually found in the metaphysis proximal to the epiphyseal plate and is **eccentric with respect to the medullary portion** of the bone.

The overlying cortex is usually thin and the internal aspect of the tumor usually has a scalloped and slightly sclerotic margin.

The usual inner pattern is that of coarse trabeculation.

Solitary Bone Cyst (Figure 9–13). The solitary bone cyst is a thin, sharply demarcated metaphyseal lesion accompanied by expansion and thinning of the bony cortex, and consisting of a central portion of either sanguineous or chocolate-colored fluid. There is *usually a thin fibrous capsule*. The preferred sites for involvement are the proximal metaphyses of the femora, humeri, and tibiae.

Radiographic Findings

The lesion is **sharply circumscribed** by a **thin sclerotic linear margin** and the cortex overlying the cyst appears thinned-out.

The lesion is centrally located in the metaphysis usually, or **appears to have been bypassed in the metaphysis** during the growth of the child.

It usually **does not cross the epiphyseal plate** into the epiphysis (unlike the chondroblastoma).

It may contain a single cavity or very fine trabeculations.

When fractured by minor trauma a **fragment of the wall of the cyst will often protrude into the cyst** (Figure 9–13), or **fall by gravity to the bottom of the cyst,** further suggesting the liquid content of the cyst ("falling fragment sign").

The solitary bone cyst may be differentiated from the giant cell tumor in

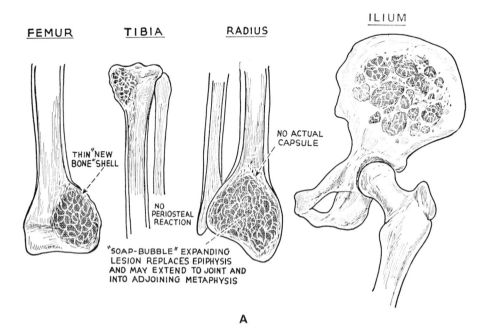

A

Figure 9–14 Giant cell tumor of the sacrum. *A*. Tracings showing pertinent features.

Figure 9–14 continued on opposite page.

B

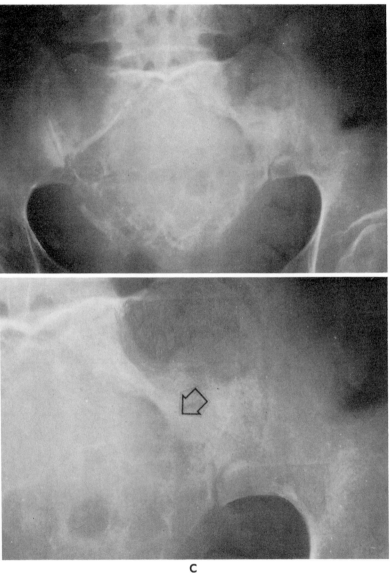

C

Figure 9–14 *(Continued).   B.* View of the entire sacrum showing the lack of sharp margination and the foamy appearance of the inner architecture of the neoplasm. *C.* Close-up view to demonstrate: (1) the "bubbly" inner architectural pattern; (2) the lack of discrete margination.

Figure 9–14 continued on following page.

that the giant cell tumor (Figure 9–14) is characterized by (1) Absence of the thin sclerotic margin; (2) Absence of the bypass growth in the metaphysis and the tumor may even involve the epiphysis, having crossed the epiphyseal plate; (3) Absence of side wall internal spiculation since the giant cell tumor is a solid and not a cystic structure; (4) The patient's age, which for a giant cell tumor is rarely prior to epiphyseal closure (age 20 years).

Fibrous Dysplasia of Bone

Clinical Considerations.   Fibrous dysplasia may be monostotic or polyostotic. Any bone in the skeleton may be involved, but since the monostotic variety is more

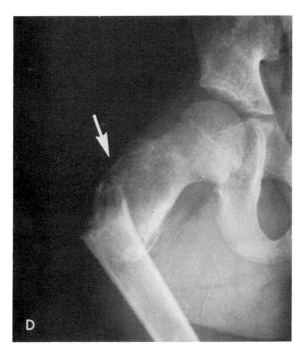

Figure 9–14 *(Continued).* *D.* Giant cell tumor of the upper metaphysis of the femur with a pathologic fracture.

common it is included in this section. The long bones of the extremities, ribs, skull, and facial bones may be especially involved.

When *polyostotic,* clinical considerations frequently conform to a syndrome described by Albright: (1) The bone lesions tend to be unilateral in distribution; (2) There are often scattered areas of melanotic pigmentation of the skin, usually on the side of the bone lesions; (3) The syndrome occurs especially in young females with precocious puberty.

Pathology

The lesions in the bone are characterized by focal areas of fibrous replacement of bone with *metaplastic* formation of irregular bone. (Fibrous dysplasia of bone closely resembles other fibrous lesions of bone, such as ossifying fibroma, nonossifying fibroma, and reparative fibrosis within a bone cyst, but it can be distinguished by the metaplastic bone formations (Reed).) Pathogenetically, the process represents a defect in the normal remodeling of bone in which resorbed bone is replaced by fibrous tissue and poorly formed woven bone. The original mass appears to extend in projecting lobules which cause deformity of the original bone.

Radiographic Findings

Because of irregular masses of poorly woven bone internal to the lesion, **fibrous dysplasia at times appears sclerotic rather than radiolucent.** (Some of the lucency may be related to coexisting arteriovenous malformations.)

Bending of the involved bone because of softening and pathologic fractures with marked proliferation of periosteal callus are common.

When the **facial bones** are involved, the **marked thickening and opacity** of the bones appear to predominate.

Encroachment upon the normal facial or cranial spaces are noteworthy.

Marked prognathism occurs with involvement of the mandible.

Exophthalmos occurs with involvement of the orbit.

Bony protuberances occur with involvement of the paranasal sinuses (see Chapter 12).

The lesions are practically always covered by a thick or thin bony cortical shell (Figure 9–15B), since the cortex of the bone appears to be eroded from within and the periosteum lays down a thin shell of bone to compensate.

Fibroxanthoma (Nonossifying Fibroma of Jaffe); Fibrous Cortical Defect (Figure 9–15)

General Considerations.   This lesion is most frequently seen in the lower part of the femoral shaft near the epiphyseal plate. Less often, it occurs in the upper shaft of the tibia, the upper or lower part of the fibular shaft, and far less frequently, in the shafts of the humerus, radius, ulna, or short tubular bones.

Radiographic Findings.   The lesion appears as a radiolucent **cortical** defect near one end of the affected bone shaft. The long axis tends to parallel the long axis of the shaft and it ranges in size from 1 to 4 cm. In some instances it appears to be lobulated. There is ordinarily a very thin reactive shell around this lesion.

Jaffe believes that the fibroxanthoma is a later stage in the development of the fibrous cortical defect.

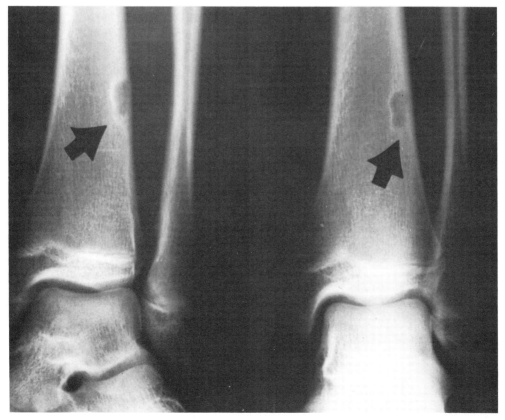

Figure 9–15 Nonosteogenic fibroma of Lichtenstein and Jaffe. (Courtesy of Colonel William L. Thompson, Armed Forces Institute of Pathology.)

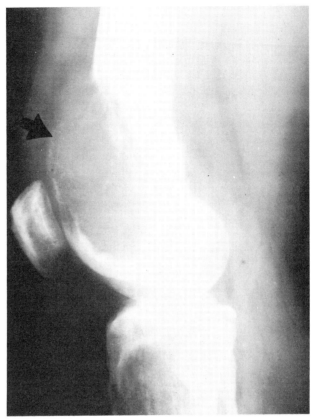

Figure 9–16 Aneurysmal bone cyst involving the distal metaphysis and epiphysis of the femur, a "blister of bone" appearance. Although this is called an aneurysmal bone cyst by many, it has also been called cystic giant cell tumor, especially with a history of injury. The thin bony roof of the lesion is noteworthy. (Courtesy of Colonel William L. Thompson, Armed Forces Institute of Pathology.)

Aneurysmal Bone Cyst (Figure 9–16)

Pathology. The cyst is a saccular protrusion of the bony cortex—a "blister of bone." Any bone of the skeleton may be involved, but about one-quarter of the cases occur in vertebrae (Aegerter and Kirkpatrick). It most often affects the ends of long bones but may affect the diaphysis, pushing the contiguous periosteum outward, which reacts by laying down a thin shell of bone. This thin shell may fracture, causing an extravasation of blood into the adjoining tissues. Occasionally the short tubular bones of the hands or feet may be affected. Children and adolescents are often affected.

Radiographic Findings. Saccular protrusion of the end of a long bone with multiple fine septae internally, and sharply demarcated, bulging, scalloped borders. It appears to begin in the cancellous bone and is surrounded by a thin identifiable cortex or periosteal new bone layer, which has a "blister of bone" appearance. In vertebrae the neural arch is usually the site of involvement.

The Benign Osteoblastoma (Giant Osteoid Osteoma, Osteogenic Fibroma)
(Lichtenstein) (Figures 9–11D and 9–17)

Radiographic Findings

Predominantly an osteolytic expanding process with evidence of cortical erosion, but there may be occasional bone production or calcification of varying degree within the tumor or around it.

A soft tissue mass arising from the eroded cortex is noted in about two-thirds of the cases.

In some cases a definite calcific shell of a characteristic nature sharply delimits the soft tissue mass. Usually an intact shell can be detected.

The tumor is usually well demarcated from the normal neighboring bone.

The tumors vary in size from approximately 2 by 1.5 cm. by 6 cm. to 10 by 6 by 6.5 cm., with an average of 2 by 3 cm.

Principal Sites of Involvement

In more than one-half of the cases, the tumor is situated in the *vertebral column.* The *neural arch* is the favorite region, and the pedicle in most instances is also invaded.

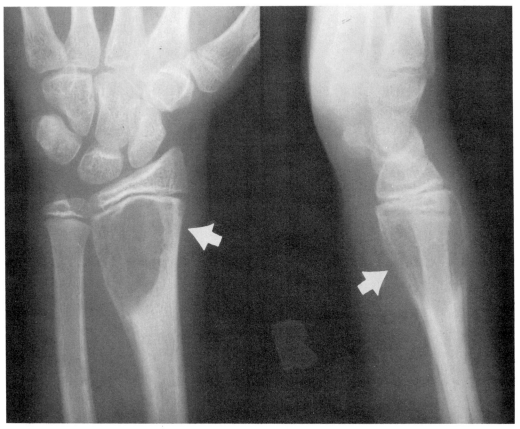

Figure 9–17   Antero-posterior and lateral views of the wrist showing a benign osteoblastoma (giant osteoid osteoma) in the distal shaft of the radius.

The second most frequent location (20 per cent) is long bone where the tumor has been identified as equally distributed between the ends and the shafts (Figure 9–17).

Many of the tumors involve small bones. Most of the time the tumor appears to have an eccentric origin.

General Comment. *Ordinarily there is no nidus which is so characteristic of osteoid osteoma and which clinically and radiographically is an entirely different type of lesion. Despite its benign nature it is an actively growing neoplasm.*

"Chondromyxosarcoma." According to Jaffe, the chondromyxoid fibroma may be misdiagnosed as a chondrosarcoma (Figure 9–12); the same author states that one should refrain from making the diagnosis of "chondromyxosarcoma." This condition, both radiographically and histologically, must not be confused with the chondrosarcoma which will be described in Chapter 10.

RADIOLUCENT DISEASES OF BONE AFFECTING THE METAPHYSIS PRIMARILY WITHOUT MARGINAL SCLEROSIS (Figure 9–18)

The diseases most frequently encountered in this category are:
1. Suppurative osteomyelitis;
2. Osteomyelitis, nonsuppurative;

AFFECTING METAPHYSIS PRIMARILY—
NO MARGINAL SCLEROSIS

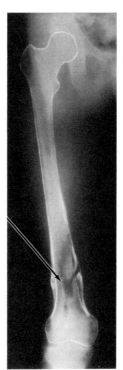

Infection
enters via
nutrient shaft

Elevation of
periosteum
by exudate

Area of
absorption
in shaft

1. INFECTION—DOES NOT PROCEED BEYOND EPIPHYSEAL LINE. NEIGHBORING BONE DECALCIFIED.
2. TUMOR—PRIMARY OR SECONDARY
    A–OSTEOSARCOMA
    B–METASTATIC TUMOR
        TO BONE

Figure 9–18 Radiolucent diseases affecting the metaphysis primarily, without marginal sclerosis. (Diagrammatic intensified radiograph.)

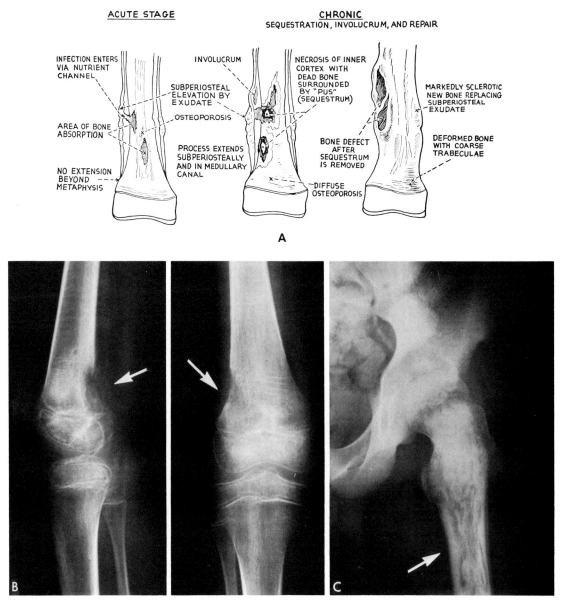

Figure 9–19 *A.* Primary hematogenous type of acute and chronic osteomyelitis demonstrating the various stages of development and pathogenesis. *B.* Acute osteomyelitis affecting the distal metaphysis of the left femur. *C.* A more advanced stage of osteomyelitis in the subchronic phase demonstrating advanced necrosis and sequestrum formation. Note that the destructive process stops at the epiphyseal line and does not cross into the epiphysis.

3. Sarcoid of bone;
4. Giant cell tumor;
5. Osteosarcoma;
6. Metastatic tumor to bone (Chapter 7);
7. Radiation osteitis.

Suppurative Osteomyelitis has been described in Chapter 8 (Figure 8–13) and is again illustrated in Figure 9–19. The radiographic stages may be summarized as follows.

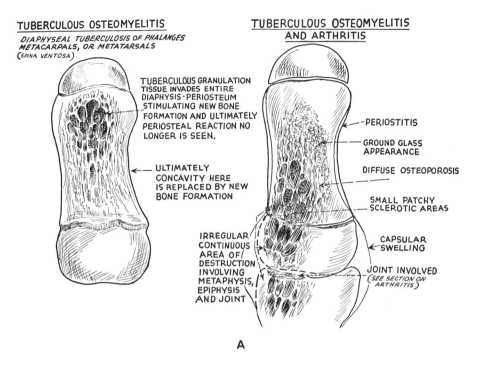

TUBERCULOUS OSTEOMYELITIS

DIAPHYSEAL TUBERCULOSIS OF PHALANGES METACARPALS, OR METATARSALS
(*SPINA VENTOSA*)

TUBERCULOUS GRANULATION TISSUE INVADES ENTIRE DIAPHYSIS-PERIOSTEUM STIMULATING NEW BONE FORMATION AND ULTIMATELY PERIOSTEAL REACTION NO LONGER IS SEEN.

ULTIMATELY CONCAVITY HERE IS REPLACED BY NEW BONE FORMATION

TUBERCULOUS OSTEOMYELITIS AND ARTHRITIS

PERIOSTITIS

GROUND GLASS APPEARANCE

DIFFUSE OSTEOPOROSIS

SMALL PATCHY SCLEROTIC AREAS

CAPSULAR SWELLING

JOINT INVOLVED
(*SEE SECTION ON ARTHRITIS*)

IRREGULAR CONTINUOUS AREA OF DESTRUCTION INVOLVING METAPHYSIS, EPIPHYSIS AND JOINT

A

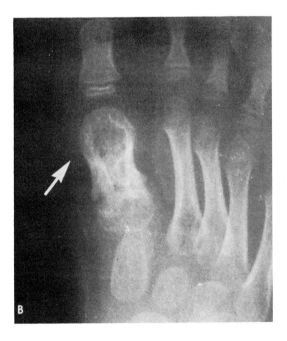

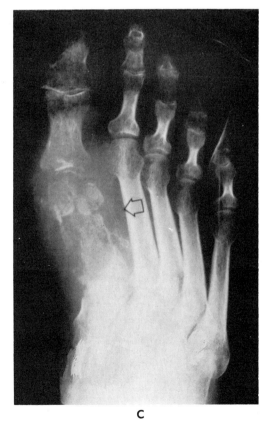

Figure 9–20 *A* and *B*. Osteomyelitis tuberculous cystic type (spina ventosa). *C*. Blastomycosis of the great toe.

C

Figure 9–20 continued on opposite page.

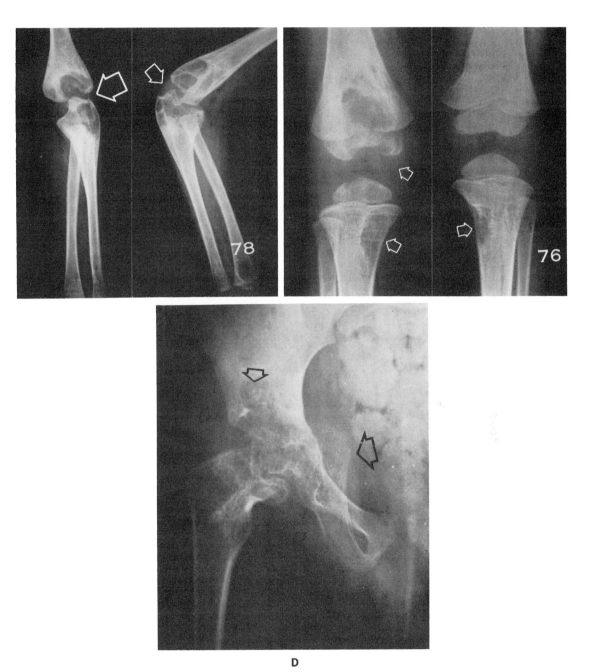

D

Figure 9–20 (*Continued*).   *D*. Tuberculosis of bones and joints. (1) Tuberculosis of the elbow; (2) The knee; (3) The hip with marked swelling of the obturator fascia and hip joint capsule. Tuberculous dactylitis is referred to as spina ventosa. (D (1) and (2) courtesy Dr. J. Johnston, Oakland, California.)

Radiographic Stages

No roentgen abnormalities usually occur until seven to ten days or longer after onset of infection.

Soft tissue swelling adjacent to the involved bone may be the earliest roentgen manifestation.

In untreated cases **small areas of rarefaction** may appear in the metaphyseal ends of the involved long bones.

The spread of the infection through the medullary bone and cortex causes **an elevation and reaction in the overlying periosteum.** Indeed, the appearance of new bone formation by such elevated periosteum may precede the roentgen observation of the lucency of the bone involved.

The **radiolucency spreads,** involving more and more of the shaft of the bone, but ordinarily **the epiphyseal plate is not crossed.** Arthritic involvement may occur if this barrier does break down.

Devitalization of the bone causes the formation of **sequestra** which can be recognized radiographically as dense osteosclerotic spicules of dead bone surrounded by a lucent zone of bone resorption.

Reactive new bone formation adjoining the destruction gives rise to the appearance of **involucra.**

EARLY ROENTGEN OBSERVATIONS IN ACUTE OSTEOMYELITIS
(Capitano and Kirkpatrick)

1. Earliest finding is a small local soft tissue swelling in the region of the metaphysis. This is shown by displacement of soft tissue planes outlined by fatty sheaths.

2. A few days later, swelling of the muscles and obliteration of the lucent planes between the muscles occur.

3. Superficial subcutaneous soft tissue edema is the last soft tissue change to be observed.

4. Although considerable bone destruction is present during this latter phase, it is still not visible roentgenographically. However, a mild local rarefaction of the metaphysis may be seen at this time.

5. The classic roentgenologic picture of bone destruction and periosteal new bone formation is not seen until 10 or 12 days after the onset of symptoms or after treatment.

6. The amount of bone destruction visible roentgenologically by the end of the second week is ordinarily far less than the actual amount of bone destruction present.

Nonsuppurative Osteomyelitis involves: tuberculosis of bone; mycotic infections of bone; fungus infections; syphilis of bone; brucella osteomyelitis; and possibly viral osteomyelitis.

Tuberculous Osteomyelitis may be classified into four types: (1) spine; (2) osteitis and arthritis combined (Figure 9–20); (3) diaphyseal tuberculosis; and (4) tuberculoid reactions in bone.

Tuberculosis of the Spine; there is usually combined destruction of the vertebral end-plates and intervertebral cartilage, with partial collapse of the vertebrae and considerable paraspinous abscess formation. These will be described more fully in Chapter 14.

Tuberculous Osteomyelitis and Arthritis. These usually coexist in long bones. The hip and knee are most commonly involved. Tuberculosis of the shoulder is shown in Figure 9–20.

RADIOGRAPHIC FINDINGS

Marked **radiolucency** and some evidence of **bone dissolution,** with minimal or **no sequestration.**

There is ordinarily **very little reactive bone formation** and **little or no periosteal reaction.**

Surrounding soft tissue atrophy results if the process is of long duration.

Diaphyseal Tuberculosis Without Adjoining Joint Involvement is rare, but extensive bone destruction with it is also rare, since this disorder heals more readily. The *greater trochanter* of the femur and the *diaphysis of the small bones of the hands* (spina ventosa) are sites of such involvement (Figure 9–20).

Tuberculoid Reactions in Bone Adjoining Tuberculous Arthritis. There is usually a disappearance of cancellous bone adjoining tuberculous arthritis.

PATHOLOGY. Replacement of cancellous bone by tuberculous granulations, but there is no actual necrosis or abscess formation. In a microscopic examination, no granulomas may be visible.

RADIOGRAPHIC FINDINGS. Severe radiolucency is manifest (Figure 9–20), with marked thinning but some preservation of the trabecular architecture. The appearance is that of severe osteoporosis.

Nocardial Osteomyelitis produces lesions in bone which are radiographically identical to those of tuberculosis.

Fungus Infections of Bone. These are usually secondary to involvement of the overlying or adjoining soft tissues, with the exception of coccidioidomycosis and blastomycosis. The latter are hematogenous in origin usually.

Actinomycosis affects the bones of the mandible, rib cage, and vertebrae especially, and is accompanied by draining sinuses. The granulomatous reaction is much like tuberculosis. Apart from *site* predilection, no special radiologic appearances can be attributed to these.

EOSINOPHILIC GRANULOMA OF BONE

1. The sites of involvement by frequency can be inferred from a report by Ochsner. He reported 20 cases as follows: skull, six; ribs and spine, each three; mastoid, pelvis, femur, each two; mandible and humerus, each one.

2. The essential roentgenographic lesion is a localized area of rarefaction which occurs in the medullary portion of the bone; it may develop a scalloped defect in the inner cortical profile as it enlarges.

3. Pathologic fracture may supervene with a periosteal reaction.

4. There is usually no sclerotic zone otherwise.

5. In the spine a single vertebral body may collapse producing a vertebra plana. This is not pathognomonic.

6. In the mandible there may be a cyst-like area around a tooth producing a "floating tooth sign" similar to histiocytosis.

7. Ribs, pelvis, and long bones do not have specific lesions otherwise.

8. Epiphyses may be affected.

9. In the lung the lesion tends to be honeycombed.

10. Gastrointestinal tract lesions may also occur, especially polypoid lesions of the stomach (Rigler et al.; Ochsner).

Blastomycosis Usually Produces a Slow Dissolution of Involved Bone and May Involve Peripheral Small Bones Especially (Figure 9–20 D). Occasionally a thick zone of sclerosis in the involved area may be identified surrounding the zone of bone dissolution.

Syphilis of Bone (Figure 9–21). This may be congenital or acquired.

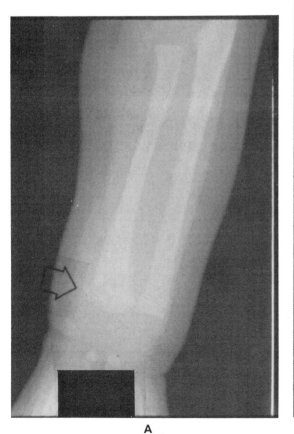
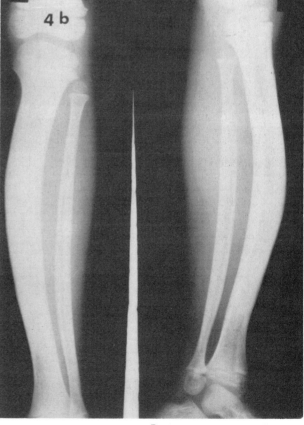

A B

Figure 9–21 Congenital syphilis involving bone. *A.* Syphilitic osteochondritis involving the distal radius in an infant with evidence also of periostitis overlying the distal radius. *B.* Congenital syphilis in an older child showing the typical saber shin bowing of the tibia.

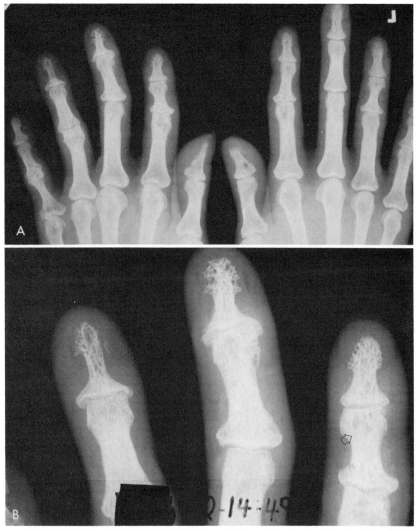

Figure 9–22   Sarcoid of the phalanges of the hand. *A*. View of the scattered and rather indiscriminate involvement of the ends of these short bones. *B*. Closeup view of several of the digits showing the cystic type resorption of the proximal and distal ends of the involved phalanges. Note also the frayed appearance of the phalangeal tufts.

Congenital Syphilis has been previously described as predominantly a metaphyseal osteochondritis and periostitis. The "saber shin" is a late manifestation (Figure 9–21; see also Chapter 8).

Acquired Syphilis of bone is a tertiary manifestation with involvement primarily of the walls of arterioles. Both long and flat bones may be involved. Necrotizing and proliferating responses in the involved sites coexist; thus, radiographically, *bone destruction and proliferation are usually found simultaneously.* There may be numerous jagged appearances with irregular subperiosteal new bone formation, imparting to the involved bone a combined lucent and sclerotic appearance. Since the sclerotic appearance may predominate, the description is placed in Chapter 10.

Brucella Osteomyelitis.   Involves the vertebrae most frequently but may involve the larger long bones or the flat bones of the pelvis.

Radiographic Appearances. Those of a suppurative osteomyelitis, with bone destruction and periosteal proliferation.

Sarcoid in Bone most frequently occurs in the small bones of the *hands and feet,* particularly the metacarpals, metatarsals, and phalanges. Any part of the reticulo-endothelial system may be involved as well. The granulomatous process in the marrow of these small bones is destructive without inner or periosteal reaction.

Radiographic Findings

Small "pseudocystic" foci of lucency are especially observed in the hands and feet, because of destruction of the small trabeculae.

A coarse reticular trabecular pattern may also be observed (Figure 9–22).

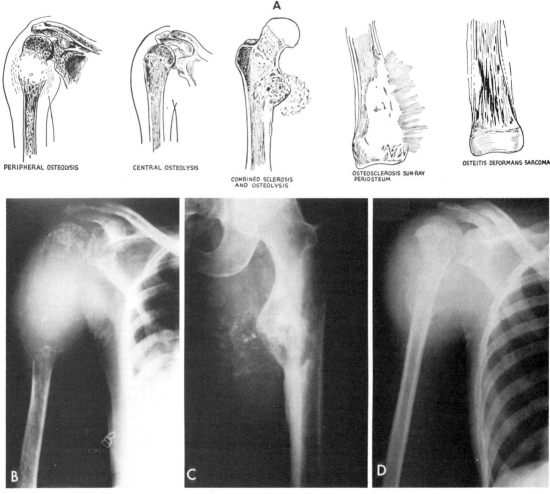

Figure 9–23 *A.* Sketches demonstrating peripheral osteolytic and central osteolytic types of osteosarcoma, combined sclerotic and osteolytic type, sclerotic sun-ray type, and type derived from osteitis deformans by malignant degeneration thereof. *B.* Radiograph demonstrating the osteolytic variety of osteosarcoma. *C.* Radiograph demonstrating the combined osteolytic and osteosclerotic type of osteosarcoma. *D.* Osteolytic variety of osteosarcoma, less advanced. (Sketches modified from Schinz-Case: Roentgen-Diagnostics.)

Figure 9–23 continued on opposite page.

The Giant Cell Tumor (Figure 9–14).   This lesion is usually situated in the end of some long tubular bone but may be situated in flat bones such as the ilium or scapula. The lower end of the femur, the upper end of the tibia, and the lower end of the radius are the three most common sites for the lesion. These account for 60 to 70 per cent of the localizations.

When there is a multiplicity of involvement, one must strongly suspect hyperparathyroidism, in which case *osteitis fibrosa cystica* may closely resemble the histologic appearance of the giant cell tumor.

Radiographic Findings

The bone cortex in the affected region is thinned and expanded and has a large "soap bubble" appearance.

There is **very little periosteal new bone formation** over the thinned and expanded cortex.

A marginal zone of sclerosis, either thick or thin, is usually not present.

It is probable that the diagnostic value of the **multilocular** appearance so frequently stressed in the past has been overemphasized, and one may be led astray if the presence of this appearance is necessarily expected in all instances.

A pathologic fracture of the thin cortex may be present.

Unfortunately, the radiographic picture of fibrosarcoma can perfectly simulate that of a giant cell tumor.

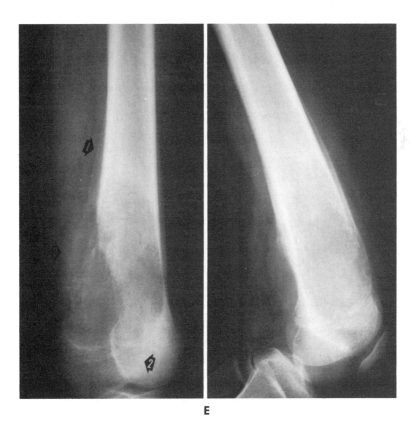

E

Figure 9–23 (*Continued*). *E.* Osteosarcoma of a lytic type involving the distal femur. (1) Oblique view shows Codman's triangle as well as the lysis and some tendency to new bone formation with invasion of the adjoining soft tissues. (2) Lateral view of the femur showing the marked lysis of the distal ends of the femur crossing into the epiphysis with the layerlike periosteal reaction on the anterior aspect of the femur. Codman's triangle is shown on the posterior aspect.

Osteosarcoma. Approximately three-quarters of osteosarcomas occur in the metaphyses of the lower femur or upper tibia in persons between 12 and 25 years of age.

Radiographic Findings. Various types of osteosarcomas are illustrated in Figure 9–23. These include primary manifestations of:

Peripheral osteolysis with a break in the cortex and a soft tissue mass.

Central osteolysis with a break in the cortex and a soft tissue mass.

Combined sclerosis and osteolysis, a break in the cortex, and a soft tissue mass.

Osteosclerosis with a sunray-type reaction of the periosteum and a soft tissue mass.

A mosaic intermixture of sclerosis and radiolucency with periosteal layering and reactions which suggest malignant degeneration from an osteitis deformans (Paget's disease of bone). The latter occurs particularly in patients over 50 years of age.

In the periosteum, Codman's triangle (the zone of reactive bone formation adjoining the tumor periosteum) is very often identified, but this may also occur with inflammatory benign lesions.

Roentgenologic Aspects of Radiation Osteitis (Bragg et al.).   In most instances the appearance suggests a loss of bone substance as well as a coarsening of the trabeculae.

Sclerosis or an associated mass is uncommon.

However, associated pathologic fractures are very common.

Occasionally, calcification within the lesion of a diffuse type may be noted.

The external diaphyseal diameter of the involved bone does not appear to change.

In the pelvis there is a tendency to mixed areas of dense sclerotic bone as well as focal loss of bone substance. Pathologic fracture is frequent. A somewhat similar appearance is noted in the ribs.

DIAPHYSEAL CORTICOPERIOSTEAL RADIOLUCENT LESIONS (Figure 9–24)

In this group of diseases one must include a number of entities which have already been described in other categories, such as:

1. Acute and chronic osteomyelitis and the mycotic infections of bone;
2. Traumatic periostitis with or without fractures;
3. Milkman's disease and associated pseudofractures (related to osteomalacia);
4. Osteosarcoma;
5. The round cell tumors, including the histiocytoses or reticuloendothelioses, solitary myeloma (of the plasma cell variety especially); Ewing's sarcoma, neuroblastoma, and reticulum cell sarcoma.

The disease entities which remain to be considered in this category are:

6. Ewing's tumor of bone;
7. Neuroblastoma;
8. Neurofibromatosis of bone;
9. Hemangioma of bone;
10. Osteomyelitis secondary to adjoining cellulitis;
11. Fibrosarcoma of bone, both of the endosteal and parosteal types.

DIAPHYSEAL CORTICO-PERIOSTEAL LESIONS

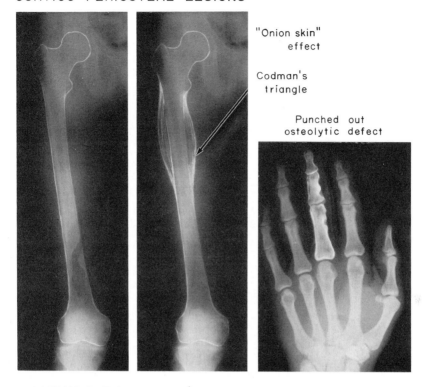

"Onion skin" effect

Codman's triangle

Punched out osteolytic defect

1. OSTEOMYELITIS   5. EWING'S TUMOR AND OTHER ROUND CELL TUMORS   6. NEUROFIBROMATOSIS

2. TRAUMATIC PERIOSTITIS AND FRACTURES

3. PSEUDOFRACTURES (MILKMAN'S DISEASE)

4. OSTEOSARCOMA

7. HEMANGIOMA

8. OSTEOMYELITIS, SECONDARY TYPE

9. FIBROSARCOMA

Figure 9–24   Diaphyseal corticoperiosteal radiolucent lesions. (Diagrammatic intensified radiographs.)

Ewing's Tumor (Endothelioma)

General Comments.   Ewing's tumor is one of the round cell tumors, which, like plasma cell myeloma and reticulum cell sarcoma, is derived from the reticulum of the bone marrow. *It is the third most common malignant primary bone tumor* and is surpassed only by plasma-cell myeloma and osteosarcoma. Virtually all patients are seen *before the age of 30.* Involvement of males is probably somewhat more frequent than females.

Principal Sites.   Most cases in younger persons begin in cylindrical bones, whereas the flat bones are more frequently involved in older patients. The tumor is situated most frequently in the femur and tibia but even the small bones of the feet, especially the os calcis, may be affected. Of the flat bones, those of the pelvic girdle are most commonly involved. Ribs and vertebrae may also, however, be affected.

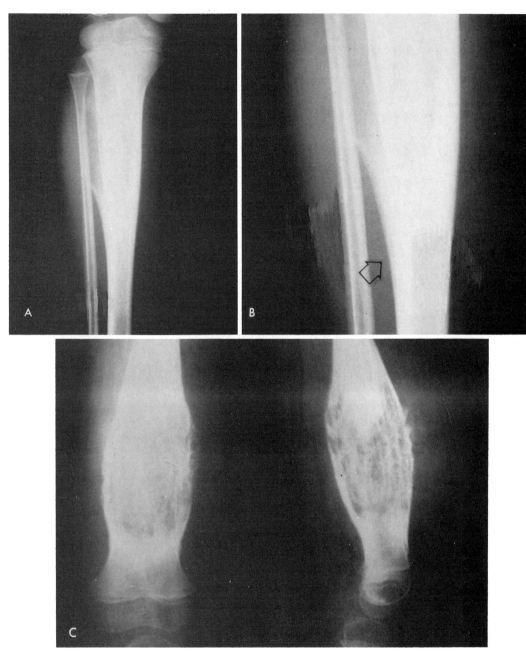

Figure 9–25   Ewing's tumor. *A.* Antero-posterior view of the upper shaft of the involved tibia, demonstrating medullary corticoperiosteal involvement. There is a lamination of the elevated periosteum. *B.* A closeup view of Codman's triangle adjoining the lesion. *C.* A different patient with Ewing's sarcoma involving the distal shaft of the femur. This view demonstrates the "onion peel" appearance of the entire destroyed portion of the distal shaft of the femur.

Radiographic Findings (Figure 9–25)

The tumor usually first involves the medullary canal, grows through the fine nutrient canals of the cortex to reach the extraosseous soft tissues. The nutrient vessels are closed to advancing tumor and the **bone undergoes necrosis. A large soft tissue mass is usually associated.**

The **periosteum is elevated in layers,** producing the so-called "onion skin" appearance.

At the extremes of the periosteal elevation there is new bone formation **(Codman's triangle).**

The metaphysis is frequently involved and even the epiphysis may occasionally be the site of origin.

Sclerosis of the bone may at times be indicated by a streaky appearance of the involved areas, and it is accentuated by radiolucency (due to the osseous destruction) of the adjoining bone.

Unfortunately, only 25 per cent of Ewing's tumors present this classic radiographic appearance (Sherman and Soong).

Also, although a diagnosis may possess a high index of suspicion, **there is a close radiographical resemblance to osteomyelitis, eosinophilic granuloma, osteosarcoma, and reticulum cell sarcoma, and biopsy is therefore essential** for definitive diagnosis.

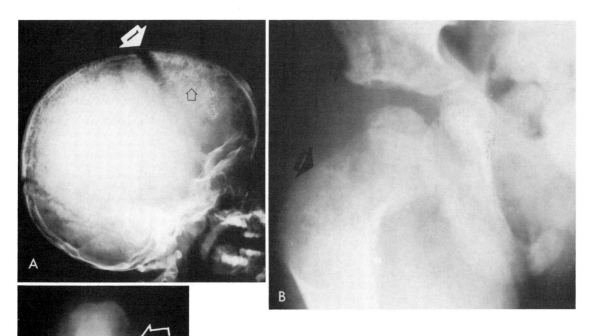

Figure 9–26 Neuroblastoma of bone. *A.* Lateral view of the skull showing diastasis of the suture with invasion of the calvarium usually from involvement of the meninges. *B.* Antero-posterior view of the right hip showing diffuse neuroblastomatous metastases involving the femur and the acetabulum. *C.* Metastases from the neuroblastoma to the os calcis in this same patient.

Neuroblastoma in Bone (Figure 9–26)

General Comments.   This tumor may arise from the sympathetic nervous system anywhere in the body, but about *half the cases have their origin in the adrenal medulla.* Characteristically, the small "round cells" of this lesion form a rosette pattern around neurofibrils. *Next to leukemia, neuroblastoma is the most common malignant disease occurring in infancy and childhood,* the onset frequently being seen *before the age of seven.*

Radiographic Findings

Bone lesions are moderately well-demarcated **osteolytic** processes with a strong tendency to symmetry of involvement. Thus the lower portions of **both** femurs are apt to be affected. Because there are often three or more bones involved simultaneously at the time of discovery, this disease entity should probably be categorized in Chapter 8 rather than here. The lesion is included here because of its corticoperiosteal appearance when an isolated lesion is seen. The **multiplicity of these lesions,** however, is noteworthy.

The **bony cortex is usually destroyed** with a periosteal reaction which may assume a **"sunburst" appearance,** although this is not pathognomonic for neuroblastoma.

In the skull there is often separation of the **skull sutures (diastasis)** due to increased intracranial pressure from metastatic tumors or meningeal involvement.

Neurofibroma (Figure 9–27)

General Comment.   Neurofibromas of bone are variable in appearance but are usually secondary to nerve involvement.

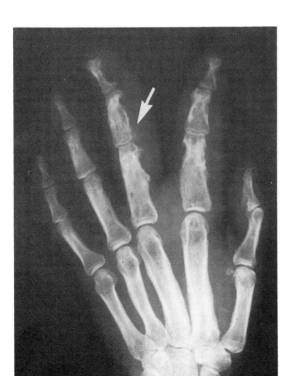

Figure 9–27 Neurofibromatosis affecting the right hand.

Radiographic Findings

The bone changes include: **scoliosis, bone atrophy, bone hypertrophy of individual bones, and skeletal anomalies. Many of the defects in the bone, but not all, apparently are the result of pressure from associated neurofibromas.**

At times only slight irregularity of bone contour is noted with cystlike cavities adjoining.

Holt and Wright reported that 29 per cent of the total group of cases studied by them showed some form of skeletal defect, and these were classified as follows:

    a. Erosive defects.
    b. Scoliosis, with dysplasia of the vertebral body.
    c. Disorders of growth, including both over- and underdevelopment.
    d. Bowing and pseudoarthrosis of the lower legs.
    e. Intraosseous cystic lesions.
    f. Numerous congenital anomalies.

Hunt and Pugh have added the following:

    g. Defects of the posterior-superior orbital wall.
    h. Disorders of growth in bone associated with elephantoid hypertrophy of overlying soft tissues.
    i. Intrathoracic meningocele.

The latter authors indicated that sarcomatous degeneration of the neurofibromas occurred in 5 per cent of the patients.

Hemangioma of Bone and Lymphangiomas of Bone (Figure 9–28)

General Comment. These lesions are usually located in the spine or skull, but other areas such as the extremities may also be involved.

Radiographic Findings

Vertebrae are involved in 10 to 30 per cent of cases, and a **characteristic vertical striated radiographic appearance may be noted** (Figure 9–28). Collapse of the involved vertebral body may result in pressure upon cord or nerve roots.

In the **extremities** there is often an **overgrowth** of the involved part. The lesion is usually corticoperiosteal with an expansion of the cortex and extension toward the medulla.

It has a multilocular appearance but the "bubbly" appearance is smaller and scattered, unlike the "soap bubble" appearance earlier described for the giant cell tumor and the aneurysmal bone cyst.

Also the lesions are usually in the diaphysis rather than in the epiphysis or metaphysis.

Massive Progressive Osteolysis of Bones, or Acro-osteolysis. This condition is related to hemangioma of bone. It may or may not be familial, and when it is acquired by adolescents and young adults, it usually follows trauma. In the few cases which have been studied, microscopic examination has usually revealed angiomas in the involved areas (Gorham et al.).

Radiographic Findings

In these affected individuals there is a progressive resorption of one or more bones in a skeletal area.

Involvement of the clavicle, scapula, jaw, pelvis, femur, and bones of the hands and feet have been reported. A major portion of an entire bone or region may generally disappear radiographically over a period of months or years (Cheney).

Osteomyelitis, Secondary Type (Figure 9–29)

General Comments. Osteomyelitis may involve bone by contiguous involvement from soft tissue infection. When this occurs there is usually an associated vascular deficiency such as occurs with peripheral arteriosclerosis or diabetes.

Most Frequent Sites are the feet. Usually the bones involved are the metaphysis and epiphysis of the distal aspects of the metatarsals or phalanges.

Radiographic Findings

The osteolytic process tends to extend irregularly in all directions from a cortical and periosteal site, but the area of maximum involvement is usually the site of soft tissue swelling.

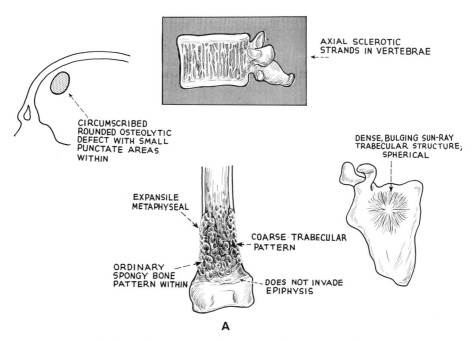

Figure 9–28   *A.* Hemangioma of bone: diagrammatic sketches illustrating the various types.

Figure 9–28 continued on opposite page.

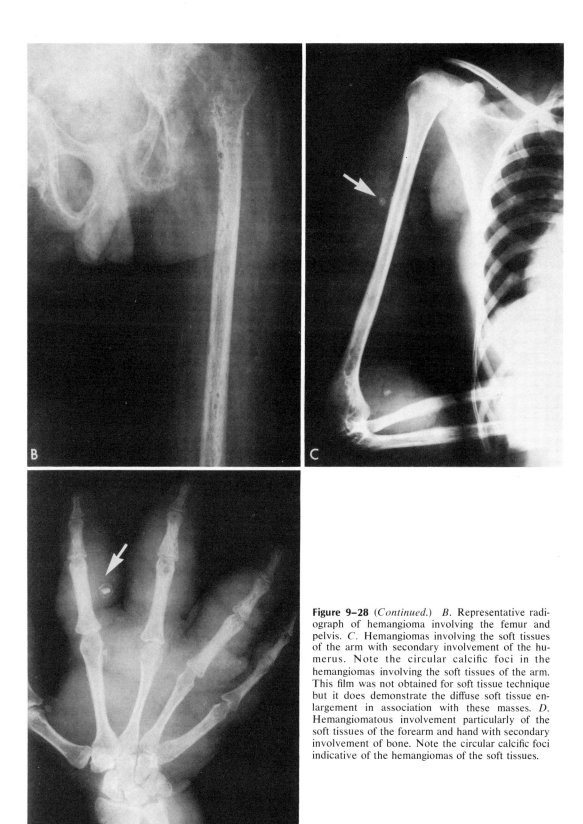

Figure 9–28 (*Continued.*) *B.* Representative radiograph of hemangioma involving the femur and pelvis. *C.* Hemangiomas involving the soft tissues of the arm with secondary involvement of the humerus. Note the circular calcific foci in the hemangiomas involving the soft tissues of the arm. This film was not obtained for soft tissue technique but it does demonstrate the diffuse soft tissue enlargement in association with these masses. *D.* Hemangiomatous involvement particularly of the soft tissues of the forearm and hand with secondary involvement of bone. Note the circular calcific foci indicative of the hemangiomas of the soft tissues.

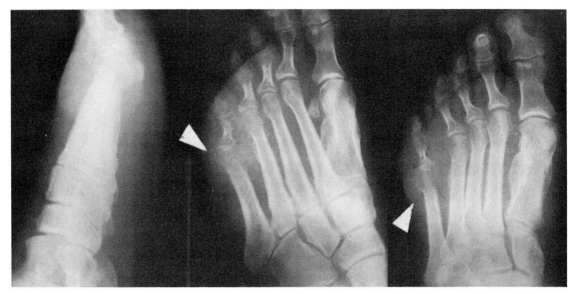

Figure 9–29   Osteomyelitis, secondary type.

The **periosteal reaction may be minimal.**
Very **little if any sequestration is ever seen.**
Very little sclerosis or evidence of new bone formation is obtained.

Fibrosarcoma of Bone (Figure 9–30)

General Comment.   Fibrosarcoma of bone is the least common of the primary malignant tumors with a probable predilection for persons in their second and third decades of life. There are two types: (1) a *medullary or endosteal variety* which arises centrally; and (2) *a periosteal type* arising in the periosteum. Both types are slow growing, and *they do not tend to metastasize until very late.* Recurrence following inadequate surgical removal is frequent.

Principal Sites are the condyle of the femur or an epicondyle of the humerus (Aegerter and Kirkpatrick). The jaw, usually the mandible, is also a frequent site of involvement.

Radiographic Findings

The periosteal variety usually appears as a **large soft tissue mass** which may **invade the underlying bone, causing lysis and radiolucency.**

The endosteal or central type fibrosarcoma destroys the trabeculae in the medullary portions of bone and later erodes the inner aspect of the surrounding cortex.

The **margins** of the tumor are **poorly defined** and usually there is **no overlying periosteal reaction,** until the entire cortex is destroyed.

Periosteal new bone may then be apparent but even it may shortly be destroyed as the tumor grows out into the adjoining soft tissues.

The primary radiographic appearance is that of radiolucency with destruction of bone and minimal or no periosteal reaction.

A
FIBROSARCOMAS OF BONE

ENDOSTEAL
OR MEDULLARY

PERIOSTEAL OR PAROSTEAL

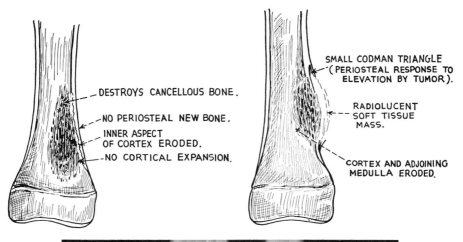

DESTROYS CANCELLOUS BONE.

NO PERIOSTEAL NEW BONE.

INNER ASPECT
OF CORTEX ERODED.

NO CORTICAL EXPANSION.

SMALL CODMAN TRIANGLE
(PERIOSTEAL RESPONSE TO
ELEVATION BY TUMOR).

RADIOLUCENT
SOFT TISSUE
MASS.

CORTEX AND ADJOINING
MEDULLA ERODED.

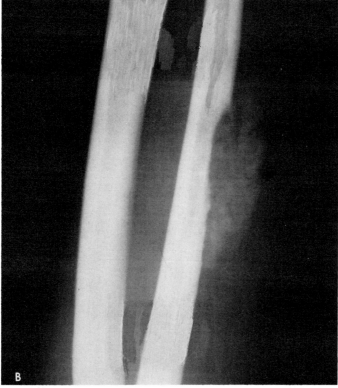

B

Figure 9–30 *A*. Endosteal or medullary fibrosarcoma involving bone: line tracings indicating the most frequent appearance of the medullary and periosteal varieties. *B*. Periosteal fibrosarcoma of the forearm involving the ulna.

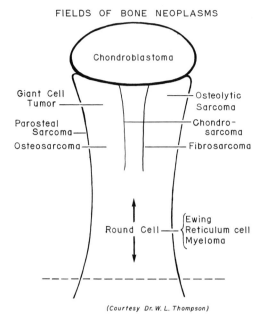

FIELDS OF BONE NEOPLASMS

(Courtesy Dr. W. L. Thompson)

Figure 9–31

Parosteal Fibrosarcoma.   This lesion is at times differentiated from the fibrosarcoma previously mentioned since it is actually an extraosseous sarcoma arising from an outer sheath of the periosteum or the nearby fibrous tissue. *It is, therefore, a soft tissue tumefaction adjacent to bone, and shows evidences of erosion of the bone. Calcification* may develop within this lesion, unlike the previously described endosteal type of fibrosarcoma. However, no portion of this lesion is actually ossified. There may be some evidence of *adjoining periosteal elevation*. The lesion is usually of a *low grade malignancy* with a good prognosis from the standpoint of survival, but local recurrences are common. Occasionally metastases to lungs and elsewhere are seen.

Localization of Bone Neoplasms.   From previous descriptions it is apparent that there are certain regions within the bone where tumors are most apt to occur, although there are exceptions. These are shown in Figure 9–31.

Questions — Chapter 9

1. What basic classification have we employed involving radiolucent bone diseases affecting a single extremity from the radiologic standpoint?

2. Which are the most significant diseases affecting the epiphyses primarily?

3. What are the major areas of involvement by osteochondroses and what are some of the common names of some of the diseases so involved?

4. What is the pathogenesis of osteochondrosis as presented in the femoral head? What are some of the clinical features of osteochondrosis of the hip (Calvé-Legg-Perthes' disease)?

5. What is meant by osteochondritis dissecans? Where is its most frequent site and where are some of the less frequent localizations of this disease process?

6. Describe the radiographic, pathologic, and clinical features of epiphyseal chondroblastoma.

7. Describe some of the clinical and radiographic features of neurotrophic osteopathy.

8. List the most important osteoporotic lesions affecting metaphyses primarily.

9. Indicate the pathogenesis and radiographic appearances of acute and chronic osteomyelitis.

10. Describe the radiographic features, pathogenesis, and some of the clinical aspects of a Brodie's abscess.

11. Describe some of the radiographic and important clinical features of tuberculous osteomyelitis.

12. Describe the important radiographic features of enchondroma. What are some of the most frequent sites of involvement?

13. Describe the most frequently affected areas by a solitary bone cyst and the important radiographic features of this entity. What are the important differential diagnoses to be considered here?

14. Describe the important clinical, pathologic and radiographic features of giant cell tumor.

15. Describe some of the important clinical and radiographic features of the nonosteogenic fibroma of Lichtenstein and Jaffe.

16. Describe the main radiographic features of osteosarcoma, indicating the several varieties of radiographic appearances which may occur. List some of the important clinical aspects of this disease.

17. List the most important disease entities affecting the diaphyses of bone predominantly.

18. List some of the important clinical and radiographic features of neurofibroma involving bone. To what other disease is neurofibromatosis very closely related?

19. Describe the important radiographic features of hemangioma of bone, indicating its several appearances in the skull, vertebrae, long bones and flat bones.

20. List those important disease entities that involve the periosteal zone primarily and the bone possibly secondarily.

21. Describe the important clinical and radiographic features of a secondary type osteomyelitis.

22. Describe the important radiographic and clinical features of parosteal or periosteal fibrosarcoma.

References

Aegerter, E., and Kirkpatrick, J. A., Jr.: Orthopedic Diseases. Second Edition. Philadelphia, W. B. Saunders Co., 1963.

Albright, F., and Reifenstein, E. C.: The Parathyroid Glands and Metabolic Bone Disease. Baltimore, Williams and Wilkins Co., 1948.

Bragg, D. G., Shidnia, H., Chu, F. C. H., and Higingotham, N. L.: Clinical and radiographic aspects of radiation osteitis. Radiology, 97: 103–111, 1970.

Capitanio, M. A., and Kirkpatrick, J. A.: Early roentgen observations in acute osteomyelitis. Amer. J. Roentgenol., 108:488–496, 1970.

Cheney, W.: Acro-osteolysis. Amer. J. Roentgenol., 94:595–607, 1965.

Codman, E. R.: Epiphyseal chondromatous giant cell tumors of upper end of humerus. Surg. Gynec. Obstet., 52:543–548, 1931.

Enna, C. D., Jacobson, R. R., and Rausch, R. O.: Bone changes in leprosy: A correlation of clinical and radiographic features. Radiology, 100:295–306, 1971.

Eyring, E. J., Bjornson, D. R., and Peterson, C. A.: Early diagnostic and prognostic signs in Legg-Calvé-Perthes disease. Amer. J. Roentgenol, 93:382–387, 1965.

Fetterman, L. E., Hardy, R., and Lehrer, H.: Clinico-roentgenologic features of Ainhum. Amer. J. Roentgenol., 100:512–522, 1967.

Feldman, F., Hecht, H. L., and Johnston, A. D.: Chondromyxoid fibroma of bone. Radiology, 94:249–260, 1970.

Fripp, A. T.: Vertebra plana. J. Bone Joint Surg., 40-B:378–384, 1958.

Gatewood, O. M. B., and Easterly, J. R.: Coexistent polyostotic fibrous dysplasia and eosinophilic granuloma of bone: A unique association. Amer. J. Roentgenol., 97:110–117, 1966.

Gorham, L. W., Wright, A. W., Schultz, H. H., and Maxon, F. C.: Disappearing bones: A rare form of massive osteolysis. Amer. J. Med., 17:674–682, 1954.

Halliday, D. R., Dahlin, D. C., Pugh, D. G., and Young, H. H.: Massive osteolysis and angiomatosis. Radiology, 82:637–644, 1964.

Holt, J. F., and Wright, E. M.: Radiologic features of neurofibromatosis. Radiology, 51: 647–663, 1948.

Hunt, J. C., and Pugh, D. G.: Skeletal lesions in neurofibromatosis. Radiology, 76:1–20, 1961.

Jaffe, H. L.: Tumors and Tumorous Conditions

of the Bones and Joints. Philadelphia, Lea & Febiger, 1958.

Jaffe, H. L., and Lichtenstein, L.: Benign chondroblastoma of bone; reinterpretation of so-called calcifying or chondromatous giant cell tumor. Amer. J. Path., *18*:969–991, 1942.

Johnson, P. M., and McClure, J. G.: Observations of massive osteolysis: A review of the literature. Radiology, *71*:28–41, 1958.

Lichtenstein, L.: Benign osteoblastoma. Cancer, *9*:1044–1052, 1956.

Lichtenstein, L.: Bone Tumors. St. Louis, C. V. Mosby Co., 1952.

De Lorimer, A. E., Moehring, H. G., and Hannan, J. V.: Clinical Roentgenology, Volume I. Springfield, Charles C Thomas, 1954.

Ochsner, S. F.: Eosinophilic granuloma of bone: Experience with 20 patients. Amer. J. Roentgenol., *97*:719–726, 1966.

Pallis, C., and Schneeweins, J.: Hereditary sensory radicular neuropathy. Amer. J. Med., *32*:116–118, 1962.

Pogonowska, M. J., Collins, L. C., and Dobson, H. L.: Diabetic osteopathy. Radiology, *89*:265–271, 1967.

Pugh, D. G.: Roentgenologic Diagnosis of Diseases of Bones. Baltimore, Williams and Wilkins Co., 1951.

Reed, R. J.: Fibrous dysplasia of bone: A review of 25 cases. Arch. Path., *75*:480–495, 1963.

Reynolds, J.: "Fallen fragment sign" in the diagnosis of unicameral bone cysts. Radiology, *92*:949–953, 1969.

Rigler, L. G., Blank, L., and Hebbel, R.: Granuloma with eosinophils: Benign, inflammatory, fibroid polyps of the stomach. Radiology, *66*:169–176, 1956.

Rosen, R. A.: Transitory demineralization of the femoral head. Radiology, *94*:509–512, 1970.

Schinz, H. R., Baensch, W. E., Friedl, E., and Vehlinger, E. (J. T. Case, translator): Roentgen-Diagnostics. New York, Grune and Stratton, 1954.

Sherman, R. S., and Soong, K. Y.: Ewing's sarcoma: Its roentgen classification and diagnosis. Radiology, *66*:529–539, 1956.

Turcotte, B., Pugh, D. G., and Dahlin, D. C.: The roentgenographic aspects of chondromyxoid fibroma of bone. Amer. J. Roentgenol., *87*:1085–1095, 1962.

Vix, V. A., and Fahmy, A.: Unusual appearance of a chondromyxoid fibroma. Radiology, *92*:365–366, 1969.

Waldenström, H.: First stages of coxae plana. J. Bone Joint Surg., *20*:559–566, 1938.

Weston, W. J., and Goodson, G. M.: Vertebra plana (Calvé). J. Bone Joint Surg., *41-B*:477–485, 1959.

10

Bone Diseases of the Extremities Characterized by Increased Density, Expansion, or Enlargement

INTRODUCTION

Bone lesions may be arbitrarily categorized as sclerotic or radiolucent, with gradations between these poles (Figure 10–1). When the bone is not uniformly sclerotic or radiolucent, the alterations in density may be further subdivided as follows:
1. *Transverse* bands, usually at the *metaphyses;*
2. *Longitudinal reticular bands,* roughly parallel to the cortex, which may be asymmetrical and corticoperiosteal;
3. *Indiscriminate, patchy* foci of lucency or sclerosis: these may be localized to epiphyses, metaphyses, or diaphyses predominantly.

As always, neighboring soft tissues and joints must be carefully noted.

This proposed classification does not necessarily refer to any particular disease. The entire concept has evolved as a method of interrelating the pathologic entity with its radiographic counterpart, so that a system of thinking and analyzing may be developed.

OSTEOSCLEROSIS AFFECTING SEVERAL EXTREMITIES

Diffuse Osteosclerosis of Several Extremities. The following classification illustrated in Figure 10–2 shows this group of diseases conforming to three general categories:

OSTEOSCLEROTIC—HYPERTROPHIC BONE DISEASE
INVOLVING SEVERAL BONES

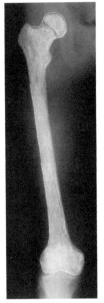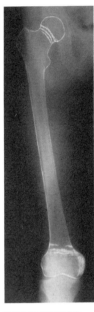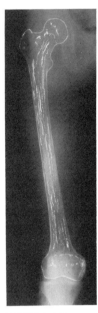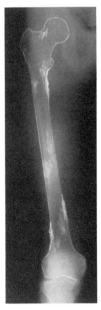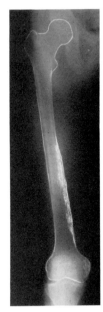

DIFFUSE   TRANSVERSE   FIBRILLAR   IRREGULAR   CORTICO-
                 BANDS   NETWORK   PATCHY   PERIOSTEAL
                                                                   INVOLVING
                                                                   SEVERAL BONES

LOCALIZED TO ONE BONE OR REGION

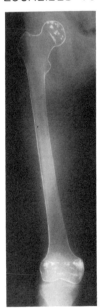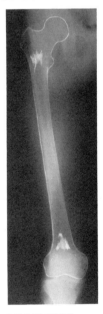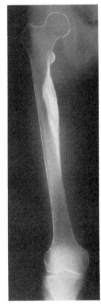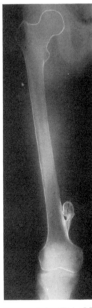

LOCALIZED   LOCALIZED   LOCALIZED   OUTGROWTH OR
EPIPHYSEAL   METAPHYSEAL   DIAPHYSEAL   OVERGROWTH
                                   PATCHY OR   (May be single or
                                   SOLID   multiple)

Figure 10–1   General spectrum of osteosclerotic or hypertrophic bone diseases involving several bones or localized to one bone or region. (Intensified radiographs.)

DIFFUSE

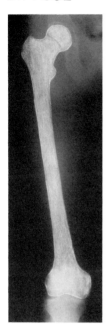
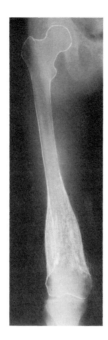
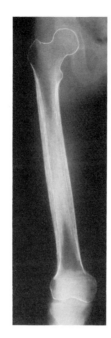

3. FLUORINE POISONING
4. JUVENILE AND TERTIARY SYPHYLIS
5. MASTOCYTOSIS URTICARIA PIGMENTOSA
6. HYPOPARATHYROIDISM
7. HYPERVITAMINOSES (A AND D)
8. PAGET'S DISEASE
9. IDIOPATHIC HYPERCAL-CEMIA OF INFANCY
10. ANEMIAS, LYMPHOMAS
11. METASTASES (CARCINOMA PROSTATE)
12. MYELOFIBROSIS OR SCLEROSIS

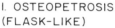

1. OSTEOPETROSIS (FLASK-LIKE)

2. ENGLEMANN'S DISEASE JUVENILE AND TERTIARY SYPHILIS

SHAFT ELLIPSOID EXPANSION

Figure 10–2   Osteosclerosis affecting several extremities of the diffuse osteosclerotic type: general categories. (Intensified radiographs.)

A. Those diseases producing dense, diffuse, sclerotic change:
  1. Osteopetrosis or marble bone disease (Albers-Schönberg disease).
  2. Engelmann's disease.
  3. Fluorine poisoning.
  4. Juvenile and tertiary syphilis.
  5. Urticaria pigmentosa (mastocytosis).
  6. Myelofibrosis or sclerosis occasionally (discussed later under Section C).
B. Those producing moderate sclerotic change:
  7. Hypoparathyroidism.
  8. Hypervitaminosis A (and D on occasion).
  9. Paget's disease (osteitis deformans) (discussed later under indiscriminate, patchy osteosclerosis).
  10. Idiopathic hypercalcemia of infancy (probably same as hypervitaminosis D).
C. Osteosclerotic marrow disorders which are in a reticulated, coarse sclerotic pattern that is often related to anemias or leukemias, or tumor invasion:
  11. Anemias, lymphomas.
  12. Metastases (carcinoma of the prostate and others).
  13. Myelofibrosis or myelosclerosis.
  14. Carcinoid metastases or carcinoid syndrome.

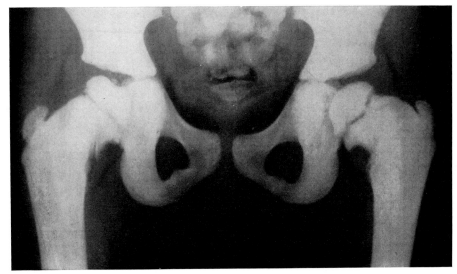

A

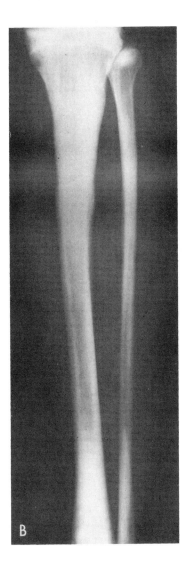

Figure 10–3 *A.* Osteopetrosis (marble bone disease). (Courtesy of L. R. Sante, M.D.) *B.* The healed fractured tibia in a patient with osteopetrosis. Note the Erlenmeyer flask deformity due to a failure of bone modeling.

Marble Bone Disease (Osteopetrosis, Albers-Schönberg Disease) (Figure 10-3)

General Comment. In this disorder there is a pronounced thickening of the bones both microscopically and radiographically. Children so affected are ordinarily retarded in physical development. The values for phosphorus and calcium are normal, but the serum phosphatase may be markedly elevated.

Radiographic Findings

The long bones are flask-shaped and broadened at both ends because the normal shaping processes brought about by osteoclasis do not occur. Growth occurs at the metaphyses without corresponding osteoclastic activity. As a result, the metaphyses are considerably broadened.

The marrow spaces are filled with bone and also appear sclerotic like very compact bone.

The bones are abnormally brittle. Fractures are common. They heal, however, thereby producing a callus which has the same abnormal features as the original bone.

The circumference of the head is abnormally large. Since the major cartilaginous growth centers are within the base of the skull, it is this area which is most extensively involved. Inadequate space for cerebrospinal fluid circulation results in hydrocephalus in many cases.

There may be inadequate room for the passage of the cranial nerves, and atrophy of the optic nerve causes failing vision with associated nystagmus and ocular palsy. Deafness and facial palsies also occur.

The teeth are small with severe caries and numerous enamel defects. Osteomyelitis and necrosis of the mandible may ensue.

The vertebrae are usually severely involved with impingement on the spinal nerves as well.

Prognosis. Myelophthisic anemia is apt to be the most troublesome complication and is frequently the cause of death. In adulthood the disease may be arrested.

Engelmann's Disease (Progressive Diaphyseal Dysplasia) (Figure 10-4)

Radiographic Findings

There is usually a homogeneous fusiform enlargement of the cortical layers of the long bones, especially in the diaphyses of the bones. The **epiphyses and metaphyses remain relatively free from involvement, in contrast to** the development in **marble bone disease.**

The base of the skull, the vertebral bodies, and the pelvis may also be involved.

Usually growth is disproportionate so that there is elongation of the extremities in comparison with the size of the trunk.

General Comment. Muscular atrophy, general wasting, and tenderness upon pressure are often associated.

Fluorine Poisoning

General Comment. Fluorine when ingested in small quantities over a period of years, leads to a great increase in the hardness and density of the skeleton.

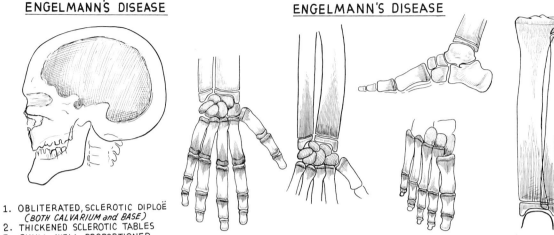

ENGELMANN'S DISEASE

1. OBLITERATED, SCLEROTIC DIPLOË
   (BOTH CALVARIUM and BASE)
2. THICKENED SCLEROTIC TABLES
3. SKULL WELL-PROPORTIONED
4. FACIAL BONES LESS FREQUENTLY
   INVOLVED

ENGELMANN'S DISEASE

1. WIDENED, MARKEDLY SCLEROTIC DIAPHYSES - NOT "CLUB SHAPED"
   AS IN OSTEOPETROSIS
2. OBLITERATED SCLEROTIC MEDULLARY PORTIONS OF LONG
   BONES; METAPHYSES LESS AFFECTED
3. EXTREMITIES ELONGATED WITH RESPECT TO TORSO
4. SKULL AND FACIAL BONES MAY ALSO BE AFFECTED;
   ALTHOUGH RARELY

Figure 10–4   Engelmann's disease.

Radiographic Findings

A general "whiteness of bone" results from an **endosteal shell-like apposition of new bone** at the expense of the medullary spongiosa.

There may also be **some periosteal bone excrescences** and some **calcification of various ligaments,** particularly the paravertebral.

The bones of the spine and pelvis are thick and dense and the contours of the vertebrae are not sharp. The transverse processes appear plump and thick.

There may be calcification of the ischiosacral ligaments.

The earliest and most subtle changes may be a thickening and roughening of the trabecular pattern of the bone, which is best seen in vertebral bodies, especially in the lateral projection. Somewhat similar changes may occur in the pelvis, clavicle, and ribs, and are accompanied by a generalized bony sclerosis, which resembles osteoblastic metastases (Morris; Soriano and Manchon).

The ribs appear to have needle like calcifications projecting into the intercostal muscular attachments.

The compact layers of bone may appear thick and the marrow cavity narrow.

The small bones of the hands and feet are less involved than the axial skeleton. The intensity of the changes is most marked in the center and less marked toward the periphery.

When fluorosis occurs during dental development a mottling of the teeth develops, caused by a hypoplasia of the enamel structure.

Urticaria Pigmentosa (Mastocytosis)

General Comment.   Apart from the characteristic skin lesions, hepatomegaly, splenomegaly, and bone lesions may be present (Sagher and Schorr; Stark et al.).

Radiographic Findings. Two different types of skeletal lesions may be associated with this disease: (1) a **diffuse sclerosis;** (2) spotted or **patchy sclerosis** resembling patchy osteoblastic metastases throughout the body.

Hypoparathyroidism

General Comment. In hypoparathyroidism there is a deficiency of parathormone production. Hypocalcemia and hyperphosphatemia result. These blood chemistry changes produce a marked increase in irritability of the musculature, lenticular opacities, and retention of calcium in the vascular walls and periarticular soft tissues, as well as in the skeleton. The blood calcium values are considerably lowered, averaging around 5 mg. per cent, and blood phosphate figures are elevated, reaching 7 mg. per cent.

"Pseudohypoparathyroidism" represents hypoparathyroidism, which is refractory to parathormone substitution therapy. These patients not only are *dwarfed with heavy stature* and round faces, but they tend to show curious deformities of the hands and feet, which may be shortened in the third, fourth or fifth metacarpals and metatarsals.

"Pseudopseudohypoparathyroidism" is a condition identical with the above except that in these patients the serum calcium and phosphorus are consistently normal. For discussion of other related conditions see Table 7–1.

Kolb and Steinbach have reported "pseudohypo-hyperparathyroidism." These patients have not only the clinical manifestations of hypoparathyroidism, but the radiographic evidence of parathyroid adenomatous effects upon the skeleton, such as subperiosteal resorption, radiolucent fine mottling of the calvarium, and absence of the lamina dura around the teeth.

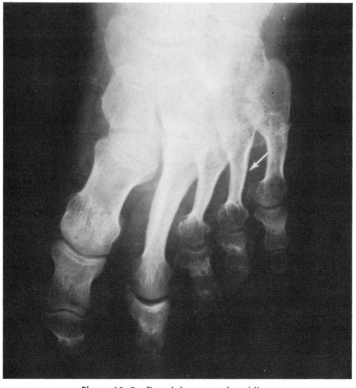

Figure 10–5   Pseudohypoparathyroidism.

Radiographic Findings (Figure 10–5)

Shortening of the metatarsals.
Hyperostosis of the bones of the calvarium.
Calcification of the intracerebral vessels and basal ganglia.
Considerable calcium deposit in the paraspinous ligaments.
Sometimes increased sclerosis of the bony structures.

Hypervitaminosis A (Figure 10–6)

Radiographic Findings. As previously indicated in Chapter 8, there is a combination of excessive metaphyseal osteoclastic activity (transverse lines of radiolucency) along with subperiosteal new bone formation and sclerosis in parallel lamellae, especially around the clavicle and ulna.

These findings are reversible when toxic doses are discontinued (Rothman and Leon; Caffey, 1951; Gribetz et al.).

General Comment and Differential Diagnosis. Vitamin A and carotene blood determination are most helpful in diagnosis (Vitamin A normally 76 to 145 units; carotene, 75 to 150 mg. per 100 cc. of plasma). This helps differentiate this condition from the infantile cortical hyperostosis of Caffey. In the latter there is an earlier appearance in infancy, the findings are much more massive, and there is a predilection for the mandible, although there may also be considerable involvement around the shoulder girdle.

Hypervitaminosis D

General Comment. Physiologically, vitamin D promotes intestinal resorption of calcium, the fixation of calcium in the skeleton, and the renal excretion of phosphate. When excessive vitamin D is administered, the clinical manifestations vary, depending upon whether the toxicity is acute or chronic. Acute vitamin D poisoning

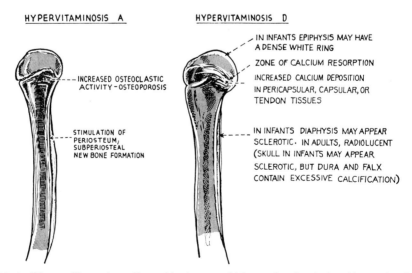

HYPERVITAMINOSIS A

INCREASED OSTEOCLASTIC ACTIVITY – OSTEOPOROSIS

STIMULATION OF PERIOSTEUM; SUBPERIOSTEAL NEW BONE FORMATION

HYPERVITAMINOSIS D

IN INFANTS EPIPHYSIS MAY HAVE A DENSE WHITE RING

ZONE OF CALCIUM RESORPTION

INCREASED CALCIUM DEPOSITION IN PERICAPSULAR, CAPSULAR, OR TENDON TISSUES

IN INFANTS DIAPHYSIS MAY APPEAR SCLEROTIC. IN ADULTS, RADIOLUCENT (SKULL IN INFANTS MAY APPEAR SCLEROTIC, BUT DURA AND FALX CONTAIN EXCESSIVE CALCIFICATION)

Figure 10–6   Diagram illustrating radiographic changes with hypervitaminosis A and hypervitaminosis D.

is characterized by evidences of gastrointestinal irritation with nausea and vomiting, and disturbances in the water balance with polydipsia and polyuria.

In the chronic form of vitamin D toxicity, hypercalcemia leads to an increased intestinal and renal excretion, and to an increased calcium deposition in the skeleton and soft tissues.

Radiographic Findings

In the growing bone there is an increased calcification in the distal metaphyses.

There may be excessive calcium deposits periosteally, giving rise to the appearance of thickening of the periosteum.

Metastatic calcium deposition occurs primarily in the kidneys, lungs, stomach, and skin.

Marrow Disorders Related to Leukemias and Anemias (see also Chapter 8)

General Comment.   Osteomyelosclerosis may occur with any of the diseases which are accompanied by hypoplasia or aplasia of the bone marrow; hence, it is particularly related to the anemias, lymphomas, and leukemias. The severity of the sclerosis depends mainly upon the metaplastic myelogenous changes in the liver and spleen and not upon the severity of the anemia, although usually the anemia will be severe.

In myelofibrosis there may not only be a progressive fibrosis of the bone marrow with myeloid metaplasia but also a leukemoid blood picture. In the peripheral blood there are two striking findings: (1) nucleated red cells, and (2) young members of the neutrophilic series. The leukocytes, when stained for alkaline phosphatase, demonstrate a high level of this enzyme in contrast to findings in myelogenous leukemia, in which the leukocyte alkaline phosphatase is abnormally depressed.

Secondary myelosclerosis may also occur in association with, or from reaction to certain toxic agents, such as irradiation and industrial solvents.

Radiographic Findings

Diffuse bone sclerosis is the end stage of the metaplastic process.

Linear longitudinal streaking and mottling due to fibrosis may precede the diffuse sclerotic process.

At times there is an irregular coarsened and somewhat reticulated pattern in these disorders because the radiolucent aspect may have been uppermost.

Sclerosis of bone is present in more than one-half the cases and is of a diffuse rather than a localized variety. There is no expansion of the bone, as in osteopetrosis or Engelmann's disease, nor is there a tendency to thickening of the individual bony trabeculae, as in Paget's disease of bone. The ribs, pelvis, vertebrae, clavicles, and scapulae are most affected. Rarely is one able to detect changes in the skull, radius, ulna, tibia, or fibula, and no changes are ordinarily found in the hands or feet.

Splenomegaly and hepatomegaly are often associated.

DIFFERENTIAL DIAGNOSIS

Metastases from carcinoma of the prostate will be manifest as a diffuse sclerosis of all the bones of the skeleton. However, since this manifestation is more likely to take on the form of indiscriminate and irregular patchy sclerosis throughout the skeleton, this disorder is described elsewhere in this text.

Marble bone disease.

Engelmann's disease.

Paget's disease of bone.

Frequency and Appearance of Osteosclerosis in Agnogenic Myeloid Metaplasia
(Pettigrew and Ward). In a group of 23 patients, osteosclerosis was present in nine,
or 40 per cent. The remainder showed bones which were normal or osteoporotic.

The typical osteosclerotic appearance was a uniform increase in density with a
so-called "ground glass" appearance.

The proximal humerus and femur were especially involved—eventually,
trabeculated bone may show a complete obliteration of the normal architecture. In
the ribs the sclerosis leads to the striking appearance described as "jail bars"
crossing the thorax.

In advanced sclerosis the trabecular pattern becomes irregular and indistinct,
and the inner margin of the cortex blends with the spongiosa. When this occurs in
vertebral bodies adjacent to end-plates, it has been called the "rugger jersey" effect
or "sandwich appearance." However, complete obliteration of the medullary space
may occur in time in both vertebrae and long bones.

Lipoatrophic Diabetes Mellitus (Lipo-skeletogenic modulation). The absence of
fat in the soft tissues of the extremities leads to a striking homogeneous soft tissue
density, and skeletal maturation is advanced. Although all the bones are increased
in density, the greatest increase is in those bones in which marrow is replaced by the
fatty marrow in adult life. This is best shown in the long tubular bones. In vertebrae,
there may be dense transverse bands of unexplained origin (Gold and Steinbach).

TRANSVERSE
BANDS

1. HEAVY, METAL POISONING

2. CRETINISM

4. DEBILITATING DISEASE WITH RECOVERY

5. HYPERVITAMINOSIS A (AND D)

6. LEUKEMIA

8. IDIOPATHIC HYPERCALCEMIA OF INFANCY
(HYPERVITAMINOSIS D)

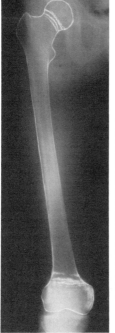

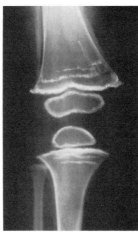

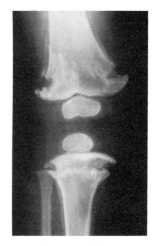

7. SCURVY

3. SYPHILIS
OSTEOPERIOSTITIS

Figure 10–7 Osteosclerosis manifested principally by transverse bands in the metaphyses: general categories. (Intensified radiographs.)

OSTEOSCLEROSIS MANIFESTED PRINCIPALLY
BY TRANSVERSE BANDS IN THE METAPHYSIS
(Figure 10–7)

The following conditions are characterized by this type of reaction:
1. Heavy metal poisoning: phosphorus osteopathy.
2. Cretinism (hypothyroidism).
3. Congenital syphilis.
4. Recovery period following debilitating disease.
5. Hypervitaminosis A and D.
6. Acute leukemia.
7. Scurvy (hypovitaminosis C).
8. Idiopathic hypercalcemia of infancy (hypovitaminosis D).

Transverse lines and bands of increased density in the metaphyses of growing bones are *usually found in children*, those apparently healthy as well as those chronically ill. When these lines occur late in the growth period, they may persist into adult life. The transverse lines are due to failure of normal resorption or removal of the calcified cartilage in the zone of provisional calcification. In the case of heavy metal poisoning, the heavy metal may be intermixed with the zone of provisional calcification.

Heavy Metal Poisoning (Figure 10–8)

Lead Osteopathy

GENERAL COMMENT.   During the growing years, if lead is taken into the body in any form, it is deposited in the skeletal system along with calcium in the zone of provisional calcification on the metaphyseal side of the epiphyseal plate. This osteosclerotic linearity in the distal metaphysis is known as "the lead line," and is histologically composed principally of *calcified cartilage intermixed with some lead elements* and an *increased number of bony trabeculae*. Lead contributes to, but is not solely responsible for, the radiopacity of the "lead line."

RADIOGRAPHIC FINDINGS

The appearance of lead osteopathy during the **growth period** consists largely of the **"lead line"** described above.

In adults the lead is diffusely distributed throughout the bone and does not create any histologic or radiographic appearance.

Metaphyseal Dysplasia Associated with Lead Poisoning in Children.   Pease et al. have reported a metaphyseal dysplasia of varying degrees in 24 out of 48 children in whom chronic lead poisoning had been demonstrated. This consisted of a *widening of the ends of the bones associated with a thinning of the cortices*. The *line of increased density* at the epiphyseal plate was also demonstrated and at times persisted in the shafts of the bones even after the intoxication phase of the disease ceased to exist. This process of increased rarefaction and widening of the ends of the bones, when congenital or inherited, is called "Pyle's disease." In patients with lead poisoning, however, the tubulation is normal prior to the acute lead poisoning phase, but is then altered by the toxic effects of the lead. On withdrawal of the lead normal tubulation may be restored. It is therefore *to be differentiated from "Pyle's disease."*

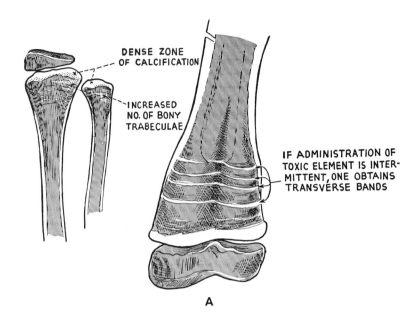

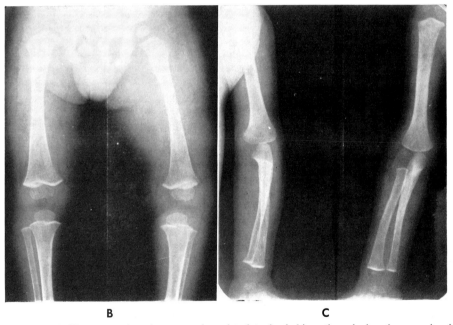

Figure 10–8 *A*. Heavy metal toxic osteopathy related to lead, bismuth and phosphorus poisoning: diagrammatic illustration of radiographic findings. No radiographic changes are seen in the adult skeletal system. *B*. A-P view of the lower extremities demonstrating lead lines. *C*. A-P views of both upper extremities demonstrating similar "lead lines," particularly in the upper end of the humerus and the lower ends of the radius and ulna.

Bismuth Osteopathy may produce findings almost identical to lead. Such intoxication was particularly prevalent when mothers and infants were treated with bismuth as a form of antiluetic therapy. In recent years such manifestations have not been seen.

Phosphorus Osteopathy is also similar to that of lead. Normal growth is resumed when the phosphorus administration is discontinued, but the phosphorus line remains

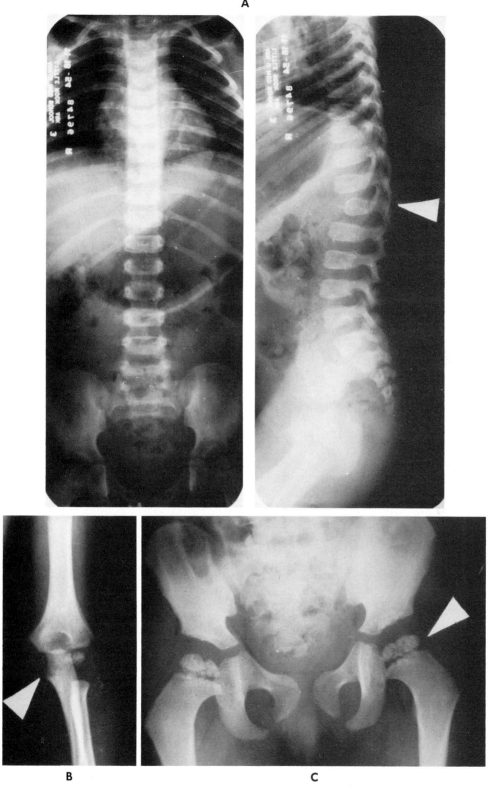

Figure 10–9 *A* to *C*. Skeletal changes in cretinism. There are a delay and irregular appearance of the ossification centers, delayed closure of the epiphyseal lines, and small punctate-type cartilaginous islands in the epiphyses of several of the long bones, particularly hips and humeri. The vertebrae tend to be flattened with increased intervertebral spaces. The illustrations show cretinism of the lower thoracic and upper lumbar spine demonstrating fragmentation in the secondary ossification centers of the endplates of vertebral bodies. This was a 32 year old female with a bone age of 10.

as a permanent indication of such intoxication. If the administration of the phosphorus is intermittent, as formerly was the case when phosphorized cod liver oil was used over a period of years, multiple transverse zones appear in the ends of the long bone, one for each winter of administration. This appearance suggests a "bone within bone" appearance.

Radium Osteopathy or radium intoxication has been traced to a number of sources but has been especially linked to those persons engaged in using radium-type paint on luminous clock dials. All recorded cases of radium poisoning have been in adults and it is particularly associated with a periostitis and osteomyelitis of the mandible.

Cretinism (Hypothyroidism) (Figure 10–9).   In infancy and childhood hypothyroidism produces cretinism. In the adult it produces myxedema. The skeletal changes are limited to the preadolescent hypothyroid group.

Clinical Features

Flat head, receding forehead, broad short face, prognathous jaw;
Thick lips, slitlike eyes;
Extremities short for trunk, but trunk is small as well (dwarfism), unlike the chondrodystrophic dwarf;
Skin is dry and hair is sparse;
Sex organs underdeveloped.

Radiographic Findings

Scanty epiphyseal growth with stippling; delayed ossification and bone age, although the epiphyses appear in normal sequence.
Sclerotic transverse striations in the metaphyses of growing long bones.
Delayed closure of the epiphyseal plate and fontanelles of the skull.
Long bones have broad, thick epiphyses, and slender diaphyses.
Vertebrae are flattened, sometimes wedged, with increased intervertebral spaces; wedged vertebrae give rise to a kyphous deformity of the spine; endplates have incompletely ossified epiphyses.
Pelvis has a coxa vara deformity; the cartilaginous junctions, especially around the acetabulum, are poorly ossified.

Zone of Metaphyseal Sclerosis Following Treatment and Improvement in Severe Debilitating Disease (Figure 10–10).   With systemic illness there may be a temporary cessation of osteoblastic activity at the zones of provisional ossification in metaphyses of long bones. Calcium deposition in the zones of provisional calcification continues. When systemic improvement ensues there is a temporary increase in osteoid deposition. The dense calcified cartilage is only partially resorbed. The new growth which bypasses these transverse calcified cartilaginous zones and transverse sclerotic lines which indicate temporary growth arrest, are shown radiographically. Aggravated forms of these transverse growth arrest lines occur in the acute leukemias.

Anticipating Meconium Peritonitis from Metaphyseal Bands. (Wolfson and Engel). There is some value in the recognition of fetal meconium peritonitis in the newborn infant who has an intestinal obstruction by the metaphyseal bands noted in the ends of the long bones. These are growth arrest zones pure and simple, but their prominence is noteworthy. The bones so affected are the iliac bones—the femurs, the scapulae, the tibia, and the proximal humeri. The intestinal obstruction may be caused by midgut volvulus, duodenal atresia, imperforate anus, or ileo or jejunal atresia and other means of small bowel obstruction, such as the meconium plug syndrome with or without cystic fibrosis. Usually these infants are very seriously ill.

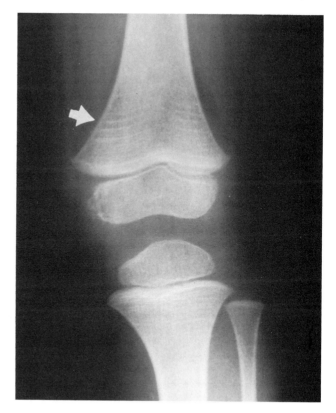

Figure 10–10 Transverse growth arrest lines around the knee.

The Roentgenologic Findings in Idiopathic Infantile Hypercalcemia

Diminution of muscle mass as measured in the midthigh and midleg (Chang et al.).

Widespread osteosclerosis, especially in the base and frontal region of the skull, mandible, vertebral bodies, epiphyses, and metaphyses of long bones; and in the pelvis especially around the acetabuli.

Faulty tubulation of the femora and sometimes osteoporosis of the metaphyses have also been described.

Nephrocalcinosis and deposits of calcium in blood vessels, brain, intramuscular planes, and bronchi.

Craniostenosis occasionally.

OSTEOSCLEROSIS MANIFESTED CHIEFLY BY LONGITUDINAL CORTICAL OR CORTICOPERIOSTEAL THICKENING OR SCLEROSIS IN MULTIPLE BONES OR REGIONS (Figure 10–11)

1. Melorheostosis leri.
2. Juvenile or tertiary syphilis.
3. Infantile cortical hyperostosis of Caffey-Silverman.
4. Hypertrophic pulmonary osteoarthropathy.
5. Blood dyscrasias: lymphomas and leukemias.
6. Chronic fungus osteomyelitis.

A

CORTICO-PERIOSTEAL (SCLEROTIC)

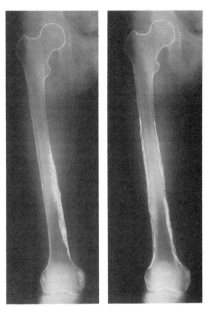

1. MELORHEOSTOSIS
2. JUVENILE AND TERTIARY SYPHILIS
3. INFANTILE CORTICAL HYPEROSTOSIS
4. HYPERTROPHIC PULMONARY OSTEOARTHROPATHY
5. ANEMIAS, LEUKEMIAS, AND LYMPHOMAS
6. FUNGUS; MANDIBLE ACTINOMYCOSIS
7. OSTEOSIS EBURNISANS UNILATERALIS
8. NEUROBLASTOMA
9. EWING'S TUMOR

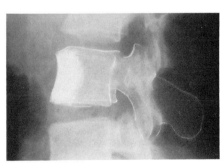

10. IDIOPATHIC VERTEBRAL (FIBROUS DYSPLASIA ?)

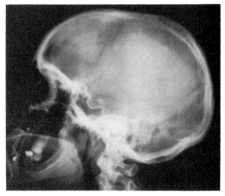

11. MENINGIOMA

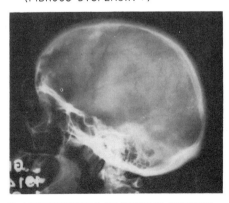

12. HYPEROSTOSIS FRONTALIS INTERNA

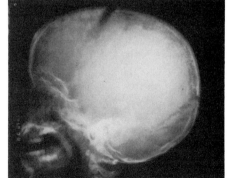

13. NEUROBLASTOMA

Figure 10–11 *A.* Diseases characterized by osteosclerosis manifested chiefly by longitudinal cortical or corticoperiosteal thickening or sclerosis in multiple bones or regions. (Intensified radiographs.)

Figure 10–11 continued on opposite page.

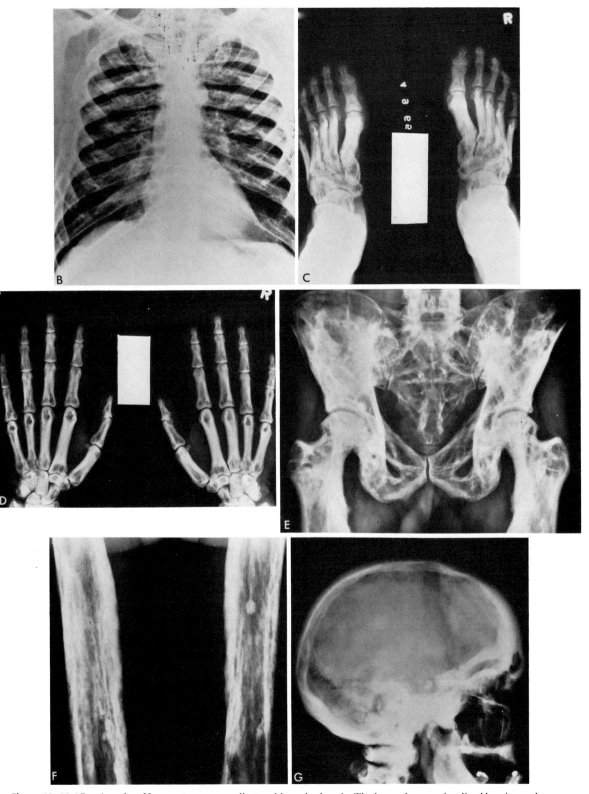

Figure 10–11 *(Continued).* Hyperostoses generalisata with pachydermia. The bony changes visualized herein are demonstrative of a coarse, longitudinal, sclerotic, reticular pattern. *B.* Rib changes in the chest. *C.* The foot. *D.* The hands. *E.* The pelvis. *F.* Closeup of the femora. *G.* Lateral view of the skull showing the calvarium to be relatively spared except in its basal portion.

7. Osteosis eburnisans unilateralis.
8. Neuroblastoma (Chapter 8).
9. Ewing's tumor (Chapter 9).
10. Fibrous dysplasia.
11. Meningioma (Chapter 13).
12. Hyperostosis frontalis interna (Chapter 12).
13. New bone formation in the collagen diseases.

Only a few of the more important of these entities will be described in the abbreviated section to follow.

Infantile Cortical Hyperostosis of Caffey-Silverman (Figure 10–12). Infantile cortical hyperostosis is a condition which appears in infants within the first five months of life and which ordinarily undergoes regression within twelve months following its initial appearance.

Clinical Features

There are local painful swellings, particularly involving the mandible, clavicles, humeri, and ribs.

The disease is acute in onset, with fever, increased erythrocytic sedimentation rate, and increased serum phosphatase.

Radiographic Findings

There is dense periosteal thickening, hyperostosis of compact portions of bone, and sclerosis of spongy portions of the diaphysis, mandible, humeri, ribs, or other long bones which may be involved.

The major involvement is in the **diaphysis** of the bone.

Lamellated periosteal reaction occurs with an uneven outer border to the periosteal reaction.

Usually the disease is unilateral, but it may be bilateral.

Clinical Course. Cortisone may hasten the resolution of this disease process. Ordinarily, the temperature returns to normal in two or three weeks. Other manifestations usually disappear in several months.

The possibility of late recurrence of infantle cortical hyperostosis was documented by Swerdloff et al., who described the apparent recurrence of infantile cortical hyperostosis in two patients, both older children, who had had this disease early in infancy.

Hypertrophic Pulmonary Osteoarthropathy (Figure 10–13)

Clinical Features. Pain and thickening of the long and short tubular bones, especially in the peripheral parts of the body. There may be an associated arthritis, and fingers appear clubbed.

Radiographic Findings. Thickening of the cortex of the small bones due to periosteal proliferation. The outermost margin of the bone is thickened and quite irregular. The ends of the bones are relatively free of involvement in comparison with the diaphyses. At the same time, the carpal and tarsal bones show a subcortical osteoporosis.

Thyroid Acropachy. Thyroid acropachy is a complication of thyroid disease and is characterized by some thickening of the cortex of the phalanges. In this

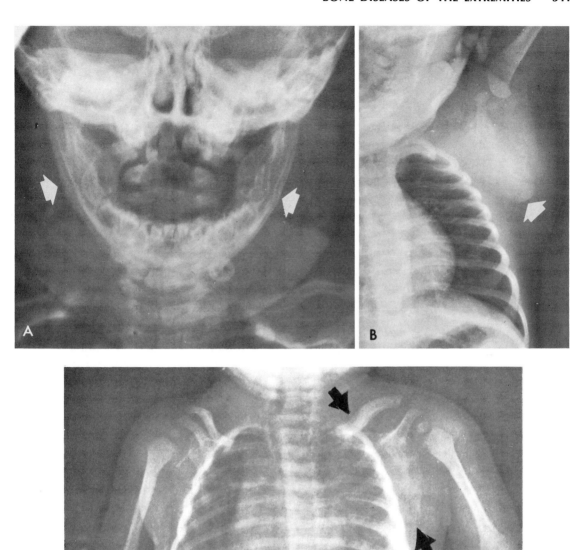

Figure 10–12   Infantile cortical hyperostosis. *A.* Mandible. *B.* Scapula. *C.* Scapula, approximately two months after *B,* showing considerable resolution of the process. At this later time, however, there is considerable involvement in the clavicle and ribs.

respect there is a close resemblance to hypertrophic pulmonary osteoarthropathy. There are, however, some differences:

1. The periosteal new bone formation in the metacarpals or the phalanges tends to be asymmetrical and somewhat "bubbled" or "lacy" in appearance. In pulmonary osteoarthropathy the cortical hyperostosis and periosteal thickening tend to be quite symmetrical.

2. In thyroid acropachy the new bone formation is diaphyseal and tends to be most marked in the midportion of the diaphysis, often giving the shaft a fusiform contour.

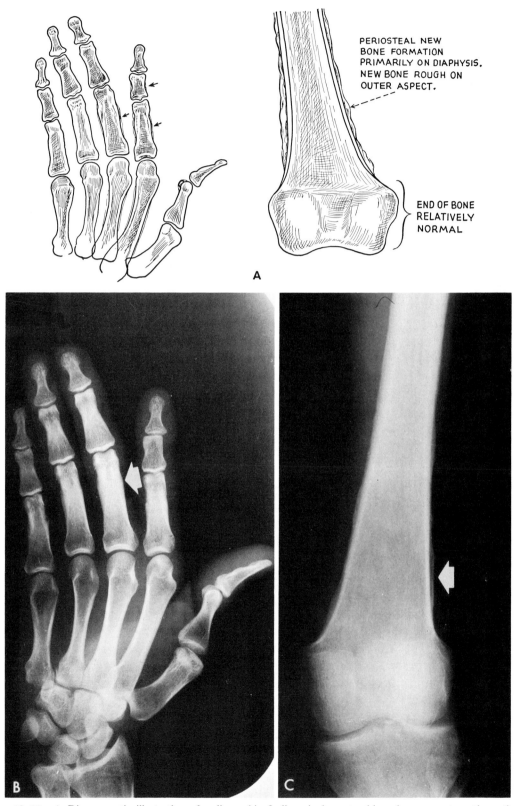

Figure 10–13 *A.* Diagrammatic illustration of radiographic findings in hypertrophic pulmonary osteoarthropathy. *B.* Hypertrophic pulmonary osteoarthropathy involving the hands. *C.* Hypertrophic pulmonary osteoarthropathy involving the distal shaft of the femur.

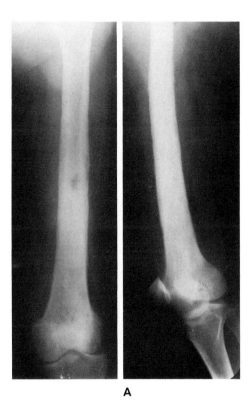

Figure 10–14 *A*. Reticulum cell sarcoma involving the shaft of the femur, showing irregular cortical and medullary sclerosis, sometimes of a linear, patchy type. In the A-P projection there is a sharply circumscribed area of diminished density due to a biopsy which was taken elsewhere prior to the time the patient appeared in our clinic for study. (Intensified radiographs.)

B. Diagrammatic illustration of radiographic findings in reticulum cell sarcoma of the bone.

A

PRACTICALLY NO
PERIOSTEAL REACTION

IRREGULAR, COARSE, JAGGED
THICKENING, WITH SLIGHT EXPANSION
OF THE BONE SHAFT

MARKED COARSE ADMIXTURE
OF OSTEOLYSIS AND OSTEOSCLEROSIS

TENDENCY TO INVOLVE METAPHYSIS
AND EPIPHYSIS IN MIDDLE-AGED
PATIENTS

B

3. The more proximal bones such as the radius and ulna or, in the case of the lower extremity, the tibia and fibula, are not involved. In this respect there is also a difference from hypertrophic osteoarthropathy (Scanlon and Clemett).

Blood Dyscrasias: Lymphomas, Leukemias and Reticulum Cell Sarcoma

Clinical Features

Lymph nodes, spleen, and occasionally liver, markedly enlarged. Fever may be cyclic, and debility is often marked.

Lymphosarcoma afflicts persons in the third, fourth, and fifth decades. Hodgkin's disease patients are about ten years younger; and reticulum cell sarcoma especially affects people 25 to 50 years of age.

Radiographic Findings

Bone involvement is found in about 30 per cent of lymphoma cases generally, with sclerosis in about 5 to 10 per cent; in the remainder of cases where bone is involved, the manifestation is usually radiolucent.

These diseases primarily affect the spine, ribs, and femora, and occasionally the proximal tibia and skull.

There are numerous intermixed radiolucent and sclerotic "blotchy" areas with a linear coarsening of the trabeculae (Figure 10–14).

Occasionally there is periosteal elevation.

Pathologic fractures are common.

Mediastinal lymph node enlargement and pleural effusion are also frequent.

There may also be erosion of bone from involvement of contiguous lymph nodes, particularly in the lumbar spine.

Chronic Fungus (Mycotic) Osteomyelitis. Mycotic disorders of bone are usually bone destructive and osteolytic; they are included here because, on occasion, there are dense sclerotic reactive zones surrounding the area of bone destruction.

In most instances there is a surrounding soft tissue swelling which aids materially in the diagnosis.

The most frequent mycoses involved are: (1) actinomycosis; (2) blastomycosis; (3) coccidioidomycosis; and (4) sporotrichosis.

Routes of Infection are: (1) by direct extension from adjoining soft tissue involvement; or (2) by hematogenous dissemination.

Differences Among Various Fungus Osteomyelitidies

ACTINOMYCOSIS usually involves the soft tissue of the head and neck, particularly the mandible, and spreads from this focus to other areas; however, it often involves the lungs (including the ribs), dorsal vertebrae, or vermiform appendix.

COCCIDIOIDOMYCOSIS is primarily a destructive process in the spongiosa of bone. New bone formation and periosteal proliferation are unusual but they may occur as a late change. There may be direct extension to the adjoining joint and involvement of both the epiphyses and diaphyses. The bones most commonly affected are the ribs and lower ends of the tibiae and fibulae.

SPOROTRICHOSIS is usually confined to the skin or subcutaneous structures, but it may involve viscera and bony structures, including joints or phalanges by extension.

BLASTOMYCOSIS may disseminate widely in any of the bones and form a local area of bone destruction usually (but not invariably) surrounded by a thick zone of reactive osteosclerosis.

New Bone Formation in the Collagen Diseases.   Several cases of polyarteritis nodosa with periosteal new bone formation in the long bones have been described. In scleroderma there has been description of new bone formation in the proximal portions of the long bone especially. Severe arthritic changes are also found with scleroderma, particularly in the hand with bony ankylosis of the finger joints. The joint changes may also be found in other collagen diseases. Juxta-articular soft tissue calcification is especially noteworthy in scleroderma also (Bjersand; Saville; Tuff-anelli and Winkelmann; Keats).

Sequestrum Formation in Fibrous Dysplasia (Pratt et al.).   Sequestrum formation has been described in two cases of proven fibrous dysplasia that were not associated with osteomyelitis. The sequestrum was seen in the medullary cavity of the tibia within a sclerotic zone of the fibrous dysplasia. (For discussion of fibrous dysplasia, see Chapters 9 and 12.)

ROENTGENOLOGIC MANIFESTATIONS OF OSTEONECROSIS
(Martel and Sitterley)

1. In 33 cases, excluding osteochondrosis of the hip, the hip was the area most frequently involved. Other joints included the shoulder, knee, ankle, wrist, and metadiaphyseal joint.
2. The associated diseases in prior steroid therapy included: lupus erythematosus, ankylosing spondylitis, dermatitis, alcoholism (with or without gout), gout, and miscellaneous others.
3. The roentgenologic features of osteonecrosis included the following:
   a. Localized rarefaction with occasional sclerosis.
   b. The "rim" sign, which is a subchondral bone fragment slightly separated from the rest of the bone.
   c. Subchondral depression of bone.
   d. Periosteal bone apposition.
   e. A mottled trabecular pattern.
   f. Other signs such as: patchy sclerosis, generalized subchondral fragmentation; acetabular protrusion; degenerative changes in the adjoining joint; the "bite sign" which is a large defect in the end of the bone giving an appearance as though a bite had been taken out of it.

MULTIPLE IRREGULAR AREAS OF OSTEOSCLEROSIS OF INDISCRIMINATE DISTRIBUTION (Figure 10–15)

The most important entities in this category are enumerated in Figure 10–15. Of these consideration will be given to:
1. Normal variant sclerotic bone islands.
2. Osteitis deformans (Paget's disease).
3. Osteosclerotic involvement from tumor metastases.
4. Osteosclerosis with parathyroid adenoma and chronic renal failure.

IRREGULAR
"PATCHY"

I. SCLEROTIC BONE ISLANDS

2. OSTEOPOIKILOSIS

3. PAGET'S DISEASE (OSTEITIS DEFORMANS)

4. OSTEOSCLEROTIC TUMOR METASTASES

5. OCCASIONAL MULTIPLE MYELOMA

6. MASTOCYTOSIS

8. OSTEOPATHIA STRIATA (VOORHOEVE)

9. OSTEOSCLEROSIS WITH PARATHYROID ADENOMA + CHRONIC RENAL FAILURE

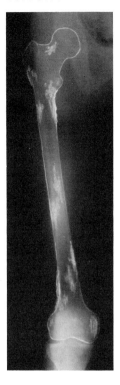

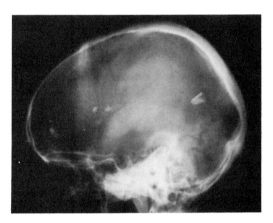

7. TUBEROUS SCLEROSIS

Figure 10–15 General categories of bone diseases characterized by multiple irregular areas of osteosclerosis of indiscriminate distribution. (Intensified radiographs.)

Normal Variant Sclerotic Bone Islands (Figure 10–16). Normal sclerotic bone islands occur frequently in the metaphyses and epiphyses of long bones, in the innominate bone, and in the short bones of the hands and feet. The upper metaphysis of the femur, the head of the humerus, the heads of the metacarpals and metatarsals, and the iliac bones are most frequently involved. These small islands of compact bone measure 3 to 5 mm. in diameter. They may or may not be symmetrical. In "osteopoikilosis" they are multiple, bilateral, and quite symmetrical, affecting peripheral small bones especially.

In certain instances differentiation from sclerotic bone metastases, particularly in the large bones, and from sesamoid bones presents the most important diagnostic problems.

Osteitis Deformans (Paget's Disease of Bone) (Figure 10–17)

Clinical Features

Possibly up to 3 per cent of the population have this disease, but it is subclinical. It may be monostotic or polyostotic.

Bone pains, headaches, and enlarging head in men, most frequently, who are more than 40 years of age.

Primary sites: spine; cranium; femora; pelvis; clavicles; ribs, tibiae; and sternum.

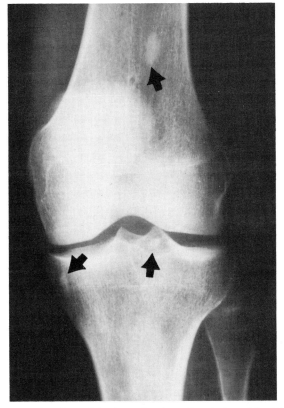

Figure 10–16   Antero-posterior view of the knee showing sclerotic bone island in the distal femur and proximal portion of the tibia.

Histologically.   Profound bone mosaic with intermixed osteoclasis and osteoblastic bone apposition.

Gross Pathology

Coarse bony trabeculation with softening of bone, widening of shaft, and bowing.

Coarse, markedly thickened spongiosa in skull and vertebrae.

Laboratory Findings

Blood calcium, phosphorus, and urinary calcium are normal.

Alkaline phosphatase is markedly elevated.

Radiographic Findings

Bones are markedly thickened, widened and bent, with coarse trabecular pattern.

Early skull: circumscribed osteoporosis (called **osteoporosis circumscripta).**

Late skull: "cotton ball" appearance.

Vertebrae: "picture frame" appearance.

Facial bones: Leontiasis ossea.

Pelvis: "sheaves of grain" appearance of trabeculae.

Course.   Progressive over years; 10 per cent develop *sarcoma.*

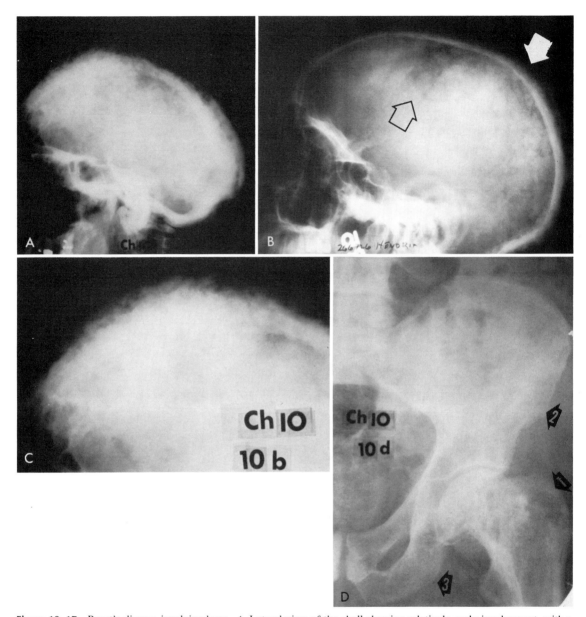

Figure 10–17 Paget's disease involving bone. *A*. Lateral view of the skull showing relatively early involvement, with a tendency toward the so-called "osteoporosis circumscripta" giving a maplike appearance to the bones of the calvarium.

B. Lateral view of the skull with late involvement of the skull showing the "cotton ball" type appearance of the bones of the calvarium.

C. Closeup view of the "cotton ball" appearance of the bones of the calvarium, showing marked involvement of all the layers of the calvarium with thickening of the diploë and marked irregularity of both the inner and outer table. The outer table at times has a shell–like appearance.

D. Antero-posterior view of the hip in Paget's disease showing a coarsened trabecular pattern not only of the ilium but also of the adjoining portions of femur and ischium.

Figure 10–17 continued on opposite page.

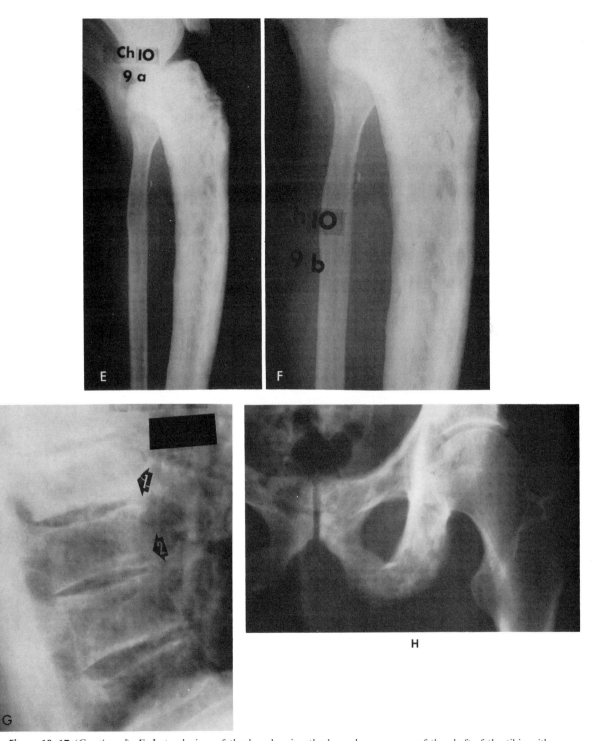

Figure 10–17 (*Continued*) *E.* Lateral view of the leg showing the bowed appearance of the shaft of the tibia with an irregular coarsened trabecular lytic process diffusely involving the entire shaft of the tibia.

F. Closeup view of the shaft of the tibia showing the irregular mosaic pattern of the trabeculae, markedly coarsened.

G. Lateral view of the thoracic vertebrae showing the boxlike, coarsened and thickened appearance of some of the vertebrae as well as a tendency to coarsened trabeculation without the boxlike appearance in others.

H. Paget's disease involving the pubis and ischium, demonstrating the coarsened trabecular pattern, some sclerosis with intermixed lucency, and some increase in dimension of the ischium.

Osteosclerotic Involvement from Tumor Metastases (Figure 10–18)

Most Frequent Origin of Tumors are the prostate, stomach, lung, pancreas and, rarely, breast and multiple myeloma. Lymphomatous tumors should also be included here. Malignant carcinoid, urinary bladder carcinoma, and mucinous adenocarcinomas of the colon, when metastatic to bone, are also especially apt to produce sclerotic metastases (Greenfield).

Carcinoma of Prostate Metastases

These may produce a diffuse chalkiness of all bones.

The earliest metastases often appear on the inner aspect of the acetabulum, passing via valveless veins (Batson's plexus), also to the sacrum and other sites in the pelvis.

The appearance may closely resemble Paget's disease of bone but can usually be differentiated on the basis of the architectural pattern.

The high serum acid phosphatase level is almost pathognomonic. It may be related to release from the prostate by disruption of its capsule.

Metastatic Foci from Carcinoma of the Breast or Other Lytic Metastases Following a Favorable Therapeutic Response. Metastatic foci which have been treated by chemotherapy, hormonal treatment, or radiotherapy, will frequently be replaced by sclerotic bone even when the primary lesion is not responsive to therapy. **Rarely the sclerosis is "ringlike" in appearance, surrounding the prior lytic foci in the bones.**

Osteosclerosis with Parathyroid Adenoma and Chronic Renal Failure. Usually primary hyperparathyroidism due to parathyroid adenoma with resulting bone disease, as well as secondary hyperparathyroidism with bony manifestations are ac-

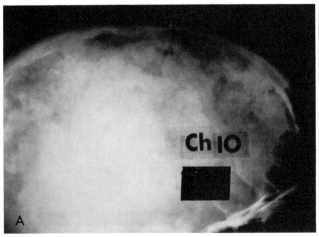
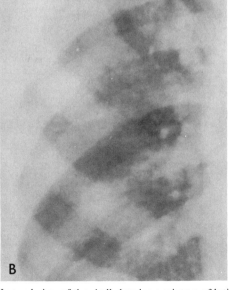

Figure 10–18 Metastases to bone from carcinoma of the prostate. *A.* Lateral view of the skull showing a mixture of lytic and osteoblastic metastases to the bones of the calvarium.
B. Metastases to the ribs showing a diffuse "whiteness" of a homogeneous type with involvement of the ribs.

companied by osteolytic radiolucencies. However, there are occasional cases of osteosclerosis reported. More frequently the bony appearance may be that of an admixture of sclerosis and lucency. The admixture of radiolucency and sclerosis often has an amorphous, homogeneous ground-glass appearance due to coarsened trabeculae and widening of the individual trabeculae.

In the thoracic and lumbar spine occasionally marked bone sclerosis affects the upper and lower thirds of the vertebral body, leaving a translucent band in the center of each vertebra (Kaye et al.; Beveridge et al.).

OSTEOSCLEROSIS OF A LOCALIZED OR REGIONAL TYPE

The main disease entities in this category are listed in Figure 10–19. Of these the most important for our present consideration are:
1. Bone infarction.
2. Osteitis condensans ilei.
3. Osteomyelitis of Garré.
4. Brodie's abscess (also see Chapter 7).
5. Osteoid osteoma.

Bone Infarction (Figure 10–20).   Two types of bone infarcts are recognized: (1) an epiphyseal type; and (2) a metaphyseal type such as occurs in caisson disease.

In the *epiphyseal* type, a dense area occurs in the cancellous bone which abuts on the joint cortex and gives rise to a snowcap appearance. The density is often patchy because of irregular replacement by new tissue. Separation of portions of the joints may occur, as in osteochondritis dissecans.

In the *metaphyseal* type, there is usually an infarct resulting from the sudden release (produced by sharp alterations in atmospheric pressure) of nitrogen into the blood. This is particularly true in fatty bone marrow, in the central nervous system, and in the mesenteric fatty tissue.

Principal Sites in Bones.   Femur, humerus, tibia, and fibula.

Radiographic Appearance.   Wedge of sclerotic bone surrounded by a narrow dense line of demarcation. The base of the wedge runs along the scar of an old epiphyseal plate but at a slight distance from it. The sides are parallel to the cortex of the shaft but separated from it by a narrow band of normal bone. Ordinarily the cortex of the bone is not affected. Sometimes the lesion takes the shape of chains or clusters of dense rings.

The bone changes in **sickle cell anemia** are often related to hemorrhagic and infarcted areas, and may resemble the findings of bone infarction.

Osteitis Condensans Ilei (Figure 10–21)

Clinical Features.   It is predominantly found in women between 20 and 40 years of age and is associated with recurrent attacks of chronic low back pain, but is apparently self-limiting in that it is seldom seen in women over 60 years of age.

Radiographic Findings.   Sclerotic appearance of the ilium adjacent to the sacroiliac joint, with a sharp demarcation between the condensed bone and the

LOCALIZED EPIPHYSEAL

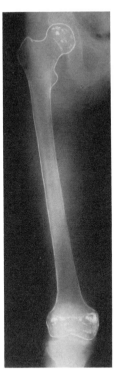

1. EPIPHYSEAL DYSPLASIA
2. HYPOTHYROIDISM
3. CONGENITAL STIPPLED EPIPHYSES
4. OSTEOCHONDROSIS
5. BONE INFARCTION (EPIPHYSEAL TYPE)

A

Figure 10–19   *A*. Osteosclerosis of a localized or regional type, predominantly epiphyseal. (Intensified radiograph.)

Figure 10–19 continued on opposite page.

adjacent normal bone, no bridging of the sacroiliac joint, and no involvement of the sacrum. Its primary importance lies in the distinction from rheumatoid spondylitis with involvement of the sacroiliac joints.

After several years, the sclerosis may disappear.

Osteomyelitis of Garré (Figure 10–22)

Clinical Features

Usually affects males less than 30 years of age.

Usually a long bone is involved in its diaphysis.

The disease is characterized by considerable pain, aching, and fever of a recurrent type at intervals of several weeks or months.

Pathologic Features.   Devascularization of the cortex of the bone with scattered small areas of necrosis. No evidence of fistula formation or suppuration.

Radiographic Findings

Principal sites are the tibia, femur, fibula, ulna, and metatarsals.

Marked layering of the periosteum with subperiosteal calcification, and marked thickening of the associated cortex, with sclerotic encroachment on the medullary portion of the bone.

One may identify small disseminated areas of rarefaction and circumscribed areas of sequestration, but no extensive necrosis and sequestration is seen.

LOCALIZED METAPHYSEAL
PATCHY OR SOLID

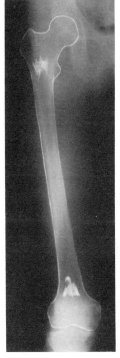

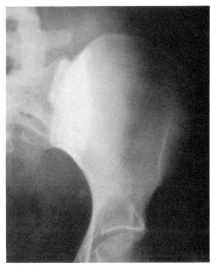

2. OSTEITIS CONDENSANS ILEI
3. LEONTIASIS OSSEI
4. OSTEOMYELITIS OF GARRÉ

B

Figure 10–19 *(Continued)* *B.* Osteosclerosis of a localized or regional type, predominantly metaphyseal. (Intensified radiographs.) *C.* Osteosclerosis of a localized or regional type, predominantly diaphyseal (corticoperiosteal). (Intensified radiograph.)

I. BONE INFARCTS

LOCALIZED DIAPHYSEAL—
CORTICO-PERIOSTEAL

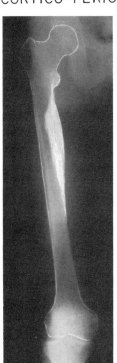

1. OSTEOID OSTEOMA
2. TRAUMATIC PERIOSTITIS

SKULL
3. HYPEROSTOSIS FRONTALIS INTERNA
4. MENINGIOMA
5. NEUROBLASTOMA
6. OSTEOMA
7. "OSSIFYING FIBROMA"

VERTEBRAL
8. FIBROUS DYSPLASIA
9. IDIOPATHIC

C

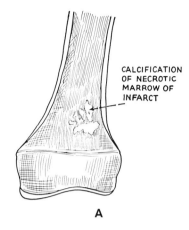

CALCIFICATION
OF NECROTIC
MARROW OF
INFARCT

A

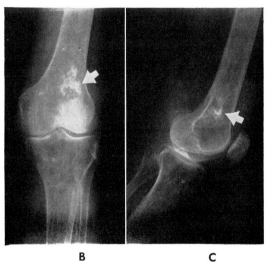

B   C

Figure 10–20 *A.* Infarction of bone as in caisson disease. *B* and *C.* A-P and lateral views of the knee demonstrating bone infarcts in the adjoining metaphyses of the femur and tibia in a patient with caisson disease.

Brodie's Abscess (Figure 10–23)

Clinical Features. Brodie's abscess is an acute suppurative osteomyelitis (see Chapter 8), which has become aborted and incarcerated so that it does not spread to large areas of adjoining cancellous tissue of the bone, nor does it usually spread to the subperiosteal region.

Pathology. A central area of suppuration and necrosis is found surrounded by a wall of granulation which collagenizes to form a thick, fibrous capsule.

Radiographic Features. A sharply **focalized area of radiolucency surrounded by a thick or thin zone of sclerosis,** most frequently in the upper shaft of the tibia, but it may in some instances occur in the ends of other long bones. At times the reactive zone of sclerosis is minimal and barely perceptible (Figure 10–23).

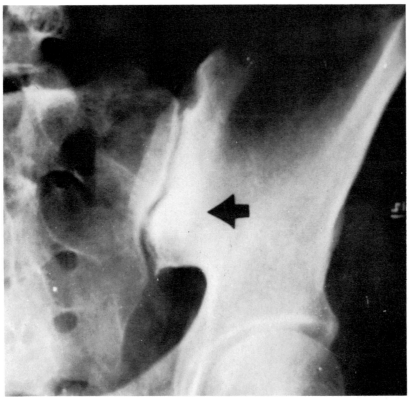

Figure 10–21   Osteitis condensans ilii. Sclerotic appearance of ilium adjacent to sacroiliac joint. Occurs mostly in women 20 to 40 years of age; may be associated with chronic low back pain, but is self-limited. Must be distinguished from rheumatoid spondylarthritis affecting sacroiliac joints.

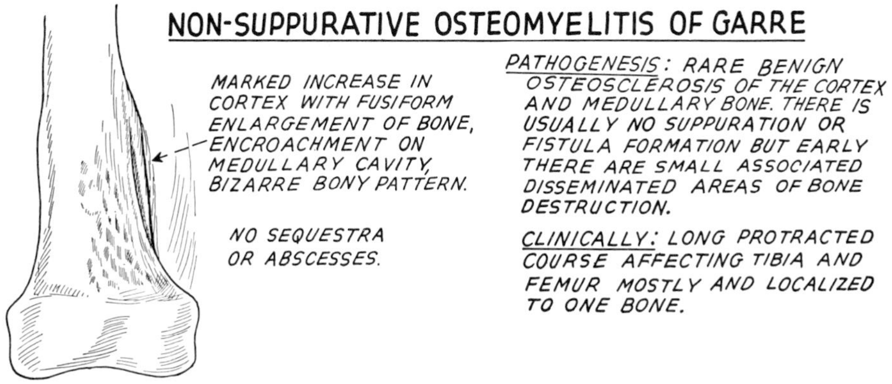

NON-SUPPURATIVE OSTEOMYELITIS OF GARRE

MARKED INCREASE IN CORTEX WITH FUSIFORM ENLARGEMENT OF BONE, ENCROACHMENT ON MEDULLARY CAVITY, BIZARRE BONY PATTERN.

NO SEQUESTRA OR ABSCESSES.

PATHOGENESIS: RARE BENIGN OSTEOSCLEROSIS OF THE CORTEX AND MEDULLARY BONE. THERE IS USUALLY NO SUPPURATION OR FISTULA FORMATION BUT EARLY THERE ARE SMALL ASSOCIATED DISSEMINATED AREAS OF BONE DESTRUCTION.

CLINICALLY: LONG PROTRACTED COURSE AFFECTING TIBIA AND FEMUR MOSTLY AND LOCALIZED TO ONE BONE.

Figure 10–22

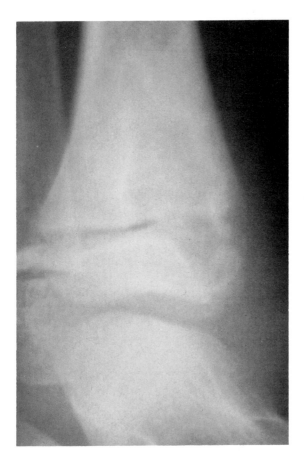

Figure 10–23   Brodie's abscess affecting the lower tibia.

Clinical Course.   Drainage is ordinarily impossible until surgical intervention has occurred. Often the offending organisms are no longer viable at the time of surgical drainage and the pus is usually found to be sterile.

Ulcer Osteomyelitis – Bone Response to Tropical Ulcer (Kolawole and Bohrer).

Devitalization of soft tissues may occur in the tropics from a number of causes; avitaminosis and malnutrition may be factors. These soft tissue changes are complicated by chronicity, recurrence, skin scarring, lymphedema, and occasionally infection due to gas gangrene and tetanus.

Roentgenologic Findings

Ulcer of soft tissues.

The ulcer is usually anterolateral in the leg.

Periosteal reaction is the earliest finding which is localized only to the bone beneath the ulcer. Occasionally it is a sunburst type. Later the periosteal new bone formation blends with the original cortex and the entire cortical bone becomes very thick, thereby giving rise to an ivory ulcer osteoma. At times the sclerotic reaction has an "onion peel" or sunburst appearance. It extends on the shaft of the bone along its margin.

Medullary changes are noted in the bones distal to the ulcer, characterized by osteoporosis and bulbous expansion of the medullary cavity toward the ulcer, while the thinning of the cortex gives rise to the cancellous ulcer osteoma.

The bones appear to bow anteriorly or laterally, with the greatest convexity under the ulcer.

Cicatrization may cause flexion deformities of the knees or feet.

Two per cent of benign tropical ulcers progress to outright malignancy with typical appearances of carcinoma. With malignant change the soft tissue swelling becomes more marked, the outline of the osteoma becomes irregular

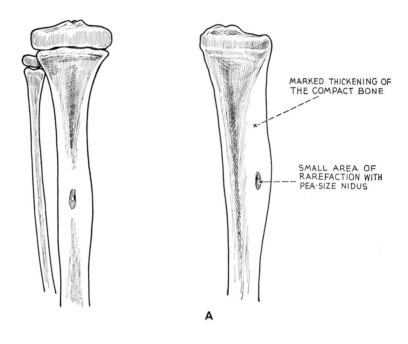

MARKED THICKENING OF THE COMPACT BONE

SMALL AREA OF RAREFACTION WITH PEA-SIZE NIDUS

A

Figure 10–24 Osteoid osteoma. *A.* Diagrammatic illustration. *B.* Radiograph. Note the small rarefied central nidus containing the sclerotic nidus. (Courtesy of E. F. Gray, M.D., and J. D. Calhoun, M.D., Little Rock, Arkansas.)

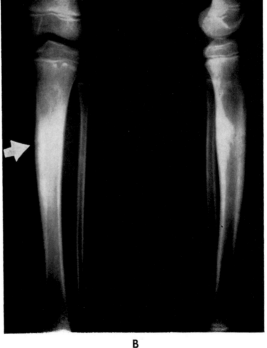

B

and hazy, and bone destruction occurs as the cortex and the medulla are eroded by the carcinoma. Fine bone spiculations can sometimes be seen at the edges of the tumor.

Osteoid Osteoma (Figure 10-24)

Clinical Features

Local tumefaction.

Extreme bone pain.

Peak incidence occurs in the second and third decades of life.

Males are affected more frequently than females.

Most frequent sites are the tibia, femur, fibula, humerus, vertebrae, and phalanges; rarely, the skull, ribs, and pelvis.

Osteoid osteoma in the femoral neck may produce a severe growth disturbance of the hip (Giustra and Feriberger).

Otherwise, when it is located near a joint it can produce both synovitis and proliferative arthritis.

When situated in a vertebra it often causes curvature of the spine—the result of muscle spasm rather than of bone deformity.

Gross Pathology. Eccentric marked cortical thickening extending inward toward cancellous structure of the bone, usually diaphyseal.

Microscopic Pathology. Cortical osteoid tissue embedded in a reticular connective tissue which forms new bone.

Radiographic Findings

Marked thickening of the compact bone.

With an overpenetrated radiograph, a **small nidus** of rarefaction measuring 3 to 5 mm. with a central sclerotic focus may be identified.

Prognosis. Good. Pain is relieved by surgical removal.

This lesion is *not to be confused* with the so-called "giant osteoid osteoma," a synonym for the "benign osteoblastoma," which it may closely resemble histologically.

DISEASES OF BONE CHARACTERIZED BY OUTGROWTH OR OVERGROWTH OF BONE
(Figure 10-25)

Diseases of bone characterized by outgrowth or overgrowth may be subdivided into those involving a single bone, and those involving several or many bones. The classification is rendered as follows:

1. Outgrowth or overgrowth of a single bone:
   a. Solitary osteochondroma.
   b. Osteoma (see Chapter 12).
   c. Osteochondromatosis or chondrocalcinosis of joints; perhaps a better term is synovial chondrometaplasia (see Chapter 11).
   d. Chondrosarcoma.

OUTGROWTH OR OVERGROWTH

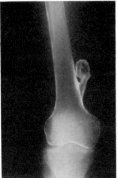

1. OSTEOCHONDROMA

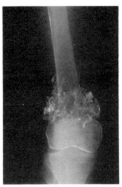

2. OSTEOSARCOMA
   SCLEROTIC TYPE

3. OSTEOCHONDROMATOSIS
   OF JOINTS

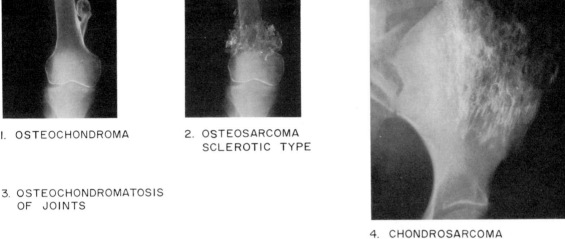

4. CHONDROSARCOMA

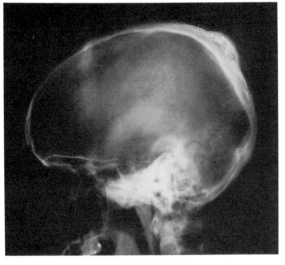

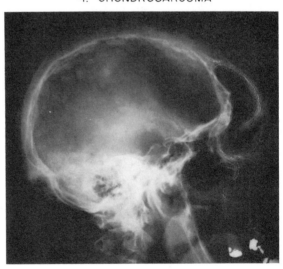

5. OSTEOMA

6. ACROMEGALY, GIGANTISM

Figure 10–25   Diseases of bone characterized by outgrowth or overgrowth of bone. (Radiographs intensified for illustrative purposes.)

> e. Osteosarcoma, sclerotic type (see Chapter 9).
> f. Localized gigantism (see Chapter 7).
> 2. Overgrowth or outgrowth involving several or many bones.
>   a. Hereditary multiple cartilaginous exostoses (multiple osteochondromas, diaphyseal aclasis).
>   b. Pituitary gigantism.
>   c. Acromegaly.
>   d. Arachnoidactyly (Marfan's syndrome) (see Chapter 7).
>   e. Engelmann's disease (see earlier in this chapter).
>   f. "Erlenmeyer flask" type failure of bone modeling: Gaucher's disease; also marble bone disease or osteopetrosis (see Chapters 7 and 8).
>   g. Pyle's disease (see Chapter 7).

Osteochondroma (Figure 10–26)

Clinical Features

Metaphyseal prominence or swelling, with no symptoms except with pressure or trauma.

Recurs unless fibrous capsule is also excised.

Malignant transformation in one to seven per cent of cases.

Maximum age incidence in first two decades.

Pathology. Mushroom shape, consisting of cancellous bone except at its base, where the bone is compact; usually there is a crown of hyaline cartilage and a fibrous capsule.

Most Frequent Sites

At sites of tendon attachment.

Lower femur, upper tibia, upper femur, upper and lower humerus, lower tibia, and pelvis.

The skull is a site for true *osteomas* rather than osteochondromas.

Osteochondromas above the knee can be responsible for the development in the popliteal space of vascular damage which produces thrombosis, false aneurysm, and arteriovenous fistula (Heilman et al.).

Radiographic Findings

Mushroom-shaped cancellous bony excrescence at sites mentioned above.

Hyaline cartilage cap is radiolucent and is not seen radiographically.

Cortex and medulla of host bone are continuous with tumor, but the compact bone is found only at the base of the lesion.

Hereditary Multiple Cartilaginous Exostoses (Diaphyseal Aclasis). This condition is familial and hereditary in about 75 per cent of cases. Cartilaginous and bony exostoses similar in appearance to those described for osteochondroma may occur at any portion of the skeleton which has been preformed in cartilage, but the localizations are *particularly frequent in the metaphyseal portions of the long bones.*

The Most Frequent Sites are the upper shaft of the humerus, hands, knee, ankle, flat bones of the pelvis, scapula, ribs, and vertebrae.

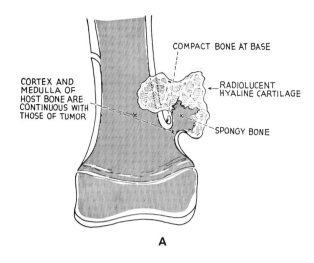

COMPACT BONE AT BASE

CORTEX AND
MEDULLA OF
HOST BONE ARE
CONTINUOUS WITH
THOSE OF TUMOR

RADIOLUCENT
HYALINE CARTILAGE

SPONGY BONE

A

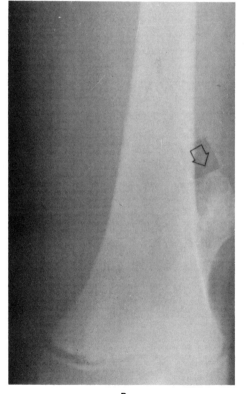

B

Figure 10–26 Osteochondroma of the femur (solitary). *A*. Diagrammatic illustration. *B*. Representative radiograph showing an osteochondroma of the distal femur.

Clinical Course. Malignant change is said to occur in about 5 per cent of the cases but otherwise the prognosis is usually considered favorable. Surgical interference is indicated only in the event that severe suffering and disturbance of function are caused by the exostoses or by the local tumor formation, or if growth in the tumor mass is recognized.

Differential Diagnosis. It is readily distinguished from chondrodysplasia (Ollier's disease), since in the latter condition an enchondromatosis appears first and the protuberant aspects of the disease come later.

Chondrosarcoma (Figure 10–27)

Clinical Features

Pain, leucocytosis, fever, local bone swelling.

Age incidence: primary type usually occurs prior to the third decade; secondary type occurs after the third decade.

Favored Sites

Fifty per cent of cases occur around knee.
Also occurs in proximal femur, pelvis, and humerus.

Pathology.   Large, lobulated mass is fixed to surrounding tissues with multiple areas of amorphous, calcified cartilage. The primary type is unassociated with pre-existing osteochondroma, but the secondary type is associated with it.

Radiographic Findings

Bone-destructive tumor mass with large, amorphous calcific foci which have a mulberry, peppery, or flocculent appearance in contrast to calcified osteoid matrix, which has a more patchy appearance. The calcium is sometimes described as "popcorn" type calcification.

Minimal periosteal reaction and Codman's triangle.

Osteolytic variety also occurs, with little or no sclerosis or calcification.

Prognosis.   The typical chondrosarcoma grows slowly and metastasizes late. If there is recurrence, excision should be repeated and even if there is metastasis, excision of both the primary lesion and the metastasis should still be considered.

Parosteal Osteoid Sarcoma (Ranniger and Altner; Edeiken et al.).   The roentgenologic features of a dense homogenous bone mass appearing outward from the parosteal surface is characteristic. Moreover the margins are lobulated and the inner portions appear to be less dense than those on the periphery. There is a fine radiolucent line which appears to separate the dense bone mass of the tumor bone from the cortex. This line runs parallel to the shaft of the bone and ends at the apparent attachment of the tumor to the shaft.

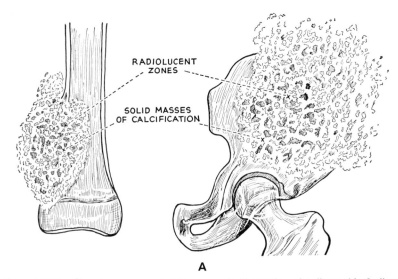

A

Figure 10–27   Chondrosarcoma. *A.* Diagrammatic illustration of radiographic findings.

Figure 10–27 continued on opposite page.

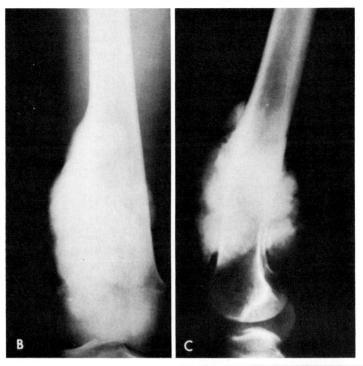

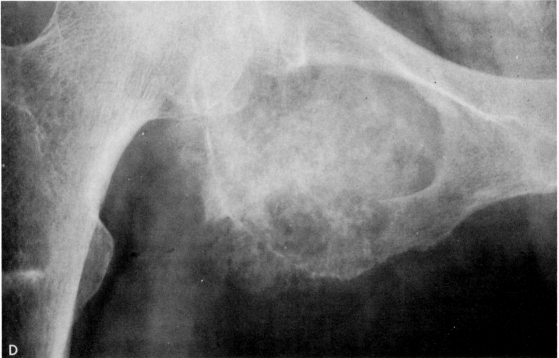

Figure 10–27 *(Continued)*   *B* and *C*. Antero-posterior and lateral views of the distal femur in a patient with an osteosarcoma of the sclerotic type for comparison. *D*. Chondrosarcoma involving the ischium and pubis.

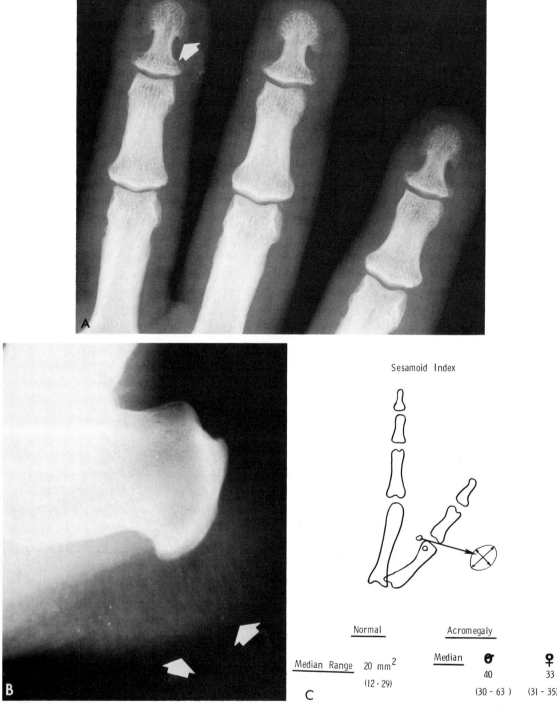

Figure 10–28 *A.* The phalanges in acromegaly. Note the typical "spade" appearance of the tufted ends of the distal phalanges with the overhanging broadened edges. Pituitary gigantism may produce a similar appearance when the individual attains adulthood.

B. Increased soft tissue width in lateral view of heel in acromegaly. The measured distance from the tuberosity of the os calcis to the adjoining skin surface usually exceeds 23 mm.

C. Method of computation of sesamoid index for diagnosis of acromegaly (Kleinberg et al.). Normally, median 20, range 12 to 29 in acromegalics. Male, median 40, range 30 to 63. Acromegalic women, median 33, range 31 to 35. The smaller indices are usually obtained from persons under 37 years of age.

Smaller tumors have a similar area of attachment to the cortex. The cortex is usually not disturbed and the architecture of the bone is intact (Wolfel and Carter).

Generalized Pituitary Gigantism. Acromegaly (Figure 10–28 A, B).

Pathology

Ordinarily this disease is related to an eosinophilic adenoma of the anterior pituitary gland in the preadolescent period or is due to a hyperplasia of the eosinophilic cells of the anterior pituitary gland.

If overproduction of hormones persists into adult life, the typical clinical picture of acromegaly is produced.

Clinical Features

History of headaches, visual disturbance, polyuria, polydipsia, disturbance of the wake-sleep rhythm, and occasionally nausea and vomiting. Pupillary dilatation, exophthalmos, and other eye signs may appear.

All the bones show an increase in growth with accelerated periosteal bone formation as well as accelerated length and growth.

Large grotesque head, with markedly prominent forehead and prognathous jaw. Mandibular angle is more obtuse than normal.

Overgrowth of mandible, lips, and nose.

Hands show considerable evidence of broadening of the shafts of the fingers and increase in their overall size. The same is true for the feet.

Excessive perspiration is likely and hair growth is usually excessive and coarse.

Pathology of Acromegaly. Eosinophilic tumors of the anterior pituitary gland account for about 30 per cent of pituitary tumors. They occur about equally among males and females and the age span between 20 and 50 years is most commonly concerned.

Radiographic Findings in Acromegaly

Skull: bony tables markedly thickened; prominent bossae; mandible markedly thickened and increased in dimension with an obtuse angle between the ramus and the body. Sella turcica: thinning of the dorsum sellae and clinoid processes with evidence of intrasellar expanding lesions often present. Increased intracranial pressure may also coexist.

Hands: shafts of phalanges are markedly thickened with an increase in the tufted ends of the distal phalanges giving a "spade" appearance (Figure 10–28 A).

Heel: the soft tissues overlying the os calcis are increased in dimension to 23 mm. or more (Steinbach) (Figure 10–28 B). All osseous trabeculations are markedly coarsened.

The product of the two greatest perpendicular diameters of the medial sesamoid bones of the first metacarpophalangeal joint (sesamoid index) (Figure 10–28 C) may also be used to identify acromegalics if it is greater than 29 for both men and women.

THE DIAGNOSTIC VALUE OF HEEL-PAD THICKNESS IN ACROMEGALY (GONTICAS ET AL.)

1. Increased heel-pad thickness was found in all acromegalic patients—therefore the diagnosis of acromegaly is questioned in the absence of this finding.

2. This sign is not pathognomonic of acromegaly since it may occur in hypo-

thyroidism and in one to two per cent of nonedematous, nonacromegalic subjects even when the results are expressed in relation to body weight.

3. The heel-pad thickness sign is still a valuable diagnostic tool in acromegaly provided that results are expressed in relation to body weight.

4. Gonticas et al. showed a normal range of 15 to 30 mm. for the thickness of the heel-pad, with a mean of 20.7 mm. (Steinbach and Russell had reported a range of 13 to 21 mm. with a mean of 17.8 mm.) There was, however, a good correlation of heel-pad thickness to body weight in kilograms. The larger heel-pads were invariably found in persons of greater than 70 kilos body weight. The heel-pad thickness in normal people was under 27 mm. in those who were 90 kilograms or less in weight.

GENERAL CONCEPTS REGARDING TUMORS OF BONE

Introduction

Despite a tremendous body of literature concerning tumors of bone, there is still considerable confusion about this important subject. A clear and concise concept of bone tumors is imperative since these tumors comprise probably the most important single group of tumors in patients under the age of 20 years, and because the therapy for these tumors when a diagnosis is rendered is often so radical.

A primary bone tumor is one that arises in one of the various tissues that compose the skeleton.

We may assume that these tissues fall into three categories:

1. *Proliferative or reactive processes,* a manifestation of *reparative proliferation;*

2. *Hamartomatous inclusions,* which are spontaneous proliferations of the cells which normally reside in a particular locus, but in which maturation is incomplete at the time of observation. These may be called *hamartomas.*

3. *A nonmaturing hyperplasia or multiplication of cells* that not only invade but also have the ability to set up independent growth; these we may call *neoplasia.*

The neoplasms of bone may be either benign or malignant.

Unfortunately, the line that separates malignant from benign tumors is not always distinct and every experienced pathologist has found that he must have all clinical and radiologic information at his disposal when he attempts to differentiate bone lesions of this or related types.

To understand the types of primary bone tumors, it is necessary to bear in mind a scheme of tissues that compose the skeleton; such a scheme may be given as follows:

The *mesoderm* gives rise to two basic elements which ultimately are found in bone: (a) the *fibroblast,* and (b) the *reticulum.*

The fibroblast, in turn, gives rise to an *osteogenic* group of cells, a *chondrogenic* group, and a *collagenic* group.

The reticulum gives rise to a *myelogenic* group.

Nervous tissue elements are also present.

We can, therefore, on this basis begin a classification of primary bone tumors into five major categories as follows:

Classification of primary bone tumors (modified from Aegerter and Kirkpatrick, 1968):

I. *Osteogenic Series*
    A. Benign
           1. Osteoid osteoma
           2. Benign osteoblastoma
           3. Osteoma
           4. Osteochondroma
    B. Malignant
           1. Osteosarcoma
           2. Periosteal sarcoma
           3. Osteoclastoma (Giant cell tumor)

II. *Chondrogenic Series*
    A. Benign
           1. Enchondroma
           2. Benign chondroblastoma
           3. Chondromyxoid fibroma
    B. Malignant
           1. Chondrosarcoma

III. *Collagenic Series*
    A. Benign
           1. Nonosteogenic fibroma
           2. Subperiosteal cortical defect
           3. Angioma
           4. Aneurysmal bone cyst
    B. Malignant
           1. Fibrosarcoma
           2. Angiosarcoma

IV. *Myelogenic Series*
    A. Malignant
           1. Plasma cell myeloma
           2. Ewing's tumor
           3. Reticulum cell sarcoma
           4. Hodgkin's disease

V. *Neurogenic Series*
    A. Benign
           1. Neurofibroma
    B. Malignant
           1. Neuroblastoma
    C. Tumors of sympathetic nerve origin, benign or malignant

Aergerter and Kirkpatrick have attempted to separate from the above groups those lesions which are neoplastic from those which are *proliferative* or *reactive*, or *hamartomatous*, and they have modified the classification as follows:

I. Reactive bone lesions
    A. Osteogenic
           1. Osteoid osteoma
           2. Benign osteoblastoma

    B. Collagenic
        1. Nonosteogenic fibroma
        2. Subperiosteal cortical defect
II. Hamartomas Affecting Bone
    A. Osteogenic
        1. Osteoma
        2. Osteochondroma
    B. Chondrogenic
        1. Enchondroma
    C. Collagenic
        1. Angioma
        2. Aneurysmal bone cyst
III. True Tumors of Bone
    A. Osteogenic
        1. Osteosarcoma
        2. Periosteal sarcoma
        3. Osteoclastoma
    B. Chondrogenic
        1. Benign chondroblastoma
        2. Chondromyxoid fibroma
        3. Chondrosarcoma
    C. Collagenic
        1. Fibrosarcoma
        2. Angiosarcoma
    D. Myelogenic
        1. Plasma cell myeloma
        2. Ewing's tumor
        3. Reticulum cell sarcoma
        4. Hodgkin's disease

As indicated above, we feel that a fifth category should be added under the true tumors of bone which would be labeled:

    E. Neurogenic
        1. Neuroblastoma
        2. Neurofibroma
        3. Tumors of sympathetic ganglion or nerve origin.

Tumors Metastatic to Bone.   The great majority of metastatic tumors in bone are of epithelial origin; however, a few sarcomas fall into this group. Ewing's tumor metastasizes to one or more bones in less than half the cases. It is usually encountered in children. Bone involvement may also be found in cases of leukemia, malignant lymphoma, and Hodgkin's disease.

Practically any tumor, with the exception of tumors of the central nervous system, may occasionally metastasize to bone. Cancers that frequently develop secondary deposits in bone are those which are primary in the *breast, prostate, thyroid, kidney,* and *lung.* Bone metastasis is also very common in *neuroblastoma.*

The thoracic vertebrae, ribs, sternum, and clavicles are most commonly involved in breast cancer; whereas lumbar and sacral vertebrae and the pelvic bones are the bones usually affected by a primary carcinoma of the prostate. Metastases in bones distal to the elbows and knees are unusual but do occur.

A primary carcinoma of the prostate, if it has grown out of the capsule of the prostate gland, will ordinarily produce an elevation of *acid phosphatase* in the blood serum. Almost any tumor, however, that destroys a considerable amount of bone and initiates osteoblastic reparative activity produces a rise in serum *alkaline phosphatase*. Elevated serum phosphatase levels may also occur with liver malfunction and disease.

Serum calcium levels may be altered in extensive skeletal metastases. High serum calcium levels may lead to metastatic calcification of soft tissues. Nephrocalcinosis may also result. Excessive osteoid production is usually induced by a malignant tumor, but irradiation and hormone therapy may also stimulate new bone formation. Sclerotic metastatic bony appearances may result in previously osteolytic areas as a result of such therapy.

The **most important functions of the radiologist** in respect to tumors of bone may be summarized as follows:
He should attempt to recognize the bone tumor type in collaboration with the pathologist.
He should attempt to label the tumor as either benign or malignant.

ROENTGEN CRITERIA FOR DIFFERENTIATION OF BENIGN FROM MALIGNANT BONE TUMOR PROCESSES

The roentgen criteria for benign versus malignant bone tumors can be described under the following headings:
1. Number of lesions—monostotic or polyostotic;
2. Size;
3. Shape;
4. Exact position of lesion or lesions—name bones and say whether in epiphysis, metaphysis, diaphysis, or a combination thereof;
5. Density—lucency, sclerosis, or a mixture of these;
6. Architecture—*internally,* and at the *margin* of the lesion or lesions;
7. Impairment of function;
8. Alterations with time;
9. Alterations with therapy.

(Function in itself may not be a very useful criterion since a pathologic fracture which seriously impairs function may occur in a benign lesion, and function in some malignant lesions may not be impaired until very late.)

Number of Lesions.   Generally a benign tumor process is a single well-circumscribed lesion of bone. There are, however, exceptions to this, since neurofibromas, for example, may be multiple; enchondromas, osteochondromas, hemangiomas, and fibrous dysplasias may also be multiple.

Size.   Size in itself is not a completely useful criterion since benign lesions may be quite large and malignant processes small. Usually the malignant processes become large during a period of several months.

Shape.   The shape of a bone lesion does not in itself help us significantly in defining it as benign or malignant.

Position.   The position of a bone lesion is of some importance, as indicated in Figure 10–29. From this illustration it is apparent that the chondroblastoma is

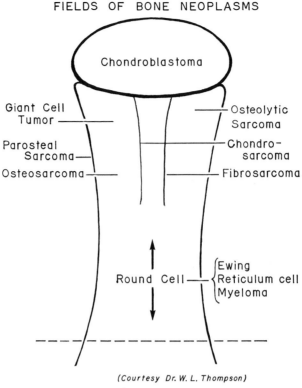

FIELDS OF BONE NEOPLASMS

(Courtesy Dr. W. L. Thompson)

Figure 10–29

most frequent in the epiphysis, while a giant cell tumor most frequently involves a metaphysis with possible extension into the epiphysis. The so-called round cell tumors (including Ewing's tumor, neuroblastoma, reticulum cell sarcoma, and the myelomas) are often medullary within the shaft of a bone, although they may be multiple or metaphyseal. The osteosarcomas, fibrosarcomas, chondrosarcomas, and periosteal sarcomas tend to be in the ends of long bones but may involve flat bones as well.

Enchondromas are particularly frequent in the small bones of the hands and feet, angiomas or hemangiomas occur frequently in vertebral bodies, and the osteosarcomas occur most often around the knee.

Density.   Primary tumors of the bone are most frequently osteolytic. Some primary bone tumors may be sclerotic, and even the lytic tumors may become sclerotic following appropriate therapy. Density of itself may help in distinguishing such processes as the benign osteoma and osteochondroma.

Architecture.   The most characteristic features of both benign and malignant tumors are found in the intimate study of the architecture of the lesions. An architectural description may include the following:

1. Presence or absence of a discrete linear or sclerotic margin.

2. A close description of the "inside" pattern of the lesion. Is it trabecular? Is it irregular? Are there vertical strands? Are there small punctate areas of calcification, or is the intricate pattern more that of "popcorn" type calcification? Is there an "onion skin" layering?

3. Is there a periosteal reaction? If so, is this periosteal reaction vertically oriented ("sunray"), layered or "onion skin-like," or irregular or lacelike?

The importance of the *outer margin* in differentiating a benign from a malignant neoplasm is illustrated in Figure 10–30. It will be noted from this illustration that, generally, malignant lesions do not have a discrete outer margin—and this includes the giant cell tumor or osteoclastoma. The thickness or thinness of this sclerotic line or margin is also important. For example, the nonosteogenic fibroma, the fibrous dysplasia, the Brodie's abscess have all rather thick margins. By contrast, the bone cyst, the angioma, and epidermoidoma have a thin discrete margin.

The "Inside" or Trabecular Pattern or Calcium Deposition in a lesion is of importance in differential diagnosis as indicated here (Figure 10–30). In fibrous dysplasia or in a Brodie's abscess, even though there are small segments of bone contained within the lesion microscopically, this ordinarily cannot be differentiated radiologically. In a fibrosarcoma the lesion is ordinarily completely lytic with no demonstrable osseous or calcium deposition within the lesion proper. This is also true of a metastatic tumor usually, particularly of the osteolytic variety.

However, small septate trabecular patterns of an irregular type may be differentiated in such lesions as the chondromyxoid fibroma, the bone cyst, the giant cell tumor, the epidermoidoma, or the angiosarcoma. The inner pattern of the vertebral hemangioma is ordinarily vertically oriented, while the inner pattern of a reticulum cell sarcoma may well be coarse, irregular "woven" trabeculations. In contrast to these, the inner pattern of an enchondroma may have punctate small foci of calcified cartilage or calcification, and the chondrosarcoma contains large clumps of "mulberry" or "popcorn-like" calcification.

The importance of the type of *periosteal reaction* in respect to a bone lesion is indicated in Figure 10–31. In these diagrams the laminated periosteal elevation of congenital syphilis, rickets, and tuberculous osteitis, is differentiated from the "onion skin" laminated periosteal elevation of a Ewing's tumor or reticulum cell sarcoma. The irregular proliferating or subperiosteal calcification of healing scurvy, chronic toxic proliferating periostitis, periostitis and osteitis secondary to chronic cellulitis, osteoperiosteal abscess, or periosteal neurofibroma are diagrammatically indicated. The "sunray" type periosteal reaction of sickle cell anemia and Mediterranean type anemias is indicated. Periosteal proliferation with new bone formation, such as is found in osteitis deformans, osteoid osteoma, the sabre shin of juvenile syphilis, osteogenic sarcoma, and the osteomyelitis of Garré is also diagrammatically indicated. It is a composite, therefore, of these major entities which helps to differentiate benign from malignant tumors and processes.

Another important feature in differentiation is the presence of a *break in the outer cortex of the bone*. Ordinarily when a break in the outer cortex of the bone occurs in the absence of pathologic fracture it spells malignant invasion of the cortex and the surrounding tissues. One must, however, be careful to determine that a pathologic fracture has not occurred which may make this kind of determination difficult.

And lastly, it is important to study the soft tissue surrounding the bone lesion very carefully. This helps to determine whether or not invasion has occurred. If invasion from the bone lesion has occurred, very often there is a notably increased density. On the other hand, inflammatory lesions may also produce soft tissue swelling and make this kind of differentiation difficult in itself.

Other points of reference for assistance in differentiation of the various tumors are indicated in Tables 10–1, 10–2, and 10–3. The age of a patient is of special importance. In the age span from birth to ten years the lesion is more apt to be a bone cyst, neuroblastoma, or Ewing's tumor; from 11 to 20 years of age, an osteogenic sarcoma or Ewing's tumor is probable, and from 21 to 30 years the giant cell

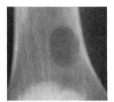

NO "RADIOLOGIC" CAPSULE

MALIGNANT TUMOR METASTASES

MULTIPLE MYELOMA

EOSINOPHILIC GRANULOMA

LIPOID DYSCRASIA

GIANT CELL
TUMOR   USUALLY
                          SOAP-
ANEURYSMAL BONE   BUBBLE
CYST   INTERIOR

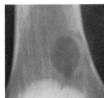

DISCONTINUOUS THIN
"RADIOLOGIC" CAPSULE

OSTEITIS FIBROSA CYSTICA
("BROWN TUMOR")

GAUCHER'S DISEASE

BRODIE'S ABSCESS

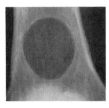

CONTINUOUS THIN
"RADIOLOGIC" CAPSULE

BRODIE'S ABSCESS

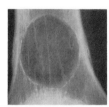

BONE CYST

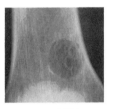

ENCHONDROMA

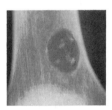

HEMANGIOMA

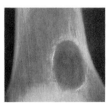

THICK "RADIOLOGIC" CAPSULE

CHRONIC GRANULOMA
OR ABSCESS

FIBROUS DYSPLASIA

BRODIE'S ABSCESS

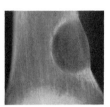

THICK "RADIOLOGIC" CAPSULE
CORTICAL

FIBROUS CORTICAL DEFECT

FIBROMAS (CHONDROMYXOID)

A

Figure 10–30   *A*. Importance of outer margin in differentiating a benign from a malignant bone tumor.
Figure 10–30 continued on opposite page.

TABLE 10–1   AGES OF OCCURRENCE OF PRIMARY BONE TUMORS

0 to 10 Years	11 to 20 Years	21 to 30 Years	31 to 70 Years
Bone cysts	Osteogenic sarcoma	Giant cell tumors (sex incidence equal)	Multiple myeloma (sex incidence equal)
Neuroblastoma	Ewing's tumor		Lymphosarcoma and reticulum cell sarcoma
Ewing's tumor			Paget's sarcoma

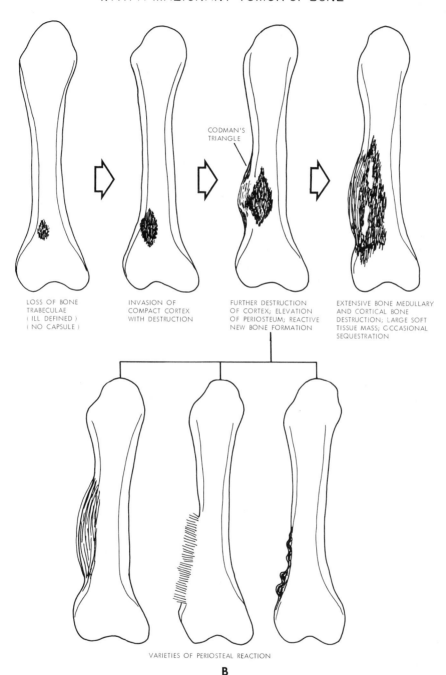

DIAGRAMMATIC RADIOGRAPHIC ALTERATIONS IN BONE
WITH A MALIGNANT TUMOR OF BONE

CODMAN'S
TRIANGLE

LOSS OF BONE
TRABECULAE
(ILL DEFINED)
(NO CAPSULE)

INVASION OF
COMPACT CORTEX
WITH DESTRUCTION

FURTHER DESTRUCTION
OF CORTEX; ELEVATION
OF PERIOSTEUM; REACTIVE
NEW BONE FORMATION

EXTENSIVE BONE MEDULLARY
AND CORTICAL BONE
DESTRUCTION; LARGE SOFT
TISSUE MASS; OCCASIONAL
SEQUESTRATION

VARIETIES OF PERIOSTEAL REACTION

B

Figure 10–30 *(Continued)*   *B.* Endosteal, cortical, and periosteal changes with a malignant tumor of bone.

Laminated Periosteal Elevation

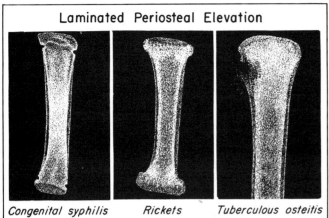

Congenital syphilis   *Rickets*   *Tuberculous osteitis*

"Onion-skin" Laminated Periosteal Elevation

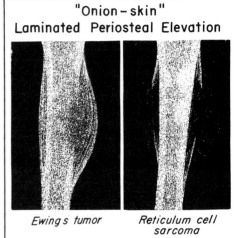

Ewing's tumor   *Reticulum cell sarcoma*

Codman's Triangle

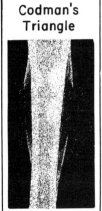

New periosteal bone formation adjoining tumor

Irregularly Proliferating or Subperiosteal Calcification

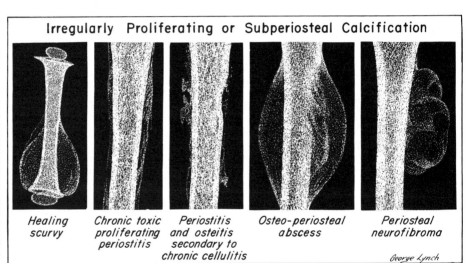

Healing scurvy   *Chronic toxic proliferating periostitis*   *Periostitis and osteitis secondary to chronic cellulitis*   *Osteo-periosteal abscess*   *Periosteal neurofibroma*

George Lynch

"Sun-ray" Type Periosteal Reaction

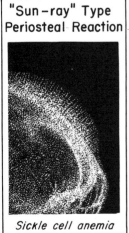

Sickle cell anemia

Periosteal Proliferation with New Bone Formation

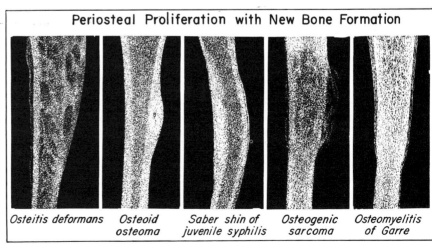

Osteitis deformans   *Osteoid osteoma*   *Saber shin of juvenile syphilis*   *Osteogenic sarcoma*   *Osteomyelitis of Garre*

Figure 10–31   Varieties of periosteal reactions.

TABLE 10–2   RELATIVE RADIOSENSITIVITY OF PRIMARY BONE TUMORS

Radiosensitive	Moderately Radioresistant	Very Radioresistant
Ewing's tumor greater than Neuroblastoma	Giant cell tumor greater than Multiple myeloma	Osteogenic sarcoma greater than Benign tumors

tumor is much more likely. In the 31 to 70 year age group, **metastatic carcinoma or sarcoma is most frequent by far;** among primary osseous tumors, multiple myeloma, lymphosarcoma, reticulum cell sarcoma, Paget's sarcoma and chondrosarcoma are most likely.

Finally, our presentation of the radiology of bone tumors has been unconventional in that the descriptive text relating to these tumors has been distributed on the basis of the most frequent objective appearances. It has been our purpose in this general summary to attempt to bring together some of the loose ends which are most important in clinical practice. It is hoped that a unified concept of the entire subject can thereby be achieved.

TABLE 10–3   ENDOCRINE ABNORMALITIES OF BONE

Endocrine	Activity +	Activity −	Growth in Length	Growth in Breadth	Epiphyseal Maturation	Increased Radiolucency	Clinical Entity	Epiphyseal line Closure	Other Features
Pituitary eosinophiles	+		++++	++++	Normal	No	Gigantism	Normal	
Pituitary deficiency		−	−	−	Normal	No	Pituitary dwarf (Loraine) Fröhlich Laurence-Moon-Biedl Simmonds	Delayed	Sexual infantilism + Preadolescent obesity + Polydactylism, mental deficiency, pigmented retina Emaciation, premature senility
Pituitary basophilism (Cushing's) adrenal cortex	+		−	−	Accelerated	Yes. Dense indented endplates of vertebrae	Cushing's syndrome	Accelerated	Premature puberty
Thyroid	+		+	+	Accelerated	Yes	Toxic thyroid	Normal	Irritability, sweating, weight loss, + + appetite
		−	−	− (slender)	Delayed (broad and thick; stippled)	No	Cretinism	Delayed	Prognathism, dry skin, sparse hair, poor intellect, brachycephalia, increased intervertebral spaces
Parathyroid	+		Normal	May be eroded	Normal	Yes. Nephrocalcinosis (occasionally osteoblastic)	Osteitis fibrosa cystica Renal rickets	Normal	Hypotonia, anorexia, polydipsia, polyuria, kyphosis
		−		No change	Normal	No (reverse)	Hypoparathyroidism	Normal	Increased irritability, lens opacity, sclerosis of bones, calc. intracerebral vessels (basal ganglia)
Adrenal cortex	+		Short	Normal	Accelerated	No		Premature	Precocious puberty, masculinization
Gonads	+		Short	Normal	Accelerated	No		Premature	
		−	++	Thinned out bones	Delayed	No		Delayed	Roughened metaphyses

Questions—Chapter 10

1. What is the general classification of the osteosclerotic and hypertrophic bone diseases of the extremities?

2. In the group of osteosclerotic diseases affecting several extremities, what general radiographic appearances that form the basis of classification are differentiated?

3. In the group of osteosclerotic diseases that are localized or regional, what are some of the main disease entities?

4. In the group of hypertrophic bone diseases representing a bone overgrowth, what are the main diseases represented?

5. In those diseases that are described as the diffuse osteosclerotic group affecting several extremities, which ones form a dense sclerosis, a moderate sclerosis, and a narrow sclerosis?

6. Describe some of the radiographic and clinical features of Engelmann's disease.

7. Describe some of the clinical and radiographic features of marble bone disease.

8. What is the characteristic radiographic and histologic pattern of fluorine poisoning involving bone?

9. Describe the clinical and radiographic features of hypoparathyroidism and indicate how these differ from pseudohypoparathyroidism and pseudopseudohypoparathyroidism.

10. What are the main diseases characterized by transverse bands of osteosclerosis, particularly in the metaphyses?

11. Describe the main clinical and radiographic features of cretinism.

12. List the main disease entities in the osteosclerotic group that are manifested chiefly by longitudinal cortical sclerosis or corticoperiosteal thickening.

13. What are the main clinical and radiographic features of infantile cortical hyperostosis?

14. Describe the main clinical and radiographic features of juvenile and tertiary syphilis of bone.

15. Describe the main clinical and radiographic features of hypertrophic pulmonary osteoarthropathy.

16. Describe the main clinical and radiographic features that are usually manifest by the blood dyscrasias.

17. Name the main osteosclerotic diseases that are characterized by multiple irregular osteosclerotic areas.

18. Describe the main clinical and radiographic features of osteitis deformans.

19. Describe the radiographic appearance of osteosclerotic tumor metastases and indicate the most frequent tumors of origin of such metastases. What is the main importance of distinguishing osteitis condensans ilii?

20. What are some of the main clinical and radiographic features of the nonsuppurative osteomyelitis of Garré?

21. What are the main radiographic features of bone infarction?

22. What are the main clinical and radiographic features of osteoid osteoma?

23. What are the main clinical and radiographic features of osteochondroma?

24. What are the main clinical and radiographic features of chondrosarcoma?

25. What are the main clinical and radiographic features of reticulum cell sarcoma of bone?

26. What is the order of frequency of the primary bone tumors?

27. Which are the bone tumors in which there is frequently multiple bone involvement?

28. Divide the various bone tumors in accordance with ages of occurrence of these primary tumors.

29. Divide the various tumors in accordance with their relative radiosensitivity.

30. Classify the primary bone tumors in relation to the principal tissues of origin.

31. Indicate the sites of predilection of the following tumors: fibrous cortical defect; aneurysmal bone cyst; giant cell tumors; chondroblastoma; giant osteoid osteoma or osteoblastoma; osteosarcoma; reticulum cell sarcoma; osteochondroma; bone cyst; endothelioma; fibrosarcoma; multiple myeloma; and parosteal bone tumors.

32. Describe the radiographic features of the following diseases: multiple cartilaginous exostoses, pituitary gigantism, acromegaly, and localized gigantism.

33. Describe some of the various representative types of periosteal elevation and subperiosteal calcification that may help differentiate such diseases as: osteosarcoma; healing scurvy; juvenile syphilis; osteoid osteoma; osteomyelitis; reticulum cell sarcoma; Ewing's sarcoma; rickets; congenital syphilis; tuberculous osteitis.

34. Describe the most important features which differentiate a benign from a malignant bone tumor.

35. Present an all-inclusive classification of bone neoplasms.

36. Describe what is meant in this text by the inside and margin architecture. How does it assist in differentiating a benign from a malignant neoplasm? What are some of the features of the margin of a lesion which help differentiate some of the benign lesions?

37. Describe the inner architectural pattern of such lesions as the vertebral hemangioma, enchondroma, chondrosarcoma, Brodie's abscess, and metastatic tumors. What is the most frequent inner architectural pattern of the giant cell tumor?

38. How would you differentiate a giant cell tumor from a benign bone cyst?

References

Aegerter, E., and Kirkpatrick, J. A., Jr.: Orthopedic Diseases. Third Edition. Philadelphia, W. B. Saunders Co., 1968.

Beveridge, B., Vaughn, B. F., and Walters, M. N. I.: Primary hyperparathyroidism and secondary renal failure with osteosclerosis. J. Fac. Radiol., 10:197–200, 1959.

Bjersand, A. J.: New bone formation and carpal synostosis in scleroderma: A case report. Amer. J. Roentgenol., 103:616–619, 1968.

Briney, A. K.: Personal communication.

Brogen, N., Duner, H., Hamrin, B., Pernow, B., Theander, G., and Waldenstrom, J.: Urticaria pigmentosa (mastocytosis). A study of nine cases with special reference to the excretion of histamine in urine. Acta Med. Scand., 163:223–233, 1959.

Bucky, N. L.: Bone infarction. Brit. J. Radiol., 32:22–27, 1959.

Burgel, E., and Oleck, H. G.: Skelett ver an der ungen bei der urticaria pigmentosa. Fortschr. Roentgenstr., 90:185–190, 1959.

Caffey, J.: Chronic poisoning due to excess of vitamin A; description of clinical and roentgen manifestations in 7 infants and young children. Pediatrics, 5:672–687, 1950; Amer. J. Roentgenol., 65:12–26, 1951.

Caffey, J.: Pediatric X-ray Diagnosis. Fourth Edition. Chicago, Year Book Medical Publishers, 1961, pp. 1014–1026.

Caffey, J., and Silverman, W. A.: Infantile cortical hyperostoses; preliminary report on new syndrome. Amer. J. Roentgenol., 54:1–16, 1945.

Chang, C. H., Gaskell, J. R., and Chun, C. S.: Abnormal muscle cylinder ratio in idiopathic infantile hypercalcemia: A new roentgen sign. Amer. J. Roentgenol., 108:533–536, 1970. (18 refs.)

Chang, C. H., Piatt, E. D., Thomas, K. E., and Watne, A. L.: Bone abnormalities in Gardner's syndrome. Amer. J. Roentgenol., 103:645–652, 1968.

Coley, B. L., and Harrold, C. S., Jr.: Analysis of 59 cases of osteogenic sarcoma with survival for 5 years or more. J. Bone Joint Surg., 32-A:307–310, 1950.

Copeland, M. M., and Geschickter, C. F.: Malignant Bone Tumors Primary and Metastatic. A Monograph for the Physician. Reprinted by American Cancer Society, Inc. From Ca-A Cancer Journal for Clinicians. Vol. 13, No. 4–6, 1963.

Edeiken, J., Farrell, C., Ackerman, L. V., and Spjut, H. J.: Parosteal sarcoma. Amer. J. Roentgenol., 111:579–583, 1971.

Engels, E. P., Smith, R. C., and Krantz, S.: Bone sclerosis in multiple myeloma. Radiology, 75:242–247, 1960.

Fairbank, T.: An Atlas of General Affections of the Skeleton. Baltimore, Williams and Wilkins Co., 1951.

Fellers, F. X., and Schwartz, R.: Etiology of the severe form of idiopathic hypercalcemia of infancy; a defect in vitamin D metabolism. New Eng. J. Med., 259:1050–1058, 1958.

Fraser, D.: Clinical manifestations of genetic aberrations of calcium and phosphorus metabolism. J.A.M.A., 176:281–287, 1961.

Giustra, P. E., and Feriberger, R. H.: Severe growth disturbance with osteoid osteoma: A report of 2 cases involving the femoral neck. Radiology, 96:285–288, 1970.

Gold, R. H., and Steinbach, H. L.: Lipoatrophic diabetes mellitus. Amer. J. Roentgenol. 101:884–896, 1967.

Gonticas, S. K., Ikkos, D. G., and Stergiou, L. H.: Evaluation of the diagnostic value of heel-pad thickness in acromegaly. Radiology, 92:304–307, 1969.

Green, A. E., Jr., Ellswood, W. H., and Collins, J. R.: Melorheostosis and osteopoikilosis, with a review of the literature. Amer. J. Roentgenol., 87:1096–1111, 1962.

Gribetz, D., Silverman, S. H., and Sobel, A. E.: Vitamin A poisoning. Pediatrics, 7:372–384, 1951.

Hasegawa, J., and Bluefarb, S. M.: Urticaria pigmentosa (mastocytosis). Arch. Intern. Med., 106:417–427, 1960.

Heilman, R. S., Topuzlu, C., and Molloy, M.: Femoral arterial injury secondary to osteochondroma of the distal femur. Amer. J. Roentgenol., *100*:533–537, 1967.

Hess, W. E., and Street, D. M.: Melorheostosis; relief of pain by sympathectomy. J. Bone Joint Surg. (Amer.), *32-A*:422–427, 1950.

Hurt, R. L.: Osteopathia striata – Voorhoeve's disease; report of a case presenting features of osteopathia striata and osteoporosis. J. Bone Joint Surg. (Brit.), *35-B*:89–96, 1953.

Isley, J. K., Jr., and Baylin, G. J.: Prognosis in osteitis condensans ilii. Radiology, *72*:234–237, 1959.

Ivins, J. C., and Dahlin, D. C.: Malignant lymphoma (reticulum cell sarcoma) of bone. Proc. Mayo Clin., *38*:375–385, 1963.

Jacobson, H. G., Fateh, H., Shapiro, J. H., Spaet, T. H., and Poppel, M. H.: Agnogenic myeloid metaplasia. Radiology, *72*:716–725, 1959.

Jensen, W. N., and Lasser, E. C.: Urticaria pigmentosa associated with widespread sclerosis of the spongiosa of bone. Radiology, *71*: 826–832, 1958.

Karpinski, F. E., and Martin, J. F.: Skeletal lesions of leukemic children treated with aminopterin. J. Pediat., *37*:208–223, 1950.

Kaye, M., Prichard, J. E., Halpenny, G. W., and Light, W.: Bone disease in chronic renal failure with particular reference to osteosclerosis. Medicine, *39*:157–190, 1960.

Keats, T. E.: Rib erosions in scleroderma. Amer. J. Roentgenol., *100*:530–532, 1967.

Kim, S. K., and Barry, W. F., Jr.: Bone island. Amer. J. Roentgenol., *92*:1301–1306, 1964.

Kleinberg, D. L., Young, I. S., and Kupperman, H. S.: The sesamoid index: an aid in the diagnosis of acromegaly. Ann. Intern. Med., *64*:1075–1078, 1966.

Kolawole, T. M., and Bohrer, S. P.: Ulcer osteoma – bone response to tropic ulcer. Amer. J. Roentgenol., *109*:611–618, 1970.

Kolb, F. O., and Steinbach, H. L.: Pseudohypoparathyroidism with secondary hyperparathyroidism and osteitis fibrosa. J. Clin. Endocrinol., *22*:59–70, 1962.

Leigh, T. F., Corley, C. C., Jr., Huguley, C. M., Jr., and Rogers, J. V., Jr.: Myelofibrosis: the general and radiologic findings in 25 proved cases. Amer. J. Roentgenol., *82*:183–193, 1959.

Lichtenstein, L.: Benign osteoblastoma; category of osteoid- and bone-forming tumors other than classical osteoid osteoma, which may be mistaken for giant-cell tumor or osteogenic sarcoma. Cancer, *9*:1044–1052, 1956.

Lott, G., and Klein, E.: Osteopetrosis: A case presentation. Amer. J. Roentgenol., *94*:616–620, 1965.

Luck, Vernon, J.: Bone and Joint Diseases. Springfield, Ill., Charles C Thomas, 1950.

Martel, W., and Sitterly, B. H.: Roentgenologic manifestations of osteonecrosis. Amer. J. Roentgenol., *106*:509–522, 1969 (45 refs.).

Martincic, N.: Osteopoikilie. Brit. J. Radiol., *25*:612–614, 1952.

Meszaros, W. T., and Sisson, M.: Myelofibrosis. Radiology, *77*:958–967, 1961.

Morris, J. W.: Skeletal fluorosis among Indians of the American Southwest. Amer. J. Roentgenol., *94*:608–615, 1965.

Mottram, M. E., and Hill, H. A.: Diaphyseal dysplasia: Report of a case. Amer. J. Roentgenol., *95*:162–167, 1965.

Norman, A., and Dorfman, H. D.: Juxta-cortical circumscribed myositis ossificans: Evolution and radiographic features. Radiology, *96*:301–306, 1970.

Pease, C. N., and Newton, G. G.: Metaphyseal dysplasia due to lead poisoning in children. Radiology, *79*:233–240, 1962.

Pettigrew, J. G., and Ward, H. P.: Correlation of radiologic, histologic and clinical findings in agnogenic myeloid metaplasia. Radiology, *93*:541–548, 1969.

Pochaczevsky, R., Yen, Y. M., and Sherman, R. S.: The roentgen appearance of benign osteoblastoma. Radiology, *75*:429–437, 1960.

Pratt, A. D., Felson, B., Wyatt, J. F., and Page, M.: Sequestrum formation in fibrous dysplasia. Amer. J. Roentgenol., *106*:162–165, 1969.

Ranniger, K., and Altner, P. C.: Parosteal osteoid sarcoma. Radiology, *86*:648–651, 1966.

Reeves, R. J., and Pederson, R.: Fungus infection of bone. Radiology, *62*:55–60, 1954.

Ribbing, S.: Hereditary, multiple, diaphyseal sclerosis. Acta Radiol., *31*:522–536, 1949.

Rothman, P. E., and Leon, E. E.: Hypervitaminosis A; report of two cases in infants. Radiology, *51*:368–374, 1948.

Sagher, F., and Schorr, S.: Short report. Bone lesions in urticaria pigmentosa: report of a central registry on skeletal x-ray survey. J. Invest. Derm., *26*:431–434, 1956.

Sankaran, B.: Osteoid osteoma. Surg. Gynec. Obst., *99*:193–198, 1954.

Saville, P. D.: Polyarteritis nodosa with new bone formation. J. Bone Joint Surg., *38B*:327–333, 1956.

Sear, H. R.: Engelmann's disease; osteopathia, hyperostica sclerotisans multiplex infantilis; report of a case. Brit. J. Radiol., *21*:236–241, 1948.

Scanlon, G. T., and Clemett, A. R.: Thyroid acropachy. Radiology, *83*:1039–1042, 1964.

Shapiro, R.: The biochemical basis of bone changes in chronic uremia. Amer. J. Roentgenol., *111*:750–761, 1971.

Shiers, J. A., Neuhauser, E. B., and Bowman, J. R.: Idiopathic hypercalcemia. Amer. J. Roentgenol., *78*:19–29, 1957.

Silverman, F. N.: Treatment of leukemia and allied disorders with folic acid antagonists; effect of aminopterin on skeletal lesions. Radiology, *53*:665–677, 1950.

Singleton, E. B.: The radiographic features of severe idiopathic hypercalcemia of infancy. Radiology, *68*:721–726, 1957.

Soriano, M., and Manchon, F.: The radiological aspects of a new type of bone fluorosis, periostitis deformans. Radiology, *87*:1089–1094, 1966.

Stark, E., Van Buskirk, F. W., and Daly, J. F.: Radiologic and pathologic bone changes associated with urticaria pigmentosa: report of a case. Arch. Path., *62*:143–148, 1956.

Steinbach, H. L.: Some roentgen features of

Paget's disease. Amer. J. Roentgenol., *86*:950–964, 1961.

Steinbach, H. L., and Russell, W.: Measurement of the Heel-Pad as an Aid to Diagnosis of Acromegaly. Radiology, *82*:418–422, 1964.

Swerdloff, B. A., Ozonloff, M. B., Gyepes, M. T.: Late recurrence of infantile cortical hyperostosis. Amer. J. Roentgenol., *108*:461–467, 1970.

Templeton, A. W., Jaconette, J. R., and Ormond, R. S.: Localized osteosclerosis in hyperparathyroidism. Radiology, *78*:955–958, 1962.

Thompson, Colonel W. L.: Personal communication.

Toomey, F. B., and Felson, B.: Osteoblastic bone metastasis in gastrointestinal tract and bronchial carcinoids. Amer. J. Roentgenol., *83*:709–715, 1960.

Tuffanelli, D. L., and Winkelmann, R. K.: Systemic scleroderma: Clinical study of 727 cases. Arch. Derm., *84*:359–371, 1961.

Van Buskirk, S. W., Tampas, J. P., and Peterson, O. S., Jr.: Infantile cortical hyperostosis: An inquiry into its familial aspects. Amer. J. Roentgenol., *85*:613–632, 1961.

Vogt, A.: Osteosklerose bei blutkrankheiten, die osteosklerotische anämie vom typus M.B. Schmidt und die osteosklerotische leukämie. Fortschr. Roentgenstr., *71*:697–717, 1949.

Wilson, T. W., and Pugh, D. G.: Primary reticulum-cell sarcoma of bone, with emphasis on roentgen aspects. Radiology, *65*:343–351, 1955.

Wolfel, D. A., and Carter, P. R.: Parosteal osteosarcoma. Amer. J. Roentgenol., *105*:142–146, 1969.

Wolfson, J. J., and Engel, R. R.: Anticipating meconium peritonitis from metaphyseal bands. Radiology, *92*:1055–1060, 1969.

Zak, S. G., Covey, J. A., and Snodgrass, J. J.: Osseous lesions in urticaria pigmentosa. New Eng. J. Med., *256*:56–59, 1957.

11

Radiology of Joints

INTRODUCTION

Anatomically, articulations between bones may be classified into three types (Figure 11–1): diarthroses, or freely movable joints; amphiarthroses, or slightly movable joints such as those which occur between vertebral bodies; and synarthroses, or immovable joints such as those which occur between the cranial bones (sutures).

In our present discussion we shall confine ourselves to the diarthrodial or synovial joints.

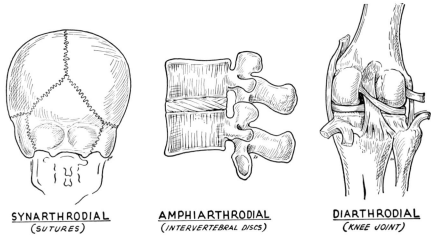

SYNARTHRODIAL
(SUTURES)

AMPHIARTHRODIAL
(INTERVERTEBRAL DISCS)

DIARTHRODIAL
(KNEE JOINT)

Figure 11–1   Classification of joints.

ROUTINE USED IN RADIOGRAPHIC INTERPRETATION OF SYNOVIAL JOINT DISEASE

A guide for routine examination of the synovial joints is presented as follows:

1. The *alignment* of the bones on either side of the joint is noted and compared with the normal alignment (Figures 11–2 through 11–10).

2. The *status of the bony structures* on either side of the joint is examined, and both epiphyses and diaphyses are noted, as well as whether or not rarefaction is present (Figure 11–11).

3. The *width of the joint space* is estimated and at the same time an estimate is made of the condition of the joint cartilage. The joint space itself is examined for loose bodies.

4. The roughness or smoothness of the *subchondral bone* is noted, together with excrescences and any rarefaction or sclerosis in the adjoining cancellous bone.

5. The *capsular and pericapsular soft tissues* may show evidence of swelling or calcium deposition in the ligamentous structures.

6. Finally, *arthrography* with air or positive contrast media offers further elucidation of pathology. A bone survey or surveys of other parts of the body may also be of assistance.

As a result of this routine, a method of analysis of joint radiographs for evidence of joint disease can be devised and is illustrated in Figure 11–11.

Ancillary Information of Importance to Radiologists

History and Physical Examination. A history is obtained, with particular attention to prior joint disease, and signs and symptoms are traced back to the origin of abnormality.

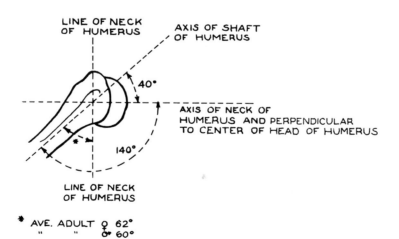

Figure 11–2   Axial relationships at the upper part of the humerus. (Modified from C. Toldt: *An Atlas of Human Anatomy for Students and Physicians.* New York, Macmillan Co., © 1926.)

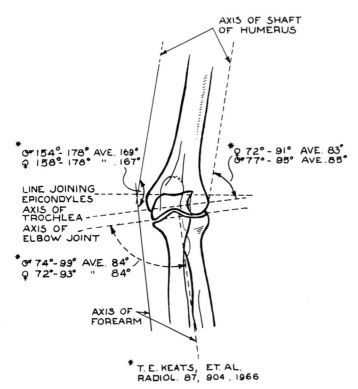

AXIS OF SHAFT
OF HUMERUS

* ♂ 154°- 178° AVE. 169°
♀ 158°- 178° " . 167°

* ♀ 72° - 91° AVE. 83°
♂ 77° - 95° AVE. 85°

LINE JOINING
EPICONDYLES
AXIS OF
TROCHLEA
AXIS OF
ELBOW JOINT

* ♂ 74°- 99° AVE. 84°
♀ 72°- 93° " 84°

AXIS OF
FOREARM

* T. E. KEATS, ET. AL.
RADIOL. 87, 904, 1966

Figure 11–3 Axial relationships of the elbow.

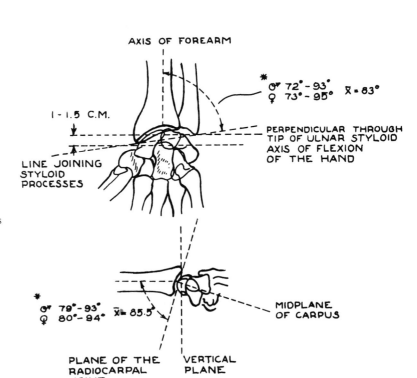

AXIS OF FOREARM

* ♂ 72° - 93° X̄ = 83°
♀ 73° - 95°

1 - 1.5 C.M.

PERPENDICULAR THROUGH
TIP OF ULNAR STYLOID
AXIS OF FLEXION
OF THE HAND

LINE JOINING
STYLOID
PROCESSES

Figure 11–4 Axial relationships of the wrist.

* ♂ 79°- 93° X̄ = 85.5
♀ 80°- 94°

MIDPLANE
OF CARPUS

PLANE OF THE
RADIOCARPAL
JOINT

VERTICAL
PLANE

* T. E. KEATS, ET AL.
RADIOL. 87: 904, 1966

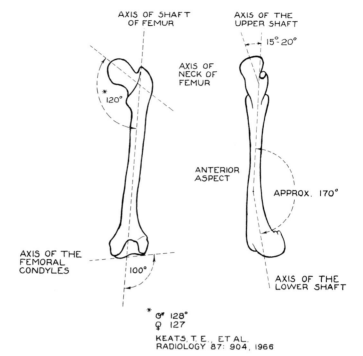

Figure 11–5 Axial relationships of the shafts of the femur, in the antero-posterior and lateral projections.

Laboratory Tests are given, such as: sedimentation rate, serology, blood count, urinalysis, blood uric acid, basal metabolic rate, antistreptolysin and antihyaluronidase titres of serum (helpful in differentiating rheumatoid arthritis); rheumatoid arthritis factor (the RA factor); bone marrow preparations for lupus erythematosus cells (helpful in differentiating lupus erythematosus and related conditions); examination of the synovial fluid, if there is any, for cell count and the differential pattern of the leukocytes; red cell agglutination test; other agglutination and complement fixation tests such as might differentiate gonorrhea, brucellosis, streptococcus, and typhoid; and adjunctive examination such as the examination of the urethral or cervical discharge, prostate discharge, synovial fluid cultures, performance of

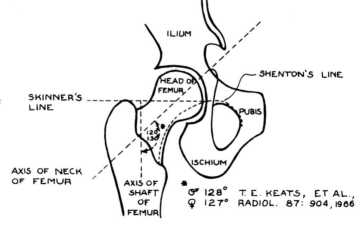

Figure 11–6 Axial relationships of the hip joint.

DISLOCATIONS OF THE HIP

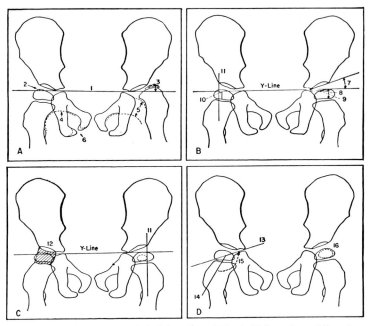

Figure 11-7   *A* to *D*. Criteria for congenital dislocation of hip. 1. Y-Symphyseal line. 2 and 3 normally are equal. 4. Shenton's line unbroken—normal. 5. Shenton's line broken—dislocation or fracture. 6. Fusion delayed, with dislocation. 7. Not greater than 34° in newborn, normally; not greater than 25° after 1 year. 8. Not less than 6 mm. normally. 9. Less than 16 mm. normally. 10. Less than one half of epiphyseal width normally. 11. Should cross epiphysis lateral to center normally. 12. Right-angled cylinder normally. 13. Line: center of acetabulum to center of head. 14. Axis of neck of femur. 15. Angle 120° to 125° normally. (Modified from Köhler, A., and Zimmer, E. A.: *Borderlands of the Normal and Early Pathologic in Skeletal Roentgenology.* English translation by J. T. Case. New York, Grune and Stratton, Inc., 1956, pp. 491–494.)

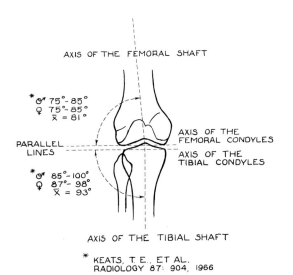

Figure 11-8   Axial relationships around the knee.

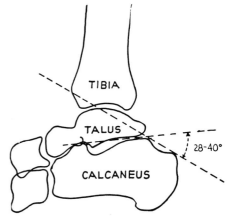

Figure 11–9 The criteria for a normal calcaneus and its proper alignment with the talus (Boehler's angle).

tuberculin tests, and blood calcium phosphorus and acid or alkaline phosphatase levels.

Associated Symptomatology which may fit into recognized syndromes includes: psoriasis; Felty's syndrome with splenomegaly and leukopenia; Still's disease in children; Reiter's syndrome with associated diarrhea, urethritis, and conjunctivitis; Sjögren's syndrome with keratoconjunctivitis sicca and xerostomia or both; Whipple's disease; colitis; skin manifestations; autoimmune (collagen) diseases.

A USEFUL CLASSIFICATION OF JOINT DISEASE FOR THE RADIOLOGIST

On the basis of the preceding analysis the radiologist, being dependent on objective signs as presented by the x-ray examination, may classify diseases according to the following characteristics:

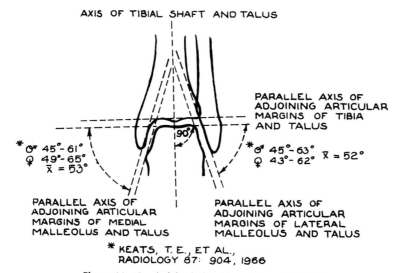

Figure 11–10 Axial relationships of the ankle joint.

ANALYSIS OF JOINT DISEASE: TISSUE PRIMARILY INVOLVED

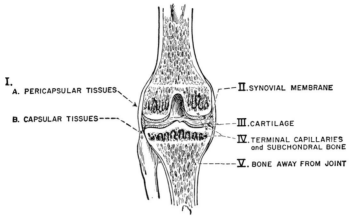

I.
  A. PERICAPSULAR TISSUES

  B. CAPSULAR TISSUES

II. SYNOVIAL MEMBRANE

III. CARTILAGE

IV. TERMINAL CAPILLARIES and SUBCHONDRAL BONE

V. BONE AWAY FROM JOINT

Figure 11–11   Method of analysis of joint radiographs for evidence of joint disease.

1. Abnormalities of alignment.
2. Diseases characterized by capsular distension without bony involvement.
   a. Simple hydrarthrosis.
   b. Idiopathic capsulitis.
   c. Acute pyogenic infection (early).
   d. Rheumatic fever (periarticular arthrosis); migratory polyarthritis.
3. Diseases characterized by subchondral and capsular proliferative response. Capsular lipping, spurring, calcification, and ossification are seen in variable degrees.
   a. Traumatic arthritis.
   b. "Hypertrophic" arthritis (also called degenerative arthritis or osteoarthritis).
   c. Hemophilic arthritis.
   d. Neurotrophic arthropathy.
4. Diseases characterized by osteoporosis of neighboring bone and narrowing of the joint space with subchondral bone resorption.
   a. Tuberculous arthritis.
   b. Rheumatoid arthritis.
   c. Pyogenic arthritis (but with somewhat less surrounding osteoporosis).
5. Diseases characterized by periarticular bone resorption without significant adjoining osteoporosis.
   a. Gout.
   b. Sarcoid.
   c. The osteochondroses (see preceding chapters on bone).
   d. The primary tumors of joints (xanthoma, synovioma-sarcoma).
6. Diseases characterized by ankylosis. This is a nonspecific late change in any destructive joint disease.
   a. Late rheumatoid arthritis.
   b. Late post-traumatic arthritis.
   c. Late pyogenic arthritis.
   d. Late tuberculosis.
7. Diseases characterized by loose bodies ("joint mice") within the joint and articular irregularities.
   a. Osteochondritis dissecans.
   b. Chondromatosis of joints (chondrocalcinosis).

c. Traumatic arthropathy (of the knee particularly, following meniscal injury).

d. Neurotrophic arthropathy.

In the case of the knee, special studies for demonstration of these loose bodies include arthrography and a special intercondyloid view of the knee joint through the flexed knee.

8. Diseases characterized by synovial, cartilaginous, capsular, pericapsular, bursal, or peritendinous calcification.

    a. Pseudogout.

    b. Peritendinitis calcarea.

    c. Pellegrini-Stieda disease (calcification of medial collateral ligament of the knee).

    d. Capsular fibrositis with calcification.

In the above classification it is noteworthy that a disease of one etiology may appear under several categories of objective radiographic appearance. *It is incumbent upon the radiologist to be thoroughly familiar with the pathogenesis of the various arthropathies.* This will require a careful analysis of the patient's history, and reconstruction of joint appearances as they probably were, as well as what they are at present. In many instances previous films will not be available for sequential interpretation. Only a careful history will supply the necessary information.

DISEASES CHARACTERIZED BY CAPSULAR DISTENTION WITHOUT BONY INVOLVEMENT

1. Simple hydrarthrosis.
2. Idiopathic capsulitis.
3. Acute pyogenic infection (early).
4. Rheumatic fever (periarticular arthrosis).

Simple Hydrarthrosis (Figure 11–12 A).   Fluid accumulation within a joint from trauma, internal derangement, or mild degenerative change. The knee is frequently affected.

Idiopathic Capsulitis (Figure 11–12 B).   Painful hip with marked disability in an infant with a mild systemic reaction. Usually a subsidence of this process ensues without sequelae after antibiotic therapy. No definite etiologic agent is isolated usually (Edwards).

Knee Joint Effusions are readily identified in lateral roentgenograms by the swelling of the suprapatellar pouch. Other signs described are anterior displacement of the patella, distention of the posterior capsule, and bulging of the infrapatellar ligament. A swelling of the suprapatellar bursa can also be demonstrated on frontal views by visualizing a semicircular lucency on each side of the distal femur at the level of the suprapatellar bursa (Harris and Hecht).

Pyogenic Arthritis (Figure 11–13)

Pathology and Pathogenesis

1. Any pus-forming organism may be involved.
2. Occasionally other organisms such as brucellosis, tularemia, typhoid or paratyphoid colon bacilli may be responsible.
3. Pathogenesis is indicated in Figure 11–13.

HYDRARTHROSIS OF THE KNEE

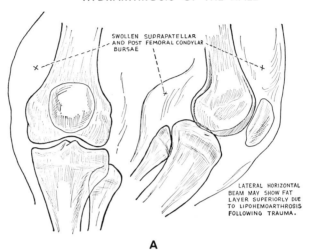

SWOLLEN SUPRAPATELLAR
AND POST FEMORAL CONDYLAR
BURSAE

LATERAL HORIZONTAL
BEAM MAY SHOW FAT
LAYER SUPERIORLY DUE
TO LIPOHEMOARTHROSIS
FOLLOWING TRAUMA.

A

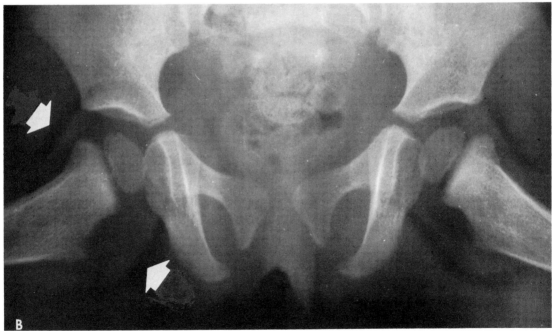

Figure 11–12   *A*. Hydrarthrosis of the knee: tracing illustrating the most important radiographic features. *B*. Idiopathic capsulitis of an infant. Painful hip with mild systemic reaction. No definite etiology known; the illness ordinarily subsides spontaneously or after antibiotic therapy. (Radiograph intensified.)

PYOGENIC ARTHRITIS
(SYNOVIAL INVOLVEMENT PRIMARILY)

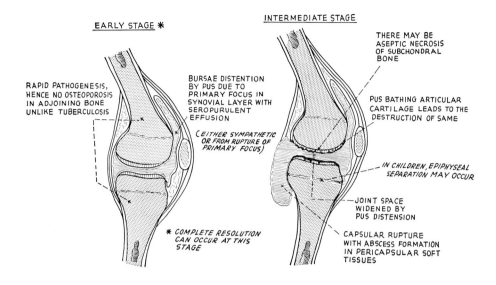

EARLY STAGE ✱

INTERMEDIATE STAGE

RAPID PATHOGENESIS, HENCE NO OSTEOPOROSIS IN ADJOINING BONE UNLIKE TUBERCULOSIS

BURSAE DISTENTION BY PUS DUE TO PRIMARY FOCUS IN SYNOVIAL LAYER WITH SEROPURULENT EFFUSION

(EITHER SYMPATHETIC OR FROM RUPTURE OF PRIMARY FOCUS)

✱ *COMPLETE RESOLUTION CAN OCCUR AT THIS STAGE*

THERE MAY BE ASEPTIC NECROSIS OF SUBCHONDRAL BONE

PUS BATHING ARTICULAR CARTILAGE LEADS TO THE DESTRUCTION OF SAME

IN CHILDREN, EPIPHYSEAL SEPARATION MAY OCCUR

JOINT SPACE WIDENED BY PUS DISTENSION

CAPSULAR RUPTURE WITH ABSCESS FORMATION IN PERICAPSULAR SOFT TISSUES

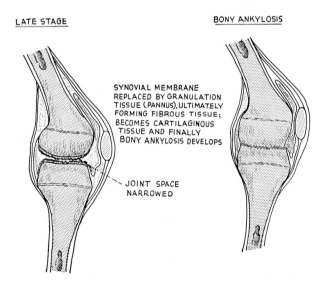

LATE STAGE

BONY ANKYLOSIS

SYNOVIAL MEMBRANE REPLACED BY GRANULATION TISSUE (PANNUS),ULTIMATELY FORMING FIBROUS TISSUE; BECOMES CARTILAGINOUS TISSUE AND FINALLY BONY ANKYLOSIS DEVELOPS

JOINT SPACE NARROWED

Figure 11–13   Diagrammatic illustration of the pathogenesis of pyogenic arthritis.

4. In children, associated dislocations and epiphyseal separations may occur.
5. Chronic alterations of the joint as illustrated in Figure 11–14 may ultimately be in evidence.
6. Occasionally, in children, a pyogenic arthritis may affect the adjoining epiphysis so that a growth disturbance may result, or a femoral head epiphysis may become necrotic because of obliteration of the blood supply.
7. Ultimately ankylosis may result. This ankylosis may be fibrous or bony. An immobile joint will ensue with thickening of the joint capsule, osteoporosis adjoining the joint, and narrowing of the joint space to complete obliteration. A contraction deformity of the extremity may result.

PYOGENIC ARTHRITIS (EARLY)

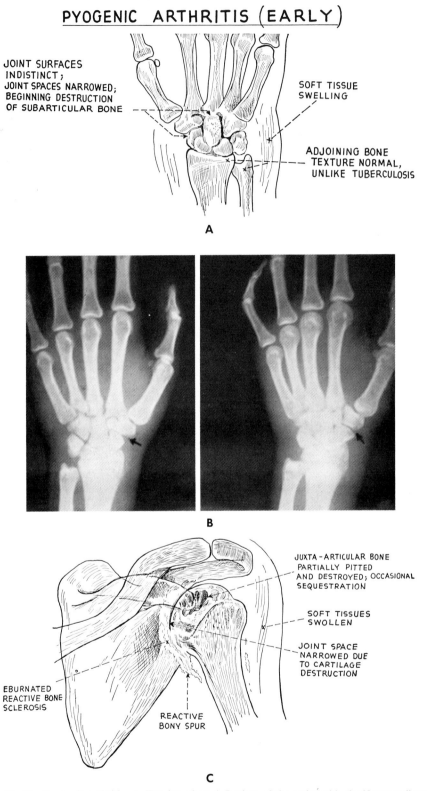

Figure 11–14   Pyogenic arthritis. *A*. Tracing of an A-P view of the wrist with significant radiographic features labeled. *B*. Radiographs of wrist and hand. *C*. Tracing of a late pyogenic arthritis of the shoulder.

Figure 11–14 continued on opposite page.

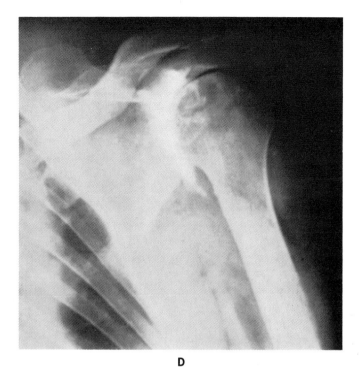

D

Figure 11–14 (*Continued*).   *D*. Radiograph of the shoulder.

8. In some instances, when fibrous ankylosis ensues, the fibrous tissue may itself be transformed into a synovialike tissue that secretes joint fluid and a small amount of motion may be restored.

Radiographic Findings

There may be an adjoining osteomyelitis—the disease under these circumstances occurs by direct subcapsular extension.

Joint distention is the earliest manifestation.

An initial increase in joint width occurs because of joint distention; later a narrowed joint space ensues as the pyogenic process becomes organized and the cartilage destroyed. This may be associated with some subarticular bone irregularity and atrophy.

In a later phase the irregular subarticular bony cortex may be more sharply demarcated.

Bony ankylosis or fibrous ankylosis may supervene.

In hip joints, apart from swelling of the hip joint capsule, there may also be swelling of the "obturator shadow." This is seen just inside the acetabulum on the inner aspect of the pelvis in the antero-posterior view (Figure 11–10).

Acute Rheumatic Fever (Figures 11–15 and 11–16).   In acute rheumatic fever there are very few radiographic manifestations.

Clinical Features

Fever, migratory articular pains, swellings of the joints which react almost specifically to salicylate therapy.

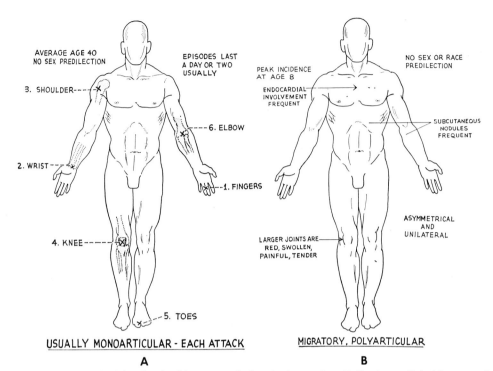

Figure 11-15 *A.* The joints involved in acute palindromic rheumatism. *B.* Pertinent clinical features of periarthritis due to rheumatic fever.

Often associated cardiac endocardial involvement.

Most cases occur prior to the age of 40, and children are often affected.

Radiographic Findings

Thickening of the periarticular soft tissues, giving the osseous structures a blurred appearance.

After joint immobilization for significant periods of time osseous atrophy may supervene.

Ordinarily, no **joint** sequelae are seen radiographically when the disease subsides.

PERIARTICULAR ARTHROSIS

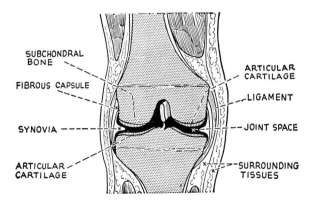

Figure 11-16 The major radiographic features in rheumatic fever. The major pathology is pericapsular swelling and not intra-articular involvement.

DISEASES CHARACTERIZED BY SUBCHONDRAL AND CAPSULAR PROLIFERATION IN ASSOCIATION WITH CARTILAGINOUS INJURY

1. Traumatic arthritis.
2. "Hypertrophic" arthritis.
3. Hemophilic arthritis.
4. Neurotrophic arthropathy.

Traumatic Arthritis (Figure 11–17)

Pathology and Pathogenesis. The pathogenesis of traumatic arthropathy is illustrated in Figure 11–17. A fracture line may penetrate into the joint cavity, with hemorrhage and distention of the joint capsule. The sequence of events which may follow is illustrated. Intermittent trauma over a period of years, possibly caused by metabolic or endocrine conditions, will cause the pathologic picture of hypertrophic arthritis illustrated next. Minor traumas associated with neurotrophic disturbances will produce one of two radiologic pictures: the spindle atrophic deformity illustrated under the neurotrophic arthropathy-atrophic type; or the features of a gross hypertrophic arthritis with subluxation illustrated under the hypertrophic variety of neurotrophic arthropathy.

Radiographic Findings (Figure 11–17 *A* and *B*)

Narrowed, irregular joint space due to cartilaginous thinning and fragmentation.

Subchondral bone is eburnated and irregular but is usually of normal or sclerotic density.

The joint, and even the extremity at the site of the joint abnormality, may be considerably deformed. Some joint motion is usually preserved, however, unless fibrous or ossific ankylosis has supervened.

Hypertrophic Arthritis (Figure 11–18)

Clinical Features

All persons beyond the second or third decade of life exhibit some degenerative changes in joints.

Weight-bearing joints are the ones most frequently involved (hips, knees, ankles, spine).

Distal interphalangeal joints of the fingers are frequently involved with associated soft tissue changes known as Heberden's nodes.

There may be precipitate episodes of pain, muscle spasm, and enforced restricted mobility.

Pathology and Pathogenesis (Figure 11–18)

Cartilaginous surfaces of joints become discolored and "fibrillate."

These fissures in the cartilage penetrate to the subchondral bone. Synovial fluid then gains access to the deeper cells, which proliferate and cause the osteophytes and exostoses characteristic of hypertrophic arthritis.

Cartilaginous fragments may separate and become loose bodies within the joint.

The joint space may be narrowed as the cartilage thins, and the capsule may become stretched, thereby permitting subluxation.

Joint effusions are frequent.

TRAUMATIC ARTHROPATHY

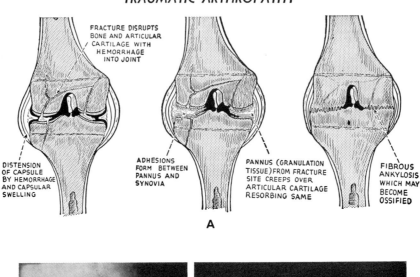

FRACTURE DISRUPTS BONE AND ARTICULAR CARTILAGE WITH HEMORRHAGE INTO JOINT

DISTENSION OF CAPSULE BY HEMORRHAGE AND CAPSULAR SWELLING

ADHESIONS FORM BETWEEN PANNUS AND SYNOVIA

PANNUS (GRANULATION TISSUE) FROM FRACTURE SITE CREEPS OVER ARTICULAR CARTILAGE RESORBING SAME

FIBROUS ANKYLOSIS WHICH MAY BECOME OSSIFIED

A

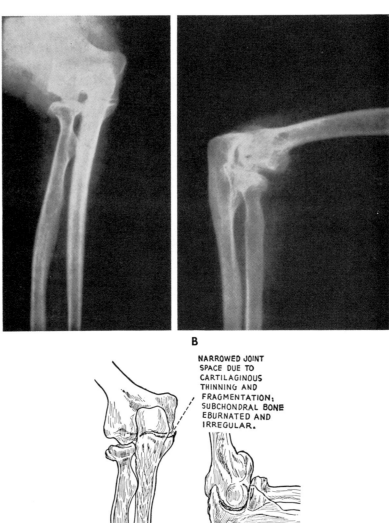

B

NARROWED JOINT SPACE DUE TO CARTILAGINOUS THINNING AND FRAGMENTATION; SUBCHONDRAL BONE EBURNATED AND IRREGULAR.

C

Figure 11–17   Traumatic arthropathy. *A*. Pathogenesis in diagram. *B*. Representative radiographs of elbow. *C*. Tracing of both antero-posterior and lateral views with appropriate areas labeled.

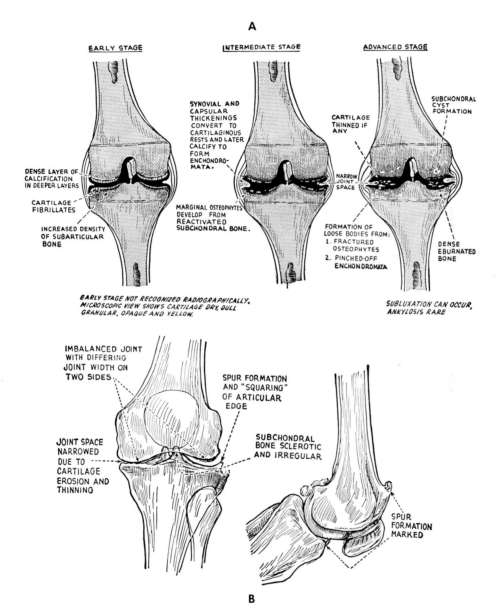

Figure 11–18 Hypertrophic arthritis. *A*. Pathogenesis in diagram. *B*. Tracing of radiographs of knee showing pertinent features.

Radiographic Findings. Weight-bearing film studies are important wherever applicable. Thinness of cartilage may not be evident in nonweight-bearing joints without "stress" film studies (Leach et al.).

At first, there is slight squaring or sharpening of the subarticular bony margins.

This sharpening may proceed to marginal osteophyte formation or bony spur formation.

The narrowing of the joint may increase and the subchondral bone may become considerably eburnated, condensed, and sclerotic.

In very advanced stages, the bony spurs may become quite large and irregular, sometimes bridging around an entire joint.

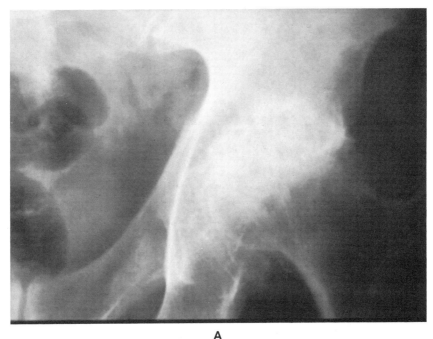

A

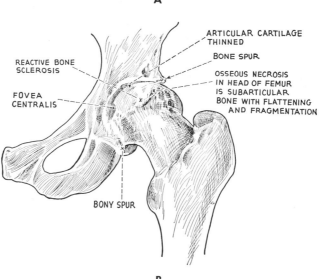

B

Figure 11–19 *A.* Malum coxae senilis of the hip. *B.* Tracing of *A*, representing principal features.

Occasionally joint mice or loose bodies may form within the joint.

In the small joints of the fingers there is frequently an associated soft tissue swelling or nodular appearance called Heberden's node.

The spine presents a particular problem. Degenerative changes occur not only in the synovial joints but in the intervertebral disks as well. The resulting changes range from various degrees of spur formation to complete bridging of the intervertebral spaces, the latter producing the condition known as "deforming spondylosis." This will be described in Chapter 14.

Malum Coxae Senilis (Morbus Coxae Senilis) (Figure 11–19).   In the hip joint, when the articular cartilage becomes very thin and the wearing process extends to the subarticular bone, osseous necrosis in the head of the femur may occur with some flattening, fragmentation, and occasionally even subluxation. Bony spur formation may supervene as in typical hypertrophic arthritis. A reactive bone sclerosis occurs, surrounding the areas of osseous necrosis in the head of the femur as well as in the acetabulum. This is the condition known as malum coxae senilis (Figure 11–19).

Otto Pelvis (Arthrokatadysis) (Figure 11–20).   Bilateral protrusion of the heads of the femora and acetabula into the pelvis is called the "Otto-Krobak pelvis." This may be (1) congenital in origin; (2) a developmental abnormality; (3) nutritional in origin; (4) traumatic, and (5) caused by rheumatoid arthritis or ankylosing spondylitis occasionally.

These protrusions of the acetabulum are usually accompanied by secondary hypertrophic arthritis of the hip joints.

Ossification of the fibrous tissue uniting the joint ends occurs and transforms the ankylosis on occasion to a bony ankylosis.

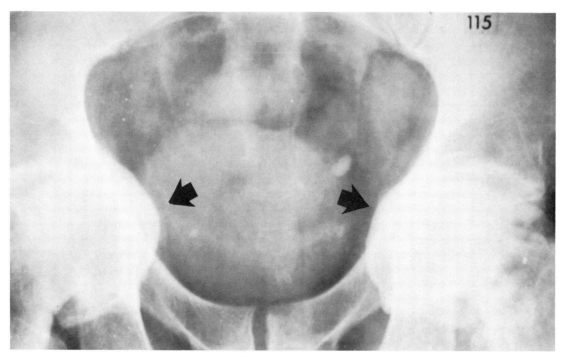

Figure 11–20   Close-up view of Otto pelvis. Note the bilateral protrusio acetabuli.

Hemophilic Arthritis (Figure 11–21)

Clinical Aspects

Periodic hemarthrosis occurs in patients with hemophilia, particularly during middle and late childhood.

Joints affected especially are knees, hips, elbows, and ankles.

Pathology and Pathogenesis (Figure 11–21)

Intra-articular hemorrhage causes considerable distention of the capsule and a temporary hyperplasia of the synovial villi.

This may resolve without further sequelae.

If particularly frequent, this hyperplasia of the synovial capsule and villi may persist with ultimate organization and fibrous ankylosis.

Radiologic Findings

Repeated hemorrhage causes a thickening of the capsule.

Deprivation of nutrition for the cartilage leads to erosion and thinning of the cartilage and narrowness of the joint space.

Subchondral bone cysts may develop.

Hypertrophic arthritis may also supervene.

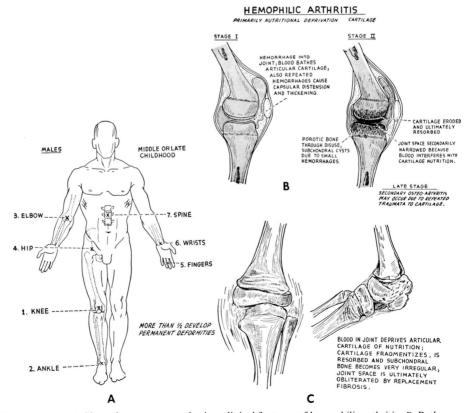

Figure 11–21 *A.* Sites of occurrence and other clinical features of hemophilic arthritis. *B.* Pathogenesis of radiographic appearances in hemophilic arthritis. *C.* Tracings of radiographs of hemophilic arthritis.

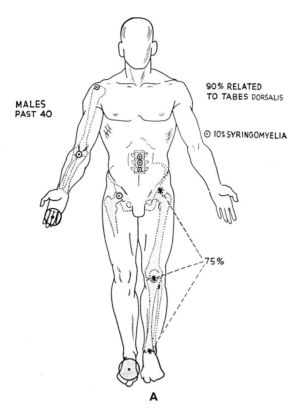

MALES
PAST 40

90% RELATED
TO TABES DORSALIS

⊙ 10% SYRINGOMYELIA

75%

A

NEURO-ARTHROPATHIES
(CARTILAGINOUS INVOLVEMENT)

(A) ATROPHIC TYPE:

   I. STAMPING GAIT, FRAGMENTATION
      OF WEIGHT-BEARING CARTILAGE,
      EXPOSED BONE WEARS DOWN

  II. SPINDLING EFFECT IS PRODUCED
      BY RESORPTION OF BONE DUE TO
      NEUROVASCULAR DISTURBANCE.

    (SEE ILLUSTRATION OF NEUROTROPHIC ARTHROPATHY)

(B) HYPERTROPHIC TYPE

    SEE OSTEO-ARTHRITIS, BUT CHANGES MORE MARKED,
    DISLOCATION MORE FREQUENT, CAPSULAR
    STRETCHING LEADING TO COMPLETE DISORGANIZATION.
    (SEE ILLUSTRATION OF CHARCOT'S JOINT)

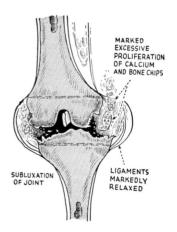

MARKED
EXCESSIVE
PROLIFERATION
OF CALCIUM
AND BONE CHIPS

SUBLUXATION
OF JOINT

LIGAMENTS
MARKEDLY
RELAXED

B

Figure 11–22 *A*. Sites of most frequent occurrence and other clinical features in neurogenic arthropathy.
B. Pathogenesis of the atrophic and hypertrophic types of neurogenic arthropathy. (See also Chapter 9.)

Neurogenic Arthropathy (Figures 11–22 and 11–23)

Clinical Features

Approximately 90 per cent are related to tabes dorsalis, but only 5 to 10 per cent of tabetic patients develop these arthropathies.

Usually there is a painless "sack of bones" at joint sites.

Rigid pupils and absent knee jerks are characteristic.

Blood serology is negative in as many as 55 per cent of cases; spinal fluid serology is negative in 30 per cent.

Pathology and Pathogenesis

Loss of deep sensation and relaxation of ligaments plus trauma leads to stretching of joint capsule and fragmentation of bone and cartilage.

This in turn leads to extensive destruction and degenerative change.

If the destruction is very rapid there may be no evidence of new bone formation.

Radiographic Findings. Two types have been described, a hypertrophic variety and an atrophic type.

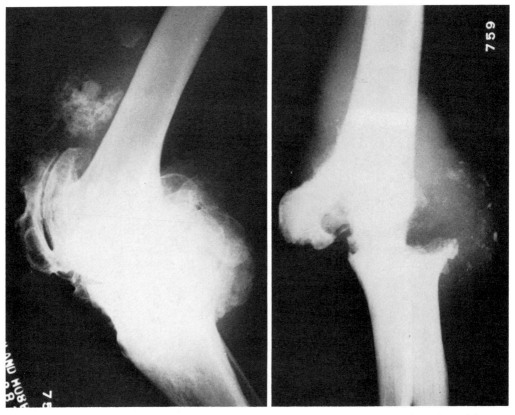

Figure 11–23 Charcot joints. *A.* Lateral view of the knee. *B.* Antero-posterior view of the elbow. In each instance note the marked periarticular bony proliferation, the articular cartilaginous and osseous destruction, and in the case of the elbow, the subluxation. (Courtesy of Dr. James Johnston.)

The Hypertrophic Type is characterized by numerous para-osseous new bone formations and subluxation.

Children with spina bifida and underlying spinal cord abnormalities who are not fully paralyzed are prone to suffer repeated injuries resulting in bizarre skeletal changes at the metaphyseal-physeal junctions of their lower extremities.

Roentgenologically, these changes are best seen in the ankle and knee joint after prolonged weight bearing. The changes may be grouped into the following categories: (1) irregular, dense, slightly widened metaphyses; (2) widened cartilaginous epiphyseal plates; and (3) subperiosteal new bone formation.

The secondary ossification centers are usually intact, although osteoporosis is marked in some cases (Gyepes et al.).

The Atrophic Type is marked by the apparent disappearance of the metaphysis of a bone which adjoins a joint (especially the small joints of the hands and feet in leprosy).

DISEASES CHARACTERIZED BY OSTEOPOROSIS OF THE NEIGHBORING BONES AND NARROWING OF THE JOINT SPACE WITH SUBCHONDRAL BONE RESORPTION

1. Tuberculous arthritis.
2. Rheumatoid arthritis.
3. Pyogenic arthritis (less surrounding osteoporosis than with the first two).

TUBERCULOUS ARTHRITIS
(SUBCHONDRAL, CHONDRAL AND SYNOVIAL INVOLVEMENT PRIMARILY)

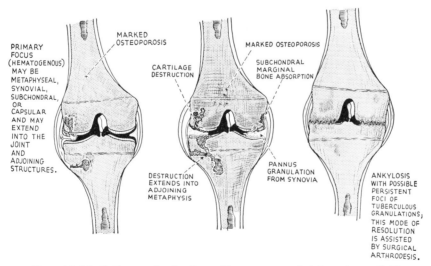

Figure 11–24 Pathogenesis of radiographic appearances in tuberculous arthritis.

General Comments

Essential lesion in this group of pathologic states is the "pannus."

This develops from a vascular synovial membrane and proceeds to grow over the avascular joint cartilage, depriving it of its proper nutrition.

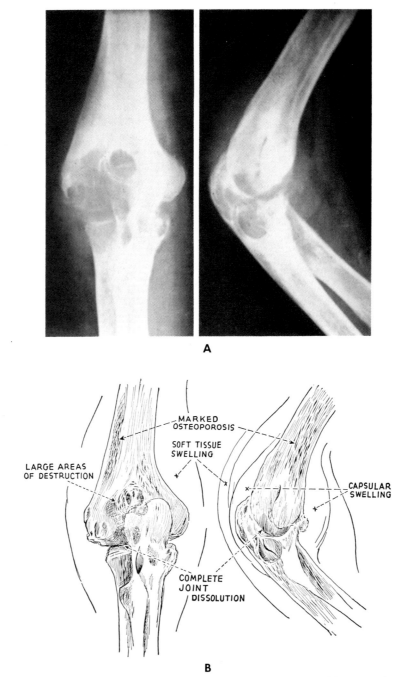

Figure 11–25 *A.* Radiographs of elbow of patient with tuberculous arthritis. *B.* Tracings of *A.*

This granulation tissue resorbs the cartilage to the underlying subchondral bone and tends to resorb the bone as well, producing small pseudocystic areas.

These subchondral cysts are typical of tuberculosis or rheumatoid arthritis.

Replacement by fibrous tissue may occur and this in turn leads to ankylosis. Bony ankylosis may ultimately occur, bridging the joint space.

Tuberculous Arthritis (Figures 11–24 and 11–25)

Clinical Features

Almost always hematogenous and at least 75 per cent are secondary to pulmonary tuberculosis in the first three decades of life.

Most frequent sites are the spine (one-third of cases); hip (one-sixth of cases); knee, elbow, wrist, and shoulder.

It is extremely disabling and painful in children.

Bony involvement is more extensive in children.

Pathology

Tuberculous granulation tissue invades the cartilage and subchondral bone with marked rarefaction ("tuberculous sicca").

Profound secondary widespread osteoporosis.

Caseation may occur commonly in spine and hip with typical "cold abscess" along muscle planes.

Sequestration is common with caseation.

Radiographic Features

Osseous changes: profound osteoporosis, minimal subarticular reactive zone of sclerosis may occur.

Interarticular space narrowness.

Subarticular bone destruction.

Articular capsule swelling and haziness.

Periarticular, paravertebral, or psoas abscess.

Changes of form or position of the affected part (flexion, kyphosis).

Rheumatoid Arthritis (Figure 11–26)

Clinical Features

Chronic polyarticular arthritis, affecting persons younger than age 40 primarily; females are more frequently affected than males; any joint may be involved but especially the small joints of the hands and feet.

In the hands, the earliest affected joints are the metacarpophalangeal joints in most instances.

The juvenile form of this disease is called Still's disease.

RADIOLOGIC MANIFESTATIONS OF THE RHEUMATOID DISEASES

1. Pulmonary manifestations.
2. Cardiac alterations.
3. Peptic ulcers and other visceral gastrointestinal changes.
4. Cricoarytenoid involvement and impairment of swallowing mechanism.
5. Joint manifestations.

RHEUMATOID ARTHRITIS

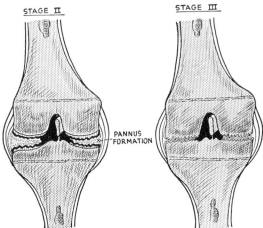
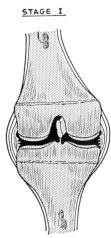

STAGE I

CHRONIC AND INFLAMMATORY
RESPONSE OF SYNOVIA TO
UNKNOWN ETIOLOGICAL FACTOR.
1. HYPEREMIA OF SYNOVIA WITH
   EDEMA AND INCREASE IN SYNOVIAL
   FLUID.
2. ENLARGEMENT AND MULTIPLICATION OF
   SYNOVIAL VILLI.
3. HYPERPLASIA OF ALL CAPSULAR ELEMENTS.
4. GRANULATIONS, FIBROSIS REPLACE SUBCHONDRAL
   BONE, PRODUCING EARLY OSTEOPOROSIS.

STAGE II

PANNUS FORMATION

1. PANNUS FORMATIONS (GRANULATION
   TISSUE PROTRUSIONS FROM SYNOVIAL
   FRINGE) ABSORB CARTILAGE,
   ACCOUNT FOR NARROW JOINT
   SPACE.
2. SUBCHONDRAL PSEUDOCYSTIC
   BONE ABSORPTION AND MORE
   MARKED OSTEOPOROSIS.

STAGE III

FIBROUS ANKYLOSIS WHICH
BECOMES TRABECULATED
TO FORM BONY ANKYLOSIS.
OFTEN ASSOCIATED WITH
CONTRACTURES.

A

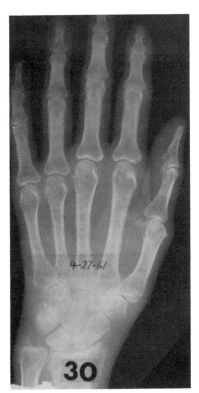
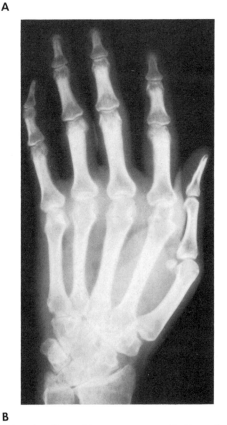

B

Figure 11–26 Rheumatoid arthritis. *A.* Pathogenesis of radiographic appearances. *B.* Examples of moderate and severe rheumatoid arthritis of the hand and knee.

Figure 11–26 continued on opposite page.

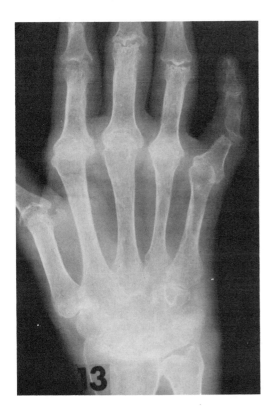
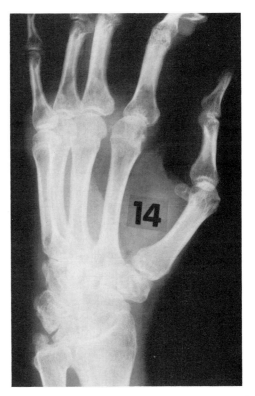

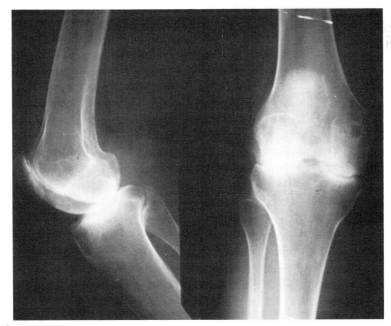

Figure 11–26   *B (Continued).*

Figure 11–26 continued on following page.

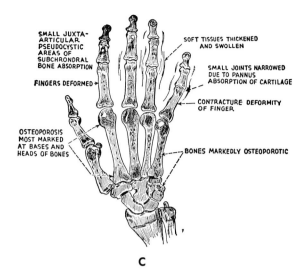

C

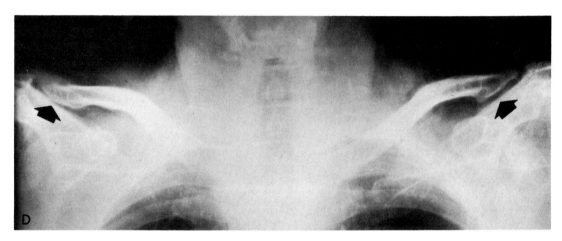

D

Figure 11–26 *(Continued).* *C.* Tracing. *D.* Resorption of the distal ends of the clavicle in a patient with rheumatoid arthritis involving the joints of the extremities.

RADIOGRAPHIC FINDINGS IN JUVENILE RHEUMATOID ARTHRITIS

1. Periarticular soft tissue swelling.
2. Local osteoporosis.
3. Periosteal thickening adjoining the joints involved.
4. Cortical erosion.
5. Destruction of joint cartilage and bone (late).
6. Growth disturbances (accelerated skeletal maturation, enlargement and ballooning of epiphyses, compression fractures of epiphyseal centers, decrease in width of shaft and osteoporosis).
7. Spondylitis is frequent, generally upper cervical, with ankylosis of apophyseal joints. Paraspinous ossification is rare as in sacroiliac involvement.
8. Occasionally there are subluxations with an overgrowth of adjoining margins of the bone, resembling the overgrowth which occurs in the shelving portion of the acetabulum.

DIFFERENTIAL FEATURES BETWEEN RHEUMATIC FEVER AND JUVENILE RHEUMATOID ARTHRITIS

1. Neck pain is frequent in juvenile rheumatoid arthritis.

2. Skin rash has a different distribution and appearance; the rash is primarily evanescent and nocturnal in juvenile rheumatoid arthritis.

3. There is a persistent elevation of red cell sedimentation rate despite adequate treatment.

4. Typical fever of juvenile rheumatoid arthritis is unattended by sweating and prostration.

5. Serial x-rays are particularly helpful. In rheumatoid arthritis there is almost always a progression; in rheumatic fever there is a relative absence of roentgen evidence in bone.

6. Distal femoral epiphysis adjoining an involved knee may be as much as 30 per cent larger than the uninvolved one in juvenile rheumatoid arthritis. This appears as early as one year after onset of the disease and usually disappears within 18 months following cessation of the disease activity.

7. Slow disappearance of disparity of leg length with femoral epiphyseal involvement in about two years.

Pathology and Pathogenesis (Figure 11–26)

Synovitis with edema and hyperplasia of synovial villi and increase in synovial fluid.

This is replaced or accompanied by granulation tissue (pannus) which grows over the cartilage and destroys it, and the granulation tissue extends into the subchondral bone, producing "cystic" resorption.

Immobilization from discomfort gives rise to a diffuse osteoporosis.

Fibrous tissue may replace the pannus and ankylosis results.

Bony ankylosis may ensue.

Subcutaneous nodules may appear and persist.

The vascular changes in the immediate vicinity of joints affected by rheumatoid arthritis has been reported by Marshall. These include occlusive changes, narrowness of digital arteries, and hyperemic changes near areas of bone erosion and in the region of synovial proliferation.

Radiographic Findings (Figure 11–26 B, C, D)

Thickened swollen joint capsules. In the hand the earliest joints to be affected are usually the metacarpophalangeal joints, particularly of the fourth and fifth fingers. An ulnar deviation of these two fingers results early, with some deformity of the hands.

The earliest roentgenologic changes in polyarthritis of the rheumatoid type consist of very slight indistinctness of the outlines of the bone corresponding with the insertion of the joint capsule, dorsoradially on the proximal end of the first phalanx of the four ulnar fingers. The bone trabeculae are thinner and are partly destroyed, although not to the point of producing a cystlike lucency (Norgaard; Martel et al.).

The proximal and middle interphalangeal joints, along with the small joints of the wrist, are next to be involved. The distal interphalangeal joints are ordinarily not involved until late in the disease. In psoriatic arthritis the converse is more often true—the distal interphalangeal joints are involved early in the course of the disease.

Marked deformity of the fingers results, with ulnar deviations, partial sub-luxations, and "cystic" resorption in the subchondral bone.

Ankylosis may supervene.

Special Comments Relating to the Spine

(For further description, see Chapter 14.)

Two types of spine involvement related to rheumatoid arthritis are differentiated: (1) ankylosing spondylitis, with primary involvement of the synovial intervertebral joints; and (2) rheumatoid arthritis, with primary involvement of the vertebral bodies per se by typical rheumatoid nodules.

Ankylosing spondylitis (Marie-Strümpell's disease, ankylosing spondylarthritis, or spondylitis rhizomélique) ordinarily begins in the lower lumbar apophyseal joints or in the sacroiliac joints and ascends the spine (Figure 11–27). The involvement of the intervertebral synovial joints histo-pathologically resembles rheumatoid arthritis. Simultaneously, there is an ascending calcification of the anterior and later-

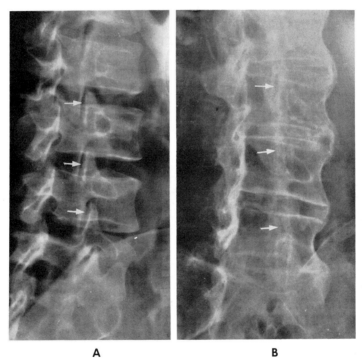

A   B

Figure 11–27 Apophyseal joints in normal adult spine and in ankylosing spondylitis. *A*. Oblique view of a normal spine discloses normal apophyseal joints (*arrows*). The joint spaces are regular, and the articular margins are smooth and distinct.

B. Oblique view of a patient with advanced ankylosing spondylitis demonstrates virtual obliteration of the apophyseal joint spaces (*arrows*), which have become ankylosed. The articular facets have all but disappeared. This is ligamentous calcification and bone demineralization—the bamboo spine.

The apophyseal joints become involved in ascending order following sacroiliac joint changes. The apophyseal joints are not uniformly affected, but almost all the joint spaces become hazy and ill defined, with many progressing to complete ankylosis and obliteration. (From Teplick, G. J., and Haskin, M. E.: *Roentgenologic Diagnosis*, 2nd Ed. Philadelphia, W. B. Saunders Co., 1971.)

Figure 11–27 continued on opposite page.

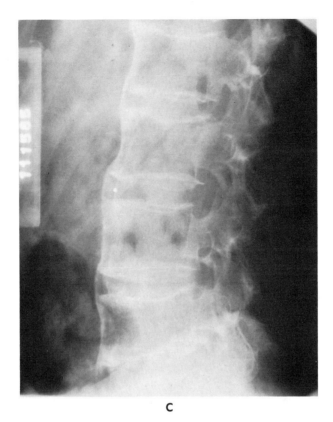

C

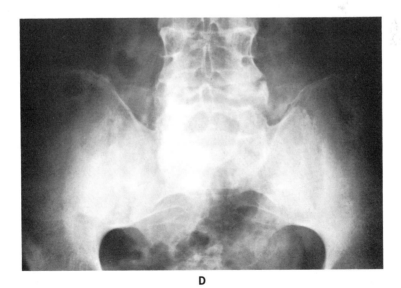

D

Figure 11–27 *(Continued).* *C.* Lateral lumbar spine with advanced ankylosing spondylitis, showing the paraspinous ligamentous calcification characteristic of this disorder. *D.* Sacroiliac joints in ankylosing spondylitis, showing obliteration of these joints.

al vertebral ligaments, leading to a "bamboo" or rigid spine in kyphosis. The costo-vertebral joints become ankylosed also, producing a rigid thoracic cage. Persons so affected are predisposed to pneumonia. The cervical spine is affected late, there is usually a lack of subcutaneous nodules, and the rheumatoid (RA) factor is usually negative.

The rheumatoid arthritis affecting vertebral bodies often begins in the cervical spine (Figure 11–28), with erosion and replacement of the bone. The end-plates adjoining involved vertebrae become irregular. Erosion of the odontoid process may

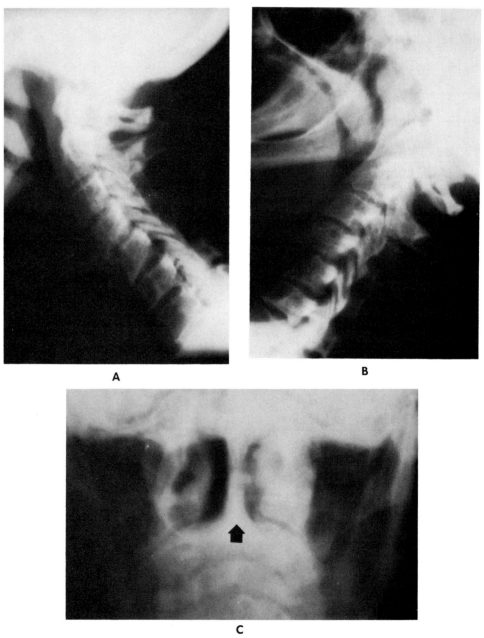

Figure 11–28 *A, B,* and *C.* Rheumatoid arthritis involving the cervical spine. In *A,* note the subluxation of C-4 in respect to C-5 which is slightly aggravated in flexion (*B*). Note also the irregular nature of the apophyseal joints. In *C,* note the resorption of much of the odontoid process.

occur. Subluxation at the atlantoaxial joint, as well as at the fourth, fifth, or sixth cervical levels may occur. The RA factor is usually present and there is involvement of peripheral joints of the body by rheumatoid arthritis in about one-half of these cases (Epstein).

The Positive Elbow Fat Pad Sign in Rheumatoid Arthritis (Jackman and Pugh).   A true lateral view of the elbow with 90 degrees of flexion must be obtained for analysis of the fat pads. The anterior and posterior fat pads are found adjacent to the distal portion of the humerus and are within the fibrous capsule of the joint space outside the synovial lining (Chapter 5). The largest fat pad lies posteriorly deep in the olecranon fossa. It is pressed into the fossa by the triceps brachii muscle during flexion and is therefore not normally seen in the lateral view. A posterior fat pad that can be distinctly seen is abnormal and is considered a positive sign. The anterior fat pad is normally visible in the lateral view as a radiolucent triangle adjacent to the humerus. There are two anterior fat pads superimposed anatomically that occupy the anterior coronoid and radial fossae. During extension they are pressed into these shallow fossae by the brachialis muscle. The anterior fat pad can be as thick as 6 or 7 mm. roentgenologically. Rarely it is too thin to be seen. To determine whether the anterior fat pad is elevated, the displacement in its distal end from the bone is of more importance than is the thickness of the pad. An anterior fat pad elevated from the bone is considered a positive sign.

Psoriatic Arthritis

Roentgenologic Features

This condition resembles rheumatoid arthritis in the small joints of the hands and feet, but in this instance the earliest joints to be affected are the distal interphalangeal joints. Occasionally, there may also be involvement of the knees and other joints such as the ankles and wrists. The RA factor is usually absent.

The five roentgenological signs of greatest importance for recognition of psoriatic arthritis are:
1. Destructive arthritis, especially of the distal interphalangeal joints.
2. Bony ankylosis of the interphalangeal joints of the hands and feet.
3. Destruction of the interphalangeal joints of the hands and feet with abnormally wide joint spaces, and sharply demarcated adjacent bony surfaces.
4. Destruction of the interphalangeal joints of the great toe with bony proliferation at the base of the distal phalanx.
5. Resorption of the tips of the distal phalanges of the hands and feet.

ACCESSORY SIGNS

1. Absence of osteoporosis.
2. Lack of ulnar deviation of the fourth and fifth fingers.
3. Lack of a positive RA factor in most instances.

In possibly as many as 10 per cent of patients, arthritis is present for a period varying from six months to as long as 25 years before the psoriasis is recognized dermatologically.

Felty's Syndrome.   It is now generally believed that the association of *rheumatoid arthritis, leukopenia, and splenomegaly* is a variant of rheumatoid arthritis. This was originally described as a syndrome by Felty in 1924.

Sjögren's Syndrome.   This syndrome may be defined as rheumatoid arthritis combined with keratoconjunctivitis sicca or xerostomia or both. In some patients

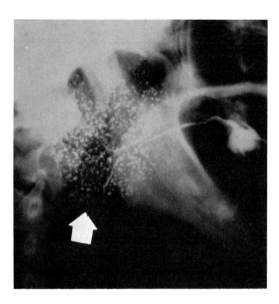

Figure 11–29 Sialograms of the parotid duct demonstrating the "pruned tree" appearance and glandular ectasia of Sjögren's disease.

there may be other associated phenomena, such as hepatomegaly, splenomegaly, congestive heart failure, leukopenia, and multiple serologic abnormalities including hyperglobulinemia.

In some patients the disease follows a rapid course indistinguishable from scleroderma or systemic lupus erythematosus.

Sialography in these patients usually demonstrates dilatation of the salivary ducts with small grapelike distentions which produce a characteristic roentgen picture (Figure 11–29).

Thyroid enlargement is not very common.

Unlike patients with rheumatoid arthritis, these patients practically never exhibit leukocytosis. Also, the incidence of a positive rheumatoid factor and lupus erythematosus cell test is not greater than in patients with rheumatoid arthritis alone.

Although the roentgenographic evidence of Sjögren's syndrome has generally been limited to its characteristic sialographic findings of ectasia and the well-known features of rheumatoid arthritis, there are some other notable roentgenographic manifestations. These include osteoarthritis in some patients with hand and wrist involvement, vascular calcification in some patients with involvement by rheumatoid arthritis of the ankles and feet, chondrocalcinosis, and occasionally osteoarthritis with involvement of the shoulder.

In the spine there are at times evidences of atlantoaxial separation, apophyseal joint destruction, osteoarthritis, sacroiliac arthritis, and rheumatoid arthritis of the hips (Silbiger and Peterson).

Arthritis with Ulcerative Colitis. This represents a form of arthritis which occurs in approximately 10 per cent of patients with ulcerative colitis in which the histologic lesion obtained in synovial biopsy resembles rheumatoid arthritis.

There is a close temporal relationship between the attacks of colitis and arthritis and the joint symptoms improve following surgical treatment for the colitis.

Usually the sedimentation erythrocyte agglutination test is negative in all patients by both agglutination and inhibition methods.

Reiter's Syndrome. This syndrome consists of urethritis, polyarthritis, and conjunctivitis.

The joints most frequently affected by rheumatoid arthritis in Reiter's syndrome are (1) the metatarsophalangeal; (2) the sacroiliac; (3) the proximal interphalangeal and the interphalangeal joint of the great toe; (4) the knee; and (5) the ankle. Many other joints are also affected but in a lesser frequency (Sholkoff et al; Mason et al.). (6) The heel pad is often involved with bilateral calcaneal spurs, with a florid periostitis of the calcaneus.

Arthritis in the Collagen Diseases. Joint disease frequently constitutes an important aspect of several of the collagen diseases, including (1) ninety per cent of cases of lupus erythematosus; (2) serum sickness; (3) dermatomyositis; (4) erythema nodosum; (5) a small percentage of cases of scleroderma and polyarteritis nodosa.

Cortisone Therapy Arthropathy (Figure 11–30). The continued injection of cortisone or related compounds brings on the typical changes of Cushing's disease.

Roentgenologic Aspects

Cases of complete joint destruction have been encountered in association with such therapy.

Massive joint lysis and dramatic spur formation typical of the Charcot joint may be produced.

Areas of aseptic necrosis with marked disruption of the normal architecture and surrounding sclerosis may result (Figure 11–30).

Steroid therapy may be responsible also for collapse of vertebral bodies with increased kyphosis.

Osteoarthropathy in Idiopathic Hemochromatosis. Osteoarthropathy has been reported by a number of investigators in association with hemochromatosis (Ross and Wood). The joint changes resemble rheumatoid arthritis closely in that there is joint space narrowness, irregularity of the articular surface, sclerosis, and subarticular cyst formation. Osteophyte formation is rarely seen but may be identified in the metacarpophalangeal and proximal interphalangeal joints. Osteoporosis may be present and chondrocalcinosis is frequently seen. When seen it is most frequent in the menisci of the knees. Ordinarily the joint involvement in the hand in hemochromatosis is more limited than in most cases of rheumatoid arthritis and there is less soft tissue swelling. Also hemochromatosis arthritis rarely affects the ulnar styloid process or radiocarpal joint. The bone density in hemochromatosis may be normal or is more uniformly diminished than in rheumatoid arthritis.

DISEASES CHARACTERIZED BY PERIARTICULAR BONE ABSORPTION WITHOUT SIGNIFICANT ADJOINING OSTEOPOROSIS

1. Gout.
2. Sarcoid.
3. The osteochondroses (see bone section, Chapter 9).
4. The primary tumors of the joints (xanthoma, synovioma).
5. Tuberous sclerosis.
6. Villonodular synovitis.

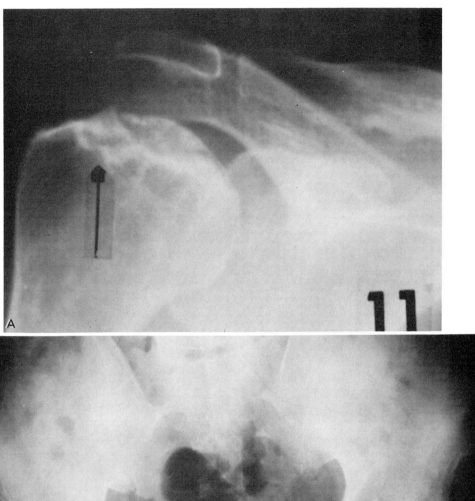

Figure 11–30 Arthropathy resulting from steroid therapy with aseptic necrosis of involved epiphysis. *A.* Shoulder joint with head of humerus undergoing aseptic necrosis. *B.* Hip joints with heads of femora undergoing aseptic necrosis.

Figure 11–30 continued on opposite page.

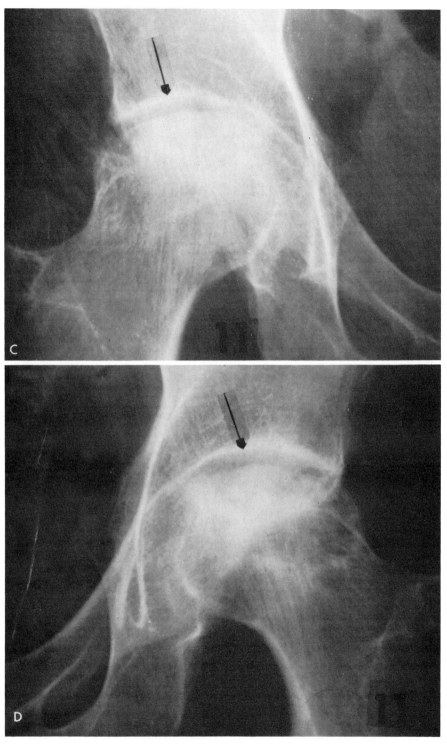

Figure 11–30 (*Continued*).   *C* and *D*. Magnified views of *B*.

General Comments.   Gout, sarcoid, tumors of joints, and villonodular synovitis will be described in this section.

The osteochondroses have been considered with the aseptic necroses of bones (Chapter 9).

The neurofibromatoses and tuberous sclerosis have been considered with osteolytic bone diseases (Chapter 8) and also with congenital bone disease (Chapter 7).

Gout (Figure 11–31)

Clinical Aspects

Mostly in men over 30 years of age.

Most frequently found in great toe but may occur elsewhere, especially around other small joints.

Markedly painful, red, and swollen, with pain recurring at night especially.

Joint may return to normal between attacks.

Laboratory Findings

Serum uric acid is elevated to as high as 25 mg. per cent (the normal value is 1 to 4 mg. per cent).

Urine uric acid is normal or only slightly elevated.

Pathology

Deposition of monosodium urate crystals in the bone in the immediate neighborhood of joints.

Urate crystal deposits may also occur in cartilage of ears, tendons, bursae, muscles, and heart valves.

Low-grade inflammation around urate tophi resembles foreign body reaction, with edema, giant cells, lymphocytes, and monocytes.

Occasionally there is pannus formation in the joint.

GOUT

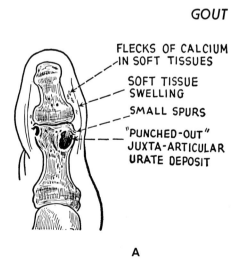

FLECKS OF CALCIUM IN SOFT TISSUES

SOFT TISSUE SWELLING

SMALL SPURS

"PUNCHED-OUT" JUXTA-ARTICULAR URATE DEPOSIT

A

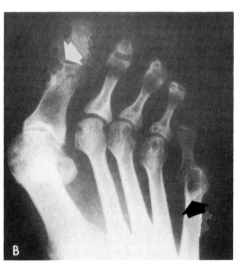

Figure 11–31   Gout. *A.* Tracing of a great toe affected by gouty arthritis. *B.* Radiograph demonstrating advanced gouty change.

Sodium biurate crystals may deposit anywhere within or outside a joint. Granulation tissue or pannus extends around the deposit, resorbing contiguous structures.

Radiographic Aspects

Changes noted in only one-third of cases.

Asymmetrical **periarticular** swelling with small, punched-out, joint marginal defects, especially of the first metatarsophalangeal joint.

Occasionally these areas are partially infiltrated with calcium.

The roentgenologic features of secondary and primary gouty arthritis are indistinguishable. Secondary gout is most often associated with blood dyscrasias and bone marrow disorders. Rare causes, however, are glycogen storage disease (von Gierke's disease) and uremia (Smith et al.).

Pseudogout (Figure 11–32 A and B). This entity is unrelated to gout and is believed to be a disorder of calcium metabolism. Calcified menisci and articular cartilage result from the deposition of calcium pyrophosphate, causing chondrocyte death, cartilage degeneration, and calcium deposition.

Juxta-Articular Cystic Lesions of Bone from Intraosseous Ganglia. Intraosseous ganglia are benign cystic lesions of bone found in the distal metaphyses of long bones of young and middle aged adults. The lesions are in a juxta-articular position, most frequently involving the medial malleolus of the tibia (Mainzer and Minaj).

Bone and Joint Lesions in Primary Amyloidosis (Grossman and Hensley). There is a striking predilection for involvement by lucent bone lesions in the proximal humerus and in the femoral neck.

There is also an increased soft tissue density representing capsular and pericapsular infiltration uniformly noted in major joints.

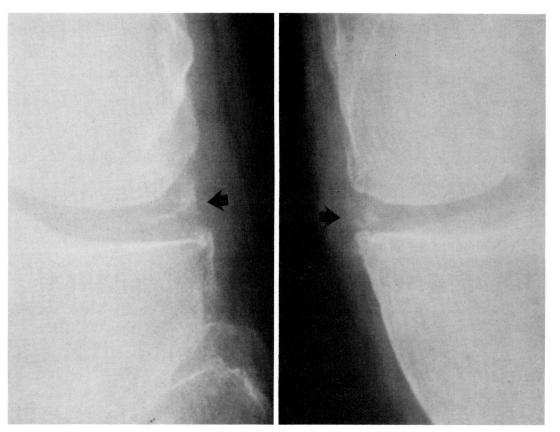

Figure 11–32 Pseudogout.

Articular Cartilage Calcification and Primary Hyperparathyroidism (Dodds and Steinbach).   Cartilage calcification has been noted in approximately 17 per cent of patients with primary hyperparathyroidism and is most frequently found in the knee and wrist. The cartilage calcification is most apt to be either punctate or linear in

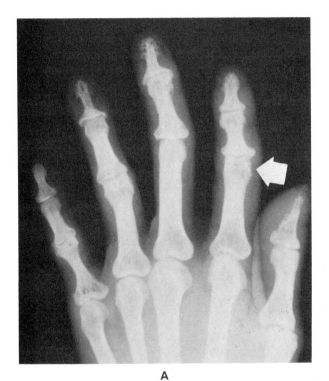

A

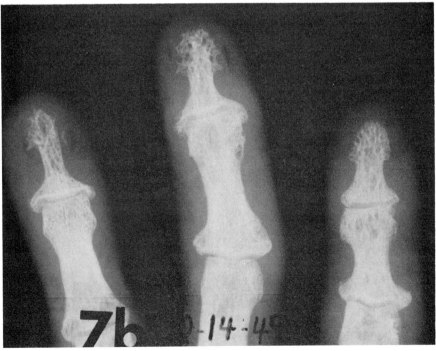

B

Figure 11–33   *A* and *B*. Hand and close-up view of phalanges in sarcoidosis. (Courtesy of Dr. James Marr, Winston-Salem, N.C.)

character. Osteitis fibrosa occurs in approximately 50 per cent of those with cartilage calcification and in only 27 per cent of those without such calcification.

Sarcoid (Figure 11–33)

Clinical Aspects.   Symptoms are variable and relatively negligible. There is an
anergy to tuberculin.
Laboratory Findings.   (1) Hypercalcemia, (2) Hyperglobulinemia.
Pathology.   (1) It is a granulomatous affection resembling tuberculosis but there
is no caseation. (2) Any organ may be affected, especially the skin, lungs (mediastinum), uveal tract of the eyes, parotid glands, and the bones (the adrenals and the
digestive tract are usually spared).

Roentgenologic Aspects

There are three types of bone manifestations:
> (a) A reticular or honeycomb structure of the spongiosa. This is
> the most frequent bony manifestation.
> (b) Round or ovoid, cystlike, punched-out lesions in the distal
> ends of the phalanges, with a thin sclerotic margin.
> (c) A mutilating form, in which the cystlike areas coalesce, forming
> large areas of destruction (Greenfield et al.; Edeiken and
> Hodes).

Enlarged mediastinal lymph nodes are often associated.
Resembles rheumatoid arthritis (but with less osteoporosis) and tuberculosis cystica multiplex.

Prognosis.   It is progressive in about 25 per cent of the cases.

TUMORS OF JOINTS

Benign Tumors

Xanthomatous Giant Cell Tumors of Joints

Clinical Aspects.   Pain, distention of the joints, elevated cholesterol in fluid
of joints.
Pathologic Aspects.   (1) The major site of involvement is the knee. (2) Tumor
may be a single pedunculated one or multiple pedunculated lesions.

Radiologic Findings.   Only a soft tissue tumor may be identified but contrast
studies of the joints are usually necessary for demonstration.

Malignant Tumors

Synovioma (Synoviosarcoma) (Figure 11–34)

Clinical Aspects.   (1) Sites of involvement are the knee, ankle, and metatarsals
most frequently, but occasionally the fingers. (2) Pain and hemarthrosis.
Pathologic Aspects.   (1) Tumor mass is usually adjacent to the joint in a neighboring bursa or tendon sheath. (2) Histologically, the tumor simulates fibrosarcoma.

SYNOVIOMA
("FIBROSARCOMA" OF SYNOVIAL OR CAPSULAR ORIGIN)

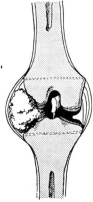

TUMOR INVADES AS IT GROWS AND DESTROYS ALL CONTIGUOUS TISSUES. ANAPLASTIC SPINDLE CELLS, SIMULATING FIBROSARCOMA, AND CUBOIDAL AND COLUMNAR CELLS SECRETING ACIDOPHILIC MUCINOUS MATERIAL.

YOUNG ADULTS
MALES:FEMALES = 3.2

LOWER EXTREMITY 79%
UPPER EXTREMITY 21%

JOINT INVOLVED = KNEE (50%)
ANKLE AND METATARSALS NEXT

1. ORIGIN MAY BE TENDON SHEATH, BURSA, OR JOINT. SYNOVIAL ORIGIN MAY BE UNPROVED.

2. PROGNOSIS: GRAVE
   5 YEAR: 20%
   10 YEAR: 0
   METASTASIZE LATE

Figure 11–34   Diagram illustrating pertinent features regarding synovioma.

Radiographic Aspects

Usually only a soft tissue mass is identified early.

Occasionally the sarcoma will have invaded the adjoining bone, producing bone destruction very much like fibrosarcoma of bone elsewhere.

Prognosis.   Prognosis is poor. Twenty per cent survive five years, but there are no ten year survivals; radiotherapy is usually of value for relief of pain only.

Chondrosarcoma.   This is an extremely rare primary tumor of a joint which usually ruptures through the joint capsule and has the same characteristics as chondrosarcoma occurring in bones elsewhere.

Villonodular Synovitis (Figure 11–35)

Synonyms are xanthoma, xanthogranuloma, giant cell tumor of tendon sheath, xanthomatous giant cell tumor, giant cell fibroangioma, and benign synovioma.

The cells contain hemosiderin pigment both within and outside the cells — hence the lesion has often been called a "pigmented tumor."

Pathologic Aspects

It is probably an inflammatory involvement of unknown cause of the synovial membrane, producing a nodular thickening of the synovia. Hemorrhage in the nodule produces the characteristic pigmentation.

Size varies from pea-sized nodules to large ones which fill an entire joint.

Most lesions are situated in the soft tissues adjoining the joint; only a few are situated within the joint. In some instances the lesions are located within the bone itself.

Most frequent site is the knee, followed by the hips, elbows, ankles, and shoulders.

Radiographic Aspects

Intra- and para-articular soft tissue masses are combined with joint effusions and erosions in bone that are smoothly outlined, homogeneous, and do not contain calcium.

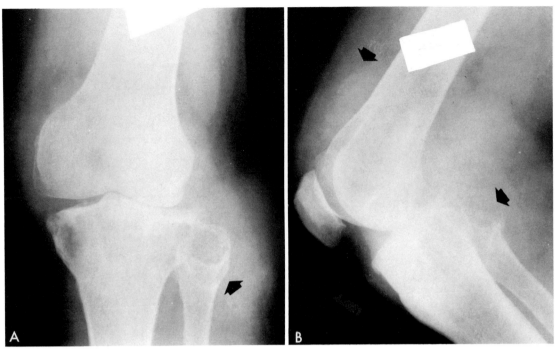

Figure 11–35 *A* and *B*. Antero-posterior and lateral views of a knee demonstrating the radiographic appearance of villo-nodular synovitis. The character of the resorption of bone, the location, and the soft tissue proliferation and increased density are characteristic. (Courtesy of Colonel William L. Thompson, Armed Forces Institute of Pathology.)

These cystlike lesions of the bone have a sharply circumscribed, thin sclerotic margin.

The bone between the lesions and in the subchondral region does not appear to be involved.

Both sides of the joint are usually involved, but the joint itself is spared.

Periosteal changes do not occur ordinarily.

Erosion of the articular cartilage may occur with resulting arthritic changes.

DISEASES CHARACTERIZED BY LOOSE BODIES IN THE JOINTS

1. Traumatic arthritis.
2. Neurotrophic arthritis.
3. Osteochondritis dissecans (see Chapter 9).
4. Chondromatosis with synovial chondrometaplasia (chondrocalcinosis).
5. Pseudogout syndrome.
6. Osteomatoses.

Of these, the synovial chondrometaplasia (chondrocalcinosis) will be discussed here.

Chondrocalcinosis (synovial chondrometaplasia); (chondromatosis)
(Figure 11–36)

Pathologic Aspects

Occasionally segments of synovial membrane become cartilaginous and ultimately ossify or calcify.

Synovial chondromas thereafter hang from the synovial membrane by a narrow vascular pedicle and sometimes they are completely separated, becoming free joint bodies ("joint mice").

In some instances these cartilaginous masses undergo central calcification of endochondral ossification.

Clinical Aspects.   The disease ordinarily affects young and middle aged adults. The joint may be swollen and somewhat painful.

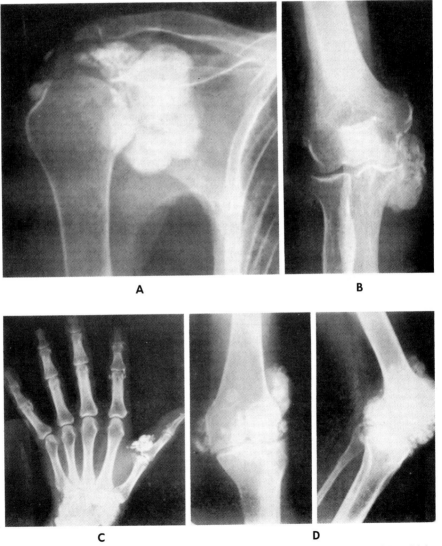

Figure 11–36 *A* to *D*. Radiographs of the shoulder, elbow, hand and knee of a patient with multiple areas of chondromatosis of the joints. (Courtesy of C. S. Pool, M.D.)

Radiographic Aspects. Calcified large or small irregular ovoid amorphous circular masses may be identified within the joint space (Figure 11–36). These appear to be bursal in location and do not appear to affect the bone significantly.

Treatment is by surgery, with removal of the synovial membrane and all accessible joint bodies.

DISEASES CHARACTERIZED BY CAPSULAR, PERICAPSULAR, OR BURSAL CALCIFICATION

1. Peritendinitis calcarea.
2. Pellegrini-Stieda disease (calcification of medial collateral ligament of knee).
3. Capsular fibrositis with calcification.

A

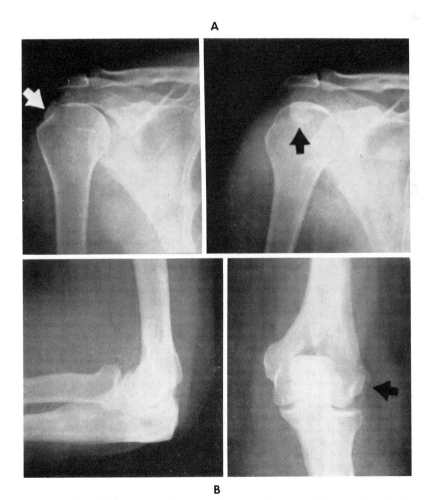

B

Figure 11–37 *A*. Peritendinitis calcarea of the shoulder. Note that rotated views are required to show the calcium, which may be obscured in one or the other of the views. *B*. Peritendinitis calcarea of the elbow.

Peritendinitis Calcarea (Figure 11–37)

General Comments

It may occur in any joint but is most frequent in the shoulder, the elbow, hip, and knee.

It is often associated with some strain on the joint and may be related to small tendinous or capsular tears.

An acute inflammatory episode occurs when the calcium irritates or breaks loose into the joint.

Roentgenologic Aspects

The calcification may be granular, amorphous, or plaquelike and may be obscured, unless rotated views are obtained with no obscuring artefacts.

Roentgen therapy may be of considerable benefit in the acute phase but recurrences are common.

Pellegrini-Stieda Disease (Figure 11–38)

This is a disease characterized by calcification of the medial collateral ligament of the knee, and is often associated with pain.

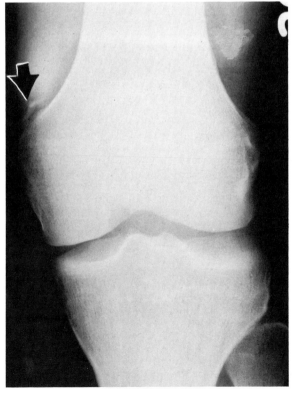

Figure 11–38 Pellegrini-Stieda disease.

ISOLATED MISCELLANEOUS JOINT DISEASES

Arthrogryposis Multiplex Congenita.   Disease present at birth characterized by flexion contractures of a few or many joints of the extremities.

Bone, Joint, and Soft Tissue Changes Following Paraplegia.   The radiographic findings in bones and joints with paraplegia are not specific as far as the joints are concerned but consist largely of erosion of bone at pressure points, periarticular rigidity, and periarticular calcification and even ossification. Pathologic fractures may ensue. Pain with gradual onset is often associated.

Alkaptonuria with Ochronosis and Arthritis.   This is a hereditary, metabolic defect in which phenylalanine and tyrosine cannot be degraded beyond homogentisic acid. The urine becomes dark on standing. The cartilage is degenerate and becomes calcified throughout the body. Ankylosis and joint degeneration are often associated.

Ochronosis is due to the ectopic deposits of brown, grayish-blue, or pigmented black material in the cartilage, tendons, and intima of blood vessels throughout the body. The joints most frequently affected are those of the spinal column, the shoulder, the knee, and the hips (Figure 11–39).

Radiographic Findings.   The appearances suggest combined atrophic and hypertrophic joint changes and in the spine there is calcification of the intervertebral disks. In other joints the cartilage becomes degraded, friable, and compressed.

Hypertrophic Pulmonary Osteoarthropathy (see Chapter 10)

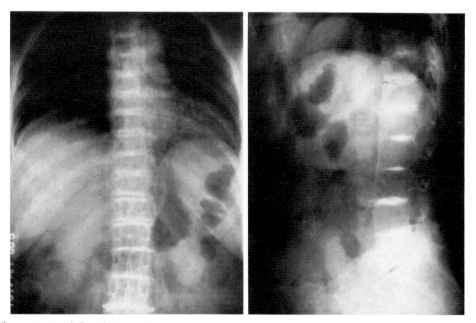

Figure 11–39   A-P and lateral views of the lower thoracic and lumbar spine in a patient with ochronosis. (Courtesy of Walter Reed Army Hospital.)

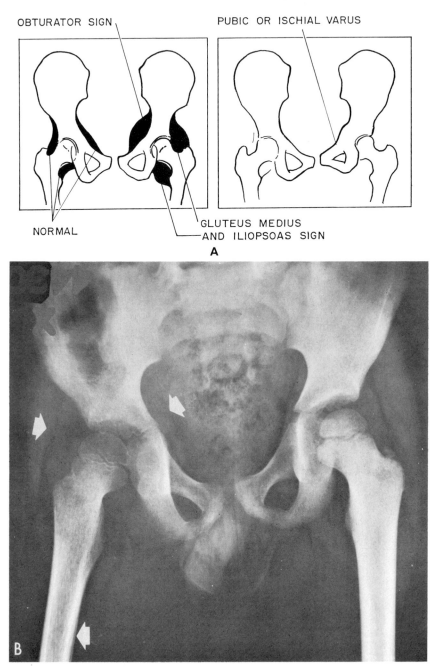

Figure 11–40 *A*. Left, diagram illustrating obturator sign; also gluteus medius and iliopsoas sign by comparison with the normal. Right, pubic or ischial varus, by comparison with normal on opposite side. *B*. Antero-posterior view of the pelvis in a patient with tuberculosis of the hip. Note the positive obturator sign and marked swelling of the capsule structures surrounding the right hip joint. Note also the periosteal elevation over the involved femur and the marked osteoporosis of all the bones of this region.

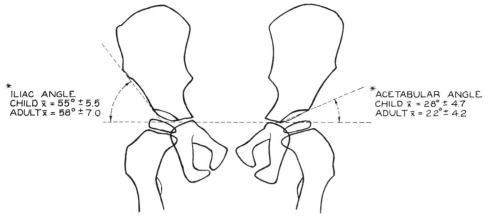

Figure 11–41   Diagram illustrating the method of measuring the iliac and acetabular angles. (From Caffey, J., and Ross, S.: Amer. J. Roentgenol., *80*:458, 1958.)

MUSCLE GROUP SIGNS AS A MANIFESTATION OF HIP DISEASE IN CHILDREN

The Obturator Sign (Figure 11–40) refers to a swelling of the obturator fascia seen on antero-posterior film studies of the pelvis. Swelling of the gluteus medius, minimus, and iliopsoas muscles have also been described as evidence of synovitis of the hip joint. This sign has also been called "the iliopsoas sign."

The "Pubic" or "Ischial Varus" Sign is a further manifestation of hip disease in children. There is a relative iliac flare and apparent widening of the sacrosciatic notch.

Kohler's "Teardrop" Sign refers to an asymmetry of the acetabular contour as it is reflected beneath the head and upper neck of the femur laterally.

The Acetabular Index — a Measure of Acetabular Cover (Beals). The acetabular index, a measure of the acetabular cover of the femoral head, is shown in the accompanying illustration (Figure 11–41). Femoral inclinations and femoral anteversion are also illustrated. Data were collected by Beals from the literature in respect to the normal values, and comparisons were made in a group of 40 patients with spastic paraplegia and diplegia. The angle of inclination was usually normal in these spastic children but anteversion was markedly increased. Decrease in the acetabular index in these children was related to the duration of ambulation. Neither anteversion nor the angle of inclination correlated with lateral displacement of the femoral head until 40 per cent or more of the femoral head was displaced beyond the bony acetabulum. With subluxation of 40 per cent or more anteversion and femoral inclination increased proportionately.

CLASSIFICATION OF JOINT DISEASES

The following is a clinical classification by the American Rheumatism Association:

1. Arthritis due to specific infection (organism specified).
2. Arthritis due to rheumatic disease.
3. Rheumatoid arthritis (specifying whether multiple or localized to the spine). Related diseases affecting joints include disseminated lupus

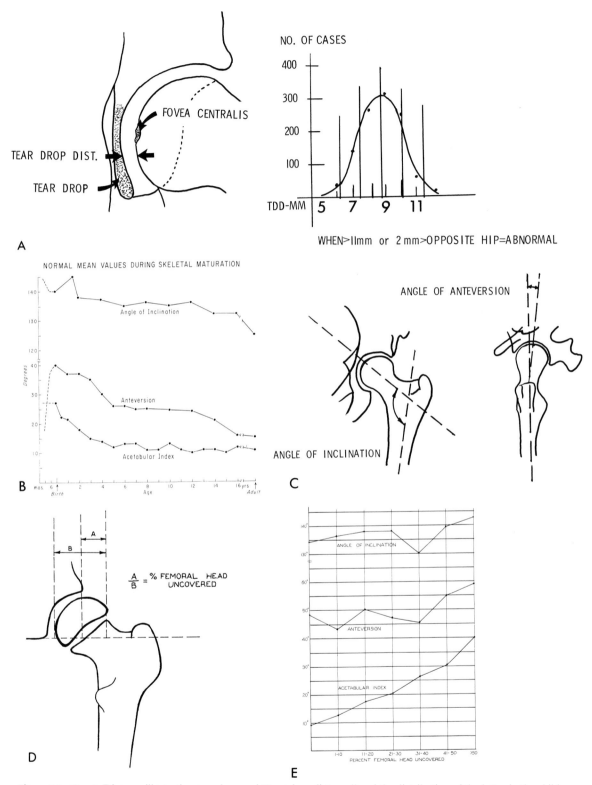

Figure 11–42 *A.* Diagram illustrating tear drop and "tear drop distance" and the distribution of the latter in the children studied. (From Eyring, E. J. et al.: Amer. J. Roentgenol., *93*:382, 1965.) *B.* Normal mean values of angle of inclination and anteversion for acetabular index (Beals). *C.* Diagram illustrating angles of anteversion and inclination. *D.* Diagram illustrating the acetabular index. *E.* Graphic relationships of acetabular cover (acetabular index) to anteversion and angle of inclination (Beals).

erythematosus, dermatomyositis, erythema multiforme exudativum, erythema nodosum, scleroderma, Reiter's disease, Sjögren's syndrome, and Felty's syndrome.

4. Arthritis due to direct trauma (specifying the joint involved).

5. Neurogenic arthropathy (specifying the joint involved).

6. Arthritis due to gout (specifying joint).

7. New growth of joints (specifying joint and neoplasm). In addition to osteochondromatosis and synoviosarcoma, one might also include here cysts of the menisci of the knee most frequently involving the lateral meniscus and the ganglion.

> (a) Villonodular synovitis—giant cell tumor of synovial and tendon sheath origin—is probably an inflammatory involvement of the synovial membrane having an unknown cause and producing a nodular thickening of the synovia.

8. Degenerative joint disease (called arthroses or osteoarthritis).

9. Hydrarthrosis, intermittent (specifying joint). This might include joint manifestations with serum sickness and the hemarthroses which accompany hemophilia and purpura of various types.

10. Periarticular fibrositis (specifying joint).

11. Diseases in which arthritis, arthropathy, or arthralgia are frequently associated. Such diseases may include acromegaly, drug intoxication, ochronosis, psoriasis, pulmonary osteoarthropathy, and Raynaud's disease.

12. Miscellaneous disturbances of the joints which may be caused by postural strain; they may be secondary to bone lesions, associated with loose bodies, or psychogenic in origin. Such arthritic manifestations may accompany osteochondritis dissecans, hysteria, and psychoneuroses.

Questions—Chapter 11

1. What are the three anatomical types of joints?

2. Outline a method of analysis of joint radiographs for evidence of joint disease.

3. Indicate the main headings of radiographic abnormalities of joint disease.

4. What are the main diseases characterized by capsular distention without bony involvement?

5. What are the main diseases characterized by capsular and subchondral proliferation?

6. What are the main diseases characterized radiographically by subchondral bone resorption with a narrowed joint space?

7. What are the main diseases characterized radiographically by sharply demarcated periarticular bone resorption?

8. What are the main diseases characterized by ankylosis?

9. What are the main diseases characterized radiographically by loose bodies within a joint ("joint mice")?

10. What are the main diseases characterized radiographically by capsular, pericapsular, bursal, or peritendinous calcification?

11. In diagrammatic fashion, indicate the axial relationships at the upper part of the humerus, at the elbow, in the knee, and in the ankle. What is meant by the critical angle in relation to the os calcis and how would this angle be measured?

12. Draw a diagram showing the important axial relationships of the wrist in both the antero-posterior and lateral projections.

13. Draw a diagram showing the important axial relationships of the hip joint. Indicate particularly the significance of Skinner's line and Shenton's line.

14. What are the important radiographic characteristics of hydrarthrosis of the knee?

15. What is meant by idiopathic capsulitis of the hip?

16. What are the major radiographic features in rheumatic fever?

17. Outline the pathogenesis of the radiographic findings in traumatic arthropathy.

18. Outline the main radiographic involvement in the pathogenesis of degenerative arthritis (hypertrophic arthritis).

19. Outline the main radiographic findings that occur in the pathogenesis of hemophilic arthritis.

20. What are the main types of neuroarthropathies?

21. What are the main radiographic features of each of the two types of neurogenic arthropathy?

22. Outline the main radiographic findings in the pathogenesis of rheumatoid arthritis.

23. What are some of the special aspects of rheumatoid arthritis of the spine?

24. What is the radiographic appearance of psoriatic arthritis?

25. Outline the main radiographic findings in the pathogenesis of tuberculous arthritis. What are the main categories of radiographic change?

26. Outline the main radiographic findings in the pathogenesis of pyogenic arthritis.

27. Outline the main radiographic findings in gout.

28. What are the main radiographic features of sarcoidosis of the small joints of the hand?

29. Classify tumors of joints.

30. What are the main radiographic features of synovioma of joints?

31. Describe the pertinent radiographic features of osteochondritis dissecans.

32. Describe the pertinent radiographic features of chondromatosis, involving joints.

33. Describe the pertinent radiographic aspects of peritendinitis calcarea.

34. Describe important clinical and radiographic features of ochronosis.

35. What is meant by the obturator sign? iliopsoas sign? and ischial varus sign in reference to the hip disease in children? What is meant by Köhler's teardrop sign?

References

Aegerter, E., and Kirkpatrick, J. A., Jr.: Orthopedic Diseases. Second Edition. Philadelphia, W. B. Saunders Co., 1963.

Albert, J., Bruce, W., Allen, A. C., and Blank, H.: Lipoid dermato-arthritis. Reticulohistiocytoma of the skin and joints. Amer. J. Med., 28: 661–667, 1960.

Alpert, M., and Meyers, M.: Osteolysis of the acromial end of the clavicles in rheumatoid arthritis. Amer. J. Roentgenol., 86:251–259, 1961.

American Rheumatism Association: Primer on the Rheumatic Diseases. J.A.M.A., 139:1068–1076; 1139–1146; 1268–1273, 1949.

Arcomano, J. P., Stunkle, G., Barnett, J. C., and Sackler, J. P.: Muscle group signs and pubic varus as a manifestation of hip disease in children. Amer. J. Roentgenol., 89:966–969, 1963.

Avila, R., Pugh, D. J., Slocumb, C. H., and Winkelmann, R. K.: Psoriatic arthritis, a roentgenologic study. Radiology, 75:691–702, 1960.

Barnett, J. C., and Arcomano, J. P.: Hip arthrography in children with Renografin. Radiology, 73:245–249, 1959.

Bauer, W., Bennett, G. A., and Zeller, J. W.: The pathology of joint lesions in patients with psoriasis and arthritis. Transactions Amer. Assoc. Physicians, 56:349–352, 1941.

Beals, R. K.: Developmental changes in the femur and acetabulum in spastic paraplegia and diplegia. Develop. Med. Child. Neurol. 11:303–313, 1969.

Berens, D. L., Lockie, L. M., Lin, R., and Norcross, B. M.: Roentgen changes in early rheumatoid arthritis: wrist-hands-feet. Radiology, 82:645–654, 1964.

Bledsoe, R. C., and Izenstark, J. L.: Displacement of fat pads in disease and injury of the elbow: a new radiographic sign. Radiology, 73:717–724, 1959.

Breimer, C. W., and Freiberger, R. H.: Bone lesions associated with villonodular synovitis. Amer. J. Roentgenol., 79:618–629, 1958.

Brogdon, B. J., and Crow, N. E.: Little leaguer's elbow. Amer. J. Roentgenol., 83:671–675, 1960.

Bundens, W. D., Jr., Brighton, C. T., and Weitzman, G.: Primary articular cartilage calcification with arthritis (pseudogout syndrome). J. Bone Joint Surg., 47A:111–122, 1965.

Currarino, G., Tierney, R. C., Giesel, R. G., and Weihl, C.: Familial idiopathic osteoarthropathy. Amer. J. Roentgenol., 85:633–644, 1961.

Del Buono, M. S.: Die Doppel kontrast arthrographie des Elbogens. Schweiz Med. Wschr., 91:1466–1470, 1961.

den Herder, B. A.: Arthrography of shoulder joint. Arch Chir. Neerl., 11:254–260, 1959.

Dodds, W. J., and Steinbach, H. L.: Primary hyperparathyroidism and articular cartilage calcification. Amer. J. Roentgenol., *104*:884–892, 1968.

Drey, L.: Roentgenographic study of transitory synovitis of the hip joint. Radiology, *60*:588–591, 1953.

Edeiken, J., and Hodes, P. J.: *Roentgen Diagnosis of Diseases of Bone.* Baltimore, Williams and Wilkins Co., 1967.

Edling, N. P. G., Ohlson, L., and Swensson, A.: Rheumatoid pneumoconiosis (Caplan's disease): Acta Radiol. (Diagnosis), *8*:168–177, 1969.

Edwards, E. G.: Transient synovitis of the hip joint in children: Report of 13 cases. J.A.M.A., *148*:30–34, 1952.

Elson, M. W.: The syndrome of exophthalmos, hypertrophic osteoarthropathy, and pretibial myxedema. Amer. J. Roentgenol., *85*:114–118, 1961.

Epstein, B. S.: Radiographic identification of arthrogryposis multiplex congenita in utero. Radiology, *77*:108–110, 1961.

Epstein, B. S.: Sternoclavicular arthritis in patients with scleroderma and rheumatoid arthritis. Amer. J. Roentgenol., *89*:1236–1240, 1963.

Felty, A. R.: Chronic arthritis in the adult associated with splenomegaly and leukopenia. Bull. Hopkins Hosp., *35*:16–20, 1924.

Ford, L. T., and Simril, W. A.: Malum gleni senilis. South. Med. J. *50*:976–981, 1957.

Gonzalez, L., Mackenzie, A. H., and Tarar, R. A.: Carotid sialography in Sjögren's syndrome Radiology, *97*:91–93, 1970.

Greenfield, G. B., Schorsch, H. A., Shkolnik, A.: The various roentgen appearances of pulmonary hypertrophic osteoarthropathy. Amer. J. Roentgenol., *101*:927–931, 1967.

Grossman, R. E., and Hensley, G. T.: Bone lesions in primary amyloidosis. Amer. J. Roentgenol., *101*:872–875, 1967.

Gyepes, M. T., Newbern, D. H., and Neuhauser, E. B. D.: Metaphyseal and physeal injuries in children with spina bifida and meningomyeloceles. Amer. J. Roentgenol., *95*:168–177, 1965.

Harris, R. D., and Hecht, H. L.: Suprapatellar effusions: A new diagnostic sign. Radiology, *97*:1–4, 1970.

Haveson, S. B., and Rein, B. I.: Lateral discoid meniscus of the knee: Arthrographic diagnosis. Amer. J. Roentgenol., *109*:581–586, 1970.

Hefke, H. W., and Turner, V. C.: Obturator sign as earliest roentgenographic sign in diagnosis of septic arthritis and tuberculosis of the hip. J. Bone Joint Surg., *24*:857–869, 1942.

Heimann, W. G., and Freiberger, R. H.: Avascular necrosis of the femoral and humeral heads after high-dosage corticosteroid therapy. New Eng. J. Med., *263*:672–675, 1960.

Hollander, J. L., ed.: Arthritis and Allied Conditions. Seventh Edition. Philadelphia, Lea & Febiger, 1966.

Holt, J. F., and Hodges, F. J.: Significant skeletal irregularities of the hands. Radiology, *44*:23–31, 1945.

Hubbard, M. J. S.: The measurement of progres-

sion in protrusion acetabuli. Amer. J. Roentgenol., *106*:506–508, 1969.

Jackman, R. J., and Pugh, D. G.: The positive elbow fat pad sign in rheumatoid arthritis. Amer. J. Roentgenol., *108*:812–818, 1970.

Jacobson, H. G., Herbert, E. A., and Poppel, M. H.: Arthrogryposis multiplex congenita. Radiology, *65*:8–17, 1955.

Jorgensen, H. G., and Petersen, O.: Bilaterale aseptische osteonekrose des kalkaneus. Fortschr. Roentgenstr. *93*:388–389, 1960.

Katz, I., and Steiner, K.: Ehlers-Danlos syndrome with ectopic bone formation. Radiology, *65*:352–360, 1955.

Kernwein, G. A., Roseberg, B., and Sneed, W. R., Jr.: Arthrographic studies of the shoulder joint. J. Bone Joint Surg. (Amer.), *39A*:1267–1279, 1957.

Klein, E. W.: Osteochondrosis of the capitellum (Panner's disease): Report of a case. Amer. J. Roentgenol., *88*:466–469, 1962.

Kunkel, H. G.: Significance of the rheumatoid factor (editorial). Arthritis Rheum., *1*:381–383, 1958.

Leach, R. E., Gregg, T., and Siber, F. J.: Weight bearing radiography in osteoarthritis of the knee. Radiology, *97*:265–268, 1970.

Levin, E. J., and Gannon, W.: Diffuse villonodular synovitis of the shoulder. Amer. J. Roentgenol., *89*:1302–1304, 1963.

Lodge, T.: Bone, joint and soft tissue changes following paraplegia. Acta Radiol., *46*:435–445, 1960.

Luck, V. J.: Bone and Joint Diseases. Springfield, Ill., Charles C Thomas, 1950.

Mainzer, F., and Minaj, H.: Intraosseous ganglion: a solitary subchondral lesion of bone. Radiology, *94*:387–389, 1970.

Marshall, T. R.: Radiographic changes in rheumatoid arthritis in digits. Radiology, *90*:121–123, 1968.

Martel, W., Champion, C. K., Thompson, G. R., and Carter, T. L.: A roentgenologically distinct arthropathy in some patients with pseudogout syndrome. Amer. J. Roentgenol., *109*:587–605, 1970 (25 references, 19 figures).

Martel, W., Hayes, J. T., and Duff, I. F.: Pattern of bone erosion in the hand and wrist in rheumatoid arthritis. Radiology, *84*:204–213, 1965.

Martel, W., Holt, J. F., and Cassidy, J. T.: Roentgenologic manifestations of juvenile rheumatoid arthritis. Amer. J. Roentgenol., *88*:400–423, 1962.

Mason, R. M., Murray, R. S., Oates, J. K., and Young, A. C.: A comparative radiologic study of Reiter's disease, rheumatoid arthritis, and ankylosing spondylitis. J. Bone Joint Surg. *41-B*:137–148, 1959.

McEwen, C., Ziff, M., Carmel, P., DiTata, D., and Tanner, M.: The relationship to rheumatoid arthritis of its so-called variants. Arthritis Rheum., *1*:481–496, 1958.

Meaney, T. F., and Hays, R. A.: Roentgen manifestations of psoriatic arthritis. Radiology, *68*:403–407, 1957.

Meschan, I., and McGaw, W. A.: Pneumoarthrography of the knee with evaluation of the procedure in 315 operated cases. Radiology, *49*:675–710, 1947.

Murray, R. S., Oates, J. K., and Young, A. C.: Radiologic changes in Reiter's syndrome and arthritis associated with urethritis. J. Fac. Radiolog., 9:37–43, 1958.

Nakata, H., and Russell, W. J.: Chest roentgenograms in rheumatoid arthritis: Hiroshima, Nagasaki. Amer. J. Roentgenol., 108:819–824, 1970.

Norgaard, F.: The earliest roentgenologic changes in polyarthritis of the rheumatoid type: rheumatoid arthritis. Radiology, 85:325–329, 1965.

Poal, J. M., Cecil, R. L., and Kemmerer, W. H.: Psoriasis and arthritis: a clinical study of 115 cases. Presented at the 7th International Congress on Rheumatic Diseases, May, 1949.

Rodko, E. A.: Alkaptonuria with ochronosis and arthritis. J. Canadian Ass. Radiol., 7:29–32, 1956.

Rogers, F. B., and Lansbury, J.: Atrophy of auricular and nasal cartilages following administration of chorionic gonadotrophins in case of arthritis mutilans with sicca syndrome. Amer. J. Med., 229:55–62, 1955.

Rokkanen, P.: Osteochondrosis of capitulum humeri (Panner's disease): Report of Case. Ann. Chir. et Gynaec. Fenniae, 47:356–361, 1958.

Ross, P., and Wood, B.: Osteoarthropathy in idiopathic hemochromatosis. Amer. J. Roentgenol., 109:575–580, 1970.

Samilson, R. L., Raphael, R. L., Post, L., Noonan, C., Siris, E., and Raney, F. L. Jr.: Shoulder arthrography. J.A.M.A., 175:773–778, 1961.

Schwarz, E., and Fish, A.: Reticulohistiocytoma: rare dermatologic disease with roentgen manifestations. Amer. J. Roentgenol., 83:692–697, 1960.

Schwarz, G. S., Berenyi, M. R., and Siegel, M. W.: Atrophic arthropathy and diabetic neuritis. Amer. J. Roentgenol., 106:523–529, 1969.

Sholkoff, S. D., Glickman, M. G., and Steinbach, H. L.: Roentgenology of Reiter's syndrome. Radiology, 97:497–503, 1970.

Silbiger, M. L., and Peterson, C. C. Jr.: Sjögren's syndrome: its roentgenographic features. Amer. J. Roentgenol., 100:554–558, 1967.

Smith, E. E., Kurlander, G. J., Powell, R. C.: Two rare causes of secondary gouty arthritis. Amer. J. Roentgenol., 100:550–553, 1967.

Thompson, M. M., Jr.: Ochronosis. Amer. J. Roentgenol., 78:46–53, 1957.

Toumbis, A., Franklin, E. C., McEwen, C., and Kuttner, A. G.: Clinical and serologic observations in patients with juvenile rheumatoid arthritis and their relatives. J. Pediat., 62:463–473, 1963.

Twigg, H. L., Zvaifler, N. J., and Nelson, C. W.: Chondrocalcinosis. Radiology, 82:655–659, 1964.

Vanselow, N. A., Dodson, V. N., Angell, D. C., and Duff, I. F.: A clinical study of Sjögren's syndrome. Ann. Intern. Med., 58:124–135, 1963.

Weldon, W. V., and Scalettar, R.: Roentgen changes in Reiter's syndrome. Amer. J. Roentgenol., 86:344–350, 1961.

Winston, J. M., and Hewson, J. S.: Early roentgen diagnosis of tuberculosis of the hip in children. Radiology, 79:241–249, 1962.

Ziff, M., Brown, P., Lospalluto, J., Badin, J., and McEwen, C.: Agglutination and inhibition by serum globulin in the sensitized sheep cell agglutination reaction in rheumatoid arthritis. Amer. J. Med., 20:500–509, 1956.

12

Roentgenology of the Skull

METHOD OF STUDY

Routine Views of the Skull. The routine views of the skull are illustrated in Figure 12–1.

Each view has a special significance and purpose.

The straight postero-anterior view will project the petrous ridges into the orbit. An optimum view of the two internal acoustic canals is obtained for comparison, but the orbital structures are partially obscured.

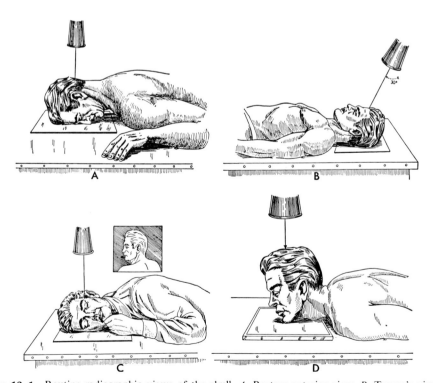

Figure 12–1 Routine radiographic views of the skull. *A*. Postero-anterior view. *B*. Towne's view. *C*. Lateral projection, to be made on both sides. *D*. Verticosubmental (axial) view.

The postero-anterior Caldwell view is best for visualization of the frontal bone and sinuses, and the petrous ridges are projected beneath the orbits, but these latter structures are not seen optimally. The ethmoid paranasal sinuses are well visualized here.

The postero-anterior Water's view is an excellent view for the facial bones as well as the orbits, but not as good for the calvarium and its contents.

The antero-posterior Towne's view is excellent for the occipital bone, the foramen magnum, the pineal gland, the petrous ridges, the zygomatic arches, and the posterolateral walls of the maxillary sinuses. The dorsum sellae is ordinarily seen well here, as projected into the foramen magnum.

The submentovertical view, or axial view, is excellent for the base of the skull and its foramina, as well as the petrous ridges, the sphenoids, and a basal view of the facial bones.

The lateral views are necessary for the lateral perspective and usually these are obtained stereoscopically.

Ideally all of these views should be obtained with the patient sitting erect or, if this is not possible, a lateral view should be obtained with a horizontal beam with the film vertical to the tabletop. This is necessary to demonstrate fluid levels and free air in the cranial cavity (Figure 12–2; communications with nose; brain abscess).

Apart from these views there are the special views for specific regions of the skull which will be described in Chapter 13.

Ideally, all of these views should be obtained for every examination of the skull.

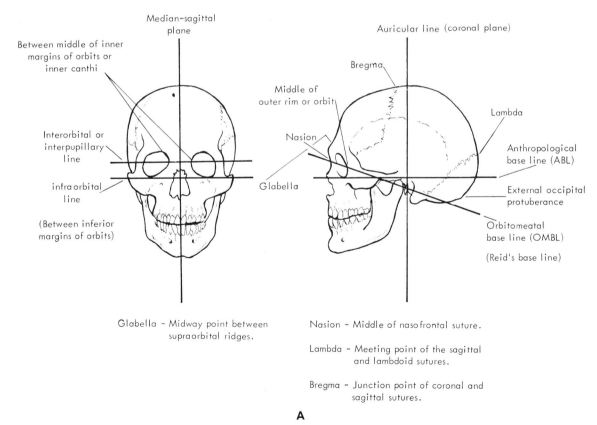

A

Figure 12–2   *A.* Commonly used reference points and lines on skull. Reid's base line, originally described as a line from the infraorbital rim to the external auditory meatus, is seldom used as a reference line because the canthomeatal line, from the outer canthus of the eye to the external auditory meatus, is more clearly defined on the patient.

Figure 12–2 continued on opposite page.

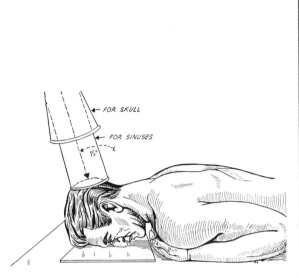

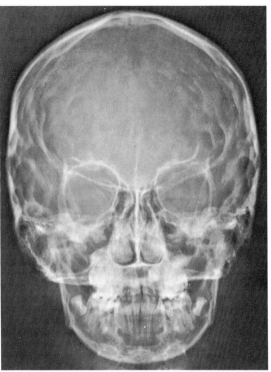

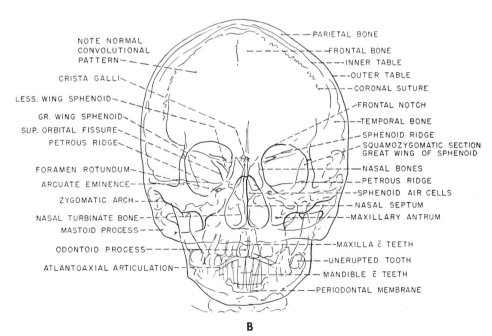

B

Figure 12–2 *(Continued)*.   *B*. Caldwell's projection of the skull: Note that patient is positioned so that the canthomeatal line is perpendicular to the film. (The original Caldwell projection for sinuses was 23 degrees with respect to the glabello-meatal line, which is the same as 15 degrees with respect to the canthomeatal line, but more variable and hence a less accurate designation.)

Figure 12–2 continued on following page.

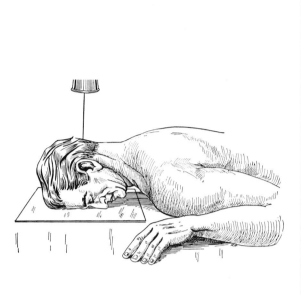

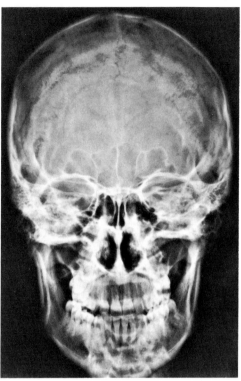

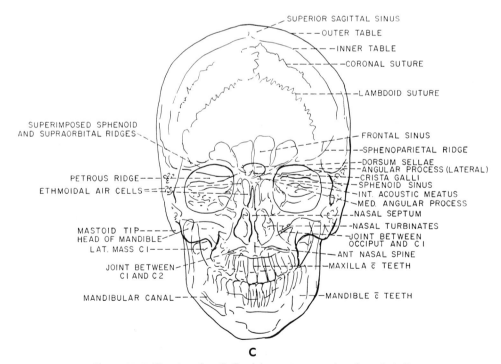

SUPERIOR SAGITTAL SINUS
OUTER TABLE
INNER TABLE
CORONAL SUTURE
LAMBDOID SUTURE

SUPERIMPOSED SPHENOID
AND SUPRAORBITAL RIDGES
FRONTAL SINUS
SPHENOPARIETAL RIDGE
DORSUM SELLAE
ANGULAR PROCESS (LATERAL)
CRISTA GALLI
SPHENOID SINUS
INT. ACOUSTIC MEATUS
MED. ANGULAR PROCESS
PETROUS RIDGE
ETHMOIDAL AIR CELLS
NASAL SEPTUM
NASAL TURBINATES
JOINT BETWEEN
OCCIPUT AND C I
MASTOID TIP
HEAD OF MANDIBLE
LAT. MASS C I
ANT NASAL SPINE
JOINT BETWEEN
C I AND C 2
MAXILLA c̄ TEETH
MANDIBULAR CANAL
MANDIBLE c̄ TEETH

C

Figure 12–2 (*Continued*).   *C. Straight postero-anterior view of skull.*

Figure 12–2 continued on opposite page.

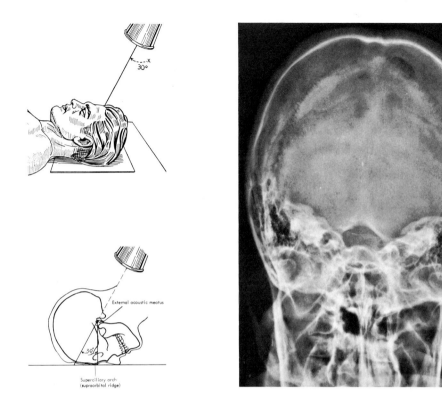

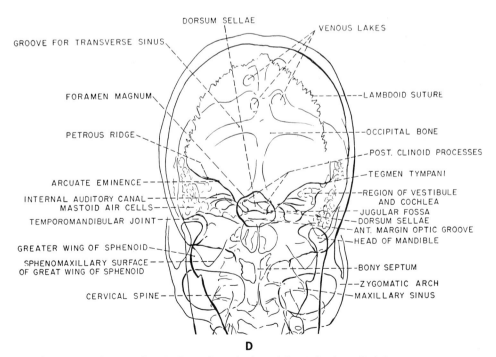

Figure 12–2 (*Continued*).   *D.* Towne's projection of the skull, also called Grashey position.

Figure 12–2 continued on following page.

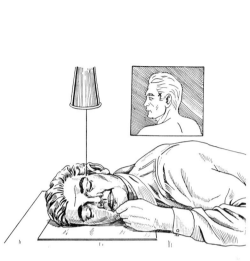

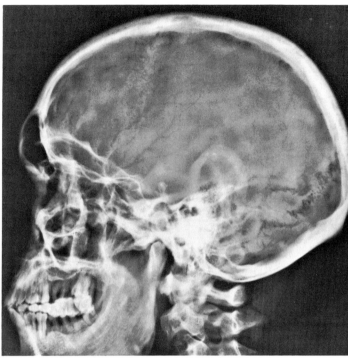

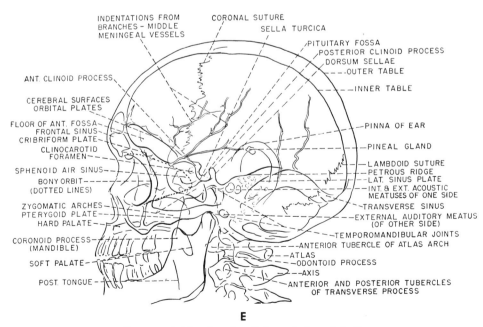

INDENTATIONS FROM
BRANCHES - MIDDLE
MENINGEAL VESSELS
CORONAL SUTURE
SELLA TURCICA
PITUITARY FOSSA
POSTERIOR CLINOID PROCESS
DORSUM SELLAE
OUTER TABLE
INNER TABLE
ANT. CLINOID PROCESS
CEREBRAL SURFACES
ORBITAL PLATES
PINNA OF EAR
FLOOR OF ANT. FOSSA
FRONTAL SINUS
CRIBRIFORM PLATE
CLINOCAROTID
FORAMEN
PINEAL GLAND
LAMBDOID SUTURE
PETROUS RIDGE
LAT. SINUS PLATE
INT. & EXT. ACOUSTIC
MEATUSES OF ONE SIDE
SPHENOID AIR SINUS
BONY ORBIT
(DOTTED LINES)
ZYGOMATIC ARCHES
PTERYGOID PLATE
HARD PALATE
TRANSVERSE SINUS
EXTERNAL AUDITORY MEATUS
(OF OTHER SIDE)
TEMPOROMANDIBULAR JOINTS
CORONOID PROCESS
(MANDIBLE)
ANTERIOR TUBERCLE OF ATLAS ARCH
ATLAS
ODONTOID PROCESS
SOFT PALATE
AXIS
POST. TONGUE
ANTERIOR AND POSTERIOR TUBERCLES
OF TRANSVERSE PROCESS

E

Figure 12–2 (*Continued*).   *E*. Lateral view of skull.

Figure 12–2 continued on opposite page.

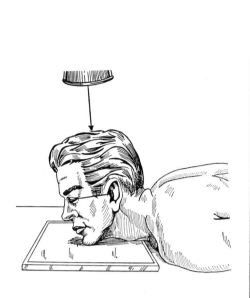

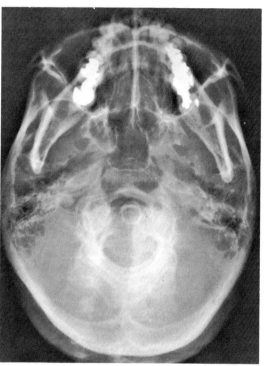

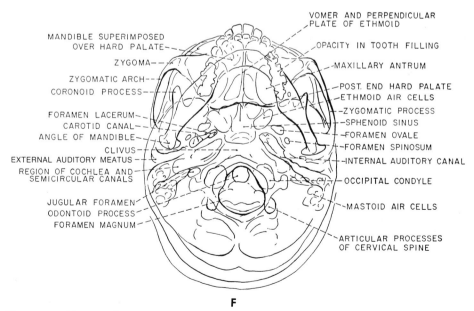

VOMER AND PERPENDICULAR
PLATE OF ETHMOID

MANDIBLE SUPERIMPOSED
OVER HARD PALATE

OPACITY IN TOOTH FILLING

ZYGOMA

MAXILLARY ANTRUM

ZYGOMATIC ARCH
CORONOID PROCESS

POST. END HARD PALATE
ETHMOID AIR CELLS

ZYGOMATIC PROCESS

FORAMEN LACERUM
CAROTID CANAL
ANGLE OF MANDIBLE

SPHENOID SINUS
FORAMEN OVALE
FORAMEN SPINOSUM

CLIVUS
EXTERNAL AUDITORY MEATUS
REGION OF COCHLEA AND
SEMICIRCULAR CANALS

INTERNAL AUDITORY CANAL

OCCIPITAL CONDYLE

JUGULAR FORAMEN
ODONTOID PROCESS
FORAMEN MAGNUM

MASTOID AIR CELLS

ARTICULAR PROCESSES
OF CERVICAL SPINE

F

Figure 12–2 (*Continued*). *F*. Axial view of skull (verticosubmental projection; Schüller position).

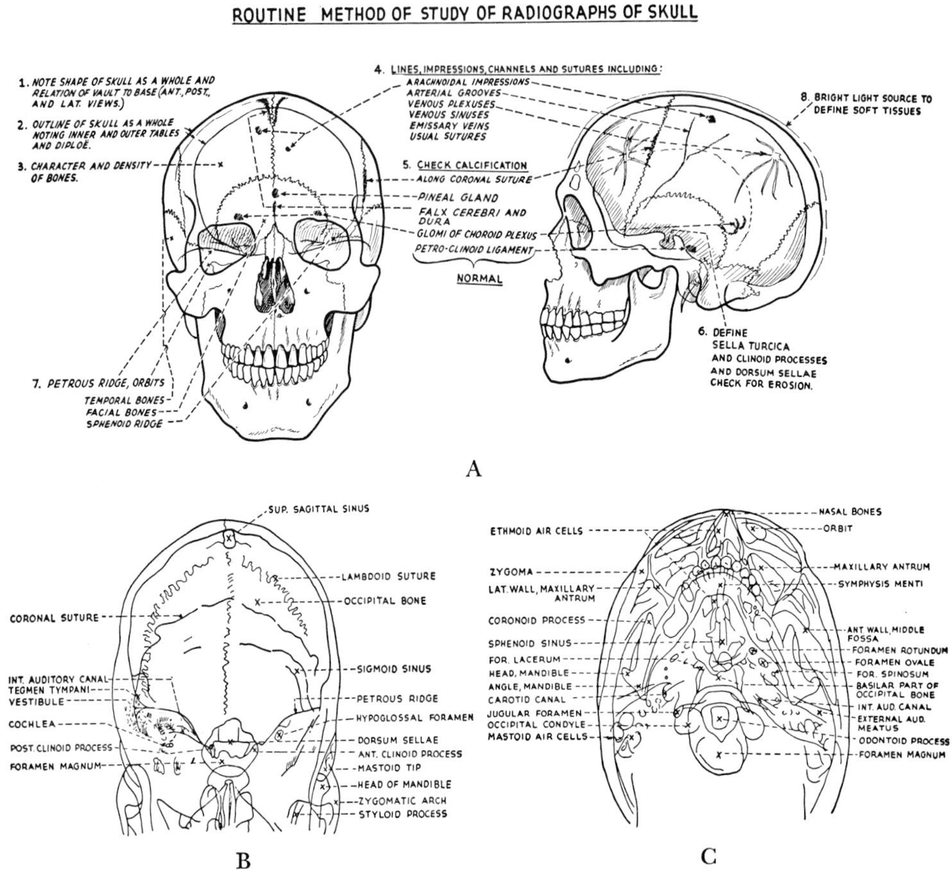

ROUTINE METHOD OF STUDY OF RADIOGRAPHS OF SKULL

A

B

C

Figure 12–3 *A.* Routine method of study of P-A and lateral radiographs of the skull. *B.* Towne's projection of the skull: labeled tracing of radiograph. *C.* Axial view of skull: labeled tracing of radiograph.

When limitations imposed by cost and radiation exposure are considered, a useful minimum would be: the postero-anterior Caldwell view (stereoscopic); the antero-posterior Towne's view; the submentovertical or axial view; both lateral views, one of which should be stereoscopic and erect (or horizontal beam study).

Additional or different views may be obtained as indicated by the clinical history and physical examination.

Routine Method of Study of Radiographs of the Skull is indicated in Figure 12–3.

There are many variations of the normal. There can be no substitute for careful attention to detail and extensive experience.

GROWTH AND AGE CHANGES IN THE SKULL AND IMPORTANT INDICES

Growth and Age Changes

The *skull is large in proportion* to the remainder of the skeleton at birth. The volume of the face in the newborn infant is only one-eighth that of the entire skull, whereas in the adult the volume occupied by the face roughly equals that occupied by the cranium. The *growth of the face and skull* is *most rapid in the first six or seven years* (see Table 12–1).

TABLE 12–1 PERCENTAGE OF ADULT FACIAL AND CRANIAL DIMENSIONS ACHIEVED AT DIFFERENT AGE LEVELS*

Age, Yr.	Cranium of Adult Dimensions				Face of Adult Dimensions			Volume Ratio
	Width	Height	Length	Bizygo-matic Width	Bigonial Width	Height	Length	Cranium Face
0				56		38	40	8 : 1
2	86	92	86	80		68	70	5 : 1
6	92	96	90	83	83	80	80	3 : 1
12	98	99	96	90	93	89	87	2.5 : 1
	max. attained by 15 yr. of age							
18	100	100	100	100	100	100	98	2 : 1

*From Watson, E. H., and Lowrey, G. G.: Growth and Development of Children. 5th Ed. Chicago, Year Book Medical Publishers, 1967.

Between seven years of age and puberty the growth of the skull is slow. *At puberty,* however, there is a second spurt in growth activity with development of the nasal accessory sinuses and further pneumatization of the mastoids. *After puberty* the skull assumes its most definitive adult appearance, except that the convolutional markings may still be present and the sella turcica may retain its infantile form until 16 to 20 years of age. (The infantile form of sella turcica will be described subsequently and is a horizontal "J" shape, with a downward concavity in the region of the limbus sphenoidale.)

Closure of the sutures of the base of the skull begins at about the age of 25 and of the cranial vault variably between the ages of 30 and 40.

The average head and chest circumferences of American children between birth and 20 years of age are shown in Table 12–2A.

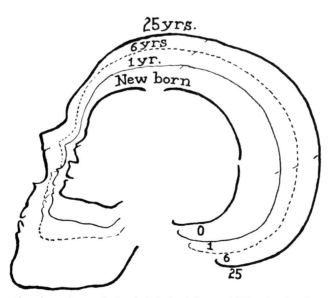

Figure 12–4 Growth and age changes in the skull during infancy, childhood and early manhood, shown in medial longitudinal section. (From Caffey, J.: *Pediatric X-ray Diagnosis*, 5th Ed. Chicago, Year Book Medical Publishers, 1967.) The skull is large in proportion to the remainder of the skeleton at birth. The volume of the face in the newborn infant is only one-eighth that of the entire skull, whereas in the adult the volume occupied by the face roughly equals that occupied by the cranium. The growth of the face and skull is most rapid in the first six or seven years.

NEWBORN SKULL

Vault is thin- measures about I mm.
in thickness

Sutures widely patent

Sella turcica still
partly cartilaginous
and "〰" shaped.

May be as much as
2-3 mm. thick in
lower frontal bone.

No pneumatization of mastoids
or paranasal sinuses.

Crowns of unerupted teeth in
alveoli identified.

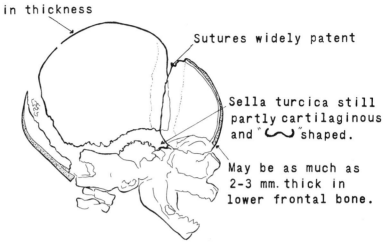

Figure 12–5   Roentgen features of the newborn skull, lateral view.

SKULL AT 2 YEARS

Assumes a more adult appearance.

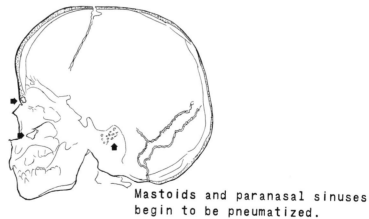

Mastoids and paranasal sinuses
begin to be pneumatized.

Until at age 7 years

Foramen magnum ⎫
Petrous bones ⎬ very much
Orbits   ⎭ like adult

Figure 12–6   Roentgen features of the skull at two years of age, lateral view.

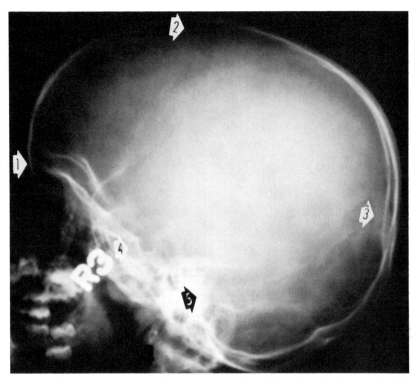

Figure 12–7 Lateral radiograph of a skull of a four year old and also that of a 13 year old with pertinent areas of growth change indicated: (1) frontal sinus region, (2) coronal sutures, (3) lambdoid sutures, (4) sella turcica, (5) mastoids. The frontal and mastoid areas become pneumatized, the sella becomes more completely ossified and the sutures become more like those of the adult. Facial changes occur in greater proportion in the 13 year old.

TABLE 12–2A AVERAGE HEAD AND CHEST CIRCUMFERENCE OF AMERICAN CHILDREN

Age	Mean Head Circumference*		Standard Deviation*		Chest Circumference*		Head-Chest Ratio
	INCHES	CM.	±INCHES	±CM.	INCHES	CM.	
Birth	13.8	35	0.5	1.2	13.7	35	1:1
1 month	14.9	37.6	0.5	1.2			
2 months	15.5	39.7	0.5	1.2			
3 months	15.9	40.4	0.5	1.2	16.2	40	1:1
6 months	17.0	43.4	0.4	1.1	17.3	44	1:1
9 months	17.8	45.0	0.5	1.2			
12 months	18.3	46.5	0.5	1.2	18.3	47	1:1
18 months	19.0	48.4	0.5	1.2	18.9	48	1:1
2 years	19.2	49.0	0.5	1.2	19.5	50	1:1
3 years	19.6	50.0	0.5	1.2	20.4	52	0.96:1
4 years	19.8	50.5	0.5	1.2	21.1	53	0.95:1
5 years	20.0	50.8	0.6	1.4	22.0	55	0.93:1
6 years	20.2	51.2	0.6	1.4	22.5	56	0.91:1
7 years	20.5	51.6	0.6	1.4	23.0	57	0.90:1
8 years	20.6	52.0	0.8	1.8	24.0	59	0.88:1
10 years	20.9	53.0	0.6	1.4	25.1	61	0.87:1
12 years	21.0	53.2	0.8	1.8	27.0	66	0.81:1
14 years	21.5	54.0	0.8	1.8	29.0	72	0.75:1
16 years†	21.9	55.0	0.8	1.8	31.0	77	0.71:1
18 years†	22.1	55.4	0.8	1.8	33.0	82	0.68:1
20 years†	22.2	55.6	0.8	1.8	34.5	86	0.65:1

*From Watson, E. H., and Lowrey, G. H.: *Growth and Development of Children,* 5th Ed. Chicago. Year Book Medical Publishers, 1967 (based on several recent sources, including Stuart and Simmons).
†Chest circumference for males only.

TABLE 12–2B CRANIAL SIZE IN CHILDREN (Cronqvist)
(after Austin and Gooding)

Age	(L + H + W) ± 2 S.D. (mm.)	Cranial Index of Cronqvist (± 2 S.D.) $\dfrac{L + H + W}{M} \times 10$
1 mo.	327 ± 26	57 ± 5
2– 3 mo.	355 ± 43	58 ± 4
4– 6 mo.	391 ± 30	57 ± 4
7– 9 mo.	421 ± 42	57 ± 5
10–12 mo.	421 ± 36	56 ± 6
1 yr.	441 ± 45	56 ± 6
2 yr.	456 ± 32	56 ± 7
3 yr.	470 ± 45	55 ± 5
4 yr.	464 ± 34	52 ± 6
5 yr.	465 ± 37	53 ± 5

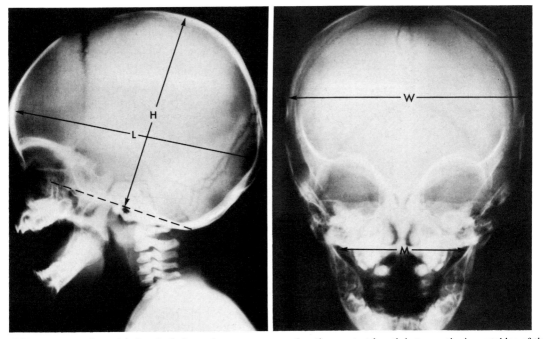

Measurements of cranial size. *Left.* Lateral roentgenogram. *L* = the greatest length between the inner tables of the skull; *H* = the greatest height, measured as the maximum perpendicular distance between the vault of the cranial cavity and a line drawn from the nasion to the posterior margin of the foramen magnum.

Right. Anteroposterior roentgenogram. *W* = the greatest width between the inner tables of the skull; *M* = the maximum distance between the inner margins of the two necks of the mandible. (From Austin, J. H. M. and Gooding, C. A.: *Radiology, 99:*642, 1971.)

Measurements.   The length, height, and breadth of the skull are shown and defined in Figure 12–8. The skull is described as a short skull when the length is short in respect to the breadth (*brachycephalic* skull); a long skull (*dolichocephalic*) when the length is great in respect to the breadth; a turrethead (*turricephaly*) when the height is great in respect to the breadth and length; a scaphoid head (*scaphocephaly*) when the head is canoe-shaped with an indentation in the region of the junction of the lambdoid or coronal and sagittal suture; and *plagiocephaly*, when the skull grows asymmetrically because of premature synostosis of sutures of half of the skull. Upon the side of suture obliteration, the growth of the skull is retarded but there is a compensatory expansion of the skull on the opposite side.

In addition, identification should be made of *microcephaly*, in which the skull is very small in size, and *macrocephaly*, in which the skull is markedly enlarged. The latter is most often caused by hydrocephalus, which is a dilatation of the cerebral ventricles.

Structurally, the skull may be divided into its cranial or "neural" and facial components. Changes in the volume of the calvarium are closely related to the growth of the neural mass, consisting of brain, cerebrospinal fluid, and meninges.

Microcephaly is often associated with small brain size (microencephaly), but may be due to other factors such as premature closure of the sutures, or prenatal infections such as cytomegalic inclusion disease, toxoplasmosis, or rubella.

Macrocephaly, although it is most often associated with hydrocephalus, may be secondary to subdural hematoma, acute meningitis, acute lead poisoning, and metastatic neuroblastoma to the meninges.

Disproportionate enlargement of the cranium in relation to the face ("pseudo-hydrocephalus") may be seen in premature infants, hypopituitarism, and hypothyroidism (Howell).

Area and volume relations of the cranium and face as projected on the lateral skull films of infants and children are reproduced from Watson and Lowery in the section below.

Normal Skull Size.   The measurements of the average Caucasian skull (Broca, quoted by Schwartz and Collins) are as follows:

Mean	*Males*	*Females*
Length	182 mm.	174 mm.
Breadth	145 mm.	135 mm.
Height	132 mm.	125 mm.

Welcker (quoted by Schwartz and Collins) gives the following figures for the capacity of the adult Caucasian skull (tables taken from Piersol):

	Mean	*Maximum*	*Minimum*
Males	1450 cc.	1790 cc.	1220 cc.
Females	1300 cc.	1550 cc.	1090 cc.

Roentgenologic Evaluation of Cranial Size in Children (Cronqvist).   The distance between the two necks of the mandible increases with skull size to the age of three years and then slowly up to the age of eight years. The indices of length, height, and width of the skull may be compared to this distance (M). The sum of length, height, and width related to M has been used as a C index and according to Cronqvist gives an accuracy of diagnosis up to 93 per cent in the determination of abnormal skull size (Table 12–2 B).

Table 12–2 A may also be used for comparative purposes.

(*Text continued on page 451*)

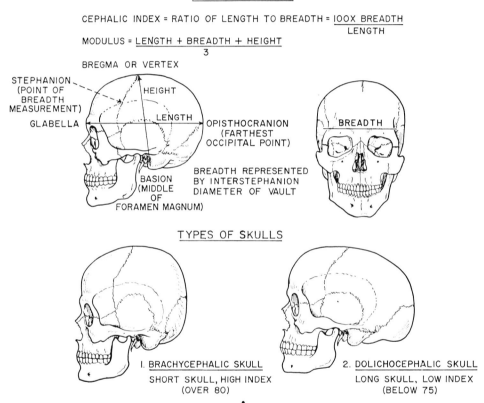

CRANIAL INDICES

CEPHALIC INDEX = RATIO OF LENGTH TO BREADTH = $\dfrac{100 \times \text{BREADTH}}{\text{LENGTH}}$

MODULUS = $\dfrac{\text{LENGTH} + \text{BREADTH} + \text{HEIGHT}}{3}$

BREGMA OR VERTEX

STEPHANION (POINT OF BREADTH MEASUREMENT)

HEIGHT

GLABELLA

LENGTH

OPISTHOCRANION (FARTHEST OCCIPITAL POINT)

BASION (MIDDLE OF FORAMEN MAGNUM)

BREADTH REPRESENTED BY INTERSTEPHANION DIAMETER OF VAULT

BREADTH

TYPES OF SKULLS

1. BRACHYCEPHALIC SKULL
SHORT SKULL, HIGH INDEX
(OVER 80)

2. DOLICHOCEPHALIC SKULL
LONG SKULL, LOW INDEX
(BELOW 75)

A

Figure 12–8 *A*. Important cranial indices and types of skulls.

Figure 12–8 continued on opposite page.

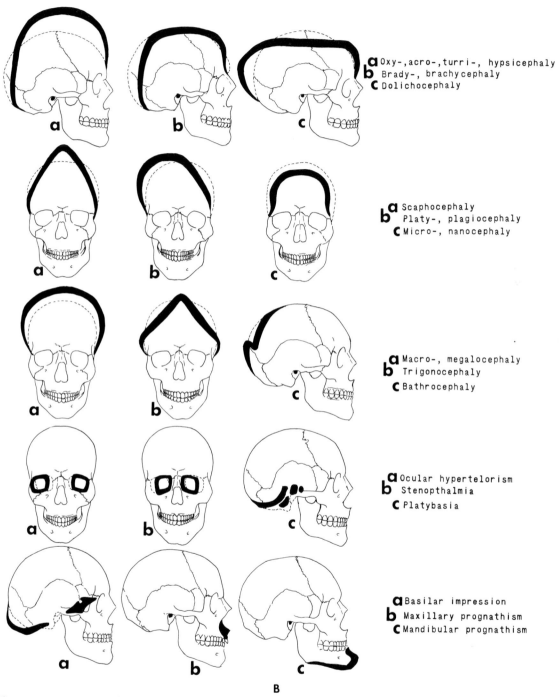

a Oxy-, acro-, turri-, hypsicephaly
b Brady-, brachycephaly
c Dolichocephaly

a Scaphocephaly
b Platy-, plagiocephaly
c Micro-, nanocephaly

a Macro-, megalocephaly
b Trigonocephaly
c Bathrocephaly

a Ocular hypertelorism
b Stenopthalmia
c Platybasia

a Basilar impression
b Maxillary prognathism
c Mandibular prognathism

B

Figure 12–8 (*Continued*). *B*. (Redrawn from similar illustrations in: Schwarz, G. S., and Golthamer, C. R.: *Radiographic Atlas of the Human Skull, Normal Variants and Pseudo-lesions.* New York and London, Hafner Publishing Co., 1965, with permission of the authors and publishers.)

Figure 12–8 continued on following page.

DANDY-WALKER CYSTS

Torcular Herophili

Sagittal sinus

Lateral sinus

Lateral sinus

POSTERO-ANTERIOR VIEW   **C**   LATERAL VIEW

Arnold-Chiari Malformation

— Lateral sinus grooves

41%

Lateral view of skull showing:

1. Flat floor of posterior fossa
2. Low lateral sinuses
3. Large foramen magnum (71 %)
4. Scalloped petrous bones (65%) **D**

Figure 12–8 (*Continued*). *C.* Posterior fossa elongation in Dandy-Walker syndrome. *D.* Changes in base of skull in Arnold-Chiari malformation. (From Kruyff, E., and Jeffs, R.: Acta Radiol. Diagnostic, *5*:18, 1966.)

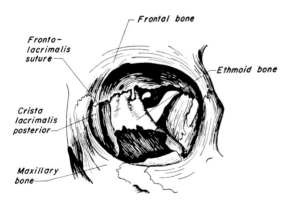

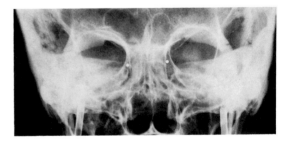

Frontal bone

Fronto-
lacrimalis
suture

Ethmoid bone

Crista
lacrimalis
posterior

Maxillary
bone

Figure 12–9 *A. Left.* Anatomy of orbit to show point of reference for measurement of interorbital distance. (Adopted from Sobotta, J.: *Descriptive Human Anatomy.* Hafner Publishing Company, Inc., New York, 1954.) *Right.* Roentgenogram of skull (anatomic specimen) with metallic markers at juncture of crista lacrimalis posterior with the fronto-lacrimalis suture. Note that the smooth curve is continuous with the medial rim of the orbital margin. The interorbital distance would be measured between the medial edges of the metallic markers. (From Gerald, B. F., and Silverman, F. N.: Amer. J. Roentgenol., *95*:154–161, 1965.

Figure 12–9 continued on opposite page.

SPHENOID ANGLE AND FACIAL ANGLE

SPHENOID ANGLE : *ANGLE BETWEEN SPHENOID AND CLIVUS (ALSO CALLED "BASAL ANGLE")*

FACIAL ANGLE : *ANGLE BETWEEN SLOPE OF FACIAL BONES AND LINE DRAWN BETWEEN ALVEOLUS AND FORAMEN MAGNUM AS SHOWN.*

NASO-PINEAL ANGLE : *ROOT OF NOSE TO MIDPOINT OF DIAPHRAGMA SELLAE AND FROM THIS TO PINEAL GLAND (NORMAL: 138.5° - 157.5°) SECOND LIMB OF ANGLE: 3.9 - 5.3 CM. (± 2 STAND. DEV.) [ISLEY ET AL]*

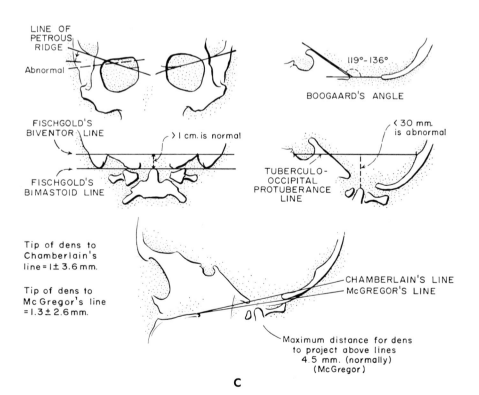

Figure 12–9 (*Continued*). *B.* The terms sphenoid angle and basal angle as defined in the text are synonymous. According to McGregor, 95 per cent of the population will have a basal angle between 122° and 148°. *C.* Various roentgen criteria for platybasia and basilar impression.

TABLE 12–3   INTERORBITAL MEASUREMENTS AT VARIOUS AGES (separating patients with mongolism from normal infants and children and having a probability of 78 per cent accuracy)

Age (Months)	Critical Level (cm.)
3	1.45
6	1.47
9	1.49
12	1.50
24	1.57
36	1.63
48	1.70
60	1.76
72	1.83
84	1.90
96	1.97
108	2.01
120	2.10
132	2.16
144	2.23

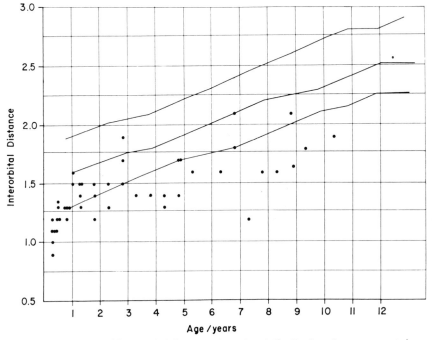

Unsmoothed curves of normal interorbital distances (in cm.) and distribution of measurements in mongols. (From Gerald, B. E., and Silverman, F. N.: Amer. J. Roentgenol., 95:154–161, 1965.)

Normal Interorbital Distances. The interorbital distance has been defined anthropologically as the maximal distance between the medial walls of the bony orbits, measured at the junction of the crista lacrimalis with the frontolacrimalis suture. There is a smooth curve continuous with the medial rim of the orbital margins at the site of measurement (Table 12–3 and Figure 12–9 A).

This graph was primarily developed to demonstrate that this distance is significantly diminished (orbital hypotelorism) in mongols (Gerald and Silverman).

This condition is indicative of hypoplasia of the bony central facial structures.

"Hypertelorism" (increased interorbital distance) is characteristic of a number of disorders of facial growth to be described later in this text.

(*Text continued on page 456*)

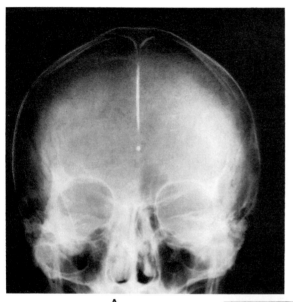

A

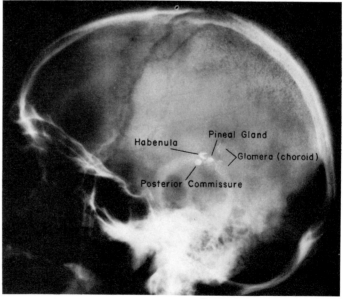

B

Figure 12–10 *A*. Radiograph demonstrating calcification in the pineal gland and falx cerebri in a postero-anterior view. *B*. Radiograph of the skull in a lateral projection demonstrating calcium deposit in the pineal gland, habenula, and glomera of the choroid.

Figure 12–10 continued on following page.

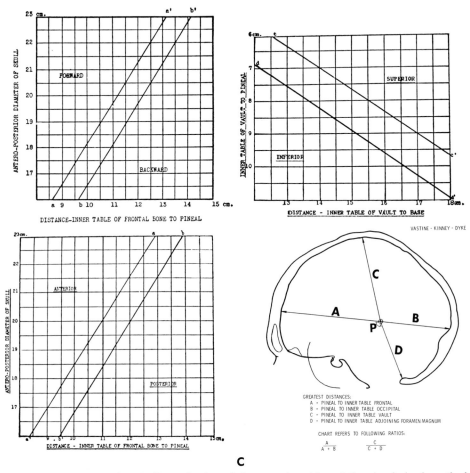

Figure 12–10 (*Continued*).   *C.* Determination of the normal position of the pineal gland: method of Vastine-Kinney, as modified by Dyke. Pineals that fall between the lines a-a' and b-b' are in the normal zone, while those that fall anterior to this zone are displaced forward and those posterior to it are displaced backward. Likewise, in the vertical plane, the normal zone lies between the lines c-c' and d-d'. When the pineal falls above it is displaced superiorly, and when it falls below it is displaced inferiorly. *Lower left.* Dyke's modification of the Vastine-Kinney graph in the antero-posterior plane. The normal zone is 4 mm. anterior to the comparable Vastine-Kinney graph. *Lower right.* Lateral view of the skull indicating points from which measurements are made to determine position of the pineal body by the Vastine-Kinney, as modified by Dyke. Pineals that fall between the lines a-a' and b-b' are in the normal their most distant points; (C) inner table of the vault and (D) inner table of the cerebellar fossa at the foramen magnum. (From Golden, R.: *Golden's Diagnostic Roentgenology.* Baltimore, Williams and Wilkins, 1936–63.)

Figure 12–10 continued on opposite page.

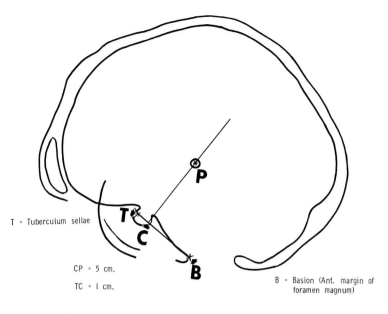

T = Tuberculum sellae

CP = 5 cm.

TC = 1 cm.

B = Basion (Ant. margin of foramen magnum)

Line PC ⊥ Line TB at C

Pineal body falls within 10 mm. of P in 98% of cases

° TFD = 70 cm. (28 inches)

D

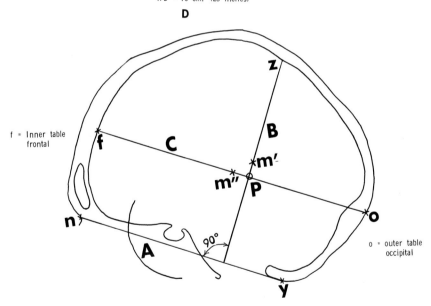

f = Inner table frontal

o = outer table occipital

y = lowermost portion of basiocciput, outer table

Line C ‖ Line A through Pineal

Line B ⊥ Line A through Pineal

m' is 1 cm. above Pineal

m' and m'' are midpoints of line B and C respectively.

m'' is 1 cm. anterior to Pineal

98.5% lie within 5 mm. of P on line C

100% lie within 5 mm. of P on line B

E

Figure 12–10 (*Continued*). *D*. Localization of the pineal gland by the method of Oon. (From Oon, C. L.: *Amer. J. Roentgenol.*, 92:1242–1248, 1964.) *E*. Localization of the pineal gland by the method of Pawl and Walter. (From Pawl, R. P., and Walter, A. K.: *Amer. J. Roentgenol.*, 105:287–290, 1969.)

Figure 12–10 continued on following page.

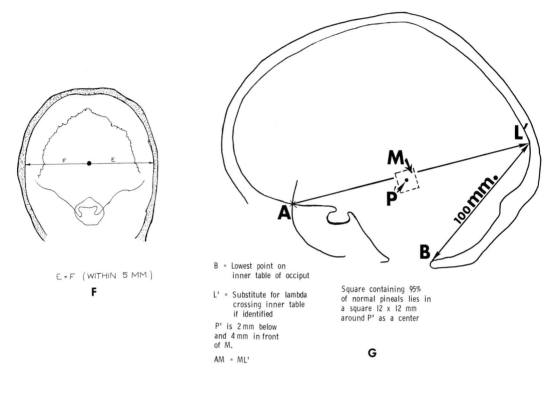

E = F (WITHIN 5 MM.)

F

B = Lowest point on
    inner table of occiput

L' = Substitute for lambda
     crossing inner table
     if identified

P' is 2 mm below
and 4 mm in front
of M.

AM = ML'

Square containing 95%
of normal pineals lies in
a square 12 x 12 mm
around P' as a center

G

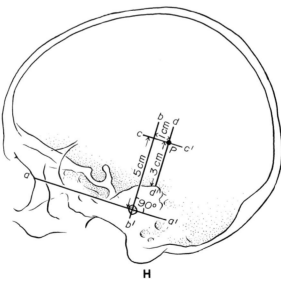

H

Figure 12–10 (*Continued*). *F.* Antero-posterior and lateral views of the skull, showing the pineal gland and the four measurements taken. *G.* Localization of the pineal gland by the method of Murase et al. *H.* Alternate technique for localization of the pineal gland in relation to the orbitomeatal line. (From Murase, Y. et al.: *Amer. J. Roentgenol.*, *110*:92–95, 1970.)

Figure 12–10 continued on opposite page.

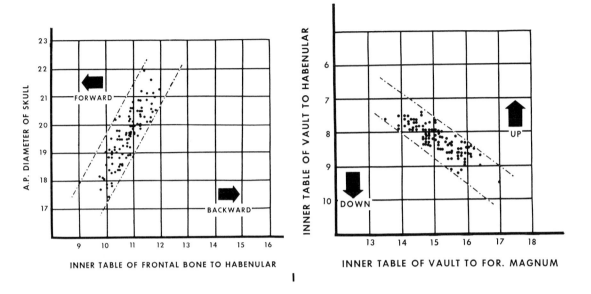

I

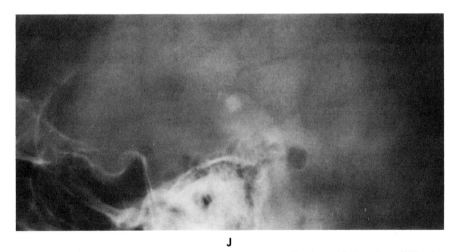

J

Figure 12–10 (*Continued*).   *I.* McCrae's graphs for normal localization of habenular calcification; and *J.* Inverted "C" appearance of habenular calcification in relation to the pineal gland calcification. (From McCrae, D. L.: *Amer. J. Roentgenol., 94*:541–546, 1965, with permission of the publishers.)

Pineal Localization. Calcification of the pineal gland is found in about half of the adult Caucasian population. Two methods of localization are illustrated in Figure 12–10. The possible limitations of pineal localization are:

Identification of the pineal gland may not be accurate. The habenular commissure, posterior commissure, and glomi of the choroid plexuses may also undergo calcification normally. The glomi may be readily differentiated on stereoscopic views, since they are situated laterally within the posterior parts of the bodies of the lateral ventricles. However, the habenular commissure which may calcify and appear as a C-shaped structure, and the posterior commissure which may appear as an amorphous area of calcification like the pineal gland both lie just anterior to the pineal gland and may be difficult to differentiate from the latter.

The films should be straight lateral and antero-posterior. It is true that rotations of even as much as 20 degrees may produce no significant change in the measured position of the pineal in the lateral projection (Agnos and Wollin), and slight rotation in the frontal projections likewise may still show the pineal to be in midline.

At best, pineal localization should be used only as a guide suggesting further investigation in respect to space-occupying lesions such as tumor, hemorrhage, or abscess; or in respect to brain atrophy which may occasionally "draw" the pineal toward the atrophic side.

Morreau has recommended an alternative method for localization of the pineal gland which he claims is more accurate.

It is distinctly unusual for the pineal gland to be calcified before the age of ten years. Calcification prior to this age suggests pinealoma.

Localization of Habenular Calcification. The localization of habenular calcification on lateral radiographs of the skull may be used in addition to localization of the pineal gland as follows:

The measurements from the inner table of the frontal bone to the apex of the C-shaped habenular calcification are made. These are compared with the antero-

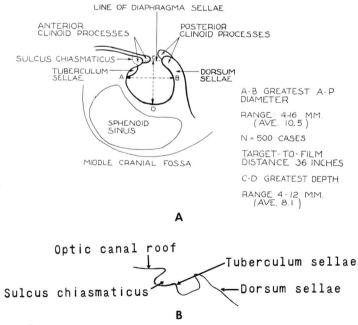

Figure 12–11 *A.* Camp's method of measuring the sella turcica in lateral view, with anatomic parts labeled. *B.* The "infantile j-shaped" sella turcica in profile. (From Kier, Amer. J. Roentgenol., *102*:747, 1968.)

Figure 12–11 continued on opposite page.

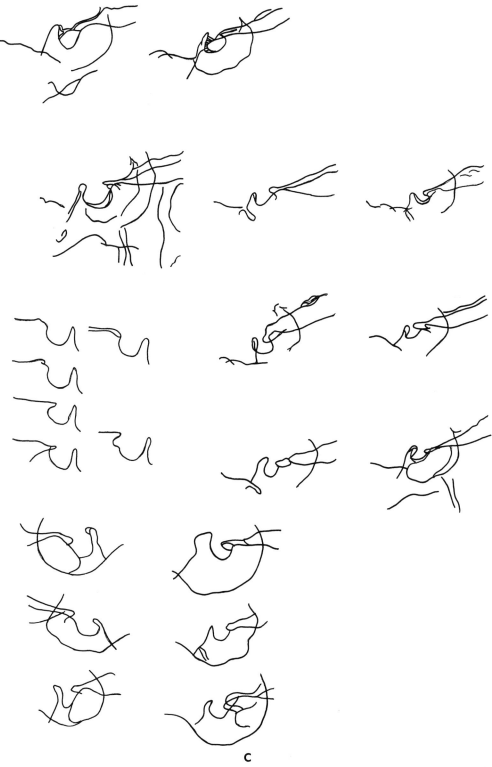

C

Figure 12–11 (*Continued*). *C*. Tracings of normal sella turcica modified from Schüller; Shapiro and Janzen; Di Chiro and Lindgren.

posterior diameter of the skull, using the outer table of the skull for this latter measurement (McRae).

McRae has considered these charts more accurate than comparable charts for localization of the pineal gland (Figure 12–10 C).

Anatomy and Measurements of the Sella Turcica (Figure 12–11). Various methods for measurement of the sella turcica have been devised, but the two most useful in our experience are those illustrated. In Camp's method, the measurement is made on the lateral film only. In the method described by Di Chiro and Nelson (Figure 12–12), a third measurement is provided which is obtained from Caldwell's projection or a suitable antero-posterior view of the skull. The "volume" of the sella turcica is calculated by dividing the product of the three dimensions by two. The mean volume was determined to be 594 cubic millimeters, with a range between 240 and 1092. Di Chiro and Nelson considered their accuracy for prediction of sellar size to be 83 per cent.

These authors also determined that the pituitary gland occupies, on the average, approximately 79 per cent of the volume of the sella, and their accuracy for prediction of pituitary size was 87 per cent. Considerable enlargement of the pituitary gland may not produce any enlargement of the sella, since lateral protrusion is possible.

The shape of the sella turcica must be assessed from the film studies quite separately from measurement of size, since asymmetrical erosion may occur, producing a "double contoured" appearance of the floor of the sella. Tomography and stereoscopic views are helpful in this regard.

In children, the region of the sella immediately adjoining the tuberculum sellae may be partially cartilaginous. The sella may appear biconcave and elongated (Figure 12–11). However, 70 per cent of the sellas in children are round in lateral view, whereas in adults only 24 per cent are round, 58 per cent are oval and 17.2 per cent are flat.

THE VOLUME OF THE SELLA TURCICA

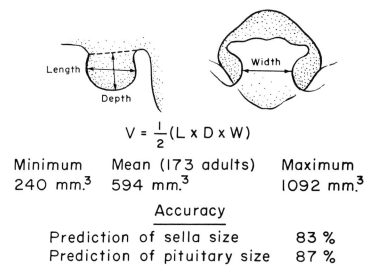

$$V = \frac{1}{2}(L \times D \times W)$$

Minimum	Mean (173 adults)	Maximum
240 mm.^{3}	594 mm.^{3}	1092 mm.^{3}

Accuracy

Prediction of sella size	83 %
Prediction of pituitary size	87 %

Figure 12–12 The volume of the sella turcica as determined by Di Chiro and Nelson.

The appearance of the *"overbridged sella"* is usually not produced by a true bony or calcific bridge replacing the diaphragma sellae (this can rarely occur), but is rather caused by the fact that the anterior interclinoid distance is wider than the posterior, and the posterior clinoids come forward beyond the interclinoid line.

The *"pneumatized dorsum sellae and posterior clinoids"* is a normal variant without pathological significance and is due to the extension of air cells from the sphenoid sinuses.

ROENTGEN SIGNS OF ABNORMALITY

General Outline. As with most other radiologic pathology, roentgen signs of abnormality of the skull can be conveniently considered under the following headings:
A. Size
    1. Abnormally small, as with microcephaly or anencephaly
    2. Abnormally large, as with hydrocephaly, or Paget's disease of bone
B. Contour
    1. Abnormality involving the bones of the vault as a whole, as with craniostenosis or trigonocephaly
        (a) There are various abnormalities in shape associated with these entities, such as brachycephaly; dolichocephaly; scaphocephaly; plagiocephaly.
    2. Localized frontal or parietal bone prominence, as with rickets or some anemias
    3. Localized bony prominences, as with osteomas and osteochondromas; meningiomas
    4. Localized soft tissue prominences, as with cephalhematoma of the scalp; encephaloceles
    5. Localized depressions in the calvarium or base of the skull, as with
        (a) Depressed skull fractures
        (b) Platybasia
        (c) Paget's disease of bone
C. Density
    1. Diffuse radiolucency, as with
        (a) Congenital disorders, such as cleidocranial dysostosis and osteogenesis imperfecta
        (b) Endocrine deficiencies, such as cretinism
        (c) Hyperparathyroidism
        (d) Neoplastic disorders, such as neuroblastoma
        (e) Nonspecific radiolucencies
    2. Demarcated single areas of radiolucency, such as
        (a) Fracture
        (b) Leptomeningeal cyst
        (c) Osteomyelitis, acute or chronic
        (d) Epidermoidoma
        (e) Hemangioma
        (f) Sinus pericranii
        (g) Dermoid cyst
        (h) Single metastasis, or invasion of the skull from a contiguous malignant neoplasm (such as one from the nasopharynx)
        (i) Invasion from a contiguous benign lesion such as the acoustic neuroma or chemodectoma

3. Multiple areas of demarcated radiolucency such as
    (a) Foramina, fenestrae, and bony thinning
    (b) Chronic infections
    (c) Craniolacunia (Lückenschädel)
    (d) Fibrous dysplasia
    (e) Hyperparathyroidism
    (f) Reticuloendothelioses (histiocytoses; eosinophilic granuloma; Hand-Schüller-Christian disease, Letterer-Siwe disease)
    (g) Metastatic malignancy
    (h) Multiple myeloma
4. Diffuse increased radiopacity as with
    (a) Osteopetrosis or Engelmann's disease
    (b) Fluorine poisoning
    (c) Marrow disorders
5. Demarcated areas of radiopacity localized to one bone, such as
    (a) Osteoma or osteochondroma
    (b) Hyperostosis frontalis interna
    (c) Meningioma
    (d) Leontiasis ossea
    (e) Fibrous dysplasia
    (f) Metastatic carcinoma
6. Demarcated areas of radiopacity, multiple, such as
    (a) Paget's disease of bone (osteitis deformans)
    (b) Metastatic carcinoma
D. Architectural abnormality in the bones of the calvarium. These have already been considered under other categories. Careful description is required in relation to the inner or outer table, or to the diploë; and distinction must be made in respect to inside architecture of a lesion as against its marginal alteration. These are largely density alterations previously considered.
E. Changes in special areas of the skull (see Chapter 13):
    1. Sella turcica
    2. Paranasal sinuses
    3. Nose
    4. Mandible and temporomandibular joints
    5. Orbits
    6. Mastoids and temporal bones
    7. Radiographic evidence of intracranial space-occupying lesions
        (a) Bony alterations
        (b) Intracranial calcification
        (c) Intracranial lucency
        (d) Special contrast studies, such as angiograms and pneumograms, and cisternomyelograms. (These are considered outside the scope of this text.)

THE CONTRACTING SKULL (Griscom and Oh et al.)

Skull film manifestations of low or decreasing intracranial tension or content.
    1. Concave fontanelle.
    2. Progressive depression of a craniotomy bone flap.

3. Overlapping or approximation of the edge of a previously diastatic fracture.

4. Sutures too narrow for the age or premature closure.

5. A smooth inner table with too few convolutional or vascular markings.

6. Thick cranial bones with endocranial laminated new bone formation. The diploic spaces may be widened and the internal diameter of the sella diminished.

7. Small cranium which is smaller than normal for the age and a low cranium-to-face ratio; a low sloping forehead.

8. A small sella turcica with massive dorsum and posterior clinoids.

9. Sinuses and mastoids hyperpneumatized with elevated petrous ridges.

10. Supraorbital ridge prominent.

11. Unilateral or local development of one or more of the above as a result of unilateral or local loss of content.

ROENTGEN SIGNS OF ABNORMALITY OF THE SKULL

The Small Skull

The *small skull* may be caused by
1. *Incomplete development of the brain* from any cause (microcrania and cerebral agenesis).
2. *Dwarfishness* (Nanosomia) of pituitary origin.
   a. Craniopharyngioma.
   b. Progeria.
3. *Craniostenosis.* When sutures are prematurely closed asymmetrically, plagiocephaly will result (see misshapen skull).

Special Radiographic Descriptions

Primary microcephaly. The superior orbital rims are high and circular in shape, the sutures are narrow but open, and the convolutional markings are decreased or absent.

Secondary microcephaly (Figure 12–13). There is a premature closure of several major sutures, and the orbits assume an ellipsoid configuration. There is a marked increase in the convolutional pattern of the cranial bones adjacent to the involved sutures.

Crouzon's dysostosis (Figure 12–14). The cranial vault is markedly distorted by premature sutural closure. The orbits are spread apart (hypertelorism), with associated exophthalmos. The maxillary facial bones are hypoplastic. The infant is mentally retarded.

The Enlarged Skull

The *enlarged skull* may be caused by:
1. *Hydrocephalus* from any cause (both obstructive and nonobstructive).
2. *Endocrine* disorders such as acromegaly.
3. *Congenital or developmental abnormalities* such as platybasia, osteogenesis imperfecta.

EFFECTS OF PREMATURE SYNOSTOSIS ON SKULL SHAPE

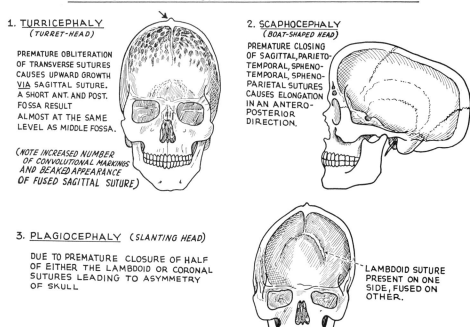

1. TURRICEPHALY
(TURRET-HEAD)

PREMATURE OBLITERATION
OF TRANSVERSE SUTURES
CAUSES UPWARD GROWTH
VIA SAGITTAL SUTURE.
A SHORT ANT. AND POST.
FOSSA RESULT
ALMOST AT THE SAME
LEVEL AS MIDDLE FOSSA.

*(NOTE INCREASED NUMBER
OF CONVOLUTIONAL MARKINGS
AND BEAKED APPEARANCE
OF FUSED SAGITTAL SUTURE)*

2. SCAPHOCEPHALY
(BOAT-SHAPED HEAD)

PREMATURE CLOSING
OF SAGITTAL, PARIETO-
TEMPORAL, SPHENO-
TEMPORAL, SPHENO-
PARIETAL SUTURES
CAUSES ELONGATION
IN AN ANTERO-
POSTERIOR
DIRECTION.

3. PLAGIOCEPHALY *(SLANTING HEAD)*

DUE TO PREMATURE CLOSURE OF HALF
OF EITHER THE LAMBDOID OR CORONAL
SUTURES LEADING TO ASYMMETRY
OF SKULL

LAMBDOID SUTURE
PRESENT ON ONE
SIDE, FUSED ON
OTHER.

A

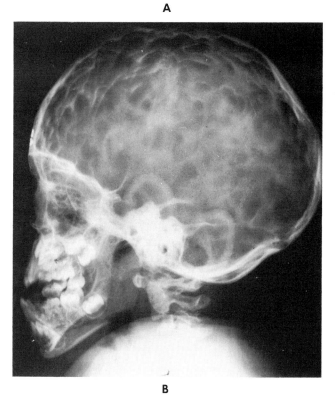

B

Figure 12–13 *A.* Effects of premature synostosis on skull shape. *B.* "Beaten brass" appearance of the skull in a patient with premature closure of sutures.

Figure 12–13 continued on opposite page.

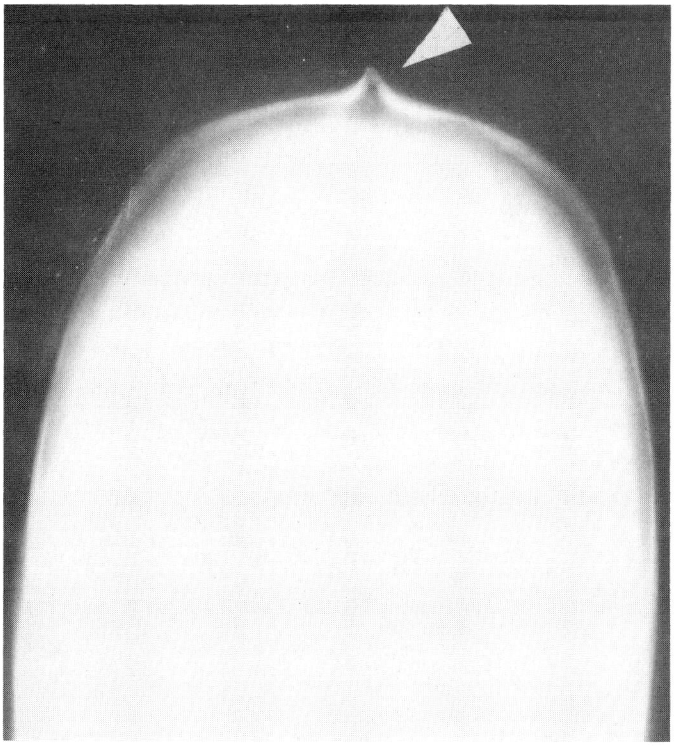

C

Figure 12–13 (*Continued*).   *C*. Coned down film of "beaked" appearance of prematurely closed sagittal suture.

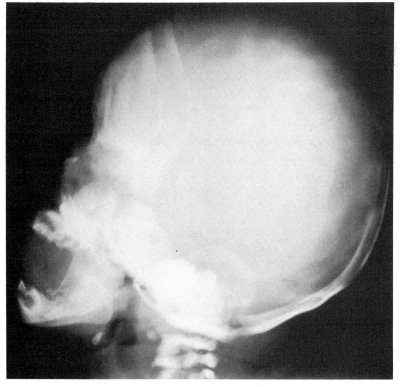

Figure 12–14   Skull in Crouzon's dysostosis.

4. *Deficiency states* such as rickets (where the skull is also deformed).
5. *Malformation of the bones* such as occurs in Paget's disease or fibrous dysplasia.
6. *Familial osteoectasia with macrocranium* (Bakwin et al.). In this syndrome the skull is markedly thickened with islands of increased density. The long bones are greatly expanded with intermixed osteoporosis and coarse trabeculation. There is a marked bowing of the lower extremities with thickened cortices on the concave aspects of the bowed bones.

Hydrocephalus

Definition.   Increased amount of cerebrospinal fluid in the ventriculo-subarachnoid pathways of the brain.

Pathogenesis.   Obstruction to flow or defective resorption of the cerebrospinal fluid. This is probably the most common cause, and the obstruction may be due to:

1. Anomalies, such as cerebral aqueduct stenosis; stenosis of the foramina of Magendie and Luschka; Arnold-Chiari malformations.

2. Infections resulting in meningitis (pyogens; tuberculosis; toxoplasmosis; torulosis).

3. Tumors.

4. Abscesses which may block the normal pathways of flow in the child or adult.

Classification

Hydrocephalus has been classified as *obstructive* when related to a specific obstructive process, and *nonobstructive* when caused by "overproduction" of cerebrospinal fluid. The latter must be exceedingly rare or nonexistent, except with choroid plexus papilloma.

Obstructive hydrocephalus has been defined as *internal* when related to obstruction within the ventricular or aqueductal system or *external* when the excess of fluid has occurred without demonstrable change in the ventricular system.

Hydrocephalus has also been called *communicating* when there is free access of fluid between the ventricles of the brain and the subarachnoid space but the fluid is prevented from circulating around the brain by the obstruction, and *noncommunicating* when the fluid is prevented from circulating around the brain as well as down the spinal subarachnoid pathway, because of an obstruction within the ventricular system, cerebral aqueduct, or the foramina of Luschka or Magendie.

Another classification recently proposed is the following (Davis and Farrell):

PRESSURE HYDROCEPHALUS

1. Decreased cerebrospinal fluid absorption.
   a. Ventricular blocks.
   b. Fourth ventricle outlet block.
   c. Incisional blocks.
   d. Brain convexity block.
   e. Arachnoid granulation block.
2. Increased cerebrospinal fluid production—rare except with choroid plexus papillomas.

NONPRESSURE HYDROCEPHALUS (hydrocephalus ex vacuo)

1. Cerebral atrophy.

Some people may have chronic hydrocephalus for many years, having achieved a dynamic equilibrium. This equilibrium may, however, be upset by any infection or metabolic disorder.

Hydrocephalus may be associated with intracranial hypertension; or even normal or low pressure. Low pressure hydrocephalus has received some attention in recent times, since it is thought to be treatable by shunting procedures (Greitz et al.).

Radiologic Features

INFANT. Before the sutures close, increased intracranial pressure produces definite expansion of the brain and the meninges, causing a marked diastasis of the sutures and enlargement of the head (Figure 12–15). The cerebral cortex and even the cranial bones may become very thin. The facial bones appear extremely small by comparison. The ventriculogram and angiogram of the brain have value in determining the cause of the hydrocephalus, and the

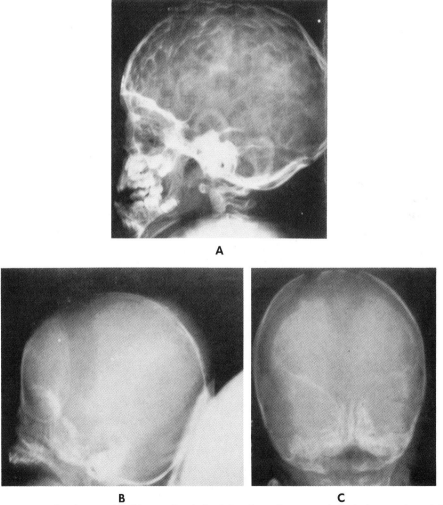

A

B   C

Figure 12–15 Craniostenosis with a turricephalic deformity and attempted surgical correction. *A*. Lateral view of skull. *B* and *C*. Lateral and A-P views of skull postoperatively with the artificial creation of expansion areas for the prematurely synostosed sutures. This child had no abnormal clinical manifestations as a result of this surgical intervention.

measurement of the thickness of the brain mantle which overlies the ventricles has value from a prognostic standpoint.

Radiographic features apart from diastasis of sutures and increased head size:

Hammered brass appearance of the bones of the calvarium (Figure 12–13). This is due to the pulsatile effect of the brain, which is under great tension. This appearance may be reversible with correction of the cause of the increased intracranial pressure. Occasionally this appearance is seen in thin skulls without hydrocephalus; or in mild form normally in young people under sixteen years of age. This appearance should not be confused with that of craniolacunia (Lückenschädel), in which there is no association with the convolutions of the brain and there is a mesodermal defect in ossification.

Abnormal vascular impressions in the bones of the calvarium.

Erosions of the calvarium, or bone replacement processes.

Elevation of the periosteum, at times producing a "sun-ray" appearance just outside the external diploë (Figure 12–17).

Abnormal calcifications within the brain or meninges may be associated (Figure 12–16).

(Ordinarily the sella turcica is not eroded in the infant, since the sutural diastasis is sufficient to make way for the bulging brain and meninges, and the sella does not undergo pressure deossification.)

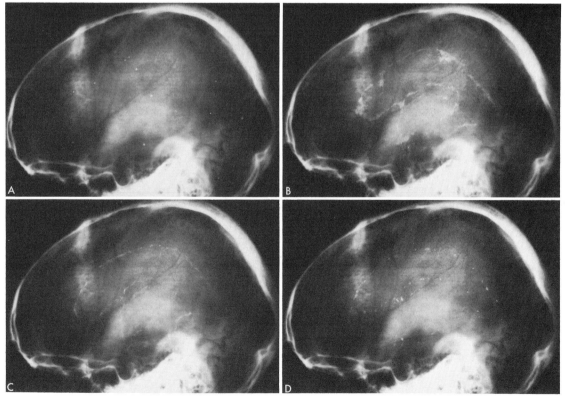

Figure 12–16 *A* to *D*. Paraventricular intracerebral calcification such as is often produced by parasitic diseases, such as toxoplasmosis, trichinosis, cysticercosis, or torulosis. (Intensified diagrammatic radiographs.)

Figure 12–16 continued on opposite page.

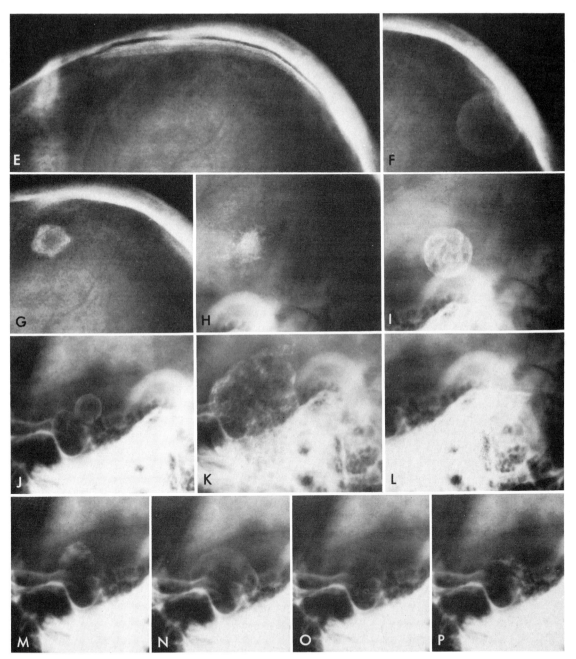

Figure 12–16 (*Continued*). Various appearances of abnormal intracranial calcification. *E.* Subdural hematoma. *F.* Calcified cysts, such as an echinococcus or hydatid cyst. *G.* Tuberculoma; also endarteritis calcificans cerebri. *H.* Astrocytoma; tuberculoma. *I.* Pinealoma. *J.* Carotid artery aneurysm. *K.* Craniopharyngioma; calcified chordoma. *L.* Coarse calcium in medulloblastoma or ependymoma of fourth ventricle. *M.* Tuberculous meningitis (nodular parasellar); craniopharyngioma. *N.* Cystlike calcium in wall of aneurysm of internal carotid artery. *O.* Intrasellar calcification, without enlarged sella; degenerate pituitary adenoma. *P.* Craniopharyngioma. (Intensified diagrammatic radiographs.)

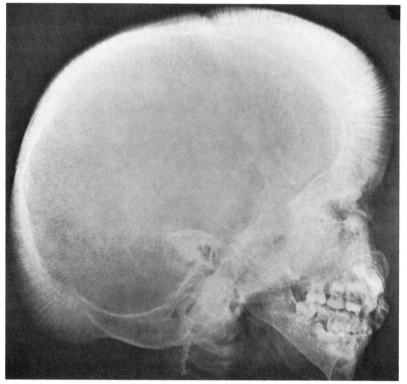

Figure 12–17 Lateral view of skull in thalassemia major, demonstrating "sun-ray" appearance just outside the external diploë.

ADOLESCENT. The hammered brass appearance may persist normally until approximately 16 years of age (Figure 12–18). In children over seven years of age sutural diastasis requires increasingly greater pressure, and erosion of the sella turcica may appear. Ordinarily the extrasellar erosion causes a gradual disappearance of the dorsum sellae, and dissolution of the posterior clinoids. Sharpening of the anterior clinoids may also result (Figure 12–19). The depth of the sella turcica may also increase, although "true ballooning" of the sella is more apt to occur with **intrasellar** expanding lesions.

ADULT. The same findings occur as those described for the infant except that:

The hammered brass appearance when it occurs is abnormal.

The pineal, being calcified in many adults, may be displaced, particularly if there is an associated tumor.

Hyperostosis may accompany the hypervascularity or erosion of the calvarium.

Elevation of the outer periosteum is less apt to occur, but may be present in local areas overlying a tumor.

Erosion of the sella turcica as described due to extrasellar pressure phenomena is more apt to occur than in the infant or young person.

Dilated ventricles may be associated with cerebral atrophy or infarction with no manifestations on plain film studies of the skull.

Abnormal intracranial calcification (see section on brain), particularly if there is an associated infectious process.

Erosion of foramina, such as optic, internal auditory, foramen ovale, jugular.

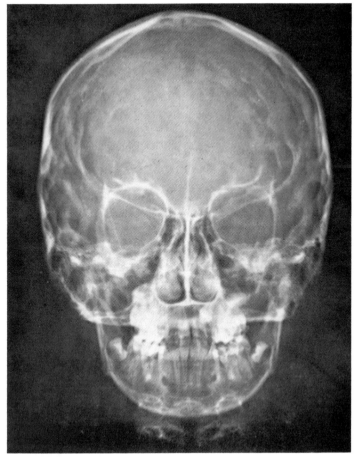

Figure 12–18   Accentuated convolutional pattern in the skull of a young person, considered to be within normal limits.

SKULL AND UPPER CERVICAL SPINE ABNORMALITIES
IN ARNOLD-CHIARI MALFORMATION (Kruyff and Jeffs)

1. Foramen magnum enlargement in 71 per cent of cases. (Kruyff and Jeffs.)

2. Scalloping of the posterior medial aspect of the petrous bases (65 per cent of cases).

3. Flatness of the floor of the posterior fossa with a shallow posterior fossa and a low position in the inion (41 per cent).

4. All three of the above occur in 39 per cent; normality occurs in 25 per cent; and 36 per cent will show one or more of the above three elements.

5. Enlarged spinal canal of C-1 and C-2 elements.

6. Vertebral artery is seen lying in a deep groove of the pons but this requires angiogram for demonstration.

7. May have scalloping of the basiocciput.

8. The transverse sinus may appear to be displaced inferiorly running near the rim of the foramen magnum.

9. For pneumographic changes see Gooding et al.

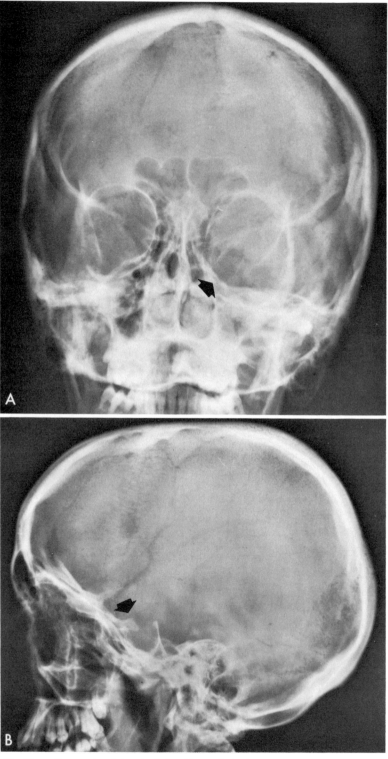

Figure 12–19 Neurofibroma involving the left orbit. *A.* P-A view of the orbit showing erosion of the orbit inferiorly with the left orbit being larger than the right. The superior orbital fissure has lost its normal anatomic demarcation. There is a tendency to sclerosis of the supraorbital ridge and thinning of the medial wall of the orbit. Note the asymmetrical appearance also of the infraorbital plates bilaterally. *B.* Lateral view of the skull demonstrating the increased depth of the sella turcica on the affected side with erosion of the anterior clinoids and some thinning of the dorsum sellae. There is some asymmetrical erosion of the sphenoid ridge on the affected side also.

NORMAL MEASUREMENTS (width and length in millimeters of the foramen magnum in normal and Arnold-Chiari skulls)
(Kruyff and Jeffs)

	Age in Years	Sex	Width	Length
Normal	1–3	Female	31 ± 3 mm.	39 ± 4.5 mm.
	1–3	Male	31 ± 2.5	40 ± 5.4
	3–7	Female	34 ± 2.4	39 ± 4.8
	3–7	Male	34 ± 2.4	43 ± 3.7
	7 and greater	Female	35 ± 2.8	44 ± 3.5
Arnold-	1–3	Female	36 ± 4	50 ± 7
Chiari	1–3	Male	38 ± 3.8	46 ± 7
	3–7	Female	43 ± 4.6	51 ± 6.4
	3–7	Male	44 ± 3	51 ± 5.3
	7 and greater	Female	46 ± 5	52 ± 4.8
		Male	46 ± 3.4	54 ± 4.8

40 degree half-axial view in supine position for the width measurement. Magnification 25 per cent. For length measurements, focus-object 75 cm. Object-film distance 15 cm. Magnification 20 per cent.

Some Disease Entities Associated with Hydrocephalus

Arnold-Chiari Malformation

Definition. Congenital elongation of the cerebellum and brain stem into the cervical spinal canal, often associated with a meningocele. The foramina of Magendie and Luschka lie below the foramen magnum, and the lumen of the fourth ventricle is almost obliterated.

Associated Lesions. Meningocele; dense fibrous adhesions binding the meningocele to a vertebral defect; hydrocephalus; microgyria; craniolacunia; hydromyelia; platybasia; cerebral aqueduct stenosis.

Radiographic Findings (Figure 12–20)

PLAIN FILMS. Nonspecific skull findings of hydrocephalus. Cervical spine shows wide upper cervical canal and a large foramen magnum.

VENTRICULOGRAMS (Gooding et al.; Davies)

Diverticulum-like structure extending anteriorly from the third ventricle. A large massa intermedia, sometimes exceeding 12 mm. in diameter.

Partial absence of the septum pellucidum, especially anteriorly, with a fusion of the lateral ventricles.

The inferior margins of the lateral ventricles at the foramina of Monro may be sharply pointed and medially directed.

ANGIOGRAMS (Scatliff et al.)

Signs related to dilated midline ventricles supratentorially: sweeping of anterior cerebral artery complex; displacement laterally of striothalamic veins with reversal of convexity.

"Fish-hook" displacement of basilar artery at its upper end posteriorly.

Arnold-Chiari Malformation

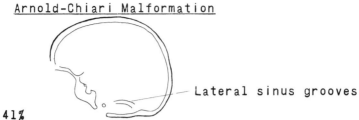

41%

Lateral view of skull showing:
1. Flat floor of posterior fossa
2. Low lateral sinuses
3. Large foramen magnum (71 %)
4. Scalloped petrous bones (65%)

A

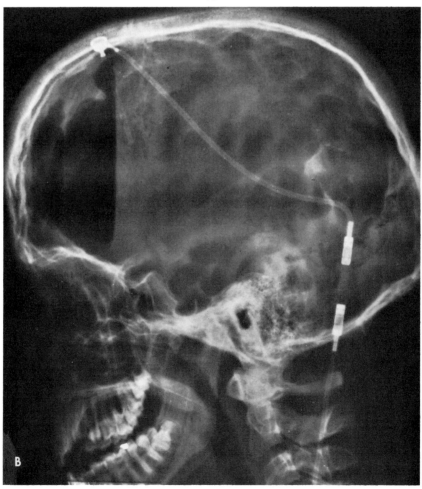

Figure 12-20   *A*. Skull in Arnold-Chiari malformation. *B*. Radiograph.

Dandy-Walker Syndrome

Definition.   Congenital malformation of the cerebellar vermis with gross dilatation of the fourth ventricle. There is nearly always an atresia of the foramen of Magendie and in many cases there is also an atresia of the foramina of Luschka.

Radiographic Findings

PLAIN FILMS.   Elevation of the transverse sinuses; outward bulging of the occipital bones with associated thinning (pressure from the dilated fourth ventricle); considerable separation of the lambdoid suture (Figure 12–21).

VENTRICULOGRAMS.   Enormous cystlike structure in the posterior fossa representing the dilated fourth ventricle. Elevation of the posterior part of the temporal horns and occipital horns of the lateral ventricles. Dilatation of the lateral and third ventricles.

ANGIOGRAMS

Signs related to dilated midline supratentorial ventricles as described previously.

Displacement of posterior fossa arteries and veins by the cystlike fourth ventricle (Huang and Wolf; Mani and Newton).

Cerebral Aqueduct Stenosis

Definition.   Stenosis of the aqueduct of Sylvius from any cause—congenital, traumatic, inflammatory, or neoplastic. It may appear early or late in life. In 88 patients reported by Schechter and Zingesser, 22 were under 5, and 19 were 31 years of age or older. Five of the patients were older than 51.

Radiographic Findings

PLAIN FILMS (Figure 12–22)

Early in life: Hydrocephalus occurs, and the head may increase in size with sudden rapidity. Sutural diastasis. After seven years of age there is erosion

(Text continued on page 478)

DANDY-WALKER CYSTS

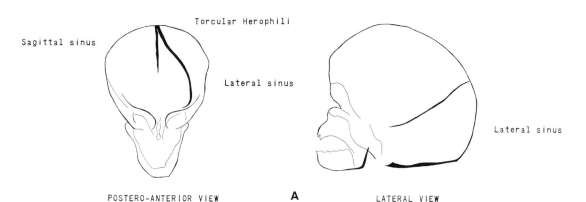

POSTERO-ANTERIOR VIEW   **A**   LATERAL VIEW

Figure 12–21   *A.* Skull in Dandy-Walker syndrome.
Figure 12–21 continued on following page.

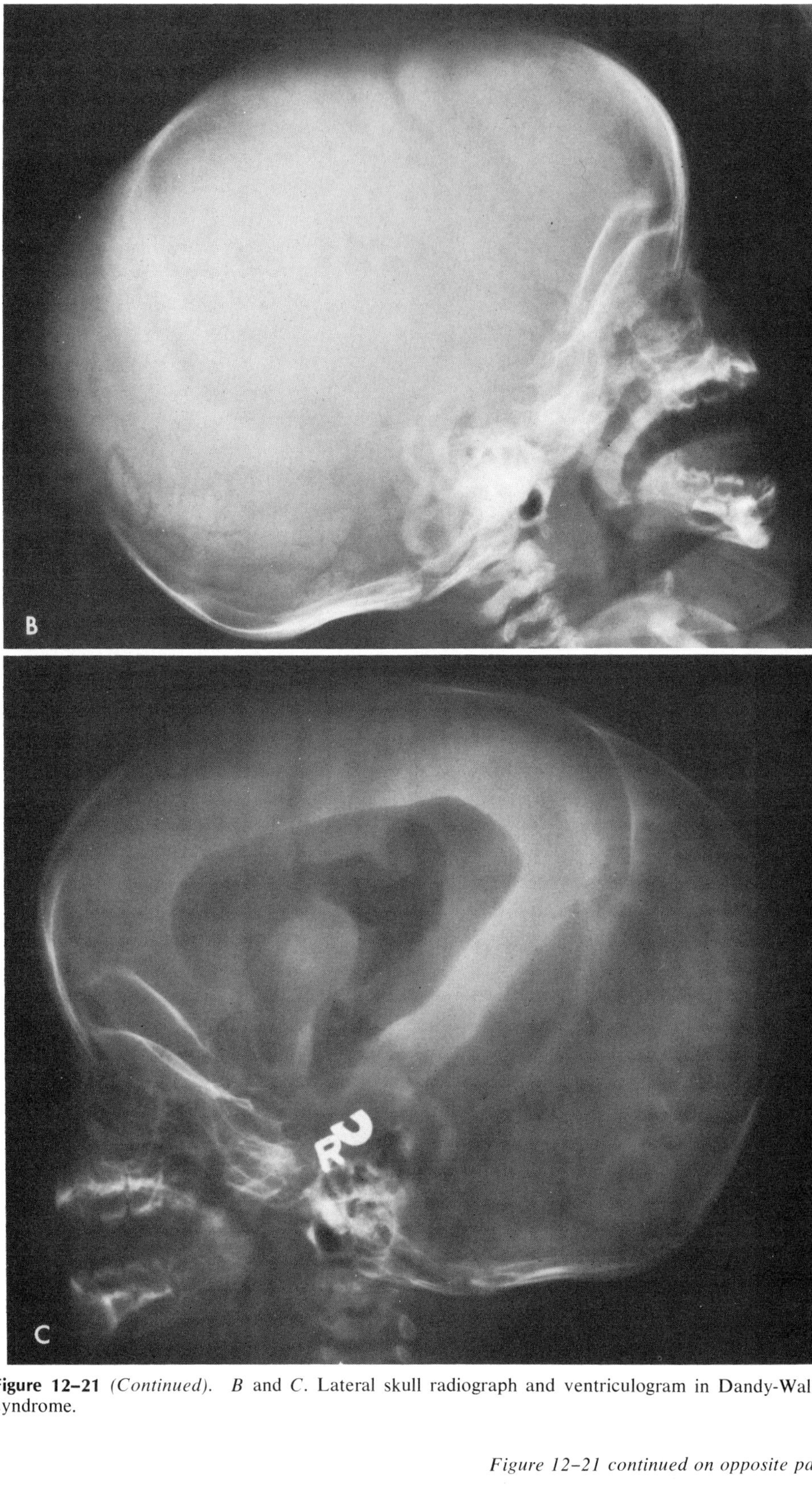

Figure 12–21 *(Continued).* *B* and *C*. Lateral skull radiograph and ventriculogram in Dandy-Walker syndrome.

Figure 12–21 continued on opposite page.

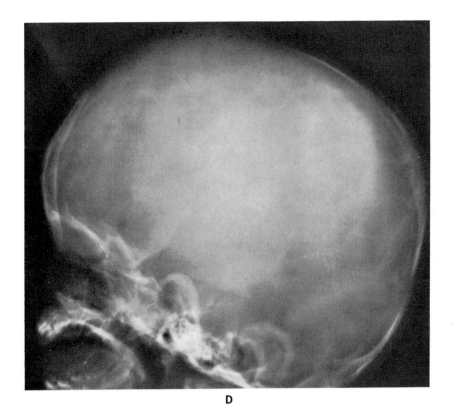

D

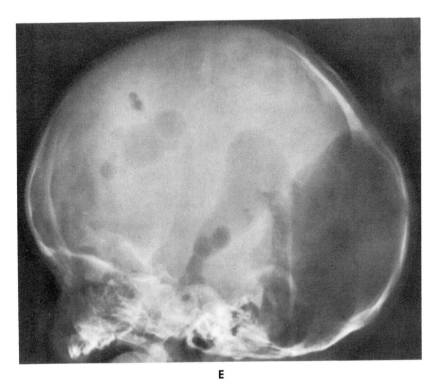

E

Figure 12–21 (*Continued*).   *D* and *E*. Skull with posterior fossa arachnoid cyst simulating Dandy-Walker syndrome, filled with air.

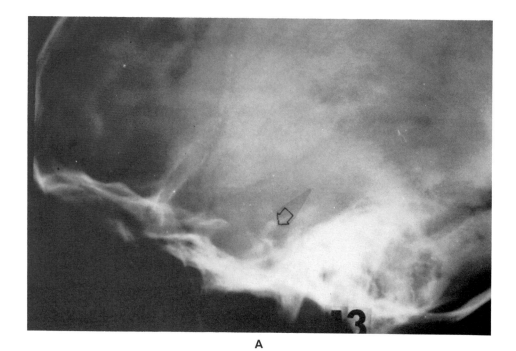

A

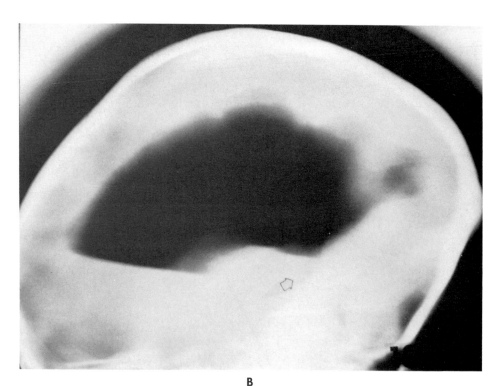

B

Figure 12–22   Cerebral aqueduct stenosis with rhinorrhea. *A*. Plain film of skull showing erosion of the dorsum and tuberculum sellae. *B*. Pneumogram showing tremendous dilatation of the lateral ventricle with very minimal air in the fourth ventricle and the cerebral aqueduct stenosis (*arrow*).

Figure 12–22 continued on opposite page.

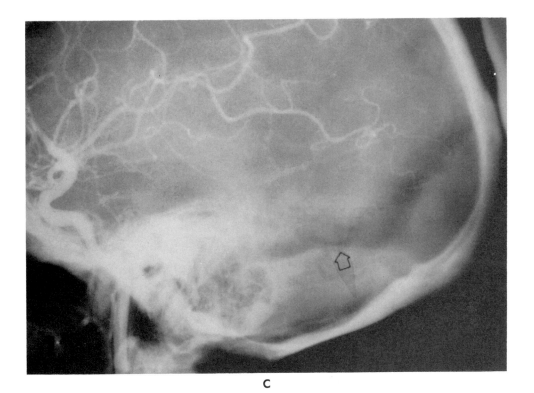

C

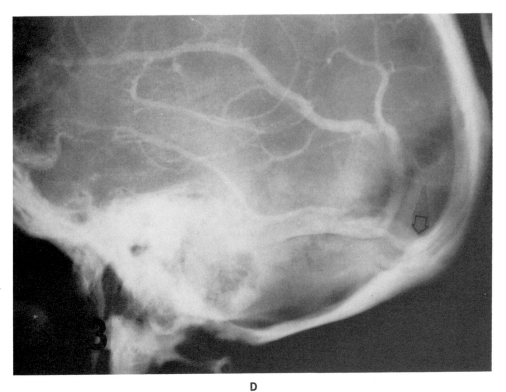

D

Figure 12–22 (*Continued*).   *C.* Arteriogram phase showing a shallow posterior fossa and the low-set internal occipital protuberance. *D.* Venogram phase showing the low-lying transverse and sigmoid sinus.

Figure 12–22 continued on following page.

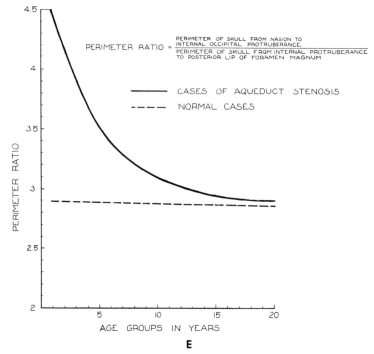

E

Figure 12–22 (*Continued*). *E.* The "perimeter ratio" as an indicator of cerebral aqueduct stenosis. (From Schechter, M. M., and Zingesser, L. H.: Radiology, *88*:905–916, 1967.)

of the dorsum sellae. Enlargement of the channel for the emissary veins in the occipital bones is frequent.

Early or late in life: The inion is at a relatively low level. The lateral and sigmoidal sinuses also appear low in position.

Calcifications: If caused by an inflammatory lesion such as toxoplasmosis, there may be paraventricular calcifications. Varix ("aneurysm") of the vein of Galen may be associated with calcification. Neoplasms impressing themselves on the cerebral aqueduct may also be calcified.

VENTRICULOGRAMS

Dilated lateral and third ventricles above the occluded or stenotic cerebral aqueduct. Air injected intraspinally will show the fourth ventricle to be small. The configurations of the cerebral aqueduct have been catalogued by Schechter and Zingesser. There is no herniation of cerebellar tonsils.

Spontaneous ventriculostomy with cerebrospinal fluid rhinorrhea may occur in the adult.

ANGIOGRAMS

Signs of dilated lateral ventricles as described previously.

Unlike Dandy-Walker syndrome, the fourth ventricle is small.

Unlike Arnold-Chiari malformation, the upper cervical spinal canal is normal in size and does not contain herniated branches of the posterior inferior cerebellar arteries.

Paget's Disease of the Skull (Osteitis deformans) (Figure 12–23)

Definition. Acquired disorder of bone characterized by destruction and the formation of bizarre replacement bone which appears *expanded,* soft, poorly mineralized, and disorganized. It may be monostotic or polyostotic.

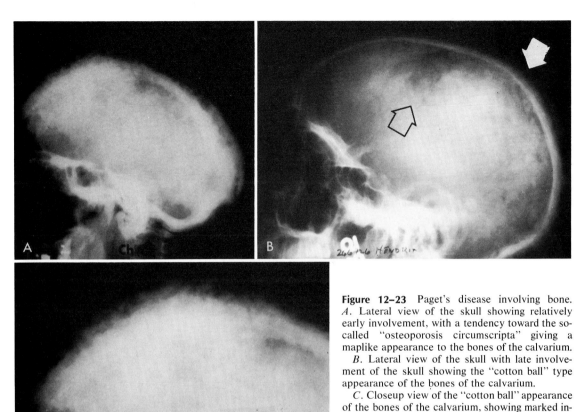

Figure 12–23 Paget's disease involving bone. *A.* Lateral view of the skull showing relatively early involvement, with a tendency toward the so-called "osteoporosis circumscripta" giving a maplike appearance to the bones of the calvarium.

B. Lateral view of the skull with late involvement of the skull showing the "cotton ball" type appearance of the bones of the calvarium.

C. Closeup view of the "cotton ball" appearance of the bones of the calvarium, showing marked involvement of all the layers of the calvarium with thickening of the diploë and marked irregularity of both the inner and outer table. The outer table at times has a shell-like appearance.

Incidence. Males to females two to one after the age of 35 years usually. Order of frequency: pelvis, skull, femur, spine, tibia, humerus, scapula, and rarely in other bones, such as mandible (Robbins).

Clinical Aspects. The involved bones tend to be enlarged and soft, bending under pressure or weight. There is a predisposition to fracture and sarcoma. Sarcoma is reported in 7.5 to 25 per cent, especially in the following locations: femur, humerus, pelvis, skull, tibia, and scapula (Freydinger et al.). There is often an increased blood flow in the involved bones, and vascular malformations may be associated, leading to cardiac hypertrophy and congestive failure in some cases (Reifenstein and Albright).

Radiologic Aspects

SKULL. Irregularly thickened, with scattered areas of involvement in the calvarium and facial bones. The outer table and diploë are most affected. There is a maplike or geographic resorption of the bone giving the appearance described as "osteoporosis circumscripta." Later the inner table may also be involved. Still later, there is a bizarre deposition of new bone in multiple, irregular patchy areas giving rise to the so-called "cotton ball" appearance. The tables and diploë ultimately become markedly thickened and the base of the skull may be so softened by the process, that a basilar impression supervenes. The sella turcica may appear small. Sarcomatous degeneration may occur.

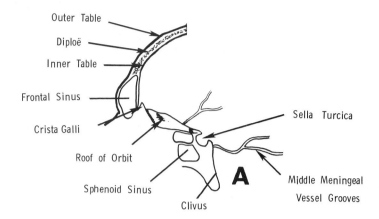

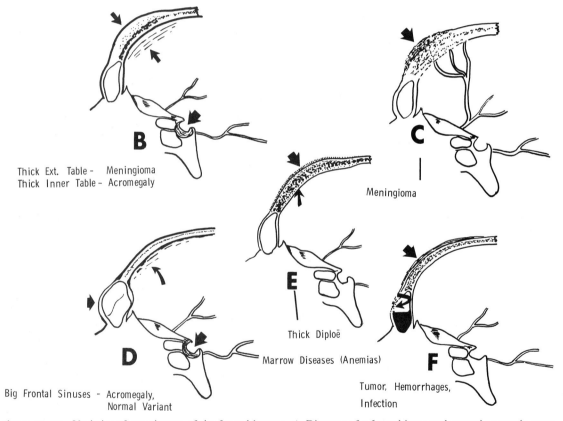

Figure 12–24   Varieties of prominence of the frontal bossae. *A.* Diagram of a frontal bone and normal anatomic parts. *B.* The thick external table as well as the internal table with erosion of the sella turcica such as might occur with either a meningioma or acromegaly. *C.* Illustrates what might occur with a meningioma. *D.* Possible results of a frontal sinus osteomyelitis. *E.* Prominence of the frontal bossae that may occur with marrow disorders such as anemia. *F.* Marked thickening of the periosteum with partial destruction of the inner or outer table (or both) resulting from hemorrhage, infection, or tumor.

Abnormalities in Contour of the Skull

LOCALIZED FRONTAL OR PARIETAL BONE "BOSSING" OR PROMINENCE
(Figure 12–24 through Figure 12–29). Some of the entities producing the roentgen appearance of undue prominence of frontal bossae are illustrated in Figure 12–24. Others in this gamut are as follows:

Thalassemia Major (plus hepato- and splenomegaly). Early, both the inner and outer tables of the skull are markedly thinned. Later, the diploë is increased in width several times, although the tables remain thin. Thin hairlike spicules of bone radiate perpendicularly to the outer table, especially in the parietal and frontal areas.

Sickle Cell Anemia. The diploë may be thickened almost to complete obliteration, but fine spicules may be seen radiating from the outer table (Figure 12–25).

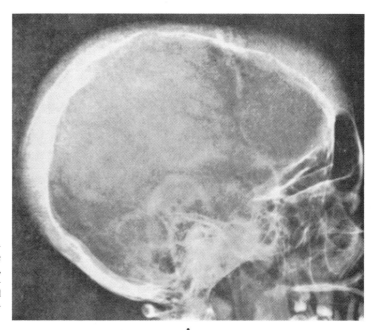

Figure 12–25 *A*. Skull in sickle cell anemia. (From Moseley, J. E.: *Bone Changes in Hematologic Disorders.* New York, Grune and Stratton, 1963.) *B*. Osteomyelitis of the frontal bone. The marked opacity of the frontal sinuses is also demonstrated.

A

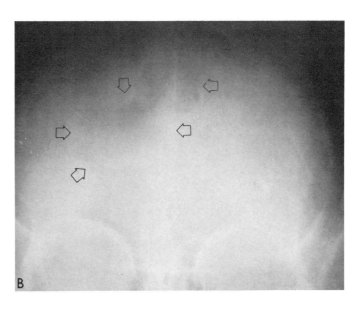

B

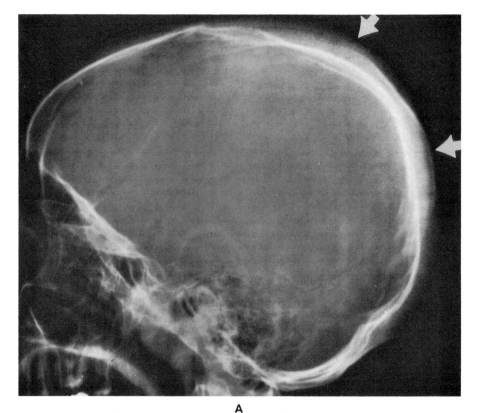

A

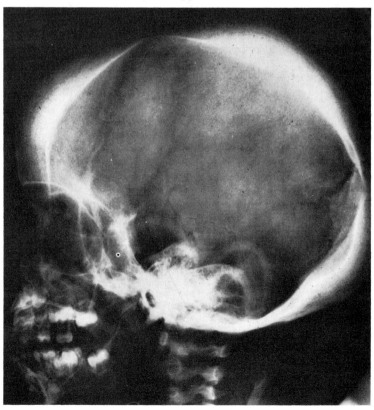

B

Figure 12–26   *A*. Lateral view of skull in hemolytic anemia. *B*. Skull in iron deficiency anemia. (Part *B* from Moseley, J. E.: Amer. J. Roentgenol., *8*:649, 1961.)

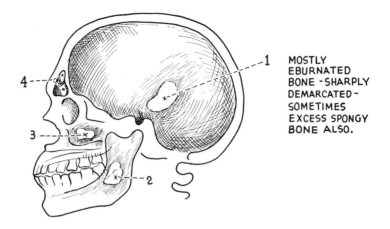

MOSTLY
EBURNATED
BONE - SHARPLY
DEMARCATED -
SOMETIMES
EXCESS SPONGY
BONE ALSO.

<u>COMMON SITES:</u>
1. CALVARIUM
2. MANDIBLE
3. MAXILLA ⎫ INCLUDING
4. FRONTAL BONES ⎭ PARANASAL
SINUSES

A

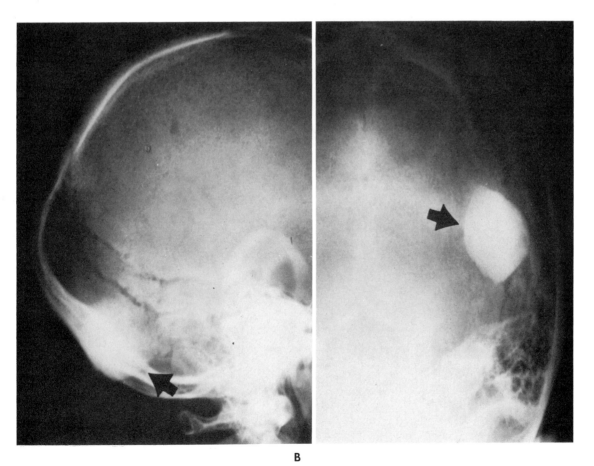

B

Figure 12–27 Osteoma of the calvarium. *A.* The most frequent sites and general appearance. *B.* Osteoma of the occipital bone as it adjoins the temporal bone.

Congenital Hemolytic Anemias in Infancy.   There is increased proliferation of the hemopoietic tissue in the skull with resultant widening of the diploë. The outer table is displaced externally and is often thin, tapering toward the edges of the frontal and parietal bones, producing a prominence of the frontal and parietal bossae. Occasionally, the diploic trabeculae assume a position perpendicular to the inner table, presenting a pattern which is referred to as a "hair-standing-on-end" appearance (Moseley) (Figure 12–26).

Erythroid Hyperplasia, with cyanotic congenital heart disease, polycythemia vera and secondary polycythemia. Somewhat similar skull changes have been reported. (See Figure 12–26.)

Gaucher's Disease.   Similar changes reported (Moseley). (See Figure 12–26.)

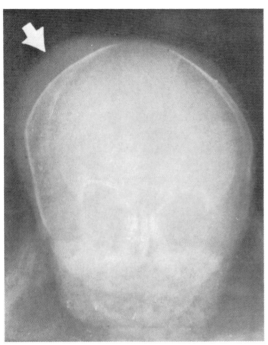

Figure 12–28   *A*. Cephalohematoma, showing soft tissue elevation of the scalp. *B*. Calcified cephalohematoma in an infant. *C*. Magnified view of previous calcified cephalohematoma.

A

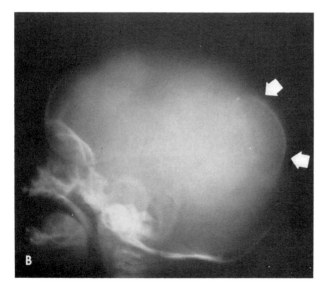

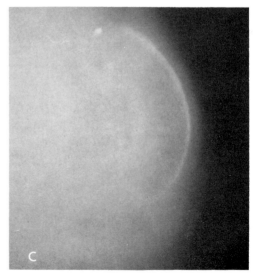

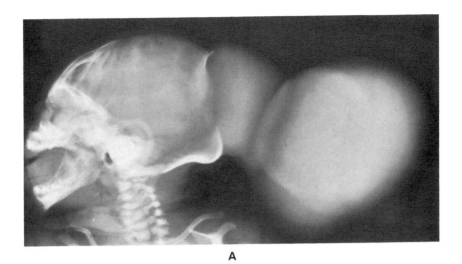

A

B

Figure 12–29 *A*. Skull with encephalocele. *B*. Caldwell view of another patient showing frontal bone defect. (Courtesy of Dr. Nitaya Suwanwela.)

Osteomas (Figure 12–27).   May involve the bones of the calvarium or face. They produce a localized prominence, protruding inward or outward.

Cephalohematoma (Figure 12–28).   An extravasation of blood between the periosteum and the external bony surface of the calvarium, especially in the newborn as the result of a traumatic delivery or hemorrhagic disease. The parietal bone is the most frequent site. Ossification of the clot may occur if it is not absorbed in two or three weeks. The underlying bone may undergo resorption which may persist throughout life.

Meningocele and Encephalocele (Figure 12–29)

Definition.   A cranial meningocele is a herniation of the meninges with associated cerebrospinal fluid through a defect in the skull. In an encephalocele there is also a herniation of the brain. It may occur anteriorly in the vicinity of the nasion, at the anterior fontanelle, in the occipital region, or rarely along the skull base.

Radiographic Findings.   Rounded soft tissue density with smooth, sharply defined borders and **an associated defect in the occipital or frontal bone.** Pneumoencephalography is valuable in demonstrating the presence or absence of subarachnoid air within the herniation.

LOCALIZED DEPRESSIONS IN THE CALVARIUM OR BASE OF THE SKULL

Depressed Skull Fracture (Figure 12–30)

Classification.   Depressed skull fractures may be either comminuted or compound but not linear.

Radiographic Findings.   Fracture lines are usually sharp and straight, unlike the tortuous appearance of sutures and the undulating appearance of vascular grooves. Overlapping bone margins of a depressed fracture usually appear "whiter" than the surrounding bone. It is well to show these in tangential view if at all possible. Stereoscopic views are also helpful. Recent fractures are characterized by their distinctness, unlike old fractures whose margins become relatively smooth. Healing is usually slow over a period of months or years. Depressed fractures usually involve both inner and outer table and diploë.

Platybasia

Definition.   Flattening of the base of the skull with an increase in the basal angle (Figure 12–31). This may coexist with a basilar impression which is a separate entity and is an anomaly of the occipitocervical junction where the upper cervical segments and foramen magnum protrude into the cranial cavity. Klippel-Feil syndrome or Arnold-Chiari malformation may coexist also.

Platybasia may be congenital or acquired as the result of rickets, Paget's disease, hyperparathyroidism, osteomalacia, or osteogenesis imperfecta.

Clinically there is a close resemblance to multiple sclerosis, spastic paralysis, syringomyelia, and adult Arnold-Chiari with adhesions.

Radiographic Findings (Figure 12–31)

In Towne's projection there is a protrusion of the occipital condyles into the posterior fossa.

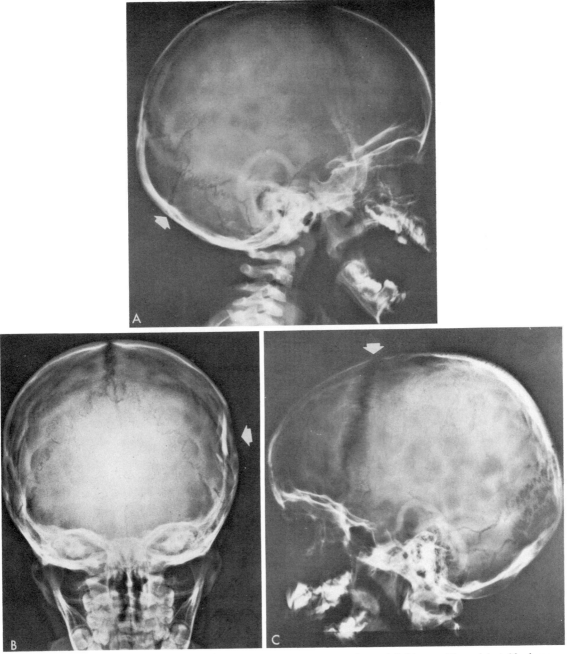

Figure 12–30 *A*. Lateral view of skull demonstrating a linear fracture of the occipital bone with no detectable depression of fragment. The appearance of the lambdoid suture for comparison is well demonstrated. *B*. Depressed fracture of the left parietal bone and adjoining squamous portion of temporal bone. A good tangential view is usually necessary to demonstrate the exact degree of depression. *C*. Lateral view of skull demonstrating diastasis of coronal suture.

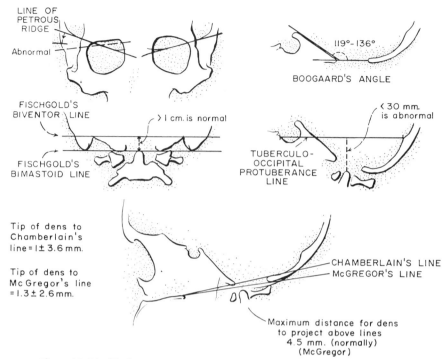

Figure 12-31 Various roentgen criteria for platybasia and basilar impression.

A straight postero-anterior view of the skull shows that a line drawn along the superior margins of the petrous ridges is angulated cephalad.

Decrease of the basal angle below 120 degrees.

Straight lateral view of the skull and upper cervical spine shows Chamberlain's line or McGregor's line (see Figure 12–31) is abnormal.

On straight postero-anterior laminograms of the skull through the mastoid process the bimastoid and biventer lines of Fischgold are abnormal (see Figure 12–31).

Unfortunately, the variations of the normal in respect to all of these lines and criteria are such as to make the diagnosis difficult at times.

Paget's Disease of Bone has been described previously.

Abnormalities of Density of the Bones of the Calvarium

DIFFUSE RADIOLUCENCY

Cleidocranial Dysostosis

Definition. Congenital deficiency in the intramembranous ossification of the bones of the calvarium, with defective formation and ossification of the clavicles.

Radiographic Appearances (Figure 12–32)

There is a defective ossification of the bones of the skull, giving rise to large fontanelles, numerous wormian bones, limited union of the frontal bone at the metopic suture, deficient ossification in the symphysis of the mandible, and diffuse radiolucency. Hypoplasia of the sinuses and prognathism are common.

Other bones are also affected as illustrated; the pubes and ischia are incompletely ossified, the clavicles are incompletely developed, the thorax is narrow, and the phalanges develop curious shapes.

Osteogenesis Imperfecta

Definition. Deficient endochondral and periosteal structure so that the long tubular bones are extremely thin, fragile, and deficient in their mineral structure. Blue sclerae and deafness from otosclerosis are often associated.

Clinical Types

Osteogenesis imperfecta congenita, with multiple prenatal as well as intrapartum fractures and failing ossification of the skull.

Osteogenesis imperfecta tarda, or osteopsathyrosis. This in turn may be of two types: (1) fractures appearing at birth and throughout life, and (2) fractures first appearing at two or three years of age, declining in frequency at puberty (Elefant and Tosovsky; McKusick).

Radiographic Appearances

The calvarium is markedly thinned and radiolucent with enlarged sutures and multiple wormian bones which give a jigsaw pattern to the skull.

The bones tend to be thin and often long, at times appearing bent and deformed from numerous fractures which have healed or are healing.

Hyperparathyroidism

Definition. Hyperactivity of the parathyroid glands with resultant hypercalcemia, excessive excretion of calcium and osteoporotic bone changes which may be localized or generalized. The bone changes range from a localized bone cyst to osteitis fibrosa cystica.

Radiographic Appearances (Figure 12–33)

As the bones of the cranial vault undergo demineralization, there is a loss of demarcation between the tables and diploë, and the bones assume a stippled appearance—"salt and pepper osteoporosis."

The lamina dura around the teeth becomes resorbed, although this finding may be caused by other diseases, such as Paget's disease, the histiocytoses, and inflammations.

The changes previously described for renal rickets develop in the long tubular bones.

With resorption of the medullary spaces and cortical bone throughout the body the bones become thin, subject to pathologic fracture, and often are the sites of cystic changes—the so-called "brown tumors" of osteitis fibrosa cystica.

Occasionally, the skull appearance is that of multiple sharply circumscribed lucencies resembling tumor metastases or multiple myeloma.

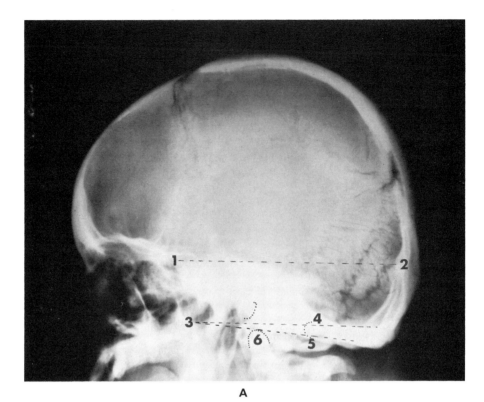

A

Figure 12–32 Radiographs of the skull in a patient with flattening of the base of the skull in cleidocranial dysostosis. Note that the Boogaard's angle of the basi-sphenoid with the foramen magnum is difficult to identify and partially reversed. Line *1–2* represents the tuberculo-occipital protuberance line and does actually lie in excess of 30 mm. above the odontoid process, *6*. Line *3–4*, Chamberlain's line, and line *3–5*, McGregor's line, are probably within normal limits, although the base of the skull appears to be flattened and overhangs posteriorly in the region of the occiput.

Figure 12–32 continued on opposite page.

Neuroblastoma (Figure 12–34)

Definition. Sympathicoblastoma originating in the cells of the sympathetic nervous system, most frequently in those from the adrenal gland.

Radiographic Appearances

The tumor metastasizes widely to the skeleton, liver, and lymph nodes. In the skull metastases are most numerous adjoining sutures. The inner and outer tables of the skull become poorly defined, so that they virtually merge.

Radiating spicules from the outer table of the skull have the appearance of "hair-on-end."

Metastases to the meninges, with invasion of the calvarium are also responsible for some of the appearance in the bones of the calvarium.

Increased intracranial pressure produces erosion of the dorsum sellae and spreading of the sutures additionally.

The metastases tend to concentrate in the ends of long bones but very rarely in the carpals or phalanges, simulating osteomyelitis.

In the bones of the pelvis the trabeculae become coarse and spongy.

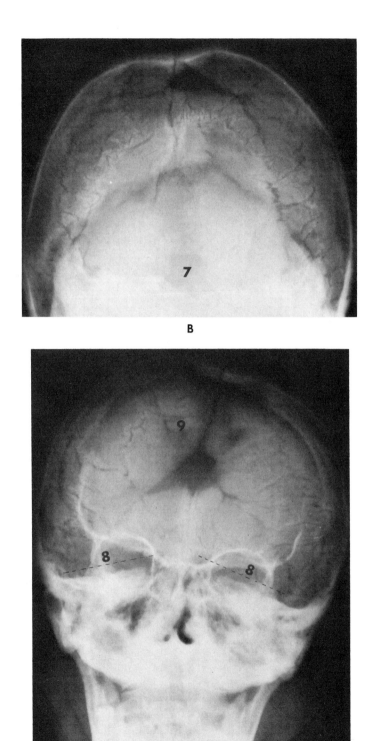

Figure 12–32 (*Continued*).   *B. 7* is the diminutive foramen magnum. *C. 8* shows the reversal of the angulation of the lines of the petrous ridges, and *9*, the innumerable wormian bones with widely patent fontanelles projected in this immediate vicinity.

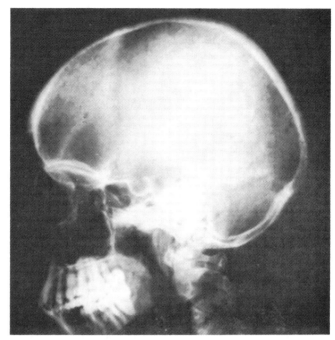

Figure 12–33   Radiograph of the skull of a patient with hyperparathyroidism due to a parathyroid adenoma. The ossification of the skull is so markedly diminished that radiography is difficult and reproduction necessarily suffers.

DEMARCATED AREAS OF RADIOLUCENCY IN THE BONES OF THE CALVARIUM

Fracture (Figure 12–30)

Classification.   Linear, compound, comminuted, depressed.

Radiographic Appearances

Jagged discontinuity in the bones of the calvarium — unlike sutures which appear serrated — and undulating vascular impressions. When a linear fracture has produced a separation of sutures it is called "diastasis of the sutures."

Multiple views of the skull are necessary for greatest accuracy, and at best fractures of the base of the skull may be very difficult to detect. Stereoscopic views are recommended.

See previous description of depressed fractures.

Leptomeningeal Cyst (Figure 12–35)

Definition.   Post-traumatic cyst of the meninges which has produced an erosion of the calvarium locally, usually in association with a fracture.

Cerebral leptomeningeal cysts may not only be of traumatic origin but of idiopathic or developmental origin as well. These are rare but do occur (Wilson and Bertan).

Radiographic Appearances.   Sharply circumscribed lucency especially involving the inner table of the calvarium first, with some persistence of the frac-

NEUROBLASTOMA

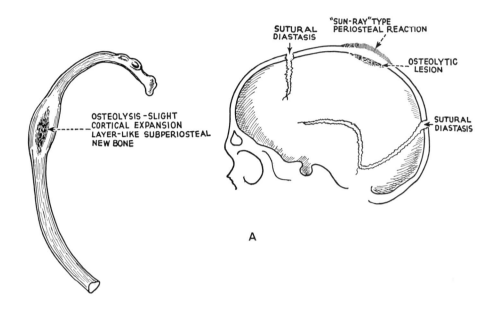

A

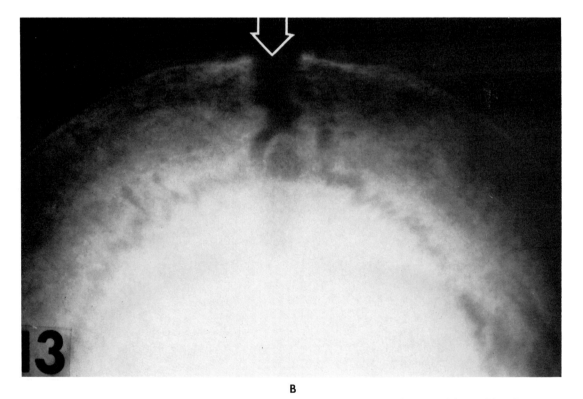

B

Figure 12–34   *A*. Salient roentgen pathologic features of neuroblastoma. *B*. Neuroblastoma of the skull in a five year old child. Close-up view to demonstrate the marked diastasis of the sutures (open arrow) and the lysis of the calvarium due to meningeal involvement by the neuroblastoma.

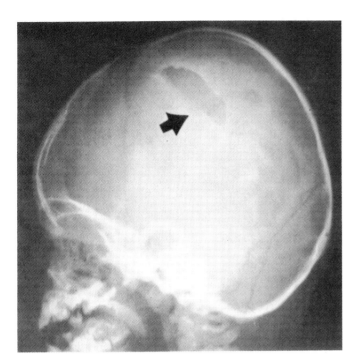

Figure 12–35 Leptomeningeal cyst. (A similar entity involving the orbit has been called a "growing fracture of the orbit.")

ture line and resorption of bone along the old disunited fracture. There is no zone of sclerosis around the lucency.

Osteomyelitis of the Bones of the Calvarium

Classification

Pyogenic (acute or chronic); syphilitic; tuberculous; or fungal (actinomycosis, coccidioidomycosis; blastomycosis; or cryptococcosis, very rarely).

Radiologic Appearances

Early: Area of diminished density with ragged, irregular outline. There is a tendency for small areas to coalesce to form larger ones. **Late:** Sclerotic areas become intermixed with the lucencies. Actinomycotic involvement is characterized by a sclerotic response predominantly. Other lesions are difficult to distinguish one from the other radiologically. (See Figure 12–38 B.)

Epidermoidoma (Figure 12–36)

Definition. A tumor formed from the inclusion of epidermal cells in the bones of the calvarium. These tumors are well encapsulated, and contain epithelial debris and cholesterol within. Although similar in composition to cholesteatomas which form in the mastoid region following chronic mastoid infection, they are of different origin and should be distinguished.

Radiographic Appearances

Well-encapsulated zone of radiolucency with a well-defined scalloped sclerotic margin.

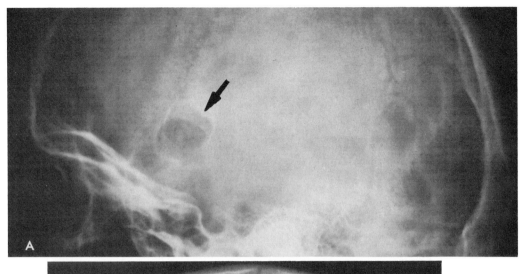

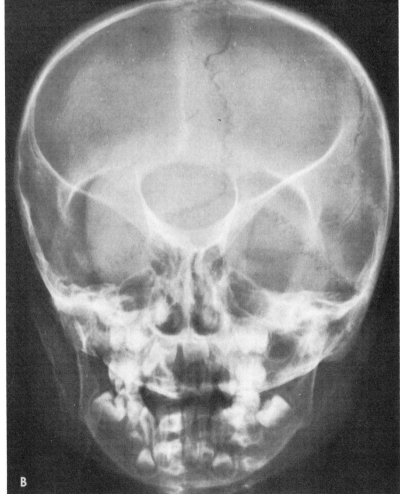

Figure 12–36   *A.* Radiograph of skull with epidermoidoma. *B.* Encephalocele defect in the frontal bone (courtesy of Dr. Nitaya Suwanwela), for comparison.

The tumor is usually situated in the diploë but involves both inner and outer table equally.

Unlike other lytic, well-encapsulated lesions of the calvarium, the central zones contain no trabeculae or foci of stippled calcification.

Hemangioma (Figure 12–37)

Definition.   Blood vessel tumor of two types, cavernous or capillary. The lesion begins in the diploë and expands the inner and outer tables in fusiform fashion.

Radiographic Appearances.   Two general types are recognized.

A LYTIC VARIETY: sharply circumscribed with a thin sclerotic zone and an inner finely reticular bony structure.

A SCLEROTIC VARIETY: bony spiculation radiating from a central point, not perpendicular to the bony tables of the skull.

DIFFERENTIAL DIAGNOSIS.   The internal trabeculation differentiates this lesion from the epidermoidoma. The lack of associated hypervascularity differentiates this from a meningioma. The leptomeningeal cyst is most apt to originate by erosion of the inner table, is often associated with disunited fracture, and is not as sharply circumscribed because of "daughter cysts" around the margin.

Sinus Pericranii

Definition.   A venous anomaly of the scalp which communicates with the intracranial venous system, most common along the midline and over the frontal bossae.

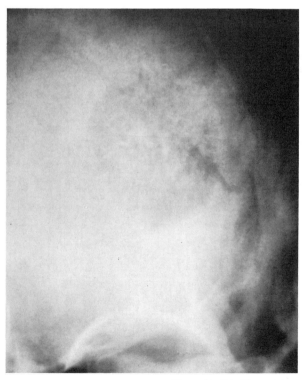
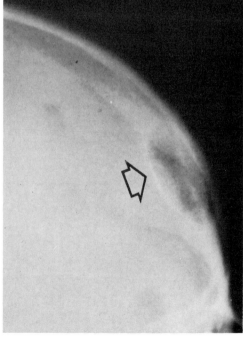

Figure 12–37   Hemangioma of the calvarium.

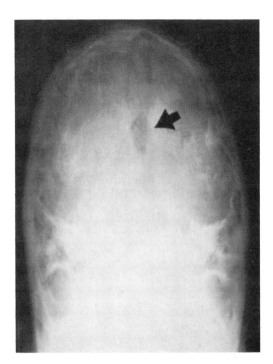

Figure 12-38   Defect in the occipital bone in association with a long-standing dermoid involving the occiput and brain.

Radiographic Appearances.   Usually there is a soft tissue mass overlying a skull defect, which in tangential view shows flattening of the underlying bone. The communication with the venous sinus may be demonstrated by injection of opaque medium into the soft tissue mass. The soft tissue mass changes in size with increased intracranial pressure or the Valsalva maneuver.

Dermoid Cyst (Teratomas) (Figure 12-38)

Definition.   Tumor derived from all three germinal layers, which may contain skin, teeth, sebaceous material, or hair.

Sites of Occurrence.   May occur anywhere in the meninges, brain, or scalp, but are most frequently situated along the midline. When they occur in the posterior fossa, increased intracranial pressure is usually associated.

Radiographic Appearances.   Usually visible as a defect in the calvarium only, unless there are associated teeth or calcified elements. There may or may not be an external palpable mass. The margin of the calvarial defect is sharp and faintly sclerotic (Figure 12-38).

CHORDOMA OF THE CLIVUS (Plaut)

Plain Roentgenographic Findings
Dense retrosellar calcification.
Bone destruction of the clivus.
Bone destruction of the dorsum sellae and petrous bone.
Calcification is of two kinds: (1) Small fragments of sequestered bone embedded in a mass. (2) Stippled calcification within the tumor tissue proper.

Vertebral Angiograms. Two different patterns are seen:

With midline tumors, backward displacement of the basilar artery with a dorsal convexity; in frontal view, minimal bowing or deviation.

Asymmetrical neoplasms show considerable displacement of the basilar artery to the opposite side with no alteration in the lateral view.

Carotid Angiograms. Depends upon how high on the clivus the neoplasm has grown. There may be a stretching of the carotid siphon. In the venous phase there may be an elevation of the basal vein of Rosenthal, with displacement of the great vein of Galen.

Pneumoencephalogram. May or may not produce signs. Fourth ventricle may be displaced backward, aqueduct may be backward and upward but pressure comes from below. Third ventricle may be deformed in its floor. There may be involvement of adjoining cistern. The cerebellar tonsils may be herniated into the foramen magnum.

Myeloencephalogram. Lateral projection may show posterior displacement of the fourth ventricle and aqueduct and possible obstruction. There may be extension toward the petrous tips or asymmetrical development of the tumor.

Invasion of the Skull by a Contiguous Benign or Malignant Neoplasm

Most Frequently Encountered Malignant Lesions

Lymphoepitheliomata and carcinomas of the nasopharynx.

Chordomas invading the base of the skull arising from remnants of the notochord. Most of these arise near the clivus and grow toward the sella turcica. They invade and destroy the adjoining sphenoid and occipital bones. They may contain amorphous calcification.

Most Frequently Encountered Benign Lesions

Tumors arising from the fifth or eighth nerves, and producing destruction of the skull in the vicinity of the foramen ovale or internal auditory meatus. (These may be neurilemmomas, endotheliomas, meningiomas, or even carcinomas.)

Chemodectomas, arising from the chemoreceptor cells occurring in the carotid or aortic bodies or glomus jugulare. They cause destruction of the contiguous bone of the middle or internal ear and extend into the cranial cavity. Approximately 80 per cent occur in females, with a familial tendency possible.

Caution in Interpretation. The two sides of the skull must be compared accurately, so that perfectly symmetrical films are necessary. At best asymmetry does occur and produces confusion, with loss of the sharp definition necessary for diagnosis.

MULTIPLE AREAS OF DEMARCATED RADIOLUCENCY

Foramina in the Base of the Skull

1. *Foramina in the Base of the Skull.*

   a. Anterior fossa. Numerous perforations in the cribriform plate on either side of the crista galli (Figure 12–39 A and B).

b. Middle fossa.
    (1) The optic foramen on each side.
    (2) Foramen rotundum on each side.
    (3) Foramen ovale on each side.
    (4) Foramen spinosum on each side.
    (5) Superior orbital fissures.
c. Posterior fossa.
    (1) Foramen lacerum on each side.
    (2) Carotid canal opening into each foramen lacerum.
    (3) Jugular foramen and canal on each side.
    (4) Hypoglossal foramen on each side.
    (5) Internal auditory meati.
    (6) Foramen magnum.
    (7) Condyloid canal on either side of the occipital condyles.
    (8) Stylomastoid foramen which transmits the facial nerve and stylomastoid artery on each side just medial and anterior to the mastoid process.
d. The cranial vault.
    (1) *Emissary veins* traverse small foramina in certain locations especially—parietal, and temporal behind the mastoid processes.

        These foramina are ordinarily less than 4 mm. in diameter. The parietal foramina may be in the midline or as much as 16 mm. lateral to the sagittal suture.

        On the average they lie 30 mm. anterior to the lambdoid suture (with extremes of 8 to 78 mm.). The distance from the coronal suture is 51 to 104 mm.

    (2) *Parietal fenestrae* or *enlarged parietal foramina do not* transmit veins and hence are not emissary foramina (Figure 12–40).

    (3) *Parietal thinness* (Figure 12–40). Two types are described, both near the midline: (a) a flat irregular triangular or quadrangular type; and (b) a sulcus or groove. Incidence is 0.4 per cent.

    (4) *Pacchionian villi* are due to pacchionian or arachnoidal granulations which produce impressions upon the calvarium. These are usually situated in a parasagittal position (Figure 12–41), with adjoining vessel channels leading to or from them.

    (5) *Venous diploë* are produced by venous channels contained within the diploë of the cranial vault. These tend to be arranged in the form of a star in the frontal and parietal bone and are sometimes referred to as "the frontal star" or "parietal star" (Figure 12–42).

    (6) *Accentuated convolutional pattern.* This is a form of thinness of the bones of the calvarium and may be within normal limits up to the age of about 16 years (Figure 12–18). When markedly accentuated they may suggest increased intracranial pressure. In older patients increased intracranial pressure should be excluded when this appearance is shown. The accentuated convolutional pattern must be distinguished from the lacunar skull (lückenschädel), which is usually unrelated to cerebral convolutions, and probably represents a mesodermal defect in ossification (Nashold and Netsky).

(Text continued on page 504)

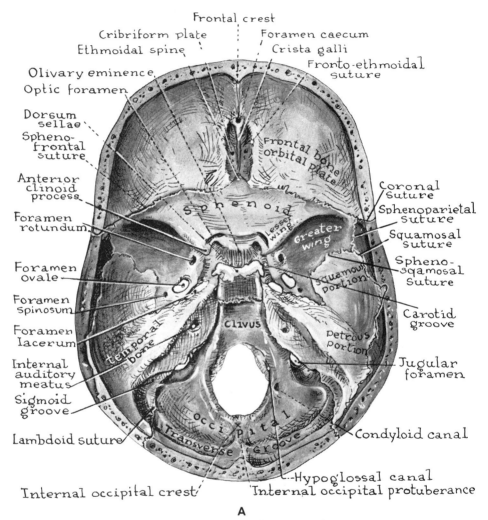

Figure 12–39 *A.* Internal aspect of the base of the skull. (From Pendergrass, E. P., Schaeffer, J. P., and Hodes, P. J.: *The Head and Neck in Roentgen Diagnosis.* 2d Ed. Springfield, Charles C Thomas, 1956).

Figure 12–39 continued on opposite page.

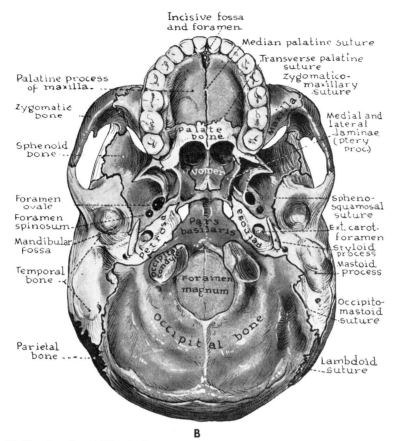

B

Figure 12–39 (*Continued*).   *B*. The skull viewed from below. (From Pendergrass, E. P., Schaeffer, J. P., and Hodes, P. J.: *The Head and Neck in Roentgen Diagnosis*. 2nd Ed. Springfield, Charles C Thomas, 1956.)

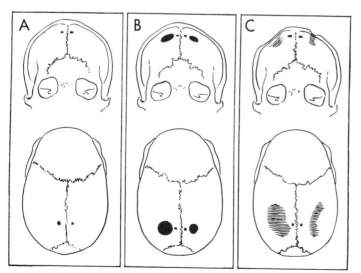

Figure 12–40   Three types of defects in parietal bone. *A*. Normal defects in parietal bone containing veins. *B*. Emissary foramina and fenestrae (enlarged parietal foramina) shown in same skull. *C*. Two forms of thinness shown, quadrangular on left and grooved on right, in association with emissary foramina. (From Nashold, B. S., Jr., and Netsky, M. G.: J. Neuropath. & Exper. Neurol., *18*:432, 1959.)

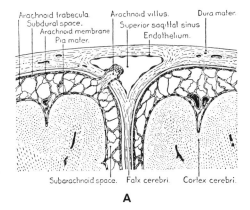

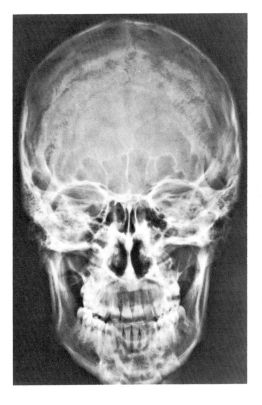
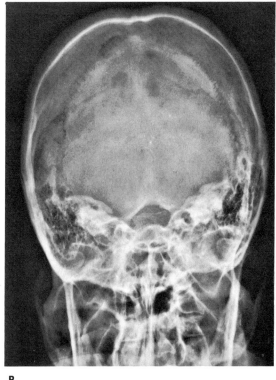

B

Figure 12–41 *A.* Schematic diagram of a coronal section of the meninges and cerebral cortex. (Weed, Amer. J. Anat.; courtesy of Wistar Institute.) *B.* Radiographs of skull demonstrating arachnoidal granulations impressing themselves upon the calvarium.

Figure 12–41 continued on opposite page.

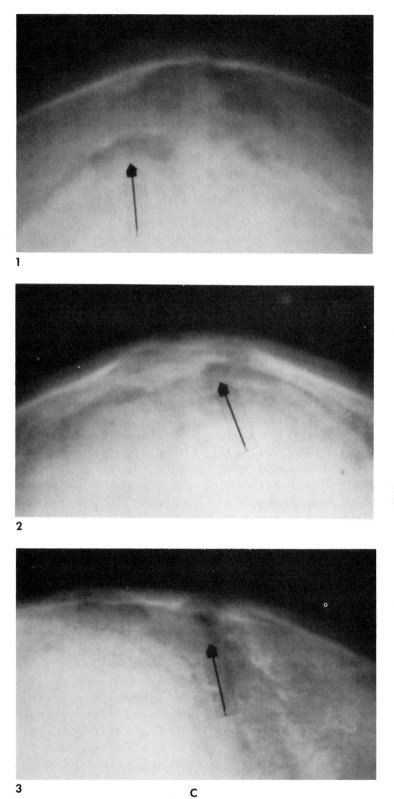

Figure 12–41 (*Continued*).   *C*. The appearance of arachnoidal granulations in close-up views. (1) On a Towne's view. (2) On a straight postero-anterior film of the skull. (3) In lateral projection.

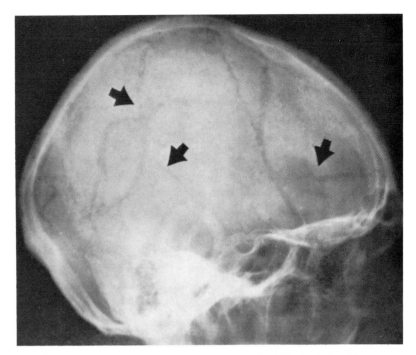

Figure 12–42 Channels in the diploë related to a venous network within the diploë. These are sometimes referred to as "parietal" and "frontal" stars respectively. (Courtesy of Chalmers S. Pool, M.D.)

Chronic Infectious Process of the Calvarium (Figure 12–43)

Classification. These include syphilis, tuberculosis, actinomycosis, blastomycosis, and coccidioidomycosis.

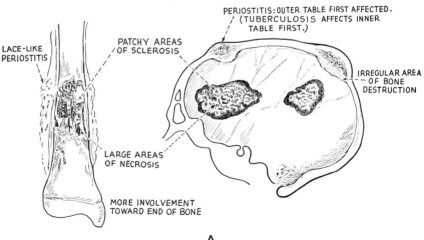

Figure 12–43 Chronic infectious processes of the calvarium. *A.* Diagrammatic illustration of the radiographic changes with acquired syphilis.

Figure 12–43 continued on opposite page.

Radiographic Appearances. Irregular areas of bone destruction giving the skull a moth-eaten appearance with small interspersed areas of sclerosis due to the contained sequestrae.

Chronic infections of the calvarium may be secondary to surgical craniotomy. A gradual lysis of bone at a surgical site is the diagnostic radiographic appearance.

Lückenschädel (Lacunar Skull, Cranial Lacunar Osteoagenesis)

Definition. Developmental disturbance of ossification of the bones of the calvarium giving rise to numerous areas of thinning in the bones of the vault, simulating

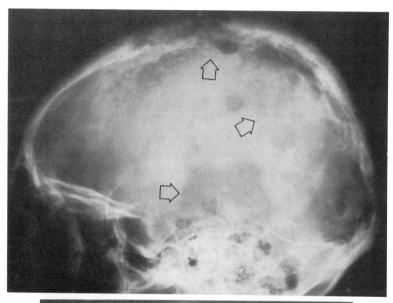

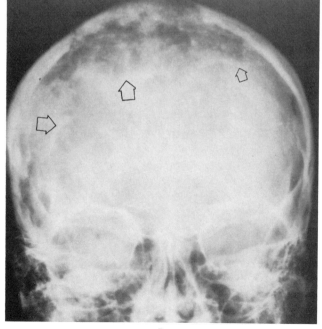

B

Figure 12–43 *(Continued).* *B.* Chronic osteomyelitis of the calvarium.

deep convolutional impressions. The defects do not correspond to the underlying brain convolutions ordinarily.

Frequently Associated Abnormalities. Spina bifida, meningocele, cleft palate, encephalocele, hydrocephalus.

Radiographic Appearances. The defects in the bones of the vault produce a honeycombed appearance, with the areas of thinness averaging about 2 cm. in diameter. There may be an associated hydrocephalus with separation or premature closure of the sutures and other anomalies. It is present at birth and invariably regresses spontaneously.

Fibrous Dysplasia

Definition. Fibroblastic proliferation within the bone, virtually replacing it, and the production of a shell of bone on the outer periphery of the lesion. There are scattered bone islands which remain within the fibroblastic proliferation.

Radiographic Appearances. An irregular radiolucency of the calvarium extending outward in projecting lobulations so that the affected bone appears scalloped and highly irregular in outline. The cortex appears to be eroded from within, while the periosteum attempts to compensate by laying down a thin shell of normal bone on the outer surface (Figure 12–44). There is usually a sclerotic zone surrounding the lytic zone within the calvarium, giving this lesion a thick outer margin.

In the skull the lesions are usually unilateral but may be bilateral.

In the paranasal sinuses, there may be an obliteration of the air space with diminution in the capacity of the adjoining orbits as the result of the marked thickening of the bony process.

The progress of the disease is variable and slow (Leeds and Seaman).

When facial bones are involved the process is called "leontiasis ossea."

Hyperparathyroidism has been previously discussed (Figure 12–45).

Reticuloendothelioses (Figure 12–46; also see Chapter 8).

Definition. This group of diseases is characterized by the abnormal appearance of lipids in reticuloendothelial cells throughout the body. As previously noted the Hand-Schüller-Christian complex consists of *histiocytosis-X, Letterer-Siwe disease* and *eosinophilic granuloma,* with the accumulation of lipids as a secondary phenomenon. *Niemann-Pick disease* and *Gaucher's disease* are due to constitutional metabolic defects in the metabolism of certain complex lipids (sphingomyelin in Niemann-Pick disease, and kerasin in Gaucher's).

In *Hand-Schüller-Christian disease,* diabetes and exophthalmos occur in about one-half of the cases and there are radiolucent bone defects principally in the skull in about 80 per cent of the cases.

Letterer-Siwe disease is a nonlipoid reticulosis, characterized by hepatosplenomegaly and lymph node enlargement. It is limited to infants and young children.

Eosinophilic granuloma occurs principally in both flat and long bones.

In *Niemann-Pick disease* the bones are involved in diffuse fashion without the focal deposits characteristic of the other entities because of reticuloendothelial involvement throughout the body. The skull is rarely affected.

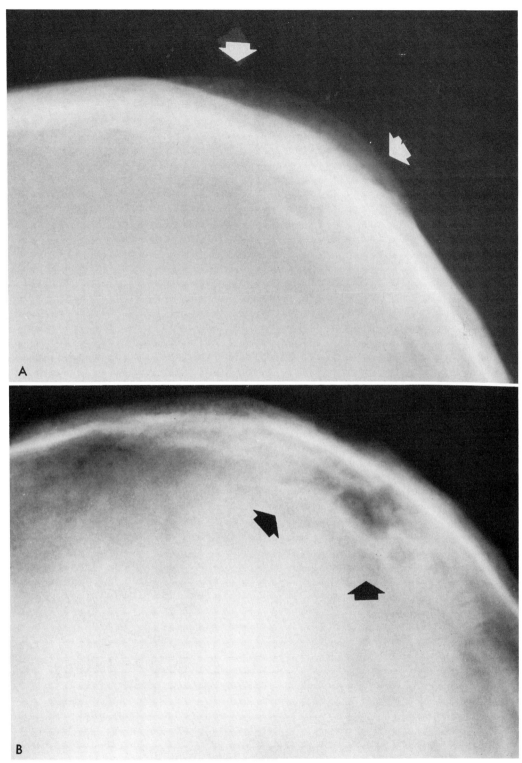

Figure 12–44   Close-up views of fibrous dysplasia of the calvarium. *A.* Soft tissue technique to demonstrate outer shell of bone (being "pushed" away from osteolytic zone). *B.* Heavier exposure, showing zone of sclerosis around radiolucent area. The relatively thick zone of sclerosis, coupled with the "shell of bone" appearance, is an important criterion for this diagnosis.

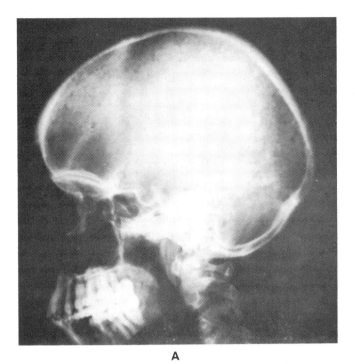

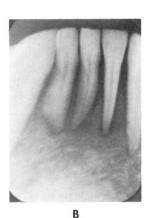

A

B

Figure 12–45 *A.* Lateral radiograph of the skull in hyperparathyroidism. *B.* Resorption of the lamina dura in hyperparathyroidism.

Figure 12–45 continued on opposite page.

Gaucher's disease is characterized by hepatosplenomegaly, skin pigmentation, and frequent hemorrhages. The skull is rarely involved.

Radiographic Appearances

Hand-Schüller-Christian disease. Skull: numerous bone defects, irregular in shape, giving the skull a map-like appearance. The edges of the defects are poorly defined with no sclerotic margin. The cranial vault, the bony orbits, and sometimes the base of the skull are affected. In the mandible, circumscribed lesions around the teeth produce the "floating tooth" sign (Figure 12–47).

Letterer-Siwe disease. Usually no bone changes are seen but occasionally the lesions of the bone will resemble Hand-Schüller-Christian disease particularly; when chronic, there is increased intracranial pressure (Feinberg and Langer).

Eosinophilic granuloma. Characteristically it occurs in the bones and does not involve the soft tissues. The appearance is the same as that of Hand-Schüller-Christian disease, although single lesions are perhaps more apt to occur and there are usually no associated systemic manifestations such as diabetes insipidus.

Niemann-Pick disease. The skull is rarely affected but the bones elsewhere may undergo resorption.

Gaucher's disease. There is a widening of the medullary cavity of the bones at the expense of the cortex, particularly toward the ends of the long bones, giving the bones an Erlenmeyer flask appearance. The skull is rarely involved.

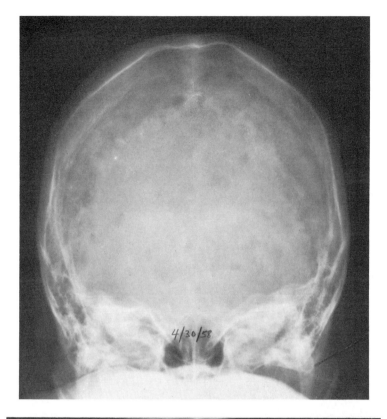

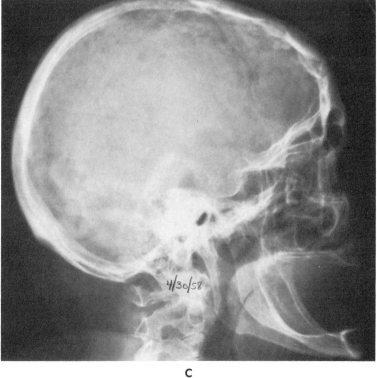

C

Figure 12–45 (*Continued*).   *C.* Skull in patient with parathyroid adenoma and hyperparathyroidism resembling metastatic tumors of the lytic type.

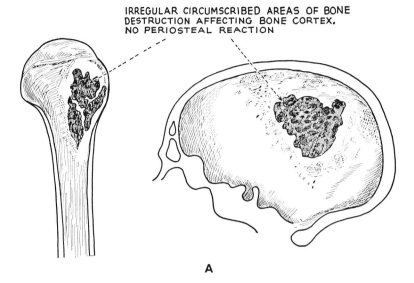

IRREGULAR CIRCUMSCRIBED AREAS OF BONE
DESTRUCTION AFFECTING BONE CORTEX,
NO PERIOSTEAL REACTION

A

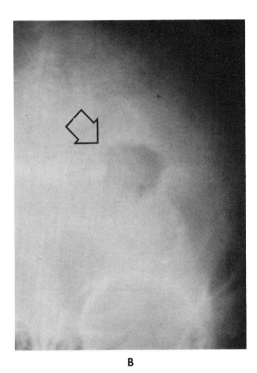

B

Figure 12–46 Representative illustration of the histiocytoses. *A.* Diagrammatic illustration of the typical radiographic appearance of eosinophilic granuloma of the bone. *B.* Eosinophilic granuloma involving the calvarium.

Metastatic Malignancy to the Skull (Figure 12–48)

Classification. These may be radiolucent (osteolytic) or hyperplastic (sclerotic).

Most Frequent Carcinomas Metastasizing to Bone are the breast, 52 per cent; prostatic carcinoma, 66 per cent; hypernephromas or clear cell carcinomas of the kidney, 35 per cent; carcinoma of the thyroid, 28 per cent; and carcinoma of the lung, approximately 25 per cent (Luck; Geschickter). Invasion of the calvarium may occur by direct extension from the scalp or the skin.

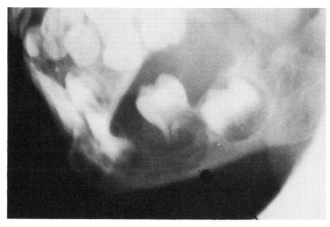

Figure 12–47   "Floating tooth" sign in reticuloendotheliosis involving the skull.

Radiographic Appearances

The osteolytic foci usually produce a punched-out appearance in the bones of the calvarium with no periosteal reaction or "radiologic capsule."

Small foci in a parasagittal situation are virtually impossible to distinguish from arachnoidal granulations except that usually small vascular channels can be identified leading into arachnoidal granulations.

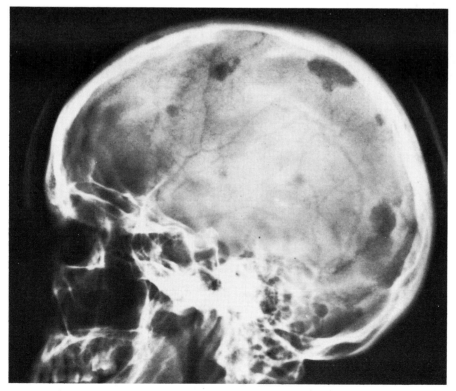

Figure 12–48   Metastatic tumors to the bones of the calvarium producing multiple osteolytic foci of a sharply circumscribed character in the bones of the calvarium.

The osteoblastic or sclerotic metastases usually have their origin in carcinoma of the prostate.

With neuroblastoma additional changes include separation of the sutures, enlargement of the head, perpendicular spiculation extending from the outer table, and patchy productive and destructive changes within the bones of the vault (Sherman and Leaming).

With Ewing's tumor additional sites apart from the skull include the vertebrae, and ribs and pelvis most frequently.

"Button sequestrum": lytic lesion with an intact central nidus of bone. It occurs in eosinophilic granuloma, calvarial tuberculosis, metastatic carcinoma, and necrosis following radiotherapy (Rosen and Nadel).

Multiple Myeloma

Definition. Malignant neoplasms arising from the hematopoietic reticulum of bone marrow characterized by innumerable foci of plasma cells. The tumor may be solitary for a period of years.

Preferential Sites. Vertebral bodies, bones of the pelvis, shoulder girdle, skull.

Radiographic Appearances (Figure 12–49)

No manifestations in approximately 25 per cent of cases.

Multiple areas of sharply defined bone destruction involving the vertebrae, pelvis, and, especially, skull and shoulder girdle.

There is often an associated generalized osteoporosis.

When the cortex is completely destroyed, a soft tissue mass may be associated.

Occasionally, the process is not sharply defined and merely appears as

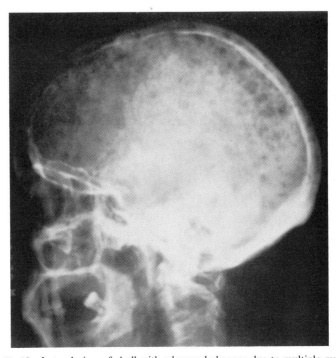

Figure 12–49 Lateral view of skull with advanced changes due to multiple myeloma.

multiple minute lytic foci throughout the bones imparting an appearance closely resembling severe diffuse osteoporosis.

Pathologic fractures are frequent.

DISEASES OF THE SKULL MANIFEST BY DIFFUSE INCREASE IN RADIOPACITY

Osteopetrosis (see Chapters 7 and 10)

Definition. Osteopetrosis or marble bone disease is a hereditary bone disorder characterized by a failure of osteoclastic resorption of the calcified matrix in the course of the normal resorption and deposition of bone. There is an associated marked anemia and brittleness of bones.

Radiographic Appearance. All of the bones of the skull, particularly those at the base, are very markedly sclerotic and thickened with complete obliteration of the diploë. The mastoids, air sinuses, and foramina at the base of the skull are small. The sella is ordinarily normal in size. The facial bones may be only minimally affected. Those bones preformed in cartilage in the base of the skull show the most extensive changes.

Engelmann's Disease (see Chapters 7 and 10)

Definition. Engelmann's disease, or progressive diaphyseal dysplasia, is a sclerotic bone disorder which affects the diaphyses of the long bones primarily. There is an increase in length of the extremities greater than that of the trunk.

Radiographic Appearance. There is a marked sclerosis of the bones at the base of the skull and of the frontal bone particularly. The mandible is not affected ordinarily.

Differentiation from osteopetrosis is especially accomplished in the bones of the extremities when the diaphysis is the primary part affected in contrast to osteopetrosis, in which the metaphyses and epiphyses tend to be club-shaped and are also affected.

Fluorine Poisoning and Marrow Disorders May Also Produce Diffuse Increased Radiopacity of the Calvarium

Metaphyseal Dysplasia (Pyle's disease; craniometaphyseal dysplasia)

Definition. Disturbance in endochondral bone formation with a failure of modelling of the cylindrical bones, resulting in an Erlenmeyer flask deformity. There appears to be a lack of osteoclastic activity in the metaphyses of the long bones producing the flaring of the metaphyses, but the cortices are thin and not thick as in osteopetrosis. There is sometimes an associated overgrowth of the skull, leontiasis ossea, which especially involves the bones of the base of the skull and facial bones (Jackson et al.).

Radiographic Appearances (pertaining to the skull)

Sclerosis of the cranial bones, especially those of the base of the skull.

The mandible and other facial bones may also appear sclerotic, as in leontiasis ossea.

Hypertelorism with overgrowth of the bridge of the nose.

These changes are associated ordinarily with the characteristic alterations described in Chapter 8 in the long bones, such as splaying of the metaphyses, thinning of the splayed cortex, and sclerosis of the diaphyseal cortex.

DISEASES OF THE SKULL MANIFEST BY MULTIPLE DEMARCATED AREAS OF RADIOPACITY

Osteitis Deformans or Paget's Disease.   See previous description and also Chapter 10 (Figure 12–23).

Metastatic Sclerotic Tumors to the Bones of the Calvarium.   Most metastases to bone originate in carcinomas and are destructive, since they produce lytic foci within the bone. These have been previously considered.

Osteosclerotic metastases are characteristic especially of certain carcinomas. Prostatic carcinoma is the most frequent primary, but others may include metastases from carcinoma of the gastrointestinal tract, thyroid, kidney, lung, breast, or carcinoid metastases.

Radiographic Appearances.   These may be single or multiple foci of sclerosis throughout the bones of the calvarium at any site. These will vary in size and circumscription. At times metastatic carcinoma of the prostate produces a diffuse sclerosis which is so densely sclerotic that it shows no definition of discrete tumor masses.

DISEASES OF THE SKULL MANIFEST BY SINGLE OR CONFLUENT DEMARCATED AREAS OF BONY SCLEROSIS

Osteoma or Osteochondroma

Definition.   Osteomas are true bone tumors consisting of dense, sclerotic, or cancellous bone. They differ from osteochondromas in respect to the cartilaginous elements and structure contained in the latter. Osteochondromas are also more apt to be pedunculated.

Sites of Predilection

Frontoethmoidal.
Orbitoethmoidal.
Parietal.
Temporal or occipital bones occasionally.
They may be exostotic or enostotic within the bone.

Radiographic Appearances (Figure 12–50).   The osteoma occurring in the vault is usually a sharply circumscribed, flat dense sclerotic area. Vessel channels may pass through the involved area without changing caliber and there is no hypervascularity. The osteochondroma may be pedunculated.

A tangential view which will demonstrate the markedly thickened circumscribed bone is recommended whenever feasible.

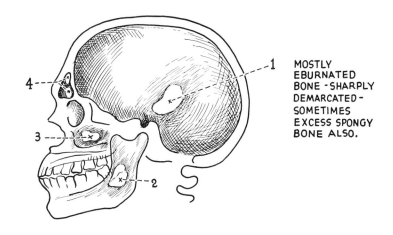

MOSTLY
EBURNATED
BONE -SHARPLY
DEMARCATED -
SOMETIMES
EXCESS SPONGY
BONE ALSO.

COMMON SITES: 1. CALVARIUM
                 2. MANDIBLE
                 3. MAXILLA   } INCLUDING
                 4. FRONTAL BONES   }   PARANASAL
                                         SINUSES
                         A

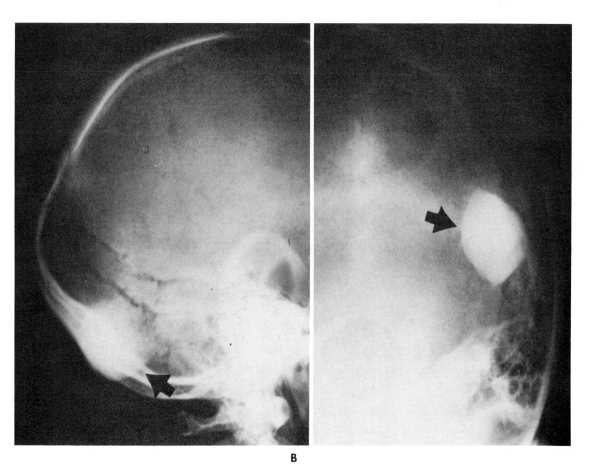

B

Figure 12–50 Osteoma of the calvarium. *A.* The most frequent sites and general appearance. *B.* Osteoma of the occipital bone as it adjoins the temporal bone.

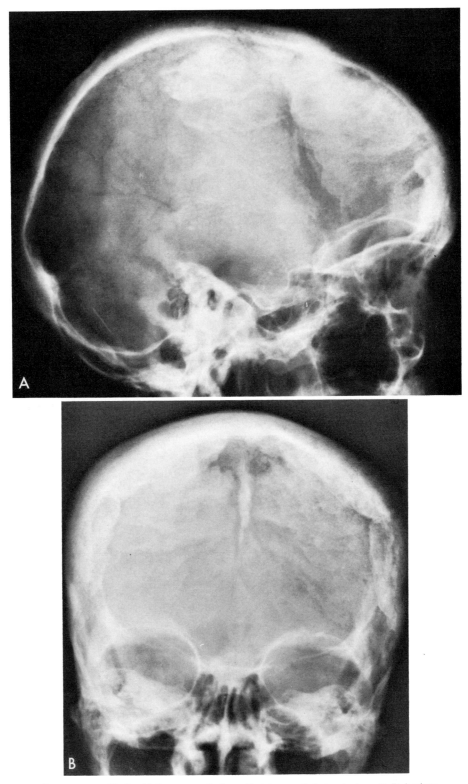

Figure 12–51   Skull with hyperostosis frontalis interna. *A*. Lateral view. *B*. P-A view.

In the orbit, if the osteoma is large, considerable deformity may result, even giving rise to exophthalmos. Differentiation from meningioma and fibrous dysplasia must be made. In meningioma there is usually associated hypervascularity and some degree of osteoporosis. In fibrous dysplasia there is an inner zone of osteoporosis with an outer shell of thick cortical bone in contrast to the diffusely dense process characteristic of osteoma.

Hyperostosis Frontalis Interna

Definition. This condition is characterized by marked hyperostotic change of the inner table of the frontal bone. It has at times been referred to as the Stewart-Morel-Moore syndrome, although it is doubtful that it represents an actual clinical entity (Salmi et al.).

The syndrome has been described as consisting of: obesity, hirsutism of the face, and occasionally other disorders suggesting a pituitary dyscrasia predominantly in females between the ages of 35 and 45. Vertigo and headaches also may be present.

Radiographic Appearance (Figure 12–51). Variable but extensive areas of sclerosis of the inner table of the frontal bone with occasional extension of the sclerotic process into the adjoining diploë of the skull. The paranasal sinuses may be large and the vascular grooves prominent. Calcification may simulate calcium deposit in the falx or dura.

Meningioma

Definition. Meningiomas or fibroblastomas are tumors which arise from the tissues surrounding the cerebrum, characterized by histological features of the meningotheliomatous and psammomatous types. They are usually of either arachnoid or dural origin.

Sites of Origin (Figure 12–52). The most frequent sites are parasagittal, the petrous ridge, sphenoidal ridge, in the region of the olfactory groove, and over the convexity of the cerebrum anterior to the fissure of Rolando. In general they originate wherever arachnoid granulations are numerous and where the cerebral veins enter the large venous sinuses.

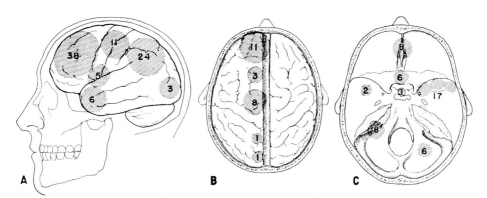

Figure 12–52 *A* to *C*. Diagrammatic sketch of the locations of intracranial meningiomas and the relative frequency of each. (From Jacobson et al.: Radiology, *72*:358, 1959.)

Radiographic Findings

PLAIN FILMS OF THE SKULL

In parasagittal meningiomas: hypervascularity, hyperostosis, and calcification within the tumor, or a combination of these appearances.

Sphenoidal ridge and olfactory groove meningiomas: very marked hyperostosis and a very dense tumor mass. There may also be an associated enlargement of the sphenoidal fissure.

Jacobson et al. found that plain films of the skull were normal in only 22.5 per cent of the cases. The roentgenologic abnormalities most frequently encountered on the plain films of the skull were as follows: localized hyperostosis, 44.1 per cent; atrophy of the dorsum sellae, 29 per cent; localized increase in vascularity, 25.8 per cent; calcification, 20.4 per cent; significant pineal shift, 19.4 per cent; localized bone resorption, 16.1 per cent; and localized spiculation, 4.3 per cent.

CEREBRAL ANGIOGRAMS. Cerebral angiograms are almost invariably abnormal (Jackson et al.). The various findings on angiography include shift of the anterior cerebral artery, new vessel formation at the site of the lesion, shift or displacement of the middle cerebral artery or other major vessels, a localized zone of avascularity, and circumferential vascular delineation of the lesion. The first three of these findings occur in approximately two-thirds of the patients.

Other angiographic findings include tumor cloud formation, and occasionally, discontinuity in the superior sagittal sinus.

PNEUMOGRAPHY OF THE BRAIN. Shift of the septum pellucidum or ventricular system was seen in 81.8 per cent of the cases (Jackson et al.) and localized deformity of a lateral ventricle in over one-half. Of 46 patients studied by pneumography of the brain, 95.7 per cent had abnormal findings.

TUMORS OCCURRING IN TEMPORAL REGION. These orginate from the dura covering the petrous pyramid or attached to the wall of the superior petrosal sinus. There may be no demonstrable associated bony change. There may, however, be unilateral atrophy of the sella turcica and the pineal gland is often displaced. Hyperostosis or osteoporosis of the adjoining bone is usually lacking. There may, however, be a small area of bony atrophy in the petrous ridge.

Occasionally, meningiomas in this location will give rise to marked hyperostosis to the extent that the lesion will be confused with an osteoma.

SPHENOID RIDGE MENINGIOMAS. Usually these produce a marked hyperostosis with an accompanying encroachment on the superior orbital fissure. The eye may be displaced. Atrophy of the sella turcica is often associated. The atrophy may be unilateral due to localized pressure. The sphenoid ridges appear asymmetrical in frontal perspective.

MENINGIOMAS INVOLVING THE OLFACTORY GROOVE. These may resemble those involving the sphenoid ridge and one may merge into the other. There is usually an overgrowth of bone.

MENINGIOMAS ARISING FROM THE WALLS OF THE LATERAL SINUSES IN THE OCCIPITAL REGION. These lesions are difficult to recognize and produce signs of increased intracranial pressure more frequently than other lesions previously mentioned. Overt evidence on the plain radiographs such as bony overgrowth, hypervascularity, or calcification may not be present, although calcification may occur.

MENINGIOMAS ORIGINATING FROM THE DURA OF THE TUBERCULUM SELLAE. These are very difficult to diagnose. Atrophy of the sella turcica is uncommon and there may only be flaky or curvilinear areas of calcification resembling the findings in an aneurysm or in craniopharyngioma.

MENINGIOMAS OCCURRING SUBTENTORIALLY. These are not usually distinguishable from any other form of intracranial tumor in a similar location. Calcification may be present and increased intracranial pressure is usually found. Subtentorial meningiomas are occasionally associated with neurofibromatosis.

MENINGIOMAS ARISING FROM THE DURAL SHEATH OF THE OPTIC NERVE. These will ordinarily produce enlargement of the optic foramen on the side affected. There may be associated bony thickenings, although this is not invariable.

MENINGIOMAS ORIGINATING WITHIN ANY OF THE VENTRICLES. There are no characteristic changes in the roentgenograms.

MULTIPLE MENINGIOMAS. These are rare but can occur. The angiographic method of demonstration is most accurate for this group of lesions.

Leontiasis Ossea

Definition. This is a descriptive term applied to cases which show an increase in density and thickness of one or more of the following: the facial bones, the base of the skull, or the frontal bones (Schwartz and Collins). The origin is usually, but not invariably, fibrous dysplasia or osteitis deformans (Paget's disease). Occasionally low grade chronic infection such as tuberculosis and syphilis may account for this appearance.

Radiographic Appearance. There is an increase in density and marked thickness of any of the facial bones, the base of the skull or the frontal bones.

Fibrous Dysplasia has been previously considered.

Questions—Chapter 12

1. Describe the routine views of the skull and indicate the special significance and purpose of each of these views in respect to the roentgenology of the skull.
2. Describe a useful routine method for study of the radiographs of the skull.
3. Describe the growth and age changes of the skull in respect to the skull and facial proportions at birth, at six or seven years of age, at puberty, and after puberty.
4. Define the following terms: brachycephalic skull; dolichocephalic skull; turricephalic skull; plagiocephalic skull.
5. What is the clinical significance of the interorbital distance? What is meant by the term "hypertelorism"?
6. Describe a method for pineal localization.
7. Where is the habenula situated in the skull? What is its significance when calcified?
8. Describe the anatomy of the sella turcica.
9. What is meant by a sella turcica that has an "infantile" shape?
10. What is meant by the term "overbridged sella"?
11. What are the general causes for a small skull?
12. What are the general causes for an enlarged skull?
13. Define hydrocephalus.
14. What different types of hydrocephalus can you name?
15. What is meant by the terms "pressure hydrocephalus" and "nonpressure hydrocephalus"?
16. Describe the radiologic features of hydrocephalus in the infant, adolescent, and adult.

17. Describe the skull and upper cervical spine abnormalities which may be noted in Arnold-Chiari malformation.

18. Define Arnold-Chiari malformation and indicate some of the lesions which are often associated.

19. Define "Dandy-Walker syndrome" and indicate the radiographic findings often found on plain films of the skull.

20. Define "cerebral aqueduct stenosis" and indicate radiographic findings which may be found on plain films early or late in life, and the significance of calcifications in the brain in respect to the above.

21. Define "Paget's disease of the skull" and describe the radiologic aspects of the skull appearances.

22. Describe the skull in thalassemia major.

23. Describe the roentgenologic appearance and localization of osteomas of the skull.

24. Define "meningocele" and "encephalocele" and indicate the radiographic findings often associated.

25. How does one demonstrate a depressed skull fracture most accurately and what is the significance of this finding?

26. Define "platybasia" and indicate the method you might employ in making the diagnosis roentgenologically.

27. How does cleidocranial dysostosis affect the radiographic appearance of the skull?

28. How does osteogenesis imperfecta affect the radiographic appearance of the skull?

29. What is the radiographic appearance of the skull in hyperparathyroidism?

30. Describe the radiographic appearances of the skull often associated with neuroblastoma.

31. What is meant by the term "leptomeningeal cyst" and under what circumstances may the lesion be found roentgenologically? What is its radiographic appearance?

32. What are the radiographic appearances of the bones of the calvarium associated with osteomyelitis affecting these bones?

33. Differentiate the radiographic appearance in the calvarium of epidermoidoma and hemangioma.

34. Where are dermoid cysts usually found in the skull, and what is the radiographic appearance often associated?

35. What are the plain roentgenographic findings in chordoma of the clivus?

36. What are the most frequently encountered benign lesions contiguous to the skull which may affect the skull's radiographic appearance?

37. What are the most frequently encountered malignant lesions contiguous with the skull which may alter the roentgen appearance of the skull?

38. What foramina occur in the base of the skull in the middle fossa and how may they be detected?

39. What foramina occur in the posterior fossa of the skull and how may they be detected?

40. What foramina occur in the cranial vault and what is their radiographic appearance?

41. What is the clinical significance of parietal fenestrae?

42. What is the clinical significance of an accentuated convolutional pattern? How does this appearance differ from lückenschädel?

43. What abnormalities are frequently associated with lückenschädel or lacunar skull?

44. Describe the radiographic appearance of a skull affected by fibrous dysplasia.

45. Classify the reticuloendothelioses. Which of these diseases are primary lipid disturbances and which are secondary?

46. What are the radiographic appearances in the skull related to the reticuloendothelioses? In which of these is the skull very rarely affected?

47. How may metastatic malignancy to the skull alter the skull appearance roentgenologically?

48. What is meant by the term "button sequestrum" and under what circumstances does it occur?

49. Describe the radiographic appearance of multiple myeloma affecting the skull.

50. Define the term "metaphyseal dysplasia" and indicate its radiographic appearance in the skull.

51. What are the most frequent sites of origin of meningioma and what are the radiographic findings in plain films of the skull?

52. Where do meningiomas originate which often do not alter the skull appearance?

53. Define "leontiasis ossea" and describe the associated radiographic appearance.

References

Agnos, J. W., and Wollin, D. G.: The effect of rotation of the skull on the measured position of the pineal gland. J. Canad. Ass. Radiol., 9:40–44, 1958.

Austin, J. H. M., and Gooding, C. A.: Roentgenologic measurement of skull size in children. Radiology, 99:641–646, 1971.

Bakwin, H., Golden, A., and Fox, S.: Familial osteoectasia with macrocranium. Amer. J. Roentgenol., 91:609–617, 1964.

Barnett, D. J.: Radiologic aspects of craniopharyngiomas. Radiology, 72:14–18, 1959.

Berg, K. J., and Lonnum, A.: Ventricular size in relation to cranial size. Acta Radiol. (Diagnosis) 4:65–78, 1966.

Brihaye, J., Mage, J., and Martin, P.: Kystes épidermigues crâniens. Acta Neurolog. et Psychiat., Belg., 58:557–596, 1958.

Britton, H. A., Canby, J. P., and Kohler, C. M.: Iron deficiency anemia producing evidence of marrow hyperplasia in the calvarium. Pediatrics, 25:621–628, 1960.

Brown, O. L., Longacre, J. J., DeStefano, G. A., Wood, R. W., and Kahl, J. B.: Roentgen manifestations of blow fracture of the orbit. Radiology, 85:908–913, 1965.

Bucy, P. C., and Capp, C. S.: Primary hemangioma of bone with special reference to roentgenologic diagnosis. Amer. J. Roentgenol., 23:1–33, 1930.

Camp, J. D.: Normal and pathologic anatomy of the sella turcica as revealed at necropsy. Radiology, 1:65, 1923.

Camp, J. D.: Normal and pathologic anatomy of the sella turcica as revealed by roentgenograms. Amer. J. Roentgenol., 12:143–155, 1924.

Carrington, K. W.: Ventriculo-venous shunt using Holter Valve as treatment of hydrocephalus. J. Mich. Med. Soc., 58:373–376, 1959.

Chamberlain, W. E.: Basilar impression (platybasia), bizarre developmental anomaly of occipital bone and upper cervical spine with striking and misleading neurologic manifestations. Yale J. Biol. Med., 11:487–496, 1939.

Cimmino, C. V., and Painter, J. W.: Iniencephaly. Radiology, 79:942–944, 1962.

Cornelius, E. A., and McClendon, J. L.: Cherubism, hereditary fibrous dysplasia of the jaws. Amer. J. Roentgenol., 106:136–143, 1969.

Cronqvist, S: Roentgenologic evaluation of cranial size in children. Acta Radiol. (Diagnosis) 7:97–111, 1968.

Currarino, G., and Silverman, F. N.: Orbital hypotelorism, arhinencephaly and trigonocephaly. Radiology, 74:206–217, 1960.

Davis, D., and Farrell, F.: Personal communication.

Davies, H. W.: Radiological changes associated with Arnold-Chiari malformation. Brit. J. Radiology, 40:262–269, 1967.

Di Chiro, G., and Nelson, K. B.: The volume of the sella turcica. Amer. J. Roentgenol., 87:989–1008, 1962 (57 ref.).

Dunn, F. H.: Apert's acrocephalosyndactylism. Radiology, 78:738–743, 1962.

Elefant, E., and Tosovsky, V.: Osteogenesis imperfecta congenita. Ann. Paediat., 202:285–292, 1964.

Eraso, S. C.: Roentgen and clinical diagnosis of glomus jugulare tumors. Four cases and a new radiographic technic. Radiology, 77:252–256, 1961.

Etter, L. E.: Atlas of Roentgen Anatomy of the Skull. Springfield, Charles C Thomas, 1955.

Feinberg, S. B., and Langer, L. O.: Roentgen findings of increased intracranial pressure in communicating hydrocephalus as insidious manifestations of chronic histiocytosis-X. Amer. J. Roentgenol., 95:41–47, 1965.

Freydinger, J. E., Duhig, J. T., and McDonald, L. W.: Sarcoma complicating Paget's disease of bone. Arch. Path., 75:496–500, 1963.

Galloway, J. R., and Greitz, T.: The medial and lateral choroid arteries: An anatomic and roentgenographic study. Acta Radiol., 53:353–366, 1960.

Gannon, W. E.: False block of internal carotid artery during angiography. Radiology, 76:748–754, 1961.

Garusi, G. F.: Hyperostosis of the vault of the skull in acromegaly. Amer. J. Roentgenol., 91:988–995, 1964 (18 refs).

Gerald, B. E., and Silverman, F. N.: Normal and abnormal interorbital distance with special reference to mongolism. Amer. J. Roentgenol., 95:154–161, 1965.

Geschickter, C. F.: Primary tumors of the cranial bones. Amer. J. Cancer, 26:155–180, 1936.

Glaser, M. A., and Blaine, E. S.: Fate of cranial defects secondary to fracture and surgery: Follow-up study of 150 patients. Radiology, 34:671–684, 1940.

Gooding, C. A., Carter, A., and Hoare, R. D.: New ventriculographic aspects of the Arnold-Chiari malformation. Radiology, 89:626–632, 1967.

Greenberg, B. E.: Epidermoid cyst of the skull: A case observed for sixteen years. Radiology, 76:107–109, 1961.

Greenwald, C. M., Eugenio, M., Hughes, C. R., and Gardner, W. J.: Importance of the air shadow of the cisterna magna in encephalographic diagnosis. Radiology, 71:695–701, 1958.

Greitz, T. V. B., Grepe, A. O. L., Kalmer, M. S. F., and Lopez, J.: Pre- and postoperative evaluation of cerebral blood flow in low-pressure hydrocephalus. J. Neurosurg., 31: 644–651, 1969.

Griscom, N. T. and Oh, K. S.: The contracting skull: inward growth of the inner table, as a physiologic response to diminution of intracranial content in children. Amer. J. Roentgenol., 110:106–110, 1970.

Haas, L. L.: Roentgenological skull measurements and their diagnostic applications. Amer. J. Roentgenol., 67:197–209, 1952.

Horrigan, W. D., and Baker, D. H.: Gargoylism: A review of the roentgen skull changes with a description of a new finding. Amer. J. Roentgenol., 86:473–477, 1961.

Howell, T. R.: Radiology of the infant's skull. South. Med. J., 64:1075–1080, 1971.

Huang, Y. P., and Wolf, B.: Angiographic features of 4th ventricle tumors with special reference to posterior inferior cerebellar artery. Amer. J. Roentgenol., 107:543–564, 1969.

Huang, Y. P., Wolf, B. S., and Okudera, T.: Angiographic anatomy of the inferior vermian vein of the cerebellum. Acta Radiol. (Diagnosis) 9:327–344, special issue, 1969.

Isley, J. K., and Baylin, G. J.: A new method for localizing the calcified pineal gland on the lateral skull roentgenogram. Amer. J. Roentgenol., 81:953–955, 1959.

Jackson, W., Albright, F., Drewry, G., Hanelin, J., and Rubin, M.: Metaphyseal dysplasia, epiphyseal dysplasia, diaphyseal dysplasia and related conditions. Arch. Intern. Med., 94:871–875, 1954.

Jacobson, H. G., Lubetsky, H. W., Shapiro, J. H., and Carton, C. A.: Intracranial meningiomas: a roentgen study of 126 cases. Radiology, 72:356–367, 1959.

Jacobson, H. G., and Shapiro, J. H.: Pseudotumor cerebri. Radiology, 82:202, 1964.

Jost, F.: Zur Klinik der basilären Impression. Wien. Klin. Wschr., 70:237–243, 1958.

Kaufman, S.: Sekundare Geschwülste der Knocken. Spez. Path. Anat., 1:954, 1922.

Klaus, E.: Roentgendiagnostik der Platybasie und basilären Impression: weitere Erfahrungen mit einer neuen Untersuchungs Methode. Fortschr. a. d. Geb. d. Roentgenstr., 86:460–469, 1957.

Kruyff, E., and Jeffs, R.: Skull abnormalities in the Arnold-Chiari malformation. Acta Radiol. (Diagnosis) 5:9–24, 1966.

Lawrence, D., Nogrady, M. B., and Cloutier, A. M.: Cherubism: A case report. Amer. J. Roentgenol., 108:468–472, 1970.

Leeds, N., and Seaman, W. B.: Fibrous dysplasia of the skull and its differential diagnosis. A clinical and roentgenographic study of 46 cases. Radiology, 78:570–582, 1962 (57 ref.).

Legre, J., Denizet, D., and Savelli, J.: Cranial lacunae secondary to trauma in infancy. J. Radiol. Electrol., 41:667–678, 1960.

Lin, J. P., Goodkin, R., Chase, N. E., and Kricheff, I. I.: The angiographic features of fibrous dysplasia of the skull. Radiology, 92:1275–1280, 1969.

Luck, J. V.: Bone and Joint Diseases. Springfield, Charles C Thomas, 1950.

Mani, R. L., and Newton, T. H.: Superior cerebellar artery: Arteriographic changes in posterior fossa lesions. Radiology, 92:1281–1287, 1969.

McGregor, M.: The significance of certain measurements of the skull in the diagnosis of basilar impression. Brit. J. Radiol., 21:171–181, 1948.

McKusick, V. A.: Heritable Disorders of Connective Tissue. Third Edition. St. Louis, C. V. Mosby Co., 1966, pp. 230–270.

McRae, D. L.: Habenular calcification as an aid in the diagnosis of intracranial lesions. Amer. J. Roentgenol., 94:541–546, 1965.

Morreau, M. H.: Radiologic localization of the pineal gland. Acta Radiol. (Diagnosis), 5: 65–67, 1966.

Moseley, J. E.: Skull changes in chronic iron deficiency anemia. Amer. J. Roentgenol., 85:649–652, 1961.

Murphy, J., and Gooding, C. A.: Evolution of persistently enlarged parietal foramina. Radiology, 97:391–392, 1970.

Müssbichler, H.: Radiologic study of intracranial calcification in congenital toxoplasmosis. Acta Radiol. (Diagnosis), 7:369–379, 1968.

Nashold, B. S., Jr., and Netsky, M. G.: Foramina, fenestrae and thinness of parietal bone. J. Neuropath. Exp. Neurol., 18:432–441, 1959.

Neuhauser, E. B. D., Schwachman, H., Wittenborg, M. H., and Cohen, J. W.: Progressive diaphyseal dysplasia. Radiology, 51:11–22, 1948.

Newton, T. H., and Potts, D. G. (eds.): Radiology of the Skull and Brain. Volumes 1 and 2. St. Louis, C. V. Mosby Co., 1971.

Oon, C. L.: The size of the pituitary fossa in adults. British J. Radiology, 36:294–299, 1963.

Palubinskas, A. J., and Davies, H.: Calcification of the basal ganglia of the brain. Amer. J. Roentgenol., 82:806–822, 1959.

Pancoast, H. K., Pendergrass, E. P., Schaeffer, J. P., and Hodes, P. J.: The Head and Neck in Roentgen Diagnosis. Second Edition. Springfield, Charles C Thomas, 1956.

Peterman, A. F., Hayles, A. B., Dockerty, M. B., and Love, J. G.: Encephalotrigeminal angiomatosis (Sturge-Weber Disease): Clinical study of 35 cases. J.A.M.A., 167:2169–2176, 1958.

Pettet, J. R., Woolner, L. B., and Judd, E. S., Jr.: Carotid body tumors (chemodectomas). Ann. Surg., 137:465–477, 1953.

Plaut, H. F., and Blatt, E. S.: Chordoma of the Clivus. Amer. J. Roentgenol., 100:639–649, 1967.

Poppel, M. H., Jacobson, H. G., Duff, B. K., and Gottlieb, C.: Basilar impression and platybasia in Paget's disease. Radiology, 61:639–644, 1953.

Reifenstein, E. C. Jr., and Albright, F.: Paget's

disease: Its pathologic physiology and the importance of this in complications arising from fractures and immobilizations. New Eng. J. Med., *231*:343–355, 1944.

Riemenschneider, P. A.: Trigonocephaly. Radiology, *68*:863–864, 1957.

Ritvo, M.: Roentgen Diagnosis of Diseases of the Skull. Annals of Roentgenology, Vol. XIX. New York, Paul B. Hoeber, Inc., 1949.

Rosen, I. W., and Nadel, H. I.: Button sequestrum of the skull. Radiology, *92*:969–971, 1969.

Rosencrantz, M.: Widened vascular grooves in fibrous dysplasia of the skull. Acta Radiol. (Diagnosis), *9*:95–101, 1969.

Russell, D. S.: Observations of the pathology of hydrocephalus. London, His Majesty's Stationery Office, Series G.B., Medical Research Council, Special Report Series No. 265, 1949.

Salmi, A., Voutilainen, A., Holsti, I. R., and Unnerus, C. E.: Hyperostosis cranii in a normal population. Amer. J. Roentgenol., *87*:1032–1040, 1962.

Saunders, W. W.: Basilar impression: The position of the normal odontoid. Radiology, *41*:589–590, 1943.

Scatliff, J. H., Kier, E. L., Zingesser, L. H., and Schechter, M. M.: Terminal basilar artery deformity secondary to suprasellar masses and third ventricular dilatation. Amer. J. Roentgenol., *101*:61–67, 1967.

Schaerer, J. P., and Whitney, R. L.: Prostatic metastases simulating intracranial meningioma. J. Neurosurg., *10*:546–549, 1953.

Schechter, M. M., and Zingesser, L. H.: The radiology of aqueductal stenosis. Radiology, *88*:905–916, 1967.

Schisano, G., and Olivecrona, H.: Neurinomas of the gasserian ganglion and trigeminal root. J. Neurosurg., *17*:306–322, 1960.

Schmitz, A. L., and Haveson, S. B.: Roentgen diagnosis of eighth nerve tumors. Radiology, *75*:531–543, 1960.

Schwartz, C. W., and Collins, L. C.: The Skull and Brain Roentgenologically Considered. Springfield, Charles C Thomas, 1951.

Schwarz, E.: Roentgen findings in progeria. Radiology, *79*:411–414, 1962.

Schwarz, E.: The skull in skeletal dysplasias. Amer. J. Roentgenol., *89*:928–937, 1963.

Scott, M. F.: Hyperostosing meningiomas of the asterion. Amer. J. Roentgenol., *87*:1041–1047, 1962.

Sherman, R. S., and Leaming, P.: Roentgen findings in hemoblastoma. Radiology, *60*:837–849, 1953.

Shopfner, C. E., Jabbour, J. T., and Vallion, R. M.: Craniolacunia. Amer. J. Roentgenol., *93*:343–349, 1965.

Steinbach, H. L., Feldman, R., and Goldberg, M. B.: Acromegaly. Radiology, *72*:535–549, 1959 (27 ref.).

Tatelman, M.: Pathways of cerebral collateral circulation. Radiology, *75*:349–362, 1960.

Taveras, J. M., and Wood, E. H.: Diagnostic Neuroradiology. Baltimore, Williams and Wilkins Co., 1964.

Watson, E. H., and Lowery, G. H.: Growth and Development of Children. Fifth Edition. Chicago, Year Book Medical Publishers, 1967.

Wilson, C. B., and Bertan, V.: Cerebral leptomeningeal cysts of developmental origin. Amer. J. Roentgenol., *98*:570–574, 1966.

Zizmor, J., Noyek, A. M., Bellucci, R. J., Gutkin, M. L., and Vermes, E.: The preoperative diagnosis of brain abscess by the roentgenologic demonstration by an air fluid level: a report of two cases. Amer. J. Roentgenol., *92*:844–849, 1964.

Zizmor, J., Smith, B., Fasano, C., and Converse, J. M.: Roentgen diagnosis of blow-out fractures of the orbit. Amer. J. Roentgenol., *87*:1009–1018, 1962.

13

Radiology of Special Areas of the Skull and Space-Occupying Lesions Within the Cranium

THE SELLA TURCICA

Normal Anatomy and Measurements (Figure 13–1).   The following anatomic parts of the sella turcica must be identified:
1. The diaphragma sellae.
2. The tuberculum sellae.
3. The hypophyseal fossa (pituitary fossa).

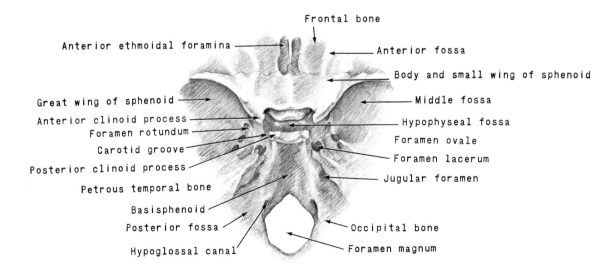

Frontal bone

Anterior ethmoidal foramina

Anterior fossa

Body and small wing of sphenoid

Great wing of sphenoid

Middle fossa

Anterior clinoid process

Hypophyseal fossa

Foramen rotundum

Foramen ovale

Carotid groove

Foramen lacerum

Posterior clinoid process

Jugular foramen

Petrous temporal bone

Basisphenoid

Posterior fossa

Occipital bone

Hypoglossal canal

Foramen magnum

Relations of the Sella Turcica

Figure 13–1   En face view of sella turcica.

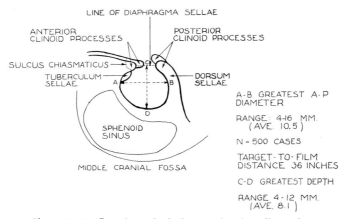

Figure 13–2   Camp's method of measuring the sella turcica.

4. The chiasmatic or optic groove.
5. The anterior clinoid processes.
6. The posterior clinoid processes.
7. The dorsum sellae.

Measurements of the sella turcica are of significance in the determination of:
1. Increased intracranial pressure.
2. Direct pressure erosion of the sella from other external causes in the immediate vicinity of the sella.
3. Intrasellar expanding lesion.

The methods for measurement have involved the following principles:
1. Antero-posterior and depth measurements (Camp) (Figure 13–2).
2. Area measurements in the lateral projection (Silverman).
3. Volume measurements (DiChiro and Nelson; Fisher and DiChiro) (Figure 13–3).

Silverman's data are based on measurements of the pituitary fossa of boys and girls one month to 18 years of age from the Fels Research Institute growth study.

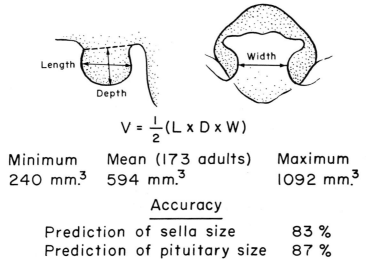

Figure 13–3   The volume of the sella turcica as determined by DiChiro and Nelson.

(The student is referred to the original data regarding this study, especially for measurement of the sella in children.)

In our practice, Camp's method has found greatest favor, although greater accuracy in doubtful cases is obtained by the volume measurements established by DiChiro and Nelson and by Fisher and DiChiro.

The measurements proposed by DiChiro and Nelson consist of length and depth, as well as width, of the sella turcica on a postero-anterior view of the sella, Caldwell view. The target-to-film distance is 28 inches. Body section radiographs may have to be employed to obtain this measurement. The width of the sella ranges between 9 and 21 mm., with a mean of 13.8 and a standard deviation of 2.1. The area of the sella turcica ranges between 47 and 129 sq. mm., with a mean of 84 and a standard deviation of 16. When corrected for magnification and empirical error, the formula for prediction of volume of the sella turcica is indicated in Figure 13–3. The data presented by DiChiro and Nelson suggest that the pituitary gland occupies approximately 79 per cent (on the average) of the volume of the sella turcica and thus considerable enlargement of the pituitary gland may not actually produce changes which can be seen on routine films of the skull. Also, the pituitary gland may be enlarged laterally without demonstrable roentgenologic changes. The accuracy for prediction of pituitary size is considered to be 87 per cent.

Hare has proposed that 130 mm.^{2} be used as a maximum area in lateral projection (Acheson).

PLAIN SKULL FILM CHANGES IN AND AROUND THE SELLA TURCICA AND THEIR SIGNIFICANCE (Weidner et al.)

1. There are great variations in the normal size and configuration of the sella turcica. This must be evaluated in at least three views: lateral; P-A for floor of sella turcica; and A-P Towne's for dorsum sellae.

2. There is no constant relationship between the size of the sella turcica and the size of the pituitary gland.

3. The best method for determination of enlargement of the sella turcica requires consideration of length, depth, and width.

4. The double contoured appearance of the floor of the sella turcica is usually evidence of intrasellar tumor with asymmetrical expansion. One must be certain, however, that the sella is not normally tilted or that other bony structures such as the sphenoid sinus and carotid sulcus may result in the false appearance of a double floor.

5. Laminography should be performed whenever the boundaries of the sella turcica are not clearly delineated on plain films.

6. Intrasellar lesions causing enlargement of the sella are usually pituitary adenomas; less commonly they are craniopharyngiomas.

a. Suprasellar or tuberculum sellae meningiomas may extend into the sella causing enlargement.

7. Unilateral enlargement of the sella turcica may be secondary to intracavernous aneurysm of the internal carotid artery.

8. Enlargement of sella is also seen with hydrocephalus when the third ventricle enlarges and bulges into the sella.

9. Adenomas of pituitary, usually arising from the anterior lobe of the pituitary, produce the following slight differences in appearance:

a. Chromophobe adenomas grow rapidly and become large with destruction and demineralization of the bony walls of the sella. There are no peripheral skeletal changes ordinarily.

b. Eosinophilic adenomas produce gigantism in the young and acromegaly in adults. They are slow-growing and the walls of the pituitary mold to conform to the configuration of a slow-growing tumor. They are well defined and the margins are well calcified usually.

c. Basophilic adenomas are tiny adenomas and rarely cause any enlargement of the sella; these patients usually have Cushing's syndrome and generalized osteoporosis. Rarely, predominantly basophilic adenomas are large expansile lesions.

10. Calcification in pituitary adenomas is rare, possibly 5 to 7 per cent (Deery).

11. Curvilinear calcification seen with chromophobe adenomas occurs in the capsule of the tumor or in the wall of the cyst. Calcification may occur in eosinophilic adenomas, called pituitary calculi.

Variations of Normal.   The sella turcica may be round or oval, deep or shallow in both children and adults. The hypophyseal fossa is highly variable in size within the limits defined previously. The clinoids are blunt protruding processes which are poorly developed in the newborn, and the middle clinoid processes are absent in some individuals.

In profile the sella at times has a somewhat biconcave appearance due to what appears to be an excavation beneath the anterior clinoids. This is without pathologic significance, but may be found more frequently in children.

The posterior clinoid processes at times participate in the pneumatization of the dorsum sellae, representing an upward extension of the air cells from the sphenoid sinuses.

Other variations of normal are illustrated in Figure 13–4. In children 70 per cent are round. In adults only 24.4 per cent are round, whereas 58 per cent are oval and 17.2 per cent are flat.

The following other *variations of normal* may be noted:

An inconstant middle clinoid process may be present on one or both sides.

The middle clinoid process may unite with either the anterior or posterior clinoid processes or both, unilaterally or bilaterally.

There may be unilateral or bilateral bridging between the anterior and posterior clinoid processes.

There may be complete or partial pneumatization of the dorsum sellae.

The dorsum sellae may grow asymmetrically on the two sides, so that the posterior clinoids do not appear parallel with one another.

The tuberculum sellae may be unduly prominent.

The sulcus chiasmatis (optic groove) may vary in depth and length, and the limbus sphenoidalis just anterior to it may be thick and knoblike.

The sella turcica varies considerably in shape, and these variations are usually without significance (flat, round, or oval).

An unusually small sella occurs in pituitary dwarfism, but ordinarily it has no pathologic significance.

There is no constant relationship between the size of the sella and the size of the hypophysis.

The Small Sella Turcica from Prolonged Cerebrospinal Fluid Shunting (Kaufman et al.).   Prolonged cerebrospinal fluid shunting procedures can cause a marked

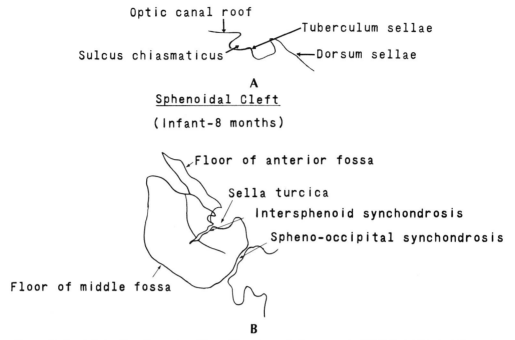

Figure 13–4   *A.* Infantile sella turcica. (From Kier, Amer. J. Roentgenol., *102*:747, 1968.) *B.* Sellar and parasellar synchondroses. (From Shopfner, C. E. et al.: Amer. J. Roentgenol., *104*:186, 1968.)

Figure 13–4 continued on opposite page.

reduction in the size of the sella turcica and a change in its configuration. Changes of the base of the skull may also be present. These include:

1. Thickening of the cribriform plate.
2. Thickening and upward bowing of the planum sphenoidale.
3. Posterior bowing of the clivus.

The bone changes are the result of remodeling and are reversible. All parts of the skull are capable of exhibiting the effects of alterations in cerebrospinal fluid pressures and pulsations. A decrease in the size of some foramina occurs. If the sella turcica is protected by the diaphragma sellae, it will not participate in the remodeling of the base and calvarium, such as occurs in the shunting procedures (Kaufman et al.).

Changes Related to Intrasellar Expanding Lesions (Figure 13–5)

Floor of sella is thinned and deepened, and may be "double contoured."

The dorsum sellae is thinned, elongated, and bent backward (Figure 13–5 A).

Ultimately, all parts may be thinned or destroyed with only anterior clinoids remaining (Figure 13–5 B).

At times erosion of the sella is asymmetrical, with one side of the hypophyseal fossa excavated more deeply than the other. This may require body section radiography for the best demonstration (both lateral and postero-anterior) (Figure 13–5 C).

Lesions

Pituitary acidophilic and chromophobic adenomas.
Occasionally, craniopharyngiomas.

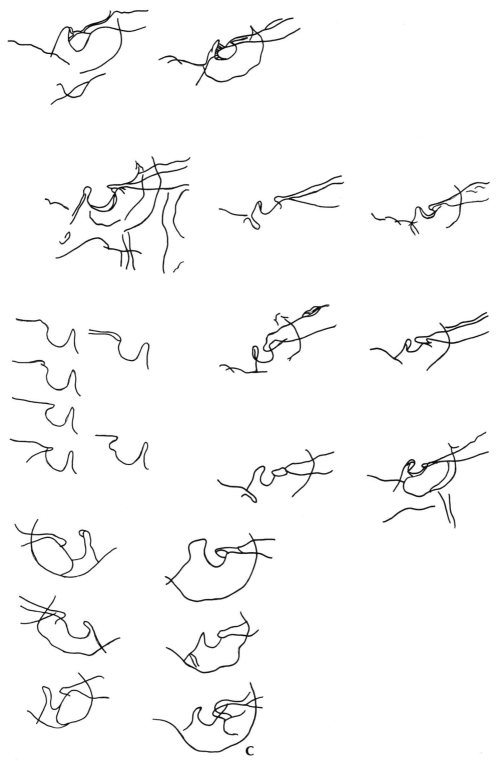

Figure 13–4 (*Continued*).   *C*. Variations in sagittal contour of the normal sella turcica.

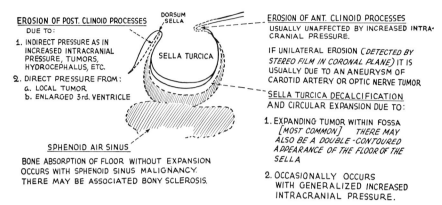

EROSION OF POST. CLINOID PROCESSES
DUE TO:
1. INDIRECT PRESSURE AS IN INCREASED INTRACRANIAL PRESSURE, TUMORS, HYDROCEPHALUS, ETC.
2. DIRECT PRESSURE FROM:
a. LOCAL TUMOR
b. ENLARGED 3rd. VENTRICLE

DORSUM SELLA

SELLA TURCICA

EROSION OF ANT. CLINOID PROCESSES
USUALLY UNAFFECTED BY INCREASED INTRACRANIAL PRESSURE.

IF UNILATERAL EROSION (DETECTED BY STEREO FILM IN CORONAL PLANE) IT IS USUALLY DUE TO AN ANEURYSM OF CAROTID ARTERY OR OPTIC NERVE TUMOR

SELLA TURCICA DECALCIFICATION AND CIRCULAR EXPANSION DUE TO:

1. EXPANDING TUMOR WITHIN FOSSA [MOST COMMON] THERE MAY ALSO BE A DOUBLE-CONTOURED APPEARANCE OF THE FLOOR OF THE SELLA

2. OCCASIONALLY OCCURS WITH GENERALIZED INCREASED INTRACRANIAL PRESSURE.

SPHENOID AIR SINUS
BONE ABSORPTION OF FLOOR WITHOUT EXPANSION OCCURS WITH SPHENOID SINUS MALIGNANCY. THERE MAY BE ASSOCIATED BONY SCLEROSIS.

Figure 13–5 Diagram illustrating the changes in the sagittal contour of the sella turcica resulting from increased intracranial pressure or an intrasellar expanding lesion.

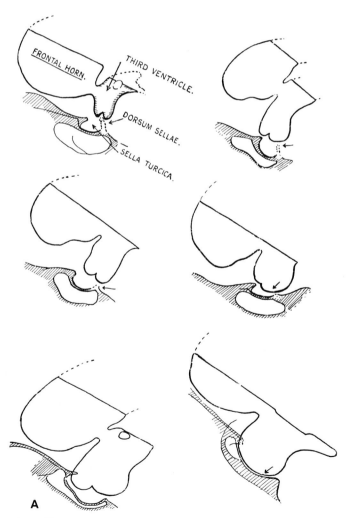

FRONTAL HORN.

THIRD VENTRICLE.

DORSUM SELLAE.

SELLA TURCICA.

A

Figure 13–6 *A.* (From Shanks, S. C., and Kerley, P.: *A Textbook of X-ray Diagnosis*, Vol. 1, 4th Ed. Philadelphia, W. B. Saunders Co., 1969.)

Figure 13–6 continued on opposite page.

B

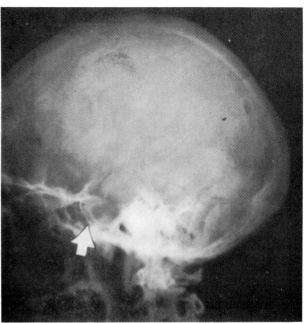

Figure 13–6 (*Continued*).   *A* and *C*. Erosion of the posterior clinoids and floor of the sella due to increased intracranial pressure from an extrasellar lesion. *B*. Double-contoured appearance of the floor of the sella due to erosion and ballooning.

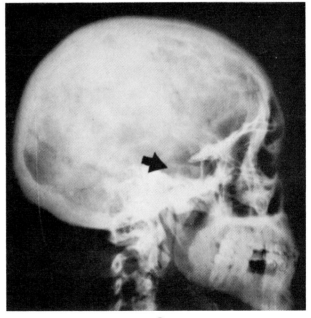

C

Changes Related to Extrasellar Intracranial Expanding Lesions (Figure 13–6)

Floor of sella is thinned but not deepened.
Dorsum sellae thinned and posterior clinoids sharpened.
Anterior clinoids sharpened.
Floor of sella tends to be like a shallow bowl rather than a deep one.

Lesions

Chronic increase in intracranial pressure from brain tumors, chronic hydrocephalus, obstructing lesions at the base of the brain.

Changes Secondary to Destructive Disease of the Sphenoid Bone

Disease Entities. Tuberculosis of the sphenoid, carcinoma of sphenoid sinus, nasopharyngeal carcinoma, chordoma, glomus jugulare tumors, metastatic tumors infiltrating the sphenoid bone, and arachnoid cysts.

Radiographic Appearances. The floor of the sella, when involved in this fashion, usually shows evidence of reaction and sclerosis as well as destruction, with indistinct outline and adjoining sphenoid destruction as well. Frequently a mass in the nasopharyngeal air space can be identified.

Pneumoencephalography may be necessary to establish the diagnosis of arachnoid cysts (Ring and Waddington).

Parasellar or Intrasellar Calcification. Calcification in or adjoining the sella turcica tends to fall into the following categories (Figure 13–7):

Flocculent (as in a craniopharyngioma—see section on brain) within the hypophyseal fossa.

Circumlinear in the arc of a circle or ellipse (also seen with craniopharyngiomas as well as with adjoining aneurysms).

Tubular, as with calcification in the carotid arteries in their cavernous portions.

Mulberry-type calcification posterior to the dorsum sellae, as seen with chronic granuloma or gliomas.

These pathological types of calcification must be differentiated from the normal calcification of the petroclinoid ligament.

Other aspects of intracranial calcification are being deferred to the discussion of the brain.

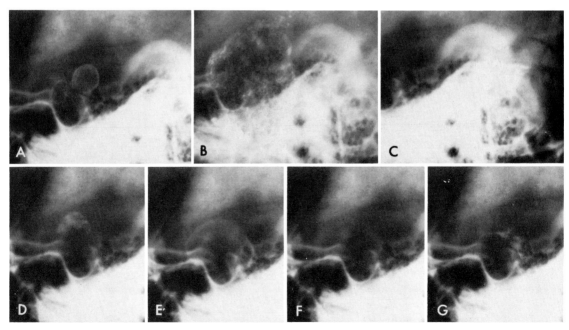

Figure 13–7   *A.* Carotid artery aneurysm. *B.* Craniopharyngioma; calcified chordoma. *C.* Coarse calcium in medulloblastoma or ependymoma of fourth ventricle. *D.* Tuberculous meningitis (nodular parasellar); craniopharyngioma. *E.* Cystlike calcium in wall of aneurysm of internal carotid artery. *F.* Intrasellar calcification, without enlarged sella; degenerate pituitary adenoma. *G.* Craniopharyngioma. (Intensified diagrammatic radiographs.)

DISEASES OF THE FACIAL BONES AND PARANASAL SINUSES

Special Views of the Face, Mandible, Nose, and Paranasal Sinuses. These are illustrated in Figures 13–8, 13–9, 13–10, 13–11.

Routine for Examination of Films Obtained in Respect to Face, Mandible, Nose, and Paranasal Sinuses. A routine for study of the films obtained of these regions is shown in Figure 13–12.

Roentgen Pathology of the Facial Bones and Paranasal Sinuses

ABNORMAL ALTERATIONS IN SIZE

Congenital Occlusion of the Nares

Hypoplasia of the Facial Bones

Pierre Robin syndrome (congenital hypoplasia of mandible) (see Chapter 7).

Mandibulofacial dysostosis (Treacher-Collins syndrome; Franceschetti's syndrome). This has been previously considered in Chapter 7 (Schwarz et al.).

Acromegaly (see Chapter 10)

(*Text continued on page 538*)

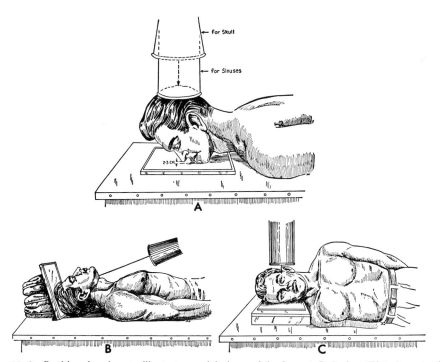

Figure 13–8 Position drawings to illustrate special views of the face. *A*. P-A view (Water's projection). *B*. Axial (submento-vertical) view. This view is utilized for visualization of the zygomatic arches, but with a lighter exposure technique than that for visualization of the other facial bones. *C*. Lateral view.

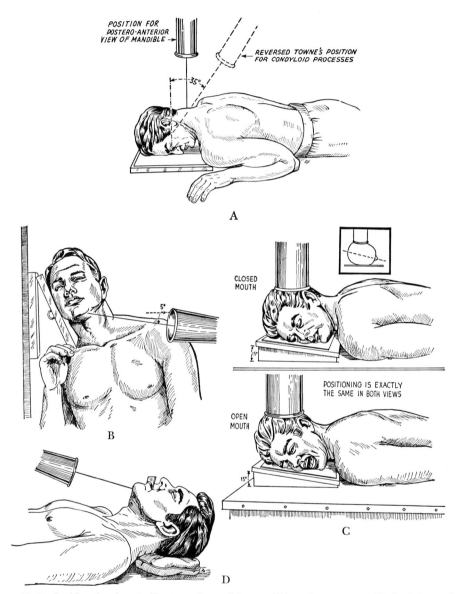

Figure 13–9 Position drawings to illustrate views of the mandible and temporomandibular joint. *A*. P-A view of the mandible. *B*. Oblique view of the mandible. *C*. Views of the temporomandibular joint with the mouth open and with the mouth closed. *D*. Intra-oral views of the body of the mandible.

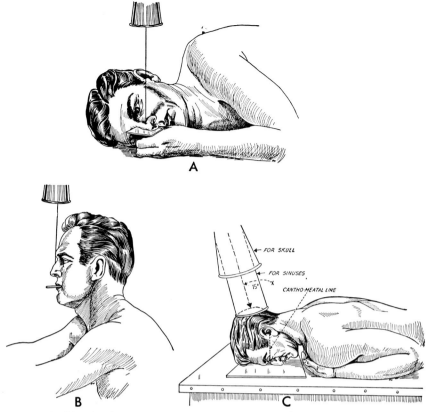

Figure 13–10 Position drawings for routine radiographic study of the nose. *A.* "Soft tissue" lateral view of the nasal bones. *B.* Tangential superior-inferior view of the nasal bones. *C.* P-A view of the nose with a 15-degree tilt of the tube caudally.

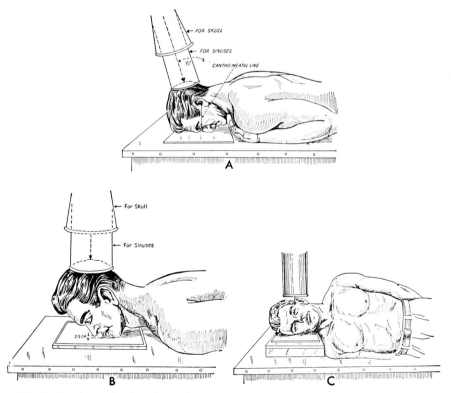

Figure 13–11 Routine projections for study of the paranasal sinuses. *A.* Caldwell's projection of the skull. *B.* P-A view with the chin on the film and the nose raised 2 or 3 cm. from the film (Water's projection). *C.* Lateral projection of the paranasal sinuses (same as lateral view of the face).

ROUTINE FOR STUDY OF PARANASAL SINUSES

I. CALDWELL'S VIEW

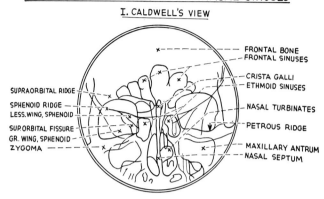

1. NOTE CLARITY AND INTEGRITY OF WALLS OF FRONTAL AND ETHMOID SINUSES.
2. NOTE FRONTAL BONE TEXTURE.
3. NOTE BONY NASAL SEPTUM AND ADJOINING TURBINATES; NOTE AERATION OF NASAL AIR PASSAGES.
4. NOTE ORBITS AND SPHENOIDAL MARKINGS THEREIN.
5. ONE CAN SEE MAXILLARY SINUSES ALSO, BUT NOT TO MAXIMUM ADVANTAGE.

Figure 13–12.

II. WATERS' VIEW, MOUTH OPEN
(a) PATIENT UPRIGHT
(b) PATIENT RECUMBENT

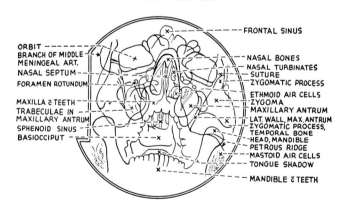

1. NOTE CLARITY OF MAXILLARY ANTRA, INTEGRITY OF ANTRAL WALLS, AND ADJOINING ZYGOMA.
2. NOTE SPHENOID SINUS.
3. OTHER SINUSES ARE ALSO SEEN, BUT NOT TO MAXIMUM ADVANTAGE.
4. NASAL BRIDGE AND SEPTUM.
5. FLUID LEVELS IN UPRIGHT FILM.

NOTE: *THIS VIEW WITH MOUTH OPEN, IN CONTRADISTINCTION TO THE ROUTINE WATERS' VIEW WITH THE MOUTH CLOSED, IS OUR INDIVIDUAL PREFERENCE, SINCE THE SPHENOID SINUS THEN COMES INTO VIEW.*

Figure 13–12 continued on opposite page.

III. LATERAL VIEW OF PARANASAL SINUSES

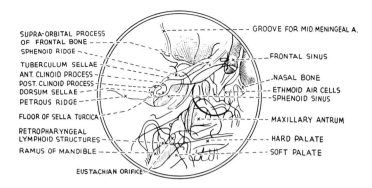

SUPRA-ORBITAL PROCESS OF FRONTAL BONE
SPHENOID RIDGE
TUBERCULUM SELLAE
ANT. CLINOID PROCESS
POST. CLINOID PROCESS
DORSUM SELLAE
PETROUS RIDGE
FLOOR OF SELLA TURCICA
RETROPHARYNGEAL LYMPHOID STRUCTURES
RAMUS OF MANDIBLE
EUSTACHIAN ORIFICE

GROOVE FOR MID. MENINGEAL A.
FRONTAL SINUS
NASAL BONE
ETHMOID AIR CELLS
SPHENOID SINUS
MAXILLARY ANTRUM
HARD PALATE
SOFT PALATE

1. NOTE FRONTAL, ETHMOID, SPHENOID AND MAXILLARY SINUSES.
2. NOTE POSTERIOR NASOPHARYNGEAL WALL.
3. NOTE SELLA TURCICA.
4. NOTE INTEGRITY OF SPHENOID RIDGE.
5. NASAL BONES MAY BE SEEN WITH BRIGHT LIGHT SOURCE.

Figure 13–12 (*Continued*).

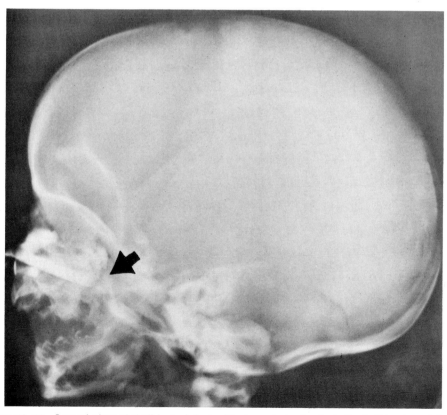

Figure 13–13 Lateral view of skull in an infant with choanal atresia. An iodized oil has been injected intranasally with complete obstruction as the result of the atresia.

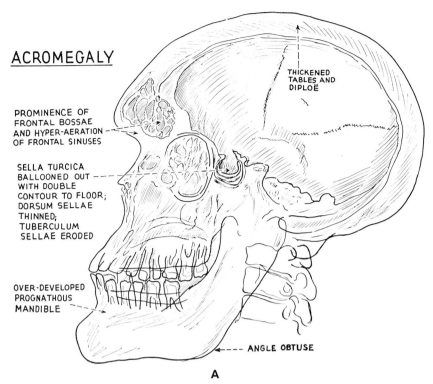

ACROMEGALY

THICKENED
TABLES AND
DIPLOË

PROMINENCE OF
FRONTAL BOSSAE
AND HYPER-AERATION
OF FRONTAL SINUSES

SELLA TURCICA
BALLOONED OUT
WITH DOUBLE
CONTOUR TO FLOOR;
DORSUM SELLAE
THINNED;
TUBERCULUM
SELLAE ERODED

OVER-DEVELOPED
PROGNATHOUS
MANDIBLE

ANGLE OBTUSE

A

Figure 13–14   *A*. Acromegalic changes in the skull and facial bones.

Hypertelorism (Greig's syndrome)

Definition.   This is a form of abnormal development of the cranial bones characterized by a great distance between the eyes, mental deficiency, brachycephaly, and a depressed nasal bridge. The condition is a result of malformation of the sphenoid bone—the greater wing being smaller, and the lesser wing larger than normal. Ocular hypertelorism occurs in conjunction with other congenital syndromes involving the face, including acrocephalosyndactyly, mongoloidism, Larsen's syndrome, craniofacial dysostosis, Hurler's syndrome, Morquio-Ullrich syndrome, basal cell nevus-jaw cyst syndrome, and pseudohypoparathyroidism.

Normal interorbital measurements for various ages are presented in Table 12–3.

Radiographic Findings

Markedly increased width between the medial margins of the orbits due to an overdevelopment of the lesser wings of the sphenoid and an underdevelopment of the greater wings.

The paranasal sinuses and mastoids tend to be quite large and the hypophyseal fossa is broad (Figure 13–15).

CHANGES IN DENSITY

Increased Density of the Paranasal Sinuses.   Representative lesions reflecting changes in aeration of the paranasal sinuses are shown in Figure 13–16. These include:

Acute and chronic sinusitis.

Thickening or edema of the mucous membrane of the paranasal sinuses.

Figure 13–14 continued on opposite page.

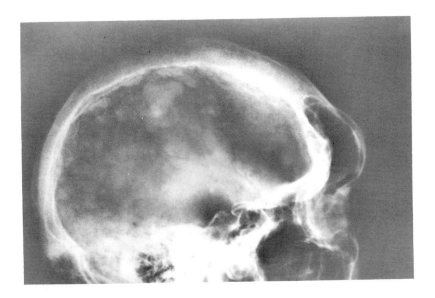

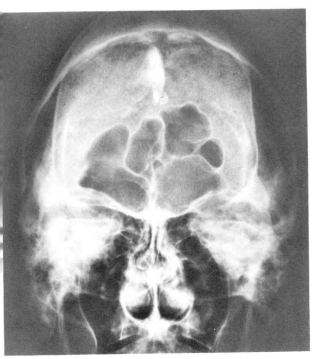

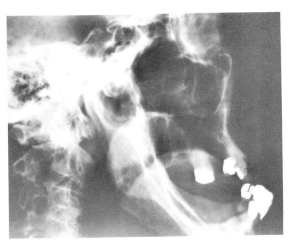

B

Figure 13–14 (*Continued*).   *B*. A lateral skull in acromegaly. Note the marked thickening of the inner and outer table of the calvarium. This is most prominent parasagittally. The frontal sinuses especially are markedly pneumatized and the mandible protrudes with the angle of the mandible more obtuse than normal. *Top*. Close-up view of the skull in the lateral projection. *Lower left*. Postero-anterior view. *Lower right*. Close-up view of the mandible in lateral projection.

HYPERTELORISM

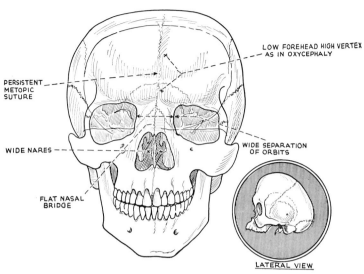

PERSISTENT METOPIC SUTURE

LOW FOREHEAD HIGH VERTEX AS IN OXYCEPHALY

WIDE NARES

WIDE SEPARATION OF ORBITS

FLAT NASAL BRIDGE

LATERAL VIEW

Figure 13–15.

Polypi.

Mucoceles.

Hemorrhage or blood clots in the sinuses.

Tumors, either primary or secondary to dental origin.

Malignant tumors originating in the epithelial lining of the paranasal sinuses (carcinomas). They may, however, on occasion be sarcomas or mixed tumors.

Foreign bodies in the sinuses.

Radiographic Appearances

Any of these lesions causes an obscuring of the normal aeration of the paranasal sinuses. If there is fluid in the sinus, a fluid level can be demonstrated in the erect position. If polypi are present rounded defects are demonstrated. In the case of benign tumors such as osteomas, dense or cancellous bone is usually shown within the sinus as a rounded, dense mass of bone arising from the anterior wall of the frontal sinus. When malignant tumors of the maxillary antrum occur, bone absorption and destruction are usually associated. This may require body section radiography for demonstration.

The mucocele occurs most frequently in the frontal sinus. The osteum of the sinus becomes blocked and there is a retention of secretions in the sinus that produces this lesion. The retained secretions produce an expansion which gradually erodes the bony walls of the sinus. The mucocele may contain some fatty substance and as a result of this diminished density it may appear somewhat less than water density. If erosion on the sinus wall has occurred, the shape of the paranasal sinus is altered accordingly with a minimal reactive zone of sclerosis.

Increased Density of the Bones of the Face

Leontiasis ossea (has been previously considered).

Osteoblastic response in relation to chronic infection or tumor metastases such as carcinoma of the prostate.

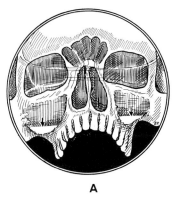

A

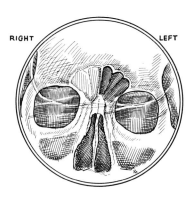

DIFFUSE THICKENING OF RIGHT
FRONTAL SINUS MUCUS MEMBRANE
PRODUCING GENERAL HAZINESS
IN THIS SINUS.

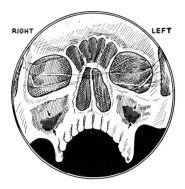

MUCOPERIOSTEAL THICKENING OF
MAXILLARY ANTRA; THE THICKENED
MUCOSAL LINE RUNS PARALLEL TO
THE ANTRAL WALL AND IS STRAIGHT;
ALLERGIC THICKENING IS OFTEN
SCALLOPED IN APPEARANCE.

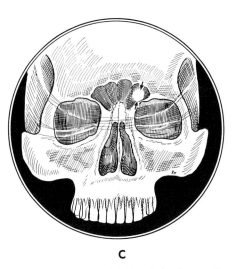

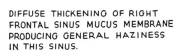

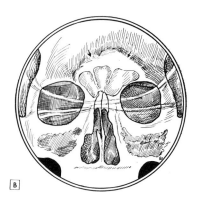

IN CONTRAST TO OSTEOMYELITIS, THIS IS PURELY
SCLEROTIC REACTION WITH NO RAREFIED AREAS
OF BONE DESTRUCTION.

C   **B**

Figure 13–16   *A.* Fluid levels in the maxillary antra demonstrated in erect film in Water's projection in a patient with acute sinusitis. *B.* Thickening of lining membrane of maxillary sinus of inflammatory or allergic origin. Sclerosis of the frontal bone surrounding the frontal sinus, indicating chronic inflammatory disease of the adjoining paranasal sinus. *C.* Osteoma of the frontal sinus.

Figure 13–16 continued on following page.

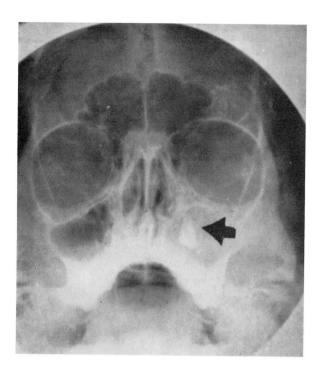

Figure 13–16 (*Continued*). *D.* Dentigerous cyst (odontoma) in the left maxillary antrum. Radiograph and tracing of a dentigerous cyst (in another patient) occupying the maxillary antrum, showing the relationship to the crown of the tooth contained within the cyst.

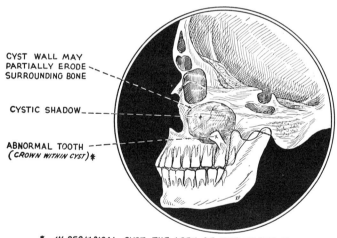

CYST WALL MAY PARTIALLY ERODE SURROUNDING BONE

CYSTIC SHADOW

ABNORMAL TOOTH (*CROWN WITHIN CYST*)*

* *IN PERIAPICAL CYST, THE APEX OF THE TOOTH IS CONTAINED WITHIN THE CYST.*

D

Figure 13–16 continued on opposite page.

A combined osteoblastic and osteolytic reaction is found in fibrous dysplasia.

Diminished Density of the Bones of the Face

Fractures

CLASSIFICATION.   Fractures are most readily classified by the major bones involved (mandible, maxilla, nose, zygoma, frontoethmoid, and mixed complex fractures).

CARCINOMA OF LEFT MAXILLARY ANTRUM

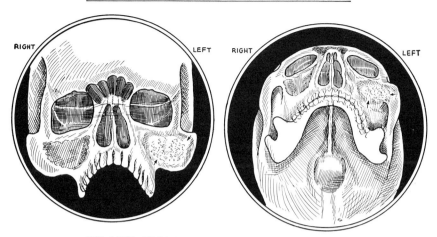

THE LEFT MAXILLARY ANTRAL RADIOLUCENCY IS COMPLETELY
REPLACED BY SOLID TUMOR WITH THE BONE SURROUNDING
THE ANTRUM INVADED AND DESTROYED; THE ANTRAL WALL
MARKINGS ARE LOST.

E

MAXILLARY ANTRAL ALLERGIC POLYP

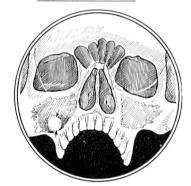

POLYPOID FILLING DEFECT IN
MAXILLARY ANTRUM, ALLERGIC
IN ORIGIN; MAY BE UNILATERAL
OR MULTIPLE; TURBINATES ARE
OFTEN SWOLLEN.

CHRONIC PANSINUSITIS

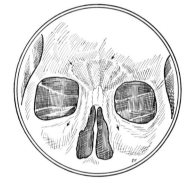

ALL OF THE SINUSES
ARE DIFFUSELY CLOUDY
AND PARTIALLY RADIO-
OPAQUE.

F

MUCOCELE OF LEFT FRONTAL SINUS

Figure 13–16 *(Continued). E to G.*

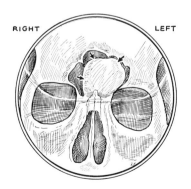

THERE IS A PRESSURE ATROPHY
OF SURROUNDING BONE CAUSED BY
A RADIOLUCENT, EXPANDING,
SHARPLY DEMARCATED LESION.

G

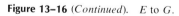

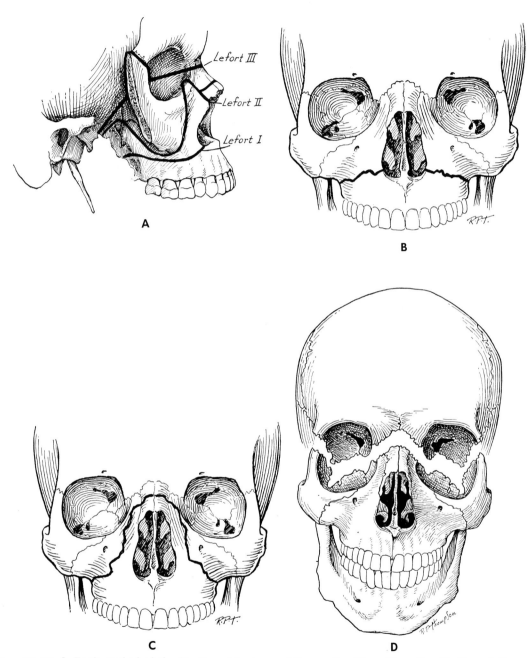

Figure 13–17 LeFort's method of classification of fractures of the maxilla. (From Kazanjian, V. H., and Converse, J. M.: *The Surgical Treatment of Facial Injuries,* 2nd Ed. Baltimore, Williams and Wilkins Co., 1959, with permission of publishers.)

FRACTURES OF THE MANDIBLE

In a study of fractures of the mandible it is important to note the relationship of the fracture line to teeth or to any underlying pathologic bony states.

The relationship of the fractures to existing teeth is important because of (a) the need to select appropriate treatment and immobilization devices, (b) the need to determine whether the fracture traverses an infectious zone in the mandible adjoining the tooth, and (c) the possibility that a devitalized tooth will act as a foreign body at the fracture site.

Fractures of the neck of the condyle are ordinarily treated best by simple methods, since the condyle is usually displaced anteriorly and medially.

Healing is very slow at first with fibrous ankylosis for a considerable time (Kazanjian and Converse).

FRACTURES OF THE MAXILLA. CLASSIFICATION.   LeFort's method of classification of fractures of the maxilla is shown in Figure 13–17.

FRACTURES OF THE BONES AND CARTILAGES OF THE NOSE.   In children the nasal bones are not fused in the midline and may be fractured independently, unlike those of the adult. Nasal bones do not fuse until adolescence. Various fractures of nasal bones are illustrated in Figure 13–18.

Radiographic Aspects.   A tangential view of the nasal bones in the fronto-mental projection should always be obtained utilizing tangential angles of anywhere from 16 to 45 degrees. The lateral view of the nose using soft tissue detail technique is also routine (Gillies and Millard).

FRACTURES OF THE ZYGOMA.   *The important anatomical considerations* may be summarized as follows: the zygoma articulates with four bones—the frontal, sphenoid, temporal, and maxilla; it participates in the formation of the lateral wall and floor of the orbital cavity, maxillary sinus, and zygomatic and temporal fossae; and it provides attachment for a number of the facial muscles.

NASAL FRACTURES

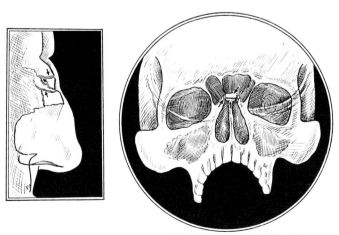

COMMINUTED FRACTURE OF NASAL BONES WITH DEPRESSION OF NASAL BRIDGE. SEPTUM IS ALSO FRACTURED.

Figure 13–18

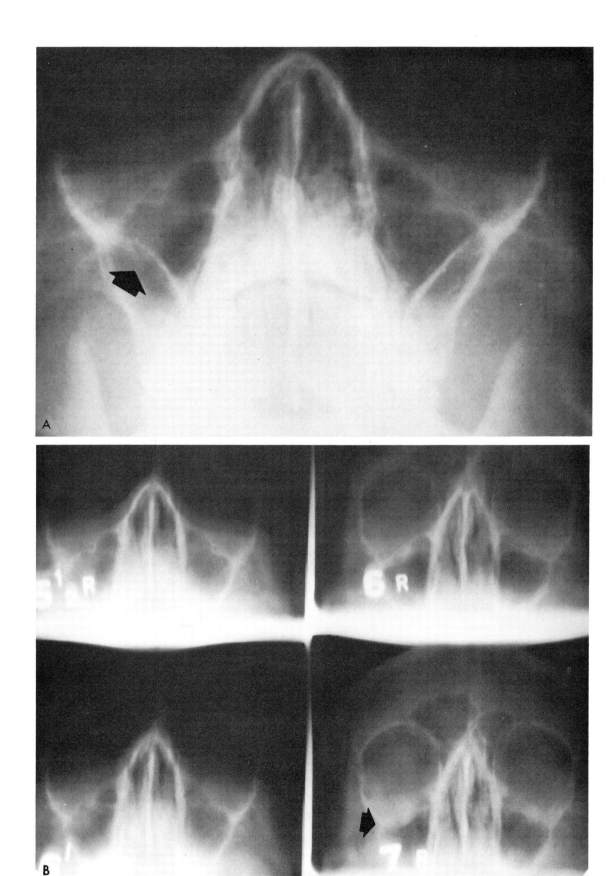

Figure 13–19 *Continued on opposite page. See opposite page for legend.*

Radiographic Considerations. Routine views obtained are (1) stereo-scopic views in Water's projection and (2) submentovertical views with particu-lar emphasis upon obtaining a tangential projection of the zygomatic processes and zygomatic arches. Body section radiography may also be indispensable when orbital fractures are suspected.

"BLOW-OUT FRACTURE" OF THE ORBIT. This is a fracture of the infraorbital plate without fracture of the infraorbital ridge. This type of fracture usually follows a direct blow to the eye. The infraorbital foramen and infraorbital nerve located close to the junction of the maxilla and zygoma may be injured as a result of a zygomatic fracture in this region, resulting in anesthesia in the distribution of the infraorbital nerve. This may be temporary or permanent. Enophthalmos may also result.

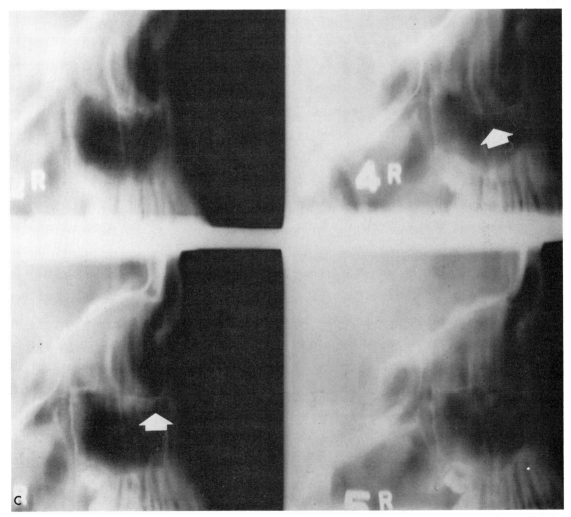

Figure 13–19 Blow-out fracture of the right orbit. *A.* Postero-anterior view of the orbits in Water's projection showing only edema around the infraorbital foramen. *B.* Body section radiographs at 5.5, 6, 6.5, and 7 cm. in Water's projection. The 7 cm. section demonstrates a definite depression of the infraorbital plate. *C.* Body section radiographs in the right lateral projection at 3.5, 4, 4.5 and 5 cm. distances from tabletop. The 4 and 4.5 cm. cuts show the depression of the infraorbital plate best.

Radiographic Findings.

The infraorbital foramen becomes cloudy.

Fragments may be identified in the maxillary sinus.

The floor of the orbit is broken into the maxillary sinus.

The maxillary sinus may be filled with orbital tissue (Figure 13–19).

FRACTURES OF THE BONES OF THE FRONTOETHMOIDAL REGION. A telescoping-type crash injury accompanied by deformity of the frontal, maxillary, and nasal bones is the type of injury which may extend into the anterior fossa of the skull and result in cerebrospinal rhinorrhea. The pointed crista galli, when fractured, may penetrate the dura.

Radiographic Considerations.

Stereoscopic views of the facial bones and skull are usually necessary.

Body section radiographs may also be required to estimate full damage.

A horizontal beam study of the skull is required to show the presence of air in the subdural subarachnoid space or ventricles, particularly if the patient is in the recumbent position. A horizontal beam study is necessary in the erect

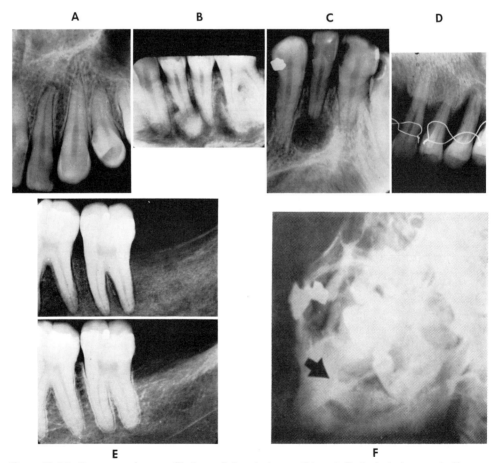

Figure 13–20 Representative mandibular and dental abnormalities. *A*. Periapical abscess. *B*. Cementoma. *C*. Dental root cysts (resemble granuloma closely). *D*. Periodontoclasia, with pyorrhea. *E*. Hyperparathyroidism (*above*). Note absence of lamina dura and return to normal following treatment (*below*). *F*. Actinomycosis. (All except *F* from Stafne, E. C.: *Oral Roentgenographic Diagnosis,* 3rd Ed. Philadelphia, W. B. Saunders Co., 1969.)

position for a similar purpose. Air may not be detected during the first 24 hours. Radiographs may be repeated if the patient shows increasing signs of frontal lobe dysfunction following such injury.

Roentgen Pathology of Paranasal Sinuses and Facial Bones: Diminished Density

Osteomyelitis

Pathogenesis. Osteomyelitis of the facial bones usually results by extension from infection in an adjoining paranasal sinus or tooth.

Radiographic Appearances. Bone resorption predominantly, with a surrounding area of bone sclerosis if the process is chronic.

The integrity of the teeth, periodontal membrane, and the lamina dura surrounding the teeth must be carefully studied. The different appearances of periodontal abnormalities are illustrated in the adjoining illustration (Figure 13–20).

Mucormycosis is a rapidly fatal important human fungal infection which may affect the paranasal sinuses especially in uncontrolled diabetics. Its roentgenologic characteristics are described as (1) nodular thickening of the soft tissue lining of many paranasal sinuses but sparing the frontal sinuses; (2) absence of fluid levels in erect roentgenograms; and (3) spotty destruction of the bony walls of the paranasal sinuses (Green et al.).

Cysts and Tumors

RADIOLOGICAL FEATURES OF DERMOID CYSTS OF THE NOSE
(Johnson, 1964)

1. Fusiform soft tissue swelling within the nasal septum.
2. Widening or disruption of the nasal vault.
3. Bifid septum.
4. Glabellar destruction and soft tissue mass.
5. Proliferation and pressure erosion of the nasal bone.
6. A large infrafrontal-interethmoid cystic space.

Classification

The *"fissural cyst."* These are found in the midline of the hard palate and cause diversion of the roots of adjoining teeth.

The *ameloblastoma* or *adamantinoma.* This tumor is usually multicystic in its appearance in the region of the angle of the mandible (Figure 13–21).

Tumors eroding the facial bones and paranasal sinuses by contiguous erosion from oral, nasal, or pituitary regions. These include carcinoma of the hard or soft palate, nasal tumors, and carcinoma or sarcoma of the paranasal sinuses. Likewise, tumors of the pituitary gland may erode downward into the sphenoid sinus.

Mixed tumors and plasma cell tumors. These are among the most frequent tumors involving the face and the adjoining bony structures.

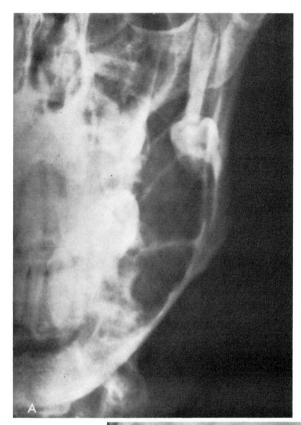

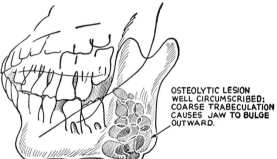

Figure 13–21   Adamantinoma involving the mandible, showing different perspectives. *A*. Postero-anterior view. *B*. Oblique view. *C*. Line diagram.

OSTEOLYTIC LESION WELL CIRCUMSCRIBED; COARSE TRABECULATION CAUSES JAW TO BULGE OUTWARD.

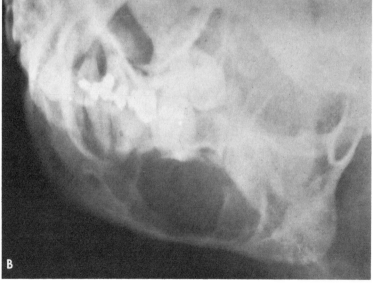

OSSIFYING FIBROMA OF THE FACE AND SKULL

1. An ossifying fibroma is frequently seen in the frontal bone at the orbital roof as an expanding lesion with a thin "eggshell" type of boundary.

2. It may appear sclerotic, produces thickened dense bone, and extends into neighboring structures, in this resembling fibrous dysplasia.

3. If it occurs in the mandible, areas of sclerosis alternate with smooth and spongy bone, producing deformity and displacement of teeth.

4. It may occur in the maxilla where it will obliterate the antral cavity and expand the bone—usually on its outer aspect—into the region of the cheek or the zygoma (Schwarz).

An inverting papilloma of the nose and paranasal sinuses may also produce opacification of the maxillary antrum to the point of destruction of its medial wall. It may cause lateral bowing and thinning of the nasal bones as well. The opacification of the maxillary antrum secondary to obstruction by an inverting nasal papilloma may be nonspecific in its appearance (Mainzer et al.).

Special Syndromes of the Temporomandibular Joints and Mandible

Costen's Syndrome. This is a dysfunction of the temporomandibular joint usually related to malocclusion of the teeth and terminating in considerable facial and head discomfort (Berlin et al.).

Fibrous Dysplasia of the Jaws (Cherubism) (Figure 13–22 *A* and *B*). This is usually a bilateral enlargement of the jaw associated with marked enlargement of adjoining lymph nodes in the submaxillary and upper jugular-carotid regions.

The affected jaw is markedly enlarged and has irregular areas of radiolucency with which are associated calcified tissue components.

The Amputated Condyloid Process of Gargoylism (Figure 13–22 *C, D*). The condyloid process may at times appear amputated in the gargoyle mandible (Hurler's disease).

MASTOIDS AND TEMPORAL BONES

Standard Positions for Radiography. The standard positions for radiography of the mastoids and temporal bones are (Figure 13–23):

Lateral oblique or Law's position.

Runström's position.

The special view of the petrous ridge in Stenver's position.

Towne's position.

The verticosubmental position or axial views.

Mayer's position on occasion.

There are other views which may be employed such as the Chausse 3 projection as shown.

Antero-posterior, lateral, and Stenver's views with polytomography.

Anatomy Portrayed on Films Obtained in the Above Positions (Figure 13–24)

(*Text continued on page 555*)

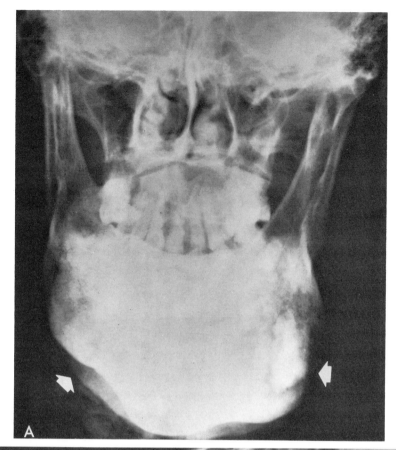

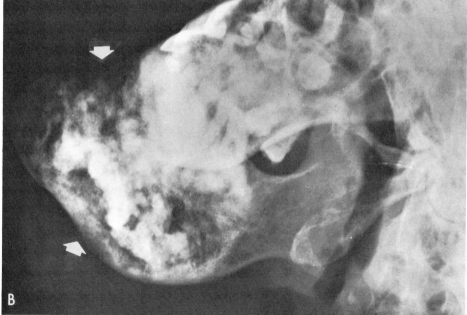

Figure 13–22   Fibrous dysplasia of the mandible (cherubism). *A*. P-A view of the mandible. *B*. Oblique view of the mandible. Note the rather characteristic appearance of the fibrous dysplasia with irregular expansion of bone, bizarre construction, and an outer shell of bone remaining intact.

Figure 13–22 continued on opposite page.

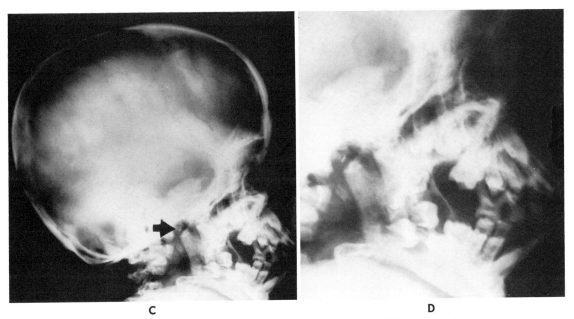

Figure 13–22 (*Continued*).   *C*. Skull in gargoylism. *D*. Mandible in gargoylism.

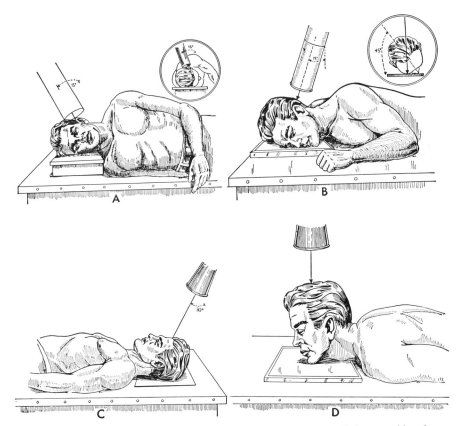

Figure 13–23 Standard positions utilized for radiographic examination of the mastoid and temporal bones. *A*. Lateral oblique projection of the mastoid process. (Runström's view: <30–35° in *A*, instead of 15°.) *B*. The special view of the petrous ridge in Stenver's position. *C*. Towne's projection. *D*. Axial or vertico-submental position used on occasion.

Figure 13–23 continued on following page.

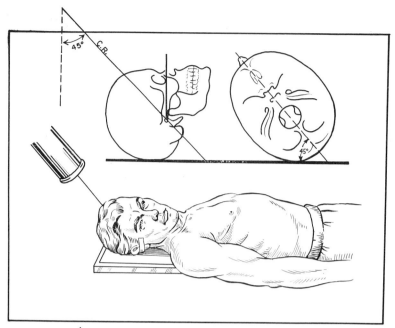

MAYER'S POSITION (FOR PETROUS RIDGE AND MASTOIDS)

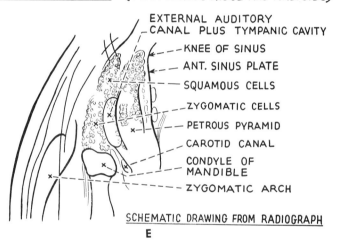

EXTERNAL AUDITORY
CANAL PLUS TYMPANIC CAVITY

— KNEE OF SINUS

— ANT. SINUS PLATE

— SQUAMOUS CELLS

— ZYGOMATIC CELLS

— PETROUS PYRAMID

— CAROTID CANAL

— CONDYLE OF
MANDIBLE

— ZYGOMATIC ARCH

SCHEMATIC DRAWING FROM RADIOGRAPH

E

Figure 13–23 (*Continued*).

CHAUSSE III PROJECTION FOR MIDDLE EAR DISEASE

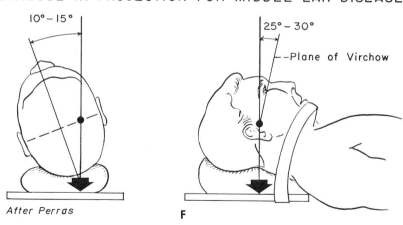

10° – 15°

25° – 30°

—Plane of Virchow

After Perras

F

Figure 13–23 continued on opposite page.

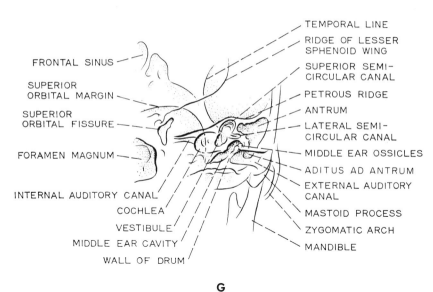

TEMPORAL LINE

RIDGE OF LESSER SPHENOID WING

SUPERIOR SEMI-CIRCULAR CANAL

PETROUS RIDGE

ANTRUM

LATERAL SEMI-CIRCULAR CANAL

MIDDLE EAR OSSICLES

ADITUS AD ANTRUM

EXTERNAL AUDITORY CANAL

MASTOID PROCESS

ZYGOMATIC ARCH

MANDIBLE

FRONTAL SINUS

SUPERIOR ORBITAL MARGIN

SUPERIOR ORBITAL FISSURE

FORAMEN MAGNUM

INTERNAL AUDITORY CANAL

COCHLEA

VESTIBULE

MIDDLE EAR CAVITY

WALL OF DRUM

G

Figure 13–23 (*Continued*). *G.* Line diagram showing the anatomy demonstrated by the Chaussé III projection.   *Figure 13–23 continued on following page.*

Classification of Radiographic Abnormalities of the Mastoids and Temporal Bones

DEVELOPMENTAL ABNORMALITIES; ABNORMALITIES OF SIZE

Atresia of the External Auditory Canal and External Meatus. Body section radiographs are especially helpful in demonstrating this abnormality and any associated abnormalities which may be present in the middle and internal ear. Careful study of the ossicles of the middle ear is especially important.

Arrested Development of the Mastoid and Petrous Air Cells

Definition. Pneumatization of the mastoid process which ordinarily begins to develop rapidly at the age of six years is arrested because of any developmental or inflammatory aberration. The cells which are ordinarily of a mixed size and variety are highly diploic and extremely small, and the bone tends to be somewhat thickened.

Radiographic Appearance (Figure 13–25). The mastoid cells are diploic and the periantral triangle is usually densely sclerotic. There is no associated bone resorption.

ABNORMALITIES IN DENSITY

Increase in Opacity of the Mastoid Air Cells With No Loss of Bone Integrity

Catarrhal mastoiditis: haziness of the mastoid region with no outright bone absorption or destruction (Figure 13–26).

Suppurative mastoiditis (Figure 13–27): may have a similar appearance to catarrhal mastoiditis except that the density may be somewhat increased. A diagnosis of suppurative mastoiditis, however, cannot be rendered radiologically unless there is outright associated bone absorption or destruction.

Chronic mastoiditis.

(*Text continued on page 566*)

ROUTINE FOLLOWED IN STUDY OF TEMPORAL BONE

I. LAW'S POSITION

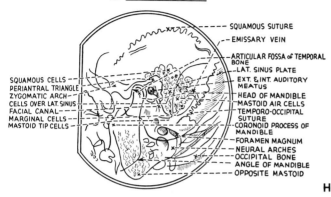

H

(1) NOTE DEGREE OF DEVELOPMENT OF PROCESS. NOTE PNEUMATIZATION OF MASTOID CELLS, WHETHER CELLS ARE MIXED OR DIPLOIC. NOTE SIZE OF CELLS. LOOK FOR EVIDENCE OF CELL NECROSIS AS INDICATED BY LOSS OF CLARITY OF CELL WALLS.

(2) FIND POSITION AND TRACE INTEGRITY OF LAT. SINUS PLATE.

(3) LOCATE AND STATE SIZE OF EMISSARY VEIN.

(4) STUDY AUDITORY MEATI FOR EROSION OR ENLARGEMENT.

Figure 13–23 (*Continued*).

II. STENVER'S POSITION

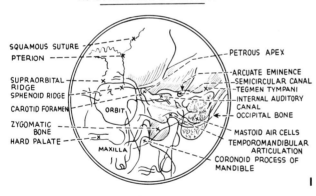

I

(1) AGAIN NOTE <u>DEGREE OF DEVELOPMENT OF PROCESS,</u> <u>PNEUMATIZATION</u> AND WHETHER CELLS ARE MIXED OR DIPLOIC. NOTE <u>SIZE</u> OF CELLS.

(2) NOTE CONTOUR OF PETROUS TEMPORAL AND INTEGRITY OF APEX AND INTERNAL ACOUSTIC MEATUS.

(3) NOTE TEGMEN TYMPANI AND INTEGRITY OF MASTOID ANTRUM UNDERLYING.

(4) NOTE INTEGRITY OF VESTIBULAR APPARATUS.

Figure 13–23 continued on opposite page.

III. VIEW OF MASTOID TIP

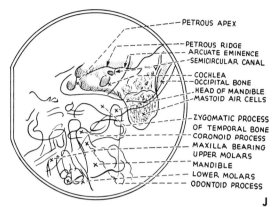

PETROUS APEX
PETROUS RIDGE
ARCUATE EMINENCE
SEMICIRCULAR CANAL
COCHLEA
OCCIPITAL BONE
HEAD OF MANDIBLE
MASTOID AIR CELLS
ZYGOMATIC PROCESS OF TEMPORAL BONE
CORONOID PROCESS
MAXILLA BEARING UPPER MOLARS
MANDIBLE
LOWER MOLARS
ODONTOID PROCESS

J

(1) NOTE <u>DEGREE OF DEVELOPMENT OF PROCESS</u>.
NOTE <u>PNEUMATIZATION</u> OF MASTOID CELLS, WHETHER
MIXED OR DIPLOIC. NOTE <u>SIZE</u> OF CELLS.

(2) NOTE CONTOUR OF PETROUS TEMPORAL AND DENSITY
OF SAME. NOTE INTEGRITY OF APEX.

IV. TOWNE'S POSITION

Figure 13–23 (*Continued*).

NOTE: THE ONLY ROUTINE VIEW WHERE A COMPARISON
OF BOTH SIDES IS POSSIBLE.

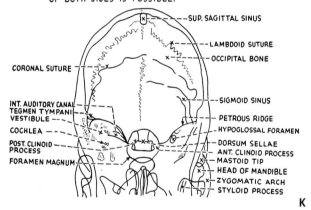

SUP. SAGITTAL SINUS
LAMBDOID SUTURE
OCCIPITAL BONE
CORONAL SUTURE
SIGMOID SINUS
INT. AUDITORY CANAL
TEGMEN TYMPANI
VESTIBULE
PETROUS RIDGE
HYPOGLOSSAL FORAMEN
COCHLEA
DORSUM SELLAE
POST. CLINOID PROCESS
ANT. CLINOID PROCESS
MASTOID TIP
FORAMEN MAGNUM
HEAD OF MANDIBLE
ZYGOMATIC ARCH
STYLOID PROCESS

K

(1) NOTE DEGREE OF DEVELOPMENT OF MASTOID PROCESSES
AND PETROUS RIDGES, PNEUMATIZATION, WHETHER DIPLOIC OR
MIXED, SIZE OF CELLS AND EXTENT OF AERATION.

(2) DELINEATE SYMMETRY OF PETROUS TEMPORAL, COMPARING RELATIVE
HEIGHT IN SKULL.

(3) NOTE INTEGRITY OF TEGMEN TYMPANI AND UNDERLYING MASTOID
ANTRUM.

(4) NOTE ARCUATE EMINENCE AND LABYRINTHINE UNDERLYING ANATOMY.

(5) NOTE INTEGRITY OF PETROUS APEX AND RELATIVE DIAMETER OF
INTERNAL ACOUSTIC MEATUS.

(6) NOTE SHAPE AND SIZE OF FORAMEN MAGNUM AND DORSUM SELLAE
PROJECTED THEREIN.

NOTE: *USUAL ROUTINE OF THE EXAMINATION OF SKULL FILM PRECEDES
USUAL EXAMINATION PROCEDURE.*

Figure 13–23 continued on following page.

V

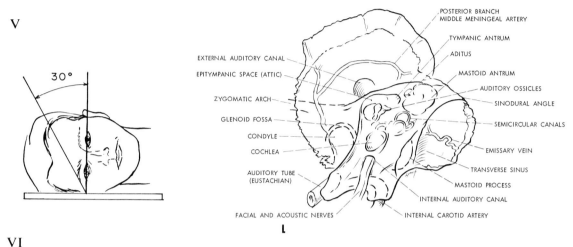

POSTERIOR BRANCH
MIDDLE MENINGEAL ARTERY

TYMPANIC ANTRUM

ADITUS

MASTOID ANTRUM

AUDITORY OSSICLES

SINODURAL ANGLE

SEMICIRCULAR CANALS

EMISSARY VEIN

TRANSVERSE SINUS

MASTOID PROCESS

INTERNAL AUDITORY CANAL

INTERNAL CAROTID ARTERY

EXTERNAL AUDITORY CANAL

EPITYMPANIC SPACE (ATTIC)

ZYGOMATIC ARCH

GLENOID FOSSA

CONDYLE

COCHLEA

AUDITORY TUBE
(EUSTACHIAN)

FACIAL AND ACOUSTIC NERVES

L

VI

SUBMENTO-VERTICAL VIEW SHOWING VARIATIONS IN ANGLE REQUIRED TO DEMONSTRATE TYMPANIC CAVITY AND OSSICLES

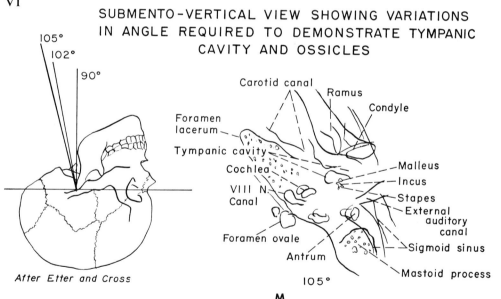

105°
102°
90°

Carotid canal

Ramus

Condyle

Foramen
lacerum

Tympanic cavity

Cochlea

VIII N.
Canal

Foramen ovale

Antrum

Malleus

Incus

Stapes

External
auditory
canal

Sigmoid sinus

Mastoid process

After Etter and Cross

105°

M

Figure 13–23 (*Continued*).

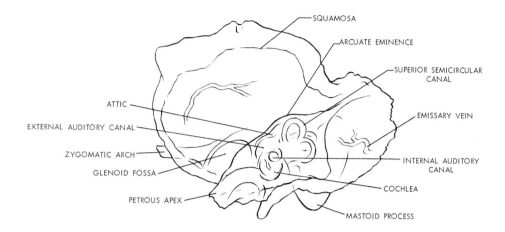

SQUAMOSA

ARCUATE EMINENCE

SUPERIOR SEMICIRCULAR CANAL

ATTIC

EMISSARY VEIN

EXTERNAL AUDITORY CANAL

ZYGOMATIC ARCH

GLENOID FOSSA

INTERNAL AUDITORY CANAL

PETROUS APEX

COCHLEA

MASTOID PROCESS

LAW'S VIEW

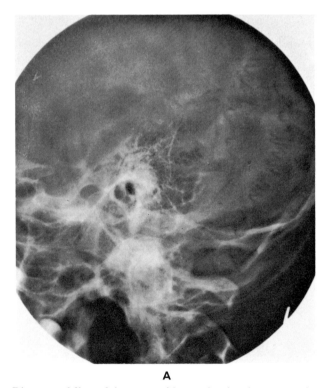

A

Figure 13–24 Diagrams of films of the temporal bones showing the anatomy in each projection.

Figure 13–24 continued on following page.

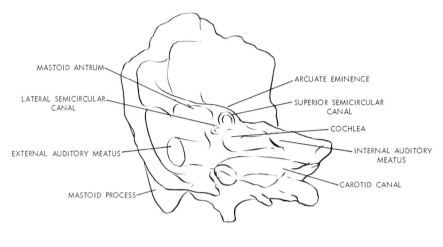

MASTOID ANTRUM

LATERAL SEMICIRCULAR
CANAL

EXTERNAL AUDITORY MEATUS

MASTOID PROCESS

ARCUATE EMINENCE

SUPERIOR SEMICIRCULAR
CANAL

COCHLEA

INTERNAL AUDITORY
MEATUS

CAROTID CANAL

STENVER'S VIEW

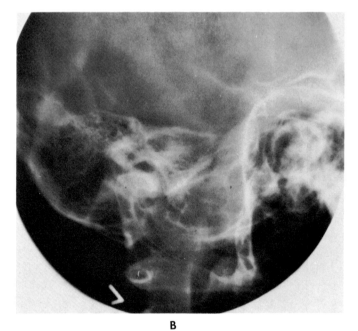

B

Figure 13–24 (*Continued*).

Figure 13–24 continued on opposite page.

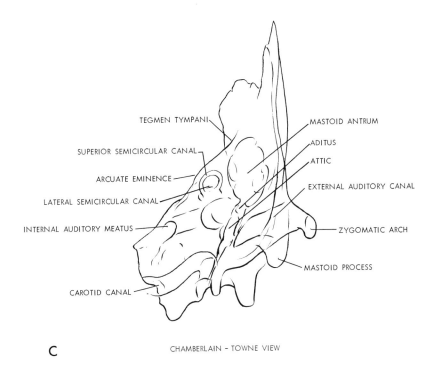

TEGMEN TYMPANI

SUPERIOR SEMICIRCULAR CANAL

ARCUATE EMINENCE

LATERAL SEMICIRCULAR CANAL

INTERNAL AUDITORY MEATUS

CAROTID CANAL

MASTOID ANTRUM

ADITUS

ATTIC

EXTERNAL AUDITORY CANAL

ZYGOMATIC ARCH

MASTOID PROCESS

C

CHAMBERLAIN - TOWNE VIEW

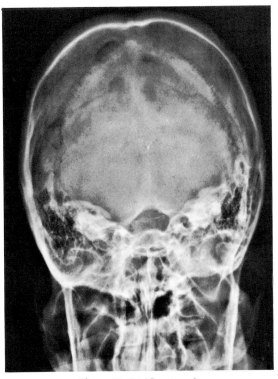

Figure 13–24 (*Continued*).

Figure 13–24 continued on following page.

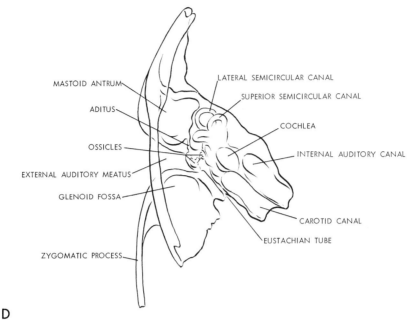

MASTOID ANTRUM

ADITUS

OSSICLES

EXTERNAL AUDITORY MEATUS

GLENOID FOSSA

ZYGOMATIC PROCESS

LATERAL SEMICIRCULAR CANAL

SUPERIOR SEMICIRCULAR CANAL

COCHLEA

INTERNAL AUDITORY CANAL

CAROTID CANAL

EUSTACHIAN TUBE

D

SUBMENTO - VERTICAL VIEW

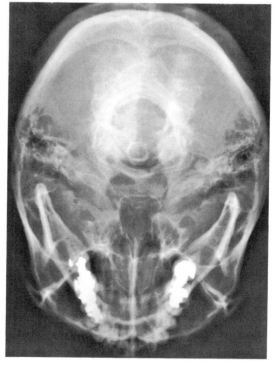

Figure 13–24 (*Continued*).

Figure 13–24 continued on opposite page.

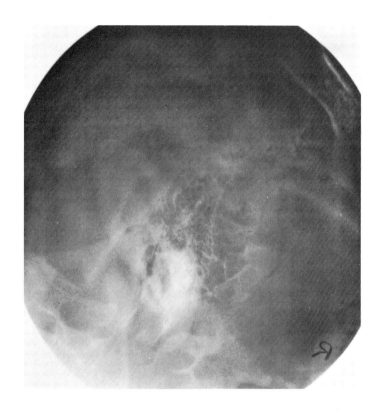

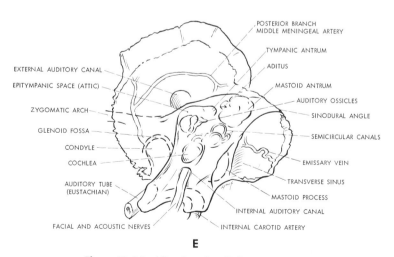

EXTERNAL AUDITORY CANAL

EPITYMPANIC SPACE (ATTIC)

ZYGOMATIC ARCH

GLENOID FOSSA

CONDYLE

COCHLEA

AUDITORY TUBE
(EUSTACHIAN)

FACIAL AND ACOUSTIC NERVES

POSTERIOR BRANCH
MIDDLE MENINGEAL ARTERY

TYMPANIC ANTRUM

ADITUS

MASTOID ANTRUM

AUDITORY OSSICLES

SINODURAL ANGLE

SEMICIRCULAR CANALS

EMISSARY VEIN

TRANSVERSE SINUS

MASTOID PROCESS

INTERNAL AUDITORY CANAL

INTERNAL CAROTID ARTERY

E

Figure 13–24   (*Continued*).   *E.* Runström view.

Figure 13–24 continued on following page.

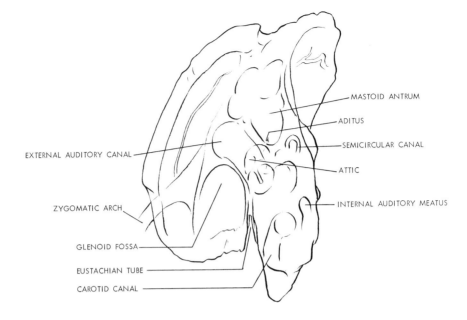

MASTOID ANTRUM

ADITUS

SEMICIRCULAR CANAL

EXTERNAL AUDITORY CANAL

ATTIC

INTERNAL AUDITORY MEATUS

ZYGOMATIC ARCH

GLENOID FOSSA

EUSTACHIAN TUBE

CAROTID CANAL

F   MAYER PROJECTION

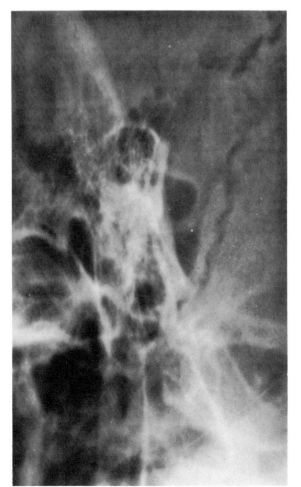

Figure 13–24 (*Continued*).

Figure 13-24 continued on opposite page.

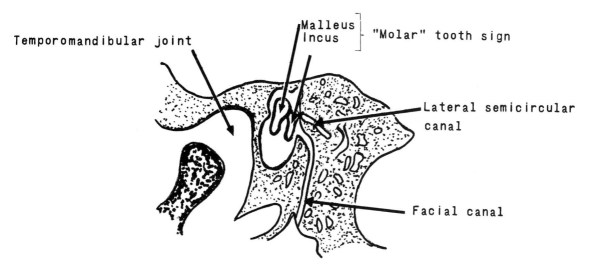

Temporomandibular joint

Malleus
Incus
} "Molar" tooth sign

Lateral semicircular
canal

Facial canal

"Molar" tooth sign

Lateral tomogram petrous pyramid
"molar tooth" sign for
identification of ossicles
(malleus and incus)

G

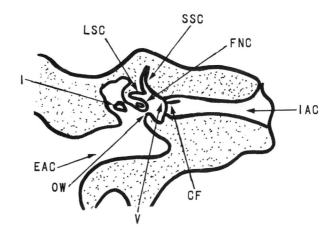

Figure 13–24 (*Continued*). *G*. Diagram of lateral basic tomogram of the middle ear at the level of the middle ear ossicles: the "molar tooth" sign. (From Potter, G. D., Amer. J. Roentgenol., *104*: 194, 1968.) *H*. Diagram of antero-posterior tomogram of the middle ear at the level of the crista falciformis. (From Valvassori, G. E.: Amer. J. Roentgenol., *94*:568, 1965.)

EAC External auditory canal
IAC Internal auditory canal
OW   Oval window
LSC Lateral semicircular canal
SSC Superior semicircular canal
V Vestibule

I Incus
FNC Facial nerve canal
CF Crista falciformis

H

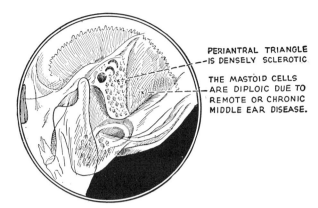

Figure 13–25 Tracing demonstrating arrested development of the mastoid air cells with marked sclerosis of the bone of the periantral triangle. This sclerotic reaction indicates remote or chronic middle ear disease.

General Radiographic Appearances

Generalized haziness of the mastoid process and cells of the petrous ridge.

The lateral sinus plate and tegmen tympani stand out by contrast more clearly.

There is a generalized increase in opacity in the affected petrous bones as well.

The cell walls become indistinct but are not resorbed or destroyed.

When the mastoid cells are diploic, only an abnormal opacity of the petrous bone and mastoid antrum is identified (Figure 13–28).

Increased Radiopacity of the Mastoids with Partial Destruction of Mastoid Cell Walls

Suppurative Mastoiditis (Figure 13–27)

PATHOGENESIS.   It is almost invariably secondary to a middle ear infectious process.

RADIOGRAPHIC APPEARANCE

Diffuse haziness of all mastoid cells and sclerosis of the periantral triangle.
Increased prominence of the lateral sinus and emissary vein.

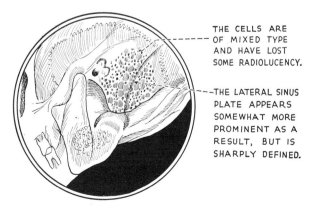

Figure 13–26 Tracing of radiograph demonstrating the radiographic findings with moderate increase in opacity of the mastoid air cells in association with catarrhal mastoiditis.

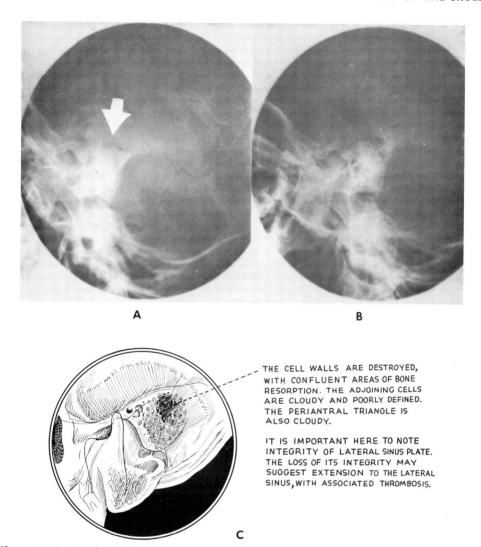

THE CELL WALLS ARE DESTROYED,
WITH CONFLUENT AREAS OF BONE
RESORPTION. THE ADJOINING CELLS
ARE CLOUDY AND POORLY DEFINED.
THE PERIANTRAL TRIANGLE IS
ALSO CLOUDY.

IT IS IMPORTANT HERE TO NOTE
INTEGRITY OF LATERAL SINUS PLATE.
THE LOSS OF ITS INTEGRITY MAY
SUGGEST EXTENSION TO THE LATERAL
SINUS, WITH ASSOCIATED THROMBOSIS.

Figure 13–27   *A* and *B*. Radiographs demonstrating suppurative mastoiditis involving the right mastoid in the region of the mastoid antrum. *C*. Diagrammatic tracing of same with pertinent radiographic features described.

SCLEROTIC MASTOIDITIS

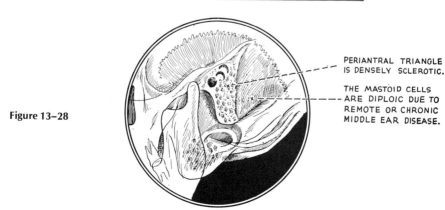

Figure 13–28

PERIANTRAL TRIANGLE
IS DENSELY SCLEROTIC.

THE MASTOID CELLS
ARE DIPLOIC DUE TO
REMOTE OR CHRONIC
MIDDLE EAR DISEASE.

Resorption of some of the cell walls, particularly in the region of the mastoid antrum so that good cellular detail is not obtained. Body section radiography assists materially in accurate diagnosis.

In the radiographic diagnosis of destruction of the temporal bone from any cause (suppurative mastoiditis, cholesteatoma, acoustic neuroma, and other tumors), tomography has proved to be the method of choice in preoperative roentgenologic diagnosis. Familiarity with the intricate detailed anatomy of the temporal bone is essential for this purpose (Figure 13–24).

It Is Important to Distinguish the large or giant air cell which is a normal variant. It is also important to know whether or not the patient has been operated upon, since the postoperative mastoid may show considerable removal and loss of cell walls, although at times occasional cells may be left behind.

THE ROENTGENOGRAPHIC DIAGNOSIS OF ACOUSTIC NEUROMA (Valvassori, 1969)

Conventional Radiographic Examination consisting of at least: P-A, lateral stereo, A-P Townes, and basal view of the skull.

Tomographic Examination of the petrous pyramids in two planes:

Frontal view shows internal auditory canal in full length.

Lateral view shows any asymmetry between the two sides outlining the cortex of the canal and the status of the porus acousticus.

Internal Auditory Canal is considered abnormal whenever:

Erosion of the cortical or capsular lines surrounding the lumen of the canal occurs.

When there is widening of two or more millimeters of any portion of the internal auditory canal by comparing it with the opposite canal.

When there is shortening of the posterior wall of the canal by at least 3 mm. in comparison with the opposite side.

When the crista falciformis runs closer to the inferior than to the superior wall of the internal auditory canal. The crista should normally be located at or above the midpoint.

Opaque Cisternography is performed as a most conclusive diagnostic study in the following situations:

When any of the preceding studies are positive.

When the audiometric tests are suggestive and the radiographic studies are inconclusive.

When there are borderline findings in the radiologic study and borderline studies in audiometric tests.

Pneumoencephalography: Air is collected in the cerebellopontine cistern and within the internal auditory canal, but positive contrast cisternography is more conclusive.

Vertebral Arteriography: The anterior inferior cerebellar artery often loops within the internal auditory canal and the superior cerebellar artery loops toward it, but variations are significant and great. The petrosal vein may also drain from this area but this too is inconclusive.

Brain Scan: A positive scan is obtained when the tumor is large and highly vascular but negative scans are not conclusive.

THE DIAGNOSIS OF OTOSCLEROSIS BY ROENTGENOLOGIC MEANS

1. Findings in petrous pyramids (Compere, 1960).
   a. Local overgrowth of osseous tissue anywhere in the otic capsule.
2. Apparent sclerosis of the entire labyrinthine capsule obscuring the labyrinthine system.
3. Hyperostoses of the entire petrous pyramid.
4. By special laminographic techniques the following additional information may be obtained:
   a. Obscuration of oval window, 90 per cent; round window, 40 per cent; cochlear capsule, 35 per cent; involvement of internal auditory canal, 30 per cent; semicircular canal, 15 per cent; and diffuse involvement, 10 per cent (Nylen).

Decrease in Density

Cholesteatoma (Figure 13-29)

DEFINITION. As a result of chronic otitis media the stratified squamous epithelium from the external auditory canal grows in size as suppuration persists and finally grows to a marginal perforation in the tympanic membrane. The desquamated cells, deposited in layers, form a pseudotumor that begins its destruction in the attic and spreads from there, slowly eroding and destroying the structures with which it comes in contact. It may even penetrate into the cranial cavity.

RADIOGRAPHIC APPEARANCE. Extensive total destruction of the lateral wall of the attic in any of the projections routinely obtained. Tomography of the middle ear, particularly in Runström's position, is especially valuable (Jensen et al.). Diagnostic accuracy is at least 80 per cent. Tomography will usually reveal a large antral cavity and destruction of the spur and lateral wall of the attic.

Unfortunately, where previous surgery has occurred these studies are not of great value (Brunner et al.).

Tumors in the Vicinity of the Apex of the Petrous Bone

CLASSIFICATION. These may represent tumors of the fifth, sixth, seventh, or eighth nerves, cerebellopontine angle tumors of meningiomatous origin, or other gliomas. Acoustic neurinomas constitute at least 90 per cent of the total group (Figure 13-30).

RADIOGRAPHIC APPEARANCES

Decalcification of the bony walls of the internal auditory meatus (comparison with opposite side is very important).
Expansion of the bony walls of the internal auditory meatus.
Erosion of the tip of the petrous bone.
General signs of increased intracranial pressure, late.

CHOLESTEATOMA

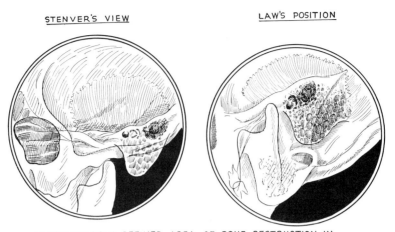

STENVER'S VIEW LAW'S POSITION

LARGE SHARPLY DEFINED AREA OF BONE DESTRUCTION IN
REGION OF MASTOID ANTRUM. IN LAW'S VIEW, THE AREA OF
DESTRUCTION IS CONTAINED WITHIN THE PERIANTRAL TRIANGLE
AND SEEMS TO IMPINGE ON ACOUSTIC MEATI.

A

Figure 13–29 *A*. Diagram showing circumscribed bone absorption in the periantral region indicating cholesteatoma formation.

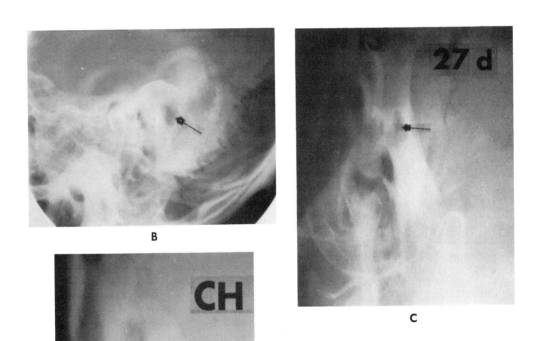

B

C

D

Figure 13–29 (*Continued*). Radiographs demonstrating cholesteatoma of the middle ear. *B*. Runström's view. *C*. Mayer's view. *D*. Close-up of Towne's view. The arrows point to the sites of bone destruction.

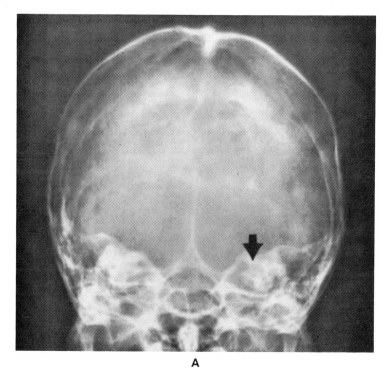

A

Figure 13–30 *A.* Acoustic neuroma on the patient's left. Note the erosion of the internal acoustic meatus by comparison with the opposite side. The film was obtained in Towne's projection. The P-A view of the skull is also valuable for this purpose.

Figure 13–30 continued on following page.

Glomus Jugularis Tumors (Riemenschneider et al.)

DEFINITION. These have frequently been called hemangio-endotheliomas of the nasopharynx. They are also called chemodectomas. They may be benign or malignant. They erode into the middle ear and may appear as a bleeding mass in the external canal. They may be accompanied by massive destruction of the petrous pyramids, involvement of the cranial nerves, pressure on the brain stem, and a mass in the nasopharynx.

CHEMODECTOMAS OF THE HEAD AND NECK
(Placios)

1. The most common location is the intratympanic (15 out of 24). Cholesteatomas, primary and secondary malignant tumors of the middle ear, and acoustic neuromas must be differentiated.

2. Glomus jugularis tumors are next in frequency, accounting for six out of 24.

3. Chemodectomas occur predominantly in females (20 out of 24) of any age group.

4. Multicentricity may occur rarely.

5. Glomus tumors in the tympanojugular area are regarded as the most common neoplasm involving the middle ear.

6. Plain roentgenograms and tomograms may show erosion and clouding of the involved area but angiography is usually necessary to establish the diagnosis beyond question.

ACOUSTIC NEUROMA

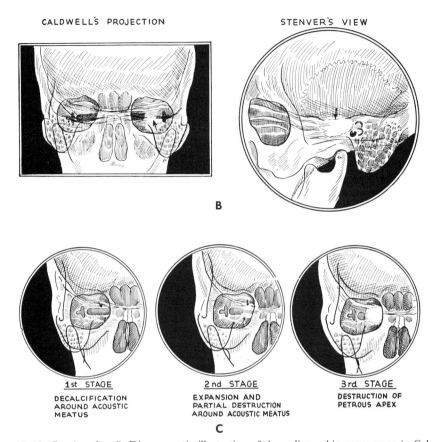

CALDWELL'S PROJECTION   STENVER'S VIEW

B

1st STAGE   2nd STAGE   3rd STAGE

DECALCIFICATION   EXPANSION AND   DESTRUCTION OF
AROUND ACOUSTIC   PARTIAL DESTRUCTION   PETROUS APEX
MEATUS   AROUND ACOUSTIC MEATUS

C

Figure 13–30 (*Continued*).   *B*. Diagrammatic illustration of the radiographic appearance in Caldwell's projection and in Stenver's view of acoustic neuroma. The internal acoustic meatus is decalcified first, then expanded and partially destroyed. The petrous apex may also be destroyed late. These changes are seen in 50 per cent of cases. (Hodes et al.) *C*. Sequential radiographic changes in association with an internal acoustic neuroma.

Figure 13–30 continued on opposite page.

RADIOGRAPHIC APPEARANCE

Minimal to massive destruction of the petrous pyramids.

The lower portion of the pyramids is first destroyed with the ridge remaining as a more or less intact shell.

Angiograms show marked abnormal vascularization in the area of destruction.

A posterior nasopharyngeal mass is usually demonstrable.

THE ORBITS

Methods of Examination (Figures 13–31, 13–32)

The routine methods of examination of the orbits include:
1. Caldwell's nose-forehead, postero-anterior projection.
2. Water's nose-chin, postero-anterior projection.

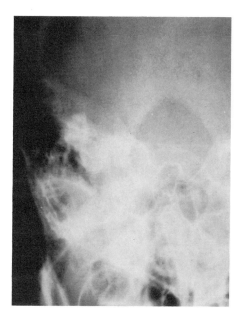

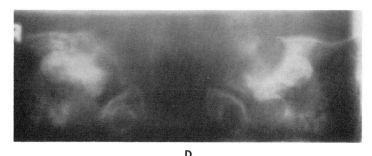

D

Figure 13–30 (*Continued*).   *D*. Petrous erosion from an acoustic neurilemmoma. *Upper*. View of petrous ridge in Towne's projection. *Lower*. Tomography showing more clearly the extent of erosion.

3. The lateral projection of the face and orbits.
4. Special views of the optic foramina.
5. Special views are thereafter obtained depending upon the specific anatomical requirements such as (Figure 13–32):
    a. The special view for each superior orbital fissure.
    b. The special view for the inferior orbital fissure.
    c. Special contrast studies with air injection into Tenon's capsule.
    d. Special views for localization of intraocular or intraorbital foreign bodies. These latter are highly specialized and the student is referred to *Roentgen Signs in Clinical Practice* for more detailed references and description.

Roentgen Signs of Abnormality

ABNORMALITIES IN CONTOUR AND SIZE

Alterations in the size of the optic canal, superior orbital fissure, and inferior orbital fissure are important radiographically. Enlargement of the optic canal is reported in tumors such as pituitary adenoma, suprasellar cholesteatoma, meningio-

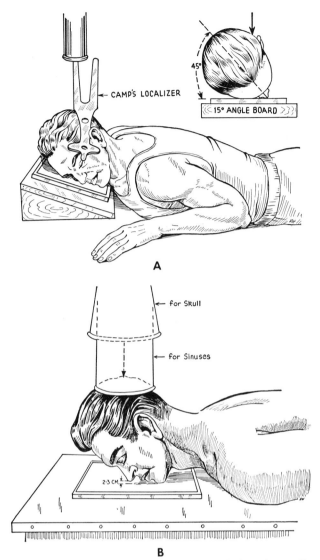

Figure 13–31   Routine study of the orbits. *A*. Special view of optic foramina. *B*. Frontal view of orbits.

mas of the sphenoid ridge, and in certain cases, opticochiasmatic cystic arachnoiditis.

Increased intracranial pressure can also cause enlargement of the optic canal just as it does of the sella turcica.

Aneurysms of the various blood vessels in the region of the optic canal, whether they are of carotid or ophthalmic arterial origin, may cause erosion.

Narrowness of the optic canal may be due to any bone disease which will produce condensation and increased thickness of bone—for example, fibrous dysplasia, meningioma, orbital hyperostosis, and Paget's disease of bone.

Asymmetries found between the two orbits are not infrequent and precautions must be exercised in interpreting such findings. Marked asymmetry may be due to enophthalmos, or enucleation of an eye very early in life (Figure 13–33).

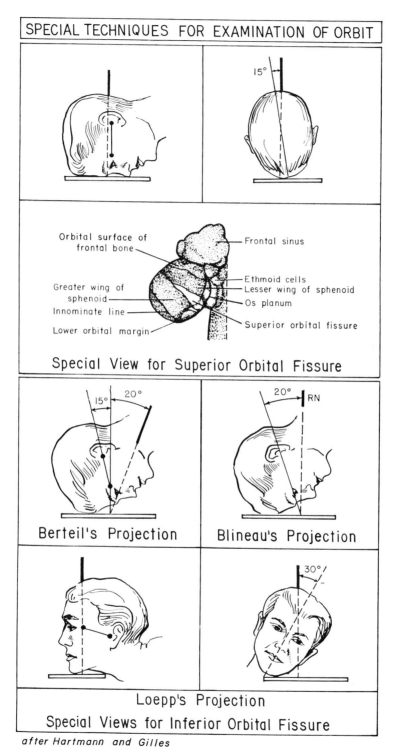

Figure 13–32   Special techniques for examination of the orbit, apart from the usual views of the facial bones previously demonstrated.

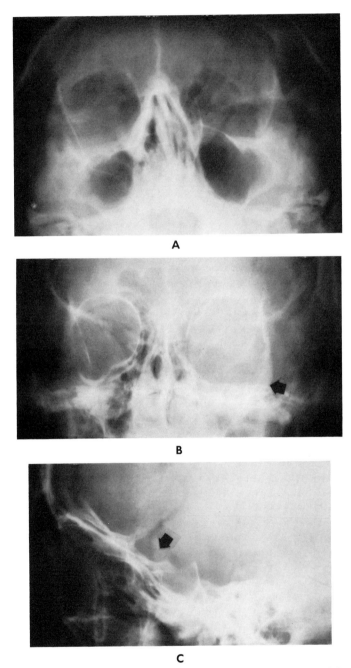

A

B

C

Figure 13–33   *A*. Asymmetry of the orbits in a child who had an enucleation on the left very early in life. *B*. Asymmetry of the orbits in an individual who has a neurofibroma of the optic nerve on the left. Postero-anterior view. *C*. Lateral view of above. Notice parasellar erosion in the optic nerve canal.

ORBITAL CHANGES IN HISTIOCYTOSIS X
(Nesbit et al.)

The roentgenologic features in a group of 14 cases:

Orbital roof lysis	12 orbits (ten of which were in five cases where both orbits were involved)
Orbital sclerosis	4 orbits
Orbital sclerosis and lysis	3 orbits

The lateral wall of the orbit was lytic in all but five cases. The lesser and greater wings of the sphenoid were lytic wherever they were involved. In most cases the predominant finding was lysis.

ALTERATIONS IN DENSITY

Intraorbital Calcification

Classification

1. Primary calcification of a neoplasm.
2. Calcification of a cataract in the optic lens.
3. Scleral calcification.
4. Corneal calcification.
5. Choroidal calcification.
6. Parasitic calcification.
7. Calcification of hematomata.
8. Fat necrosis with calcification.
9. Calcification with retrolental fibroplasia in infants.

The neoplasms which may be calcified are primarily the retinoblastoma and dermoid cysts.

ALTERATIONS IN POSITION OF THE GLOBE

LOCALIZATION OF INTRAOCULAR AND INTRAORBITAL FOREIGN BODIES

On the standard radiographs of the orbit, the presence or absence of an opaque foreign body is first established. In addition to the usual routine views, special tangential views of the anterior chamber of the globe may be obtained by inserting dental films with pressure along the inner canthus of the eye and obtaining tangential views of the anterior chamber. Superimposed frontal or lateral radiographs may also be obtained with the patient first looking up and then down, and in this fashion it may be established that the foreign body moves with movements of the globe.

Once this has been established, various methods which will facilitate removal are available for more accurate localization. These involve special localization devices, such as Sweet's apparatus and plastic localizer lenses which contain metallic markers placed in contact with the cornea.

ORBITAL TUMORS

The most frequent of these are angiomas (16.2 per cent according to Reese) and pseudotumors. Sarcomas are only slightly fewer in incidence (13 per cent).

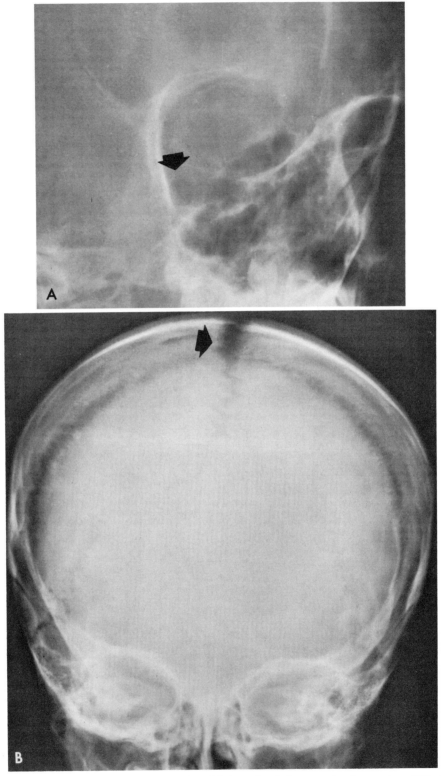

Figure 13–34   Glioma of the optic nerve. *A*. Special view of optic foramen showing erosion of this structure by the glioma. *B*. Spreading of the sutures due to increased intracranial pressure in this condition.

Pseudotumors characteristically do not cause x-ray changes of the orbital bone. Bony changes are usually present, however, in both primary and secondary orbital tumors.

Radiographic Findings in Optic Nerve Glioma (Figure 13–34)

Enlargement of the optic foramina.

The J-shaped or pear-shaped sella turcica.

Enlargement of the pituitary fossa and decalcification of the cortical bone of the sella turcica.

Shortening or truncation of the dorsum sellae.

Generalized separation of the cranial sutures.

Very prominent convolutional impressions on the calvarium in young persons from increased intracranial pressure.

Suprasellar calcification (very rare).

(Holman; Bahn; Hartmann and Gilles; *Roentgen Signs in Clinical Practice*).

RADIOLOGIC EVIDENCES OF INTRACRANIAL SPACE-OCCUPYING LESIONS

Introduction. Radiologic techniques have contributed significantly to the accurate localization and diagnosis of intracranial mass lesions. These methods, in the order of their complexity, include:

1. *Plain Films of the Skull,* including special coned-down and laminographic studies with the aid of polytomography, as described previously.
2. *Radioisotopic Studies.* These include:
    a. *Cervicocranial scintiphotograms* in rapid sequence following the intravenous injection of a bolus of radionuclide.
    b. Rectilinear scans or scintiphotos of the head in frontal, lateral, and angled posterior projections.
3. *Angiograms* of the head, which may be performed by:
    a. Four vessel arch and selective catheterization techniques.
    b. Percutaneous carotid angiograms of the neck.
    c. Percutaneous retrograde brachial angiograms—the left retrograde brachial being used for posterior fossa studies in lieu of a percutaneous left vertebral angiogram.
4. *Pneumograms of the Head.* These may be performed by:
    a. *Pneumoencephalography:* Withdrawal of fractions of cerebrospinal fluid via lumbar spinal puncture and replacement of the fluid with air or other suitable gaseous medium.
    b. *Ventriculography:* The instillation of the gaseous medium into the ventricles of the brain directly by puncture of the posterior parietal lobe of the brain through a small trephine opening in the parietal bone.
5. *Cisternomyelograms with Pantopaque:* In this technique, a small quantity of the Pantopaque is introduced into the lumbar region and carefully manipulated into each cerebellopontine angle under fluoroscopic control, and control of the patient's head.
6. *Ventriculograms with Pantopaque.*
7. *Dural Sinus Venograms,* where obstruction of a venous sinus is suspected.

8. *Instillation of Sterile Micropaque Barium into Known Abscess and Neoplastic Cavities,* in order to study the sequential diminution or enlargement of such cavities under treatment.

9. *Radioisotopic Myelocisternoencephalo Photograms:* In this technique the radioactive medium in high specific activity is injected into the lumbar region and is followed several hours later to the basal cisterns of the head; after 24 hours it is followed over the convexity of the brain. Abnormally, the radioactivated cerebrospinal fluid appears in the ventricles of the brain in certain cases of low pressure hydrocephalus.

The discussion of all these methods is outside the scope of this text except for the plain films of the skull, and it too must be outlined only in introductory fashion.

Roentgen Signs on Plain Films of the Skull Indicative of Intracranial Space-Occupying Mass Lesions

CHANGES INDICATIVE OF INCREASED INTRACRANIAL PRESSURE

These are indicated in Figure 13–35. Brief summary comment will be made about each of these basic abnormalities.

Increased Convolutional Impressions. In adults over the age of 16, the appearance of convolutional impressions upon the bones of the calvarium must arouse the suspicion of increased intracranial pressure, warranting further investigation by special diagnostic means. In younger persons it may be a normal appearance.

Separation of the Sutures. By the age of six or seven years, the sutural appearance begins to approach that which may be seen up to the age of approximately 14 or 15. Sutures begin to fuse after the age of 25 or 30.

Some sutural variations include:

1. A persistence of the metopic suture in the frontal bone which normally begins to close at the age of two and is usually obliterated by the age of four.

2. Persistence of accessory sutures, especially in the parietal bone or in the transverse occipital region.

3. A persistent suture between the inferior portion of the squamous part of the

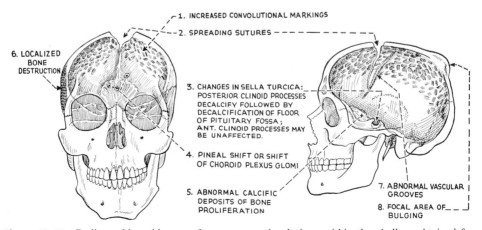

Figure 13–35 Radiographic evidences of space-occupying lesions within the skull as obtained from plain films of the skull.

temporal bone and the occipital bone adjacent to the foramen magnum, ordinarily obliterated by the second or third year of life.

4. The mendosal sutures are found in the occipital bones and usually disappear in the first year of life.

5. Sutural or wormian bones may be encountered in various suture lines in some anomalies and dysostoses of the cranium such as osteogenesis imperfecta and cleidocranial dysostosis.

Changes in the Sella Turcica (Figures 13–5 and 13–6).   These changes occur in the following sequence:

1. Atrophy and resorption of the posterior clinoid processes.

2. Atrophy, thinning, and ultimate disappearance of the upper part of the dorsum sellae and the floor of the sella turcica.

3. Sharpening and partial resorption of the anterior clinoid processes and the tuberculum sellae, the last portions of the sella turcica ordinarily to show evidence of atrophy.

At times the changes in the sella turcica produced by increased intracranial pressure simulate closely the ballooning which is characteristically produced by intrasellar expanding lesions such as pituitary adenomas. Ordinarily this ballooning is differentiated by early erosion of the floor of the hypophyseal fossa with internal erosion of the posterior clinoids and ultimately of the dorsum sellae. A double-contoured appearance of the hypophyseal fossa may be produced if the erosion is asymmetrical. Body section radiographs are helpful in ascertaining this finding beyond question.

Often with intrasellar expanding lesions calcium deposition also occurs, assisting in the differential diagnosis.

Osteoporosis of the Bones of the Skull.   This is not a dependable indication since so many systemic causes of this condition exist.

Displacement of Physiologically Calcified Intracranial Structures.   Normal calcium deposition occurs in the following structures (Figure 13–36): (1) pineal body; (2) choroid plexus; (3) falx cerebri; (4) tentorium cerebelli; (5) the walls of the longitudinal superior sinus and dura mater; (6) arachnoidal granulations; (7) habenular commissure.

Of these calcified structures, the following may be readily displaced by intracranial mass lesions: (1) the pineal body; (2) the choroid plexuses; (3) the habenular commissure. The pineal body and the habenular commissure are the most accurate signs in this regard and localization charts for this purpose have been previously submitted.

Symmetrical calcification of the cerebral basal ganglia is an abnormal finding often associated with chronic parathyroid insufficiency.

Thus, in 11 cases of basal ganglia calcification, 65 per cent showed some type of hypoparathyroidism (Hastings-James). The others were "idiopathic."

Likewise, symmetrical calcification in the cerebellum of undetermined significance may on occasion be observed. Usually this occupies the dentate nucleus.

Abnormal Vascular Grooves.   Marked localized increase in the size or number of the arterial channels in the calvarium is of importance since this may indicate the location of a neoplasm. Likewise, widening of an emissary canal or foramen may indicate increased intracranial pressure. These are seen in the midline in the region of the occipital protuberance and normally do not exceed 2 mm. in width (Chynn).

Sinus pericranii is a congenital venous anomaly on the surface of the head, communicating with the intracranial venous system. It increases in size when the intracranial pressure is raised.

Accentuation of the venous diploë in itself is without pathologic significance.

(Text continued on page 585)

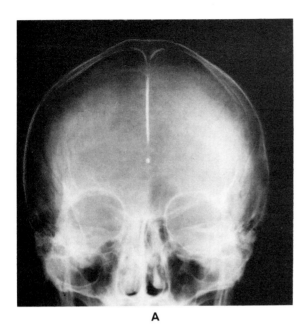

A

Figure 13–36 *A*. Radiograph demonstrating calcification in the pineal gland and falx cerebri in a postero-anterior view. *B*. Radiograph of the skull in a lateral projection demonstrating calcium deposit in the pineal gland, habenula, and glomera of the choroid plexuses (black arrow). The habenula is the U-shaped structure immediately anterior to the pineal gland (intensified).

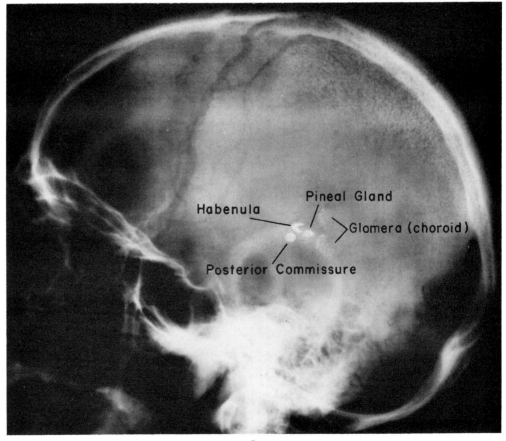

B

Figure 13–36 continued on opposite page.

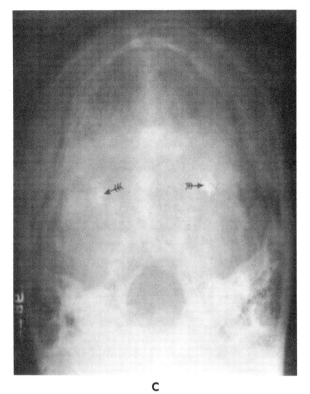

C

D

Figure 13–36 (*Continued*).   *C*. Roentgenogram in Towne's projection to show calcification in the glomera of the choroid plexuses. *D*. Radiograph to show calcification in the petroclinoid ligament in a straight lateral projection.

Figure 13–36 continued on following page.

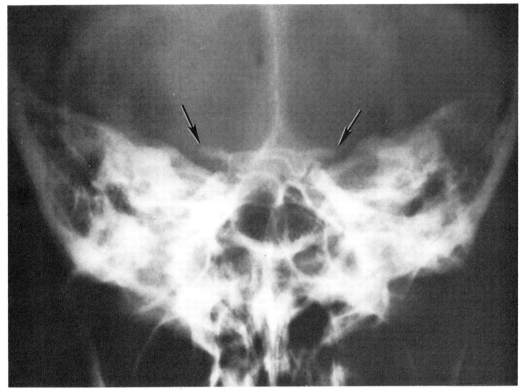

E

F

Figure 13–36 (*Continued*).   *E.* Radiograph in a slight oblique showing the configuration of the petro-clinoid ligament when the lateral is not true. *F.* Radiograph in Towne's projection showing the petroclinoid ligaments extending between the posterior clinoid processes and dorsum sellae and the petrous ridge (intensified).

Abnormal Calcium Deposits.   Abnormal calcification within the skull may be said to be either (a) non-neoplastic or (b) neoplastic in origin.

Non-neoplastic Calcification.   This may be outlined as follows:

1. Congenital and neonatal:
    a. Tuberous sclerosis.
    b. Infantile hemiplegias.
2. Parasitic diseases:
    a. Toxoplasmosis.
    b. Torulosis.
    c. Cysticercosis.
    d. Echinococcosis.
    e. Trichinosis.
3. Inflammatory processes:
    a. Tuberculous meningitis.
    b. Encephalitis.
    c. Brain abscess.
    d. Tuberculoma.
    e. Luetic gumma.
4. Vascular lesions:
    a. Arteriosclerosis.
    b. Angiomas.

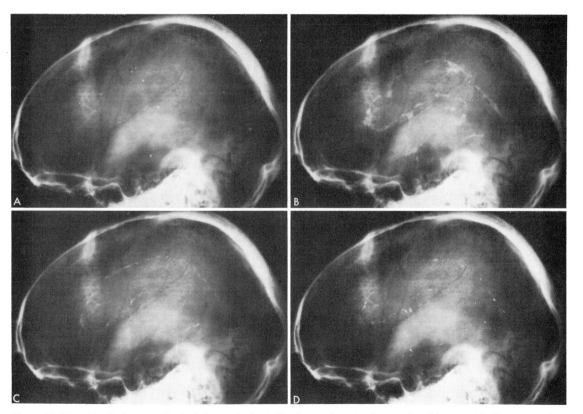

Figure 13–37   *A* to *D*. Paraventricular intracerebral calcification such as is often produced by parasitic diseases, such as toxoplasmosis, trichinosis, cysticercosis, or torulosis. (Intensified diagrammatic radiographs.)

Figure 13–37 continued on following page.

E

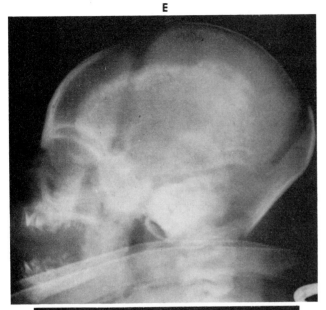

Figure 13–37 (*Continued*). Cytomegalic inclusion disease. *E*. Frontal view. *F*. Lateral view. (Courtesy of Dr. M. H. Poppel, New York, N. Y.)

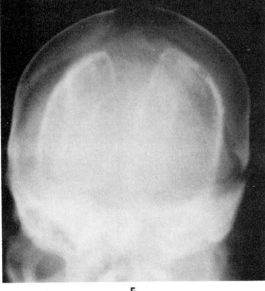

F

Figure 13–37 continued on opposite page.

    c. Sturge-Weber syndrome.
    d. Aneurysms (circle of Willis; vein of Galen).
    e. Endarteritis calcificans cerebri.
    f. Cerebral hemorrhages.
    g. Subdural hematoma.
  5. Endocrine disorders:
    Parathyroid insufficiency.
  6. X-ray injury:
    Necrosis of the brain following roentgen radiation.

    Some of these are illustrated in the accompanying figures (Figure 13–37).

    Not illustrated is the so-called **"aneurysm" of the vein of Galen,** which **may undergo calcification.** It is important to recognize the differences between

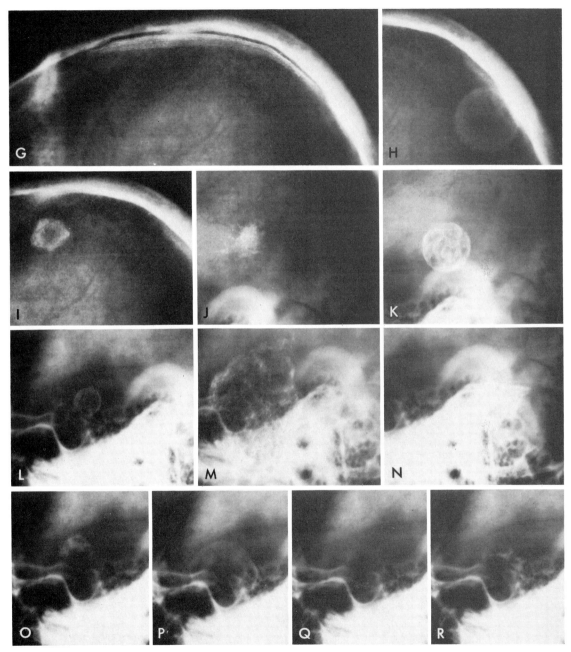

Figure 13–37 (*Continued*).   Various appearances of abnormal intracranial calcification. *G.* Subdural hematoma. *H.* Calcified cysts, such as an echinococcus or hydatid cyst. *I.* Tuberculoma; also endarteritis calcificans cerebri. *J.* Astrocytoma; tuberculoma. *K.* Pinealoma. *L.* Carotid artery aneurysm. *M.* Craniopharyngioma; calcified chordoma. *N.* Coarse calcium in medulloblastoma or ependymoma of fourth ventricle. *O.* Tuberculous meningitis (nodular parasellar); craniopharyngioma. *P.* Cystlike calcium in wall of aneurysm of internal carotid artery. *Q.* Intrasellar calcification, without enlarged sella; degenerate pituitary adenoma. *R.* Craniopharyngioma. (Intensified diagrammatic radiographs.)

Figure 13–37 continued on following page.

this entity and abnormal pineal, habenular, or neoplastic calcification in this region. The differential features may be outlined as follows:

1. The calcific deposit is thin and delicate and forms a complete or incomplete ring.

2. It is situated in the region normally occupied by the pineal gland in the lateral projection, very near or in the midline in the frontal projection where one would expect to find the vein of Galen.

3. The ring of calcification, whether complete or incomplete, is large, exceeding 2.5 cm. in diameter.

4. The patient is older than the age of nine years.

In differential diagnosis, the pineal tumors do not calcify in this manner and epidermoids in the quadrigeminal area are rare. A lipoma should contain a central zone of radiolucency (Wilson and Roy).

Neoplastic Calcification (Figure 13–38)

PATHOLOGIC TUMORAL CALCIFICATIONS. Calcification in intracranial neoplasms was reported in 13 per cent of 1,557 tumors (Martin) and occurs far more frequently in the supratentorial lesions than in infratentorial ones. It occurs primarily in the walls of blood vessels or within the tumor areas of ischemic or hemorrhagic degeneration and necrosis. It occurs also in the walls of cysts or cystic neoplasms.

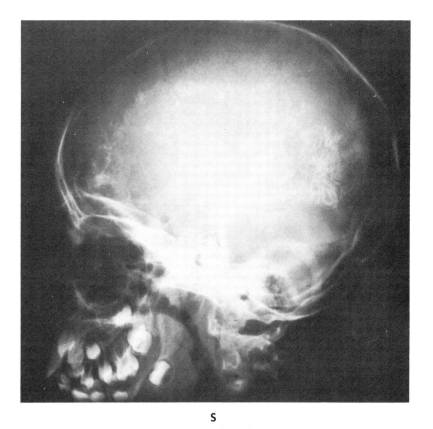

S

Figure 13–37 (*Continued*). *S*. Intracranial calcification with Sturge-Weber syndrome. Angiograms of the brain usually do not intensify these areas of calcification. Radioisotopic brain scans (99m-technetium) have been shown to be positive even when no calcification is identified.

Figure 13–37 continued on opposite page.

The tumors which are most frequently calcified are:

1. Gliomas:
   a. Oligodendroglioma.
   b. Astrocytoma.
   c. Pinealoma.
   d. Ependymoma.
   e. Spongioblastoma polare.
   f. Medulloblastoma.
   g. Glioblastoma multiforme.
2. Meningiomas.

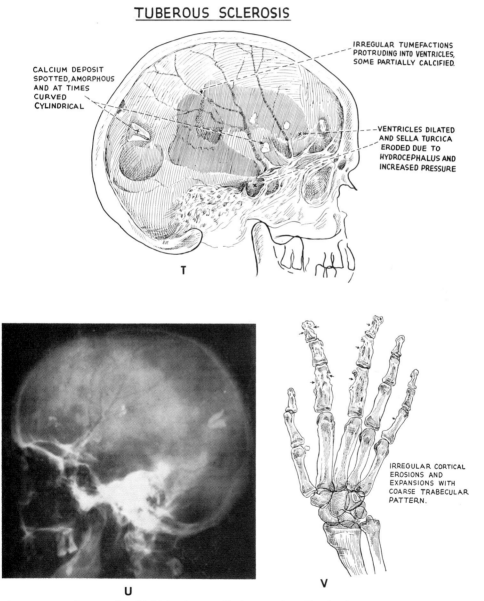

TUBEROUS SCLEROSIS

IRREGULAR TUMEFACTIONS PROTRUDING INTO VENTRICLES, SOME PARTIALLY CALCIFIED.

CALCIUM DEPOSIT SPOTTED, AMORPHOUS AND AT TIMES CURVED CYLINDRICAL

VENTRICLES DILATED AND SELLA TURCICA ERODED DUE TO HYDROCEPHALUS AND INCREASED PRESSURE

T

IRREGULAR CORTICAL EROSIONS AND EXPANSIONS WITH COARSE TRABECULAR PATTERN.

U

V

Figure 13–37 (*Continued*).   Multiple circumscribed areas of calcification in tuberous sclerosis with the changes in the hand of this patient also diagrammatically indicated. *T*. The skull, following ventriculography. *U*. Plain radiograph. *V*. The hand.

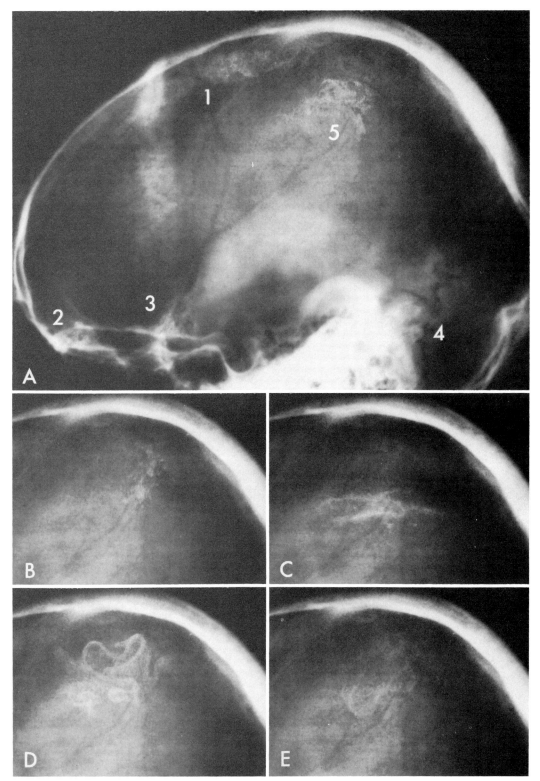

Figure 13–38 Diagrammatic illustration of various neoplastic types of intracranial calcification. *A*. Meningioma, showing usual sites of meningioma formation. 1. Parasagittal. 2. Olfactory groove. 3. Sphenoid ridge. 4. Petrous and tentorial. 5. Elsewhere in meninges. *B*. Astrocytoma. *C*. Glioblastoma multiforme. *D*. Angioma (Sturge-Weber syndrome). *E*. Oligodendroglioma.

3. Congenital tumors:
     a. Craniopharyngioma.
     b. Chordoma.
     c. Epidermoid.
     d. Lipoma.
4. Chromophobe pituitary adenoma.
5. Choroid plexus papilloma.

The gliomas constitute approximately half of the intracranial tumors. These occur more frequently in the cerebrum than in the brain stem or in the cerebellum. Approximately two-thirds of the gliomas are *glioblastomas or astrocytomas;* if the *medulloblastomas,* which occur most frequently in children, are included, these three tumor types *constitute about three-quarters of all the gliomas.*

The *oligodendroglioma and the astrocytoma are most frequently calcified,* the former far more than the latter. In the usually reported series, approximately five per cent of all gliomas show calcium deposition.

It is said that calcium deposits can be recognized in approximately 80 per cent of oligodendrogliomas.

Meningiomas may vary from single to multiple lesions and from a few cm. to 15 or 20 cm. in diameter. They constitute about 10 to 15 per cent of all intracranial tumors.

Meningiomas have certain frequent locations and some characteristic appearances which permit a fairly accurate radiographic diagnosis in approximately 75 per cent of the cases. Their most frequent anatomic sites are: parasagittal, the petrous ridge, the sphenoidal ridge, the region of the olfactory groove, and over the convexity of the cerebrum anterior to the fissure of Rolando (Figure 13–39).

Apart from the characteristic locations of meningiomas, certain other radiographic appearances draw attention to tumors of this type: localized erosion and hypervascularity of the calvarium (25 per cent of the cases); calcification within the neoplasm (10 per cent of the cases); displacement of the pineal gland (about two-thirds of the cases); and evidences of erosion of the sella turcica (about one-half of the cases) (Martin and Lemmen; Epstein and Davidoff; Jacobson et al.).

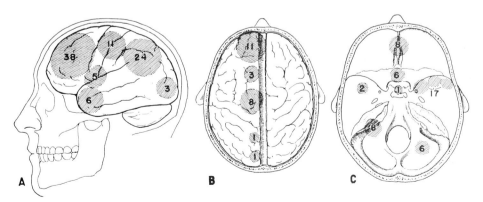

Figure 13–39   *A* to *C.* Diagrammatic sketch of the locations of intracranial meningiomas and the relative frequency of each. (From Jacobson et al.: Radiology, *72:*358, 1959.)

Figure 13–39 continued on following page.

MENINGIOMA

PUNCTATE, CONGLOMERATE AREAS OF CALCIFICATION NEAR INNER SURFACE
OF CALVARIUM OFTEN (50%) PRODUCING AN ASSOCIATED OSTEOMA IN THE
ADJOINING CALVARIUM.

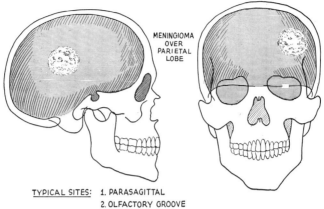

MENINGIOMA
OVER
PARIETAL
LOBE

TYPICAL SITES: 1. PARASAGITTAL
2. OLFACTORY GROOVE
3. SPHENOID RIDGE

PARASAGITTAL MENINGIOMA

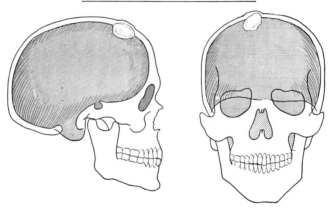

SPHENOID RIDGE MENINGIOMA

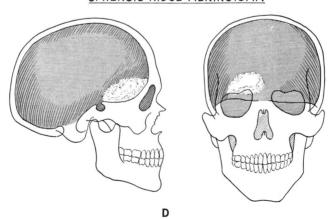

D

Figure 13–39 (*Continued*).   *D.* Calcification as observed in approximately 10 to 20 per cent of meningiomas. This is often associated with marked hyperostosis of the sphenoidal ridge, olfactory groove, or
parasagittal region, depending upon the location of the tumor.

Figure 13–39 continued on opposite page.

Local Areas of Erosion

Apart from local erosion produced by gliomas in pressing themselves upon the convexity of the calvarium and by meningiomas which are characterized by other features described above, there are certain lesions which are especially characterized by erosions in specific anatomic areas. The most important of these is the acoustic neuroma.

Acoustic Neuroma.   This is a slow-growing perineural fibroma involving the eighth nerve particularly, but occasionally it grows to such size that it involves by contiguity the seventh nerve and extends to involve the cerebellopontine angle and the fifth nerve. Ordinarily, the sixth nerve and motor division of the fifth nerve are spared.

The radiographic abnormalities which may be visualized in approximately half of these lesions include: (1) alterations in the normal shape and size of the internal auditory meatus; (2) resorption of the petrous apex; (3) resorption of the entire internal auditory canal.

Special contrast studies such as pneumograms with body section radiography and myelocisternograms are especially helpful in outlining these lesions accurately. Angiography may also be helpful by careful delineation of the arteries and veins in the immediate vicinity of the cerebellopontine angle. The acoustic neuromas are the most prominent tumors of the cerebellopontine

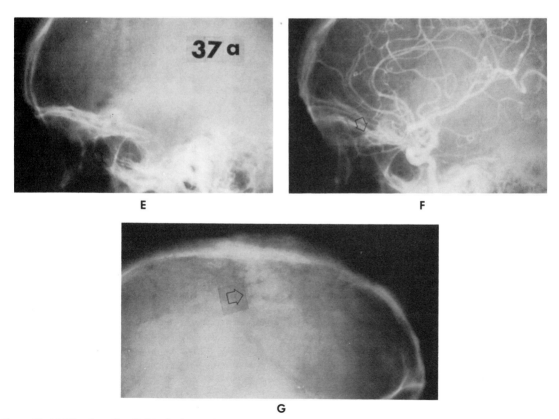

E   F

G

Figure 13–39 (*Continued*).   *E.* Meningioma with involvement of the skull. Lateral view of sphenoid ridge meningioma with marked hyperostosis and local hypervascularity, as well as some associated hyperlucency. *F.* Angiogram showing the meningeal branches supplying the meningioma area. *G.* Parasagittal meningioma likewise showing marked hyperostosis, hypervascularity and intermixed hyperlucency.

Figure 13–39 continued on following page.

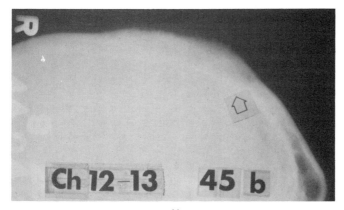

H

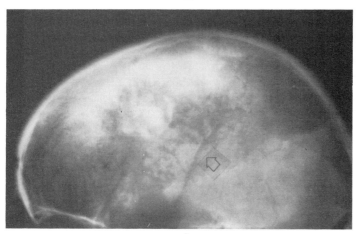

I

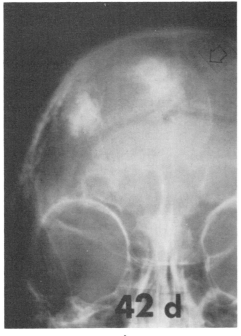

J

Figure 13–39 (*Continued*).   *H*. Close-up view to demonstrate the extensive external table hyperostotic alteration. *I*. Large meningioma encompassing much of the right frontal and parietal region in the lateral projection. *J*. Same in frontal projection. The psammomatous calcification is amorphous and at times the capsule of the lesion appears calcified.

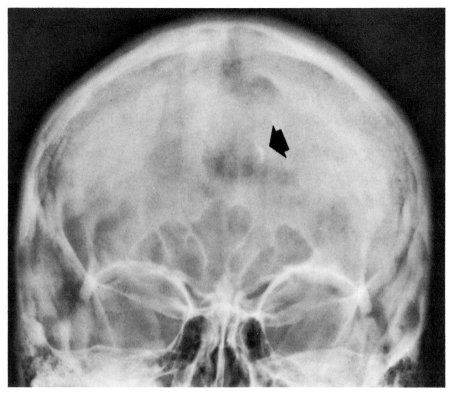

Figure 13-40   P-A view of the skull demonstrating a lipoma of the corpus callosum. Note the shell of calcification surrounding the midline area of radiolucency within the brain. This has an ovoid appearance and is situated in the region of the corpus callosum.

angle but meningiomas, cholesteatomas and gliomas can occur in this region and give similar roentgen findings (Schmitz and Haveson).

Areas of Diminished Density Within the Calvarium (Lipomas of the brain). The intracranial lipoma usually involves the corpus callosum—it may be associated with partial or total agenesis of the corpus callosum.

It is usually characterized radiographically by an ovoid lucent zone in this immediate vicinity surrounded by a thin rim of calcification. Calcium is usually situated in the tumor capsule and appears as an ovoid deposition on either side of the midline surrounding the zone of lucency (which is due to the lipoma) and giving the appearance of parentheses around the lipoma (Figure 13-40).

Alterations in the Posterior Fossa.   Radiography of the posterior fossa is also of interest in relation to developmental defects which occur in the lateral sinuses, in the inion, in the development of the occipital bone, and in the spinal canal of the upper cervical segments (Liliequist; Liliequist, Tovi, and Schisano).

Thus, in cerebral aqueduct stenosis the posterior fossa is shallow and the inion and lateral sinuses are low in position.

In the Dandy-Walker syndrome, the lateral sinuses are elevated, the inion is high, and the posterior curvature of the occipital bone appears increased in its arch.

In the Arnold-Chiari malformation, there is frequently evidence of expansion of the foramen magnum and the neural canal of the upper two or three cervical segments.

There may be evidence of atrophy of the inner table of the skull corresponding to the extent of the malformation of the cisterna magna. This entire malformation may be surrounded by a very narrow area of sclerosis of the inner table of the calvarium.

Questions—Chapter 13

1. What is the range of normal measurement for the sella turcica by Camp's method?

2. What other methods of measurement of the sella turcica have been standardized apart from the Camp technique?

3. Describe the changes which occur in and about the sella turcica in relation to intrasellar expanding lesions.

4. Describe the changes which occur in and about the sella turcica due to extrasellar intracranial expanding lesions.

5. Describe the changes which occur in and about the sella turcica in relation to destructive diseases of the sphenoid bone.

6. Describe the various types of parasellar and intrasellar calcification.

7. Which views are obtained routinely in the radiographic study of the face?

8. Which views are obtained routinely for radiographic examination of the mandible?

9. Which views are considered routine in the radiographic examination of the nose?

10. Which radiographic views are considered routine in examination of the paranasal sinuses?

11. Describe the skull in acromegaly.

12. Describe the skull in hypertelorism.

13. List five general causes for increased density of the paranasal sinuses. How may they be recognized radiographically?

14. Indicate the importance of identification of teeth in respect to fractures of the mandible.

15. Indicate the LeFort classification for fracture of the maxilla.

16. Why is it important to recognize fractures of the zygoma?

17. Describe the radiographic appearances of the "blow-out fracture" of the orbit. What bone or bones are especially fractured in this region?

18. Describe the importance of recognition of fractures of the bones of the fronto-ethmoidal region. What complications are especially important to exclude in such injuries?

19. Describe some of the radiographic appearances of peridental resorption, and the diseases recognized by such studies.

20. Describe the typical radiographic appearances of the ameloblastoma (adamantino-ma) of the mandible.

21. What is meant by "cherubism" of the jaw?

22. Describe at least four standard positions for radiography of the mastoid and temporal bone.

23. What is the significance of increase in opacity of the mastoid air cells with no loss of bone integrity?

24. What is the significance of increased radiopacity of the mastoid with destruction of mastoid air cells?

25. Describe the radiographic appearances of a cholesteatoma involving the mastoid region.

26. What are the most frequent tumors in the vicinity of the apex of the petrous bone? How do they manifest themselves radiographically?

27. Indicate some of the causes of infraorbital calcification. Note that in the text nine different causes are listed.

28. Which are the most frequent orbital tumors?

29. What are the radiographic findings with optic nerve glioma?

30. Indicate the routine and special procedures utilized for diagnosis and localization of intracranial mass lesions.

31. List the changes in the skull indicative of increased intracranial pressure.

32. Describe the changes in the sella turcica related to increased intracranial pressure.

33. List the areas of physiologic calcification within the cranium and indicate which of these are significant in respect to the localization of mass lesions within the cranial cavity.

34. What are some of the causes of non-neoplastic calcification in the cranial cavity? Describe some of their appearances.

35. Which are the most frequent calcifying tumors found within the cranial cavity? Do some of the lesions have characteristic or partially characteristic features?

36. Indicate the most frequent localization for meningioma. What are the roentgen appearances of the meningioma on plain films of the skull?

37. Describe the usual types of erosion which may be manifest on special studies of the skull with the acoustic neuroma.

38. Where is the most frequent occurrence of lipoma of the brain and what is its characteristic roentgen appearance?

39. Describe various alterations in size and contour of the posterior fossa in respect to: (1) Arnold-Chiari malformation; (2) Dandy-Walker syndrome; (3) cerebral aqueduct stenosis; (4) medulloblastoma of the posterior fossa in a child.

References

Acheson, R. M.: Measuring the pituitary fossa from radiographs. Brit. J. Radiol., 29:76–80, 1956.

Allen, J. H., Jr., and Riley, H. D., Jr.: Generalized cytomegalic inclusion disease, with emphasis on roentgen diagnosis. Radiology, 71:257–262, 1958.

Bahn, G. C., and Hauser, G.: A review of orbital tumors. South. Med. J., 51:1444–1447, 1958.

Bailey, P., and Cushing, H.: A Classification of Tumors of the Glioma Group on a Histogenic Basis with a Correlated Study of Prognosis. Philadelphia, J. B. Lippincott Co., 1926.

Bakay, L.: The Blood-Brain Barrier, With Special Regard to the Use of Radioactive Radioisotopes. Springfield, Ill. Charles C Thomas, 1956.

Baker, H. L., Jr.: Myelographic examination of the posterior fossa with positive contrast medium. Radiology, 81:791–801, 1963.

Balkissoon, B., Johnson, J. B., Barber, J. B., and Greene, C. S.: Cerebral arteriography; diagnostic value in cerebrovascular disease. J.A.M.A., 169:676–682, 1959.

Barnett, D. J.: Radiologic aspects of craniopharyngiomas. Radiology, 72:14–18, 1959.

Becker, J. A., and Woloshin, H. J.: Mastoiditis and cholesteatoma: A roentgen approach. Amer. J. Roentgenol., 87:1019–1031, 1962 (31 ref.).

Bender, M. A., and Blough, M.: Photoscanning in medical radioisotope scanning. Pp. 31–38 in Medical Radioisotope Scannings. Vienna, International Atomic Energy Agency, 1959.

Bennett, J. C., Maffly, R. H., and Steinbach, H. L.: The significance of bilateral basal ganglia calcification. Radiology, 72:368–378, 1959 (56 ref.).

Brownell, G. L.: Theory of radioisotope scanning. Int. J. Appl. Radiat., 3:181–192, 1958.

Brünner, S., Petersen, O., and Stoksted, P.: Tomography of the auditory ossicles. Acta Radiol., 56:20–29, 1961.

Brünner, S., Petersen, O., and Sandberg, L. E.: Tomography in cholesteatoma of the temporal bone. Amer. J. Roentgenol., 97:588–596, 1966.

Bull, J. W. D.: Contribution of radiology to the study of intracranial aneurysms. Brit. Med. J., 2:1701–1708, 1962.

Bull, J. W. D.: Positive contrast ventriculography. Acta Radiol., 34:253–268, 1950.

Bullock, L. J., and Reeves, R. J.: Unilateral exophthalmos; roentgenographic aspects. Amer. J. Roentgenol., 82:290–299, 1959.

Camp. J. D.: Intracranial calcification and its roentgenologic significance. Amer. J. Roentgenol., 23:615–624, 1930.

Camp, J. D.: Normal and pathologic anatomy of the sella turcica as revealed at necropsy. Radiology, 1:65, 1923.

Camp, J. D.: Pathologic non-neoplastic intracranial calcification. J.A.M.A., 137:1023–1031, 1948.

Camp, J. D.: Roentgenologic manifestations of intracranial disease. Radiology, 13:484–493, 1929.

Camp, J. D.: Significance of intracranial calcification in the roentgenologic diagnosis of intracranial neoplasms. Radiology, 55:659–667, 1950.

Camp, J. D., and Allen, E. P.: Microtia and congenital atresia of the external auditory canal: Demonstration of external auditory canal by means of tomography. Amer. J. Roentgenol., *43*:201–203, 1940.

Chynn, K. Y.: Occipital emissary vein enlargement: A sign of increased intracranial pressure. Radiology, *81*:242–247, 1963.

Cobble, S. P., and Brackett, C. E.: Changes in the ventricular size during stereotaxic surgery. Amer. J. Roentgenol., *95*:890–898, 1965. (There are excellent illustrations of the types of stereotaxis apparatus and development that we have participated in.)

Collins, E. T.: Case with symmetrical congenital notches in the outer part of each lower lid and effective development of the malar bones. Trans. Ophth. Soc. U.K., *20*:190, 1900.

Compere, W. E., Jr.: Radiographic Atlas of the Temporal Bone. Book I, American Academy of Ophthalmology and Otolaryngology, 1964.

Compere, W. E., Jr.: Radiologic findings in otosclerosis. Arch. Otolaryngol., *71*:150–155, 1960.

Converse, J. M.: Reconstructive Plastic Surgery. Philadelphia, W. B. Saunders Co., 1964.

Cronqvist, S., and Köhler, R.: Angiography in epidural hematomas. Acta Radiol. (Diag.), *1*:42–52, 1963.

Cunningham, J. D., and Marden, P. A.: Blow-out fractures of the orbital floor. Arch. Ophthal., *68*:492, 1962.

Cushing, H.: Intracranial Tumors. Notes upon a Series of 2,000 Verified Cases with Surgical-mortality Percentages Pertaining Thereto. Springfield, Ill. Charles C Thomas, 1932.

Cushing, H., and Bailey, P.: Tumors Arising from the Blood Vessels of the Brain. Angiomatous Malformations and Hemangioblastomas. Springfield, Ill., Charles C Thomas, 1928.

Dahlgren, S.: Thorotrast tumors: Review of literature and report of two cases. Acta Path. Microbiol. Scand., *53*:147–161, 1961.

Davidoff, L. M., and Dyke, C. G.: The Normal Encephalogram. Second Edition. Philadelphia, Lea and Febiger, 1946.

Dechaume, M., Grellet, M., Payen, J., Bonneau, M., Guilbert, F., and Boccara, S.: Le chérubisme. A propos de cinq nouveaux cas. Presse Méd., *70*:2763–2766, 1962.

Deery, E. M.: Note on calcification in pituitary adenomas. Endocrinology, *13*:455–458, 1929.

DiChiro, G., and Nelson, K. B.: The volume of the sella turcica. Amer. J. Roentgenol., *87*:989–1008, 1962.

Doubleday, L. C.: Roentgenologic aspects of the black eye. J.A.M.A., *179*:27–29, 1962.

Dunsmore, R. H., Scoville, W. B., and Whitcomb, B. B.: Symposium: Intracranial vascular abnormalities; complications of angiography. J. Neurosurg., *8*:110–118, 1951.

Echternacht, A. P., and Campbell, J. A.: Midline anomalies of the brain, their diagnosis by pneumoencephalography. Radiology, *46*:119–131, 1946.

Ecker, A.: The Normal Cerebral Angiogram. Springfield, Ill., Charles C Thomas, 1951.

Ecker, A., and Riemenschneider, P. A.: Angiographic Localization of Intracranial Masses. Springfield, Ill., Charles C Thomas, 1955.

Editorial: A new look in mastoids. J. Canad. Ass. Radiol., *14*:142–143, 1963.

Epstein, B., and Davidoff, L. M.: Atlas of Skull Roentgenograms. London, Kimpton, 1953.

Ernyei, S.: Mesodermal dysgenesis of cornea and iris (Rieger). Amer. J. Ophth., *59*:106–108, 1965.

Etter, L. E., and Cross, L. C.: Projection angle variations required to demonstrate the middle ear, antrum, and mastoid process. Radiology, *80*:255–257, 1963.

Figi, F. A.: Fibromas of the nasopharynx. J.A.M.A., *115*:665–671, 1940.

Fisher, D. F., and Anthony, D. H.: Intra-ocular foreign bodies: Diagnosis, complications and surgical treatment. J. Tenn. St. Med. Ass., *44*:130–136, 1951.

Fisher, R. L., and DiChiro, G.: The small sella turcica. Amer. J. Roentgenol., *91*:996–1008, 1964.

Franceschetti, A., and Klein, D.: Mandibulofacial dysostosis: A new hereditary syndrome. Acta Ophth., *27*:143, 1949.

Gaard, R. A.: Ocular hypertelorism of Greig: A congenital craniofacial deformity. Amer. J. Orthodontics, *47*:205–219, 1961.

Gillies, H. D., and Millard, D. R., Jr.: Principles and Art of Plastic Surgery. Boston, Little, Brown and Co., 1957.

Gonsette, R., Dereymaeker, A., Hou, H., and Cornélis, G.: L'iodoventriculographie. I. Technique, indications, images normates. Acta Neurol. Belg., *58*:778–796, 1958.

Gorlin, R. J., and Goetz, R. W.: Multiple nevoid basal-cell epithelioma, jaw cysts and bifid rib. A syndrome. New Eng. J. Med., *262*:908–912, 1960.

Gorlin, R. J., Yunis, J. J., and Tuna, N.: Multiple nevoid basal cell carcinoma, odontogenic keratocysts and skeletal anomalies: A syndrome. Acta Dermato Vener., *43*:39–55, 1963.

Grant, J. C. B.: An Atlas of Anatomy, Fifth Edition. Baltimore, Williams and Wilkins Co., 1962.

Green, W. G., Goldberg, H. I., and Wohl, G. T.: Mucormycosis, infection of the craniofacial structures. Amer. J. Roentgenol., *101*:802–806, 1967.

Hartmann, E., and Gilles, E.: Roentgenologic Diagnosis in Ophthalmology. Philadelphia, J. B. Lippincott Co., 1959.

Hastings-James, R.: Lenticulodentate calcification. Radiology, *97*:571–576, 1970.

Hodes, P. J., Pendergrass, E. P., and Young, B. R.: Eighth nerve tumors: Their roentgen manifestations. Radiology, *53*:633–665, 1949.

Hodges, F. J., Holt, J. F., Bassett, R. C., and Lemmen, L. J.: Reliability of brain tumor localization by roentgen methods. Amer. J. Roentgenol., *71*:624–631, 1954.

Holman, C. B.: Roentgenologic manifestations of glioma of the optic nerve and chiasm. Amer. J. Roentgenol., *82*:462–471, 1959.

Horwitz, N. H.: Positive contrast ventriculography, a critical evaluation. J. Neurosurg., *13*:388–399, 1956.

Ingalls, R. G.: Tumors of the Orbit and Allied Pseudo Tumors: An Analysis of 215 Case Histories. Springfield, Ill., Charles C Thomas, 1953.

Jacobson, H. G., Lubetsky, H. W., Shapiro, J. H., and Carton, C. A.: Intracranial meningiomas. A roentgen study of 126 cases. Radiology, 72:356–367, 1959.

Jayne, E. H., Hays, R. A., and O'Brien, F. W., Jr.: Cysts and tumors of the mandibles, their differential diagnosis. Amer. J. Roentgenol., 86:292–309, 1961 (19 ref.).

Jensen, G., Jespersen, C., and Brunner, S.: Value of different projections in diagnosing cholesteatoma. Acta Radiol., 54:177–185, 1960.

Johnson, G. F., and Weisman, P. A.: Radiological features of dermoid cysts of the nose. Radiology, 82:1016–1021, 1964.

Kaufman, B., Sandstrom, P. H., and Young, H. F.: Alteration in size and configuration of the sella turcica, as the result of prolonged cerebrospinal fluid shunting. Radiology, 97:537–542, 1970.

Kautz, F. G., and Schwartz, I.: Intra-ocular calcium shadows: choroid ossification. Radiology, 43:486–491, 1944.

Kazanjian, V. H., and Converse, J. M.: The surgical treatment of facial injuries. Baltimore, Williams and Wilkins Co., 1959.

Keirns, M. M., and Whiteleather, J. E.: The angiographic study of carotid insufficiency and cerebral ischemia. Amer. J. Roentgenol., 81:929–944, 1959.

Kruyff, E., and Munn, J. D.: Posterior fossa tumors in infants and children. Amer. J. Roentgenol., 89:951–965, 1963.

Kuhn, R. A.: Importance of accurate diagnosis by cerebral angiography in cases of stroke. J.A.M.A., 169:1867–1875, 1959.

LeFort, P.: Étude expérimentale sur les fractures de la mâchoire supérieure. Rev. Chir., 23:208, 360, 479, 1901.

Lewin, J. R., Rhodes, D. H., Jr., and Pavsek, E. J.: Roentgenologic manifestations of fracture of the orbital floor (blow-out fracture). Amer. J. Roentgenol., 83:628–632, 1960.

Liliequist, B.: Pontine angle tumors, encephalographic appearances. Acta Radiol. Supp., 186:1–96, 1959.

Liliequist, B.: The subarachnoid cisterns. An anatomic and roentgenologic study. Acta Radiol. Supp., 185:1–108, 1959.

Liliequist, B., Tovi, D., and Schisano, G.: Developmental defects of the tentorium and cisterna magna; Report of two cases diagnosed by encephalography and confirmed at operation. Acta Psychiat. Scand., 35:223–234, 1960.

Lindblom, K.: Roentgenographic study of vascular channels of the skull, with special reference to intracranial tumors and arteriovenous aneurysms. Acta Radiol. Supp., 30:1–146, 1936.

Lindgren, E.: Radiologic examination of the brain and spinal cord. Acta Radiol. Supp., 151:1–147, 1957.

List, C. F., Holt, J. F., and Everett, M.: Lipoma of corpus callosum. Clinicopathologic study. Amer. J. Roentgenol., 55:125–134, 1946.

McAfee, J. G., and Taxdal, D. R.: Comparison of radioisotope scanning, cerebral angiography and air studies in brain tumor localization. Radiology, 77:207–222, 1961.

MacKenzie, K. G. A., Preston, C. D., Stewart, W., and Haggith, J. H.: Thorotrast retention following angiography: A case with postmortem studies. Clin. Radiology, 13:157–162, 1962.

Mainzer, F., Stargardter, F. L., Connolly, E., and Eyster, E. F.: Inverting papilloma of the nose and paranasal sinuses. Radiology, 92:964–968, 1969.

Mannick, J. A., Suter, C. G., and Hume, D. M.: The "subclavian steal" syndrome: A further documentation. J.A.M.A., 182:254–258, 1962.

Martin, F. A., Webster, J. E., and Gurdjian, E. S.: Relative accuracy of electroencephalography, air studies and angiography; in series of 200 mass lesions. J. Neurosurg., 10:397–403, 1953.

Martin, F., Jr., and Lemmen, L. J.: Calcification in intracranial neoplasms. Amer. J. Path., 28:1107–1131, 1952.

Martin, H. L., and McDowell, F.: Evaluation of seizures in the adult. A.M.A. Arch. Neurol. Psychiat., 71:101–104, 1954.

Mascherpa, F., and Valentino, V.: Intracranial Calcification. Springfield, Ill., Charles C Thomas, 1959.

Masson, C. B.: The occurrence of calcification in gliomas. Bull. Neurol. Inst. New York, 1:314–327, 1931.

Matsubara, T., and Nomura, T.: Emulsified iodized oil ventriculography. Amer. J. Roentgenol., 84:48–51, 1960.

Meschan, I.: An Atlas of Normal Radiographic Anatomy. Second Edition. Philadelphia, W. B. Saunders Co., 1959.

Meyer, J. S.: Ischemic cerebrovascular disease (stroke). Clinical investigation and management. J.A.M.A., 183:237–240, 1963.

Mones, R., and Werman, R.: Pantopaque myeloencephalography. Radiology, 72:803–809, 1959.

Morris, L.: Angiography of the superior sagittal sinus and transverse sinuses. Brit. J. Radiol., 33:606–613, 1960.

Murtagh, F., and Stauffer, H. M.: Practical value of internal cerebral vein in anteroposterior phlebogram. Amer. J. Roentgenol., 80:978–981, 1958.

Nesbit, M. E., Jr., Wolfson, J. J., Kieffer, S. A., and Peterson, H. O.: Orbital sclerosis in histiocytosis X. Amer. J. Roentgenol., 110:123–128, 1970.

Norlen, G., and Wickbom, I.: The relative merits of encephalography and ventriculography for the investigation of intracranial tumors. J. Neurol. Neurosurg. Psychiat., 21:1–11, 1958.

Nylen, B.: Histopathological investigations on localization, number, activity and extent of otosclerotic fossi. J. Laryngol. and Otolaryngol., 63:321–327, 1949.

Perras, P.: The value of Chausée III and transorbital projections in middle ear disease. J. Canad. Ass. Radiol., 14:144–150, 1963.

Peterman, A. F., Hayles, A. R., Dockery, M. B., and Love, J. G.: Encephalotrigeminal angiomatosis (Sturge-Weber disease); clinical study of 35 cases. J.A.M.A., 167:2169–2176, 1958.

Pfeiffer, R. L.: Traumatic Enophthalmos. Arch. Ophthal., 30:718–726, 1943.

Philip, T., Samuel, E., and Duncan, J. G.: Reversed vertebral artery blood flow in subclavian artery obstruction (subclavian steal). Clin. Radiol., *14*:310–316, 1963.

Pico, G.: Mandibulofacial dysostosis. Amer. J. Ophth., *52*:521–526, 1961.

Poppen, J. L., and Strain, R. E.: Symposium on orthopedic surgery and neurosurgery; chronic subdural hematomas. Surg. Clin. N. Amer., *32*:791–799, 1952.

Proetz, A. W.: The displacement method of sinus diagnosis and treatment. St. Louis, Annals Publishing Co., 1931.

Ralston, B. L., Gross, S. W., and Newman, C. W.: Pantopaque ventriculography in the localization of surgical lesions of the posterior fossa. Amer. J. Roentgenol., *81*:972–983, 1959 (16 ref.).

Ray, B. S., Dunbar, H. S., and Dotter, C. P.: Dural sinus venography. Radiology, *57*:475–486, 1951.

Reese, A.: Tumors of the Eye. Second Edition. New York, Hoeber Medical Division, Harper and Row, 1963.

Reese, A. B.: Orbital tumors and their surgical treatment. Amer. J. Ophthal., *24*:386, 1941.

Reivich, M., Holling, H. E., Roberts, B., and Toole, J. F.: Reversal of blood flow through the vertebral artery and its effect on cerebral circulation. New Eng. J. Med., *265*:878–885, 1961.

Riemenschneider, P., Hoople, G. D., Brewer, D., Jones, D., and Ecker, A.: Roentgenographic diagnosis of tumors of the glomus jugularis. Amer. J. Roentgenol., *69*:59–65, 1953.

Ring, B. A., and Waddington, M.: Primary arachnoid cysts of the sella turcica. Amer. J. Roentgenol., *98*:611–615, 1966.

Ritvo, M.: Roentgen Diagnosis of Diseases of the Skull. New York, Paul B. Hoeber, Inc., 1949. Annals of Roentgenology, V. 19.

Robertson, E. G.: Pneumoencephalography. Springfield, Ill., Charles C Thomas, 1957.

Robin, P.: Glossoptosis due to atresia and hypotrophy of the mandible. Amer. J. Dis. Child., *48*:541, 1934.

Robinson, H. B. G.: Classification of cysts of the jaws. Amer. J. Orthodont. (Oral Surg. Sect.), *31*:370–375, 1945.

Robinson, H. B. G., Koch, W. E., and Kolas, S.: Differential diagnosis of cysts and tumors of the jaw. Dental Radiography and Photography, *29*:61–68, 1956.

Samuel, E.: Clinical Radiology of the Ear, Nose and Throat. New York, Paul B. Hoeber, Inc., 1952.

Schechter, M. M., and Zingesser, L. H.: The radiology of aqueductal stenosis. Radiology, *88*:905–916, 1967.

Schisano, G., and Olivecrona, H.: Neurinomas of the gasserian ganglion and trigeminal route. J. Neurosurg., *17*:306–322, 1960.

Schlesinger, E. B., DeBoves, S., and Taveras, J. M.: Localization of brain tumors using radio-iodinated human serum albumin. Amer. J. Roentgenol., *87*:449–462, 1962.

Schmitz, A. L., and Haveson, S. B.: The roentgen diagnosis of eighth nerve tumors. Radiology, *75*:531–543 1960 (27 ref.).

Schunk, H., Davies, H., Drake, M.: A study of meningiomas with correlation of hyperostosis and tumor vascularity. Amer. J. Roentgenol., *91*:431–443, 1964.

Schwartz, C. W.: Cranial and intracranial epidermoidomas from a roentgenological viewpoint. Amer. J. Roentgenol., *45*:18–26, 1941.

Schwartz, C. W.: Gliomas roentgenologically considered. Radiology, *27*:419–432, 1936.

Schwartz, C. W.: Meningiomas from the roentgenological viewpoint. Amer. J. Roentgenol., *39*:698–712, 1938.

Schwartz, C. W.: Recognition of some forms of intracranial lesions. Amer. J. Med. Sci., *190*:220–225, 1935.

Schwartz, C. W.: Tumors of the hypophysis cerebri from the roentgenologic viewpoint. Amer. J. Roentgenol., *40*:548–570, 1938.

Schwartz, C. W.: Vascular tumors and anomalies of the skull and brain from a roentgenologic viewpoint. Amer. J. Roentgenol., *41*:881–900, 1939.

Schwarz, E.: Ossifying fibroma of the face and skull. Amer. J. Roentgenol., *91*:1012–1015, 1964.

Scott, M.: Symposium on Pediatrics; diagnosis and treatment of hydrocephalus. Med. Clin. N. Amer., *36*:1739–1750, 1952.

Shy, G. M., Bradley, R. B., and Matthews, W. B., Jr.: External Collimation Detection of Intracranial Neoplasia with Unstable Nuclides. Edinburgh, Livingston, 1958.

Silverman, F.: Roentgen standards for size of the pituitary fossa from infancy through adolescence. Amer. J. Roentgenol., *78*:451–460, 1957.

Smith, A. B.: The role of radiology in the diagnosis of brain tumors. South. Med. J., *45*:388–395, 1952.

Smith, B., and Regan, W. F., Jr.: Blow-out fracture of the orbit. Mechanism and correction of internal orbital fracture. Amer. J. Ophth., *44*:733–739, 1957.

Smith, C. G.: The x-ray appearance and incidence of calcified nodules on the habenular commissure. Radiology, *60*:647–650, 1953.

Sosman, M C., and Putnam, J. J.: Roentgenological aspects of brain tumors; meningiomas. Amer. J. Roentgenol., *13*:1–10, 1925.

Steinberg, I., and Halpern, M.: Roentgen manifestations of the subclavian steal syndrome. Amer. J. Roentgenol., *90*:528–531, 1963.

Sutton, D.: The radiological diagnosis of lipoma of the corpus callosum. Brit. J. Radiol., *22*:534–539, 1949.

Sweet, W. H., Mealey, J., Jr., Brownell, G. L., and Aronow, S. P.: Arsenic-76 coincidence positron brain scanning. In Medical Radioisotope Scanning. Vienna, International Atomic Energy Agency, 1959, pp. 163–168.

Tatelman, M.: Angiographic evaluation of cerebral atherosclerosis. Radiology, *70*:801–810, 1958.

Taveras, J. M., and Poser, C. F.: Roentgenologic aspects of cerebral angiography in children. Amer. J. Roentgenol., *82*:371–391, 1959.

Taveras, J. M., and Wood, E. H.: Diagnostic Neuroradiology. Baltimore, Williams & Wilkins Co., 1964.

Tod, P. A., Thorpe, R. J., Jamieson, K. G., and Yelland, J. D. N.: The Dandy-Walker syndrome. The Journal of the College of Radiologists of Australasia, 9:111–116, 1965 (June).

Valvassori, G. E.: Abnormal internal auditory canal: acoustic neuroma. Radiology, 92:449–459, 1969.

Valvassori, G. E.: Laminagraphy of the ear. Normal roentgenographic anatomy. Amer. J. Roentgenol., 89:1155–1167, 1963.

Valvassori, G. E.: Laminagraphy of the ear. Pathologic conditions. Amer. J. Roentgenol., 89:1168–1178, 1963.

Valvassori, G. E.: Otosclerosis: a new challenge to roentgenology. Amer. J. Roentgenol., 94:566–575, 1965.

Vastine, J. H., and Kinney, K. K.: The pineal shadow as an aid in the localization of brain tumors. Amer. J. Roentgenol., 17:320–324, 1927.

Weidner, W., Rosen, L., and Hanafee, W.: The neuroradiology of tumors of the pituitary gland. Amer. J. Roentgenol., 95:884–889, 1965.

Whiteleather, J. E., and Keirns, M. M.: Present status of cerebral angiography. Angiology, 11:297–309, 1960.

Wiley, C. J.: Lipoid proteinosis—a new roentgenologic entity. Amer. J. Roentgenol., 89:1220–1221, 1963.

Williams, C. L., Scott, S. M., and Takaro, T.: Subclavian steal. Circulation, 28:14–19, 1963.

Wilson, C. B., and Roy, M.: Calcification within congenital aneurysms of the vein of Galen. Amer. J. Roentgenol., 91:1319–1326, 1964.

Wilson, M., and Snodgrass, S. R.: Positive contrast ventriculography. Radiology, 72:810–815, 1959.

Wollschlaeger, G., Wollschlaeger, P. B., Brannan, D. D., and Segal, A. J.: Lipoma of the corpus callosum. Amer. J. Roentgenol., 86:142–147, 1961 (39 ref.).

Zegarelli, E. V., and Kutscher, A. H.: Fibrous dysplasia of the jaws. Dental Radiography and Photography, 36:27–46, 1963.

14

The Radiology of the Vertebral Column

ROUTINE POSITIONS FOR EXAMINATION OF THE CERVICAL AND THORACIC SPINE
(Figures 14–1; 14–2)

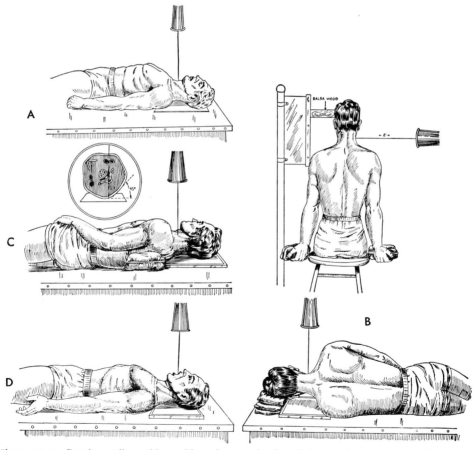

Figure 14–1 Routine radiographic positions for examination of the cervical spine. *A*. A–P view. *B*. Lateral view. *C*. Oblique view. *D*. Special view of the upper two cervical segments, taken through the open mouth. Views in flexion and extension in the lateral and oblique projections may also be employed. As an alternate to the antero-posterior views of the cervical spine shown (including the view of the odontoid with the mouth open), an antero-posterior view may be obtained with the lower jaw in slow motion. This tends to blur out the mandible so that the upper cervical segments may be visualized without interference.

602

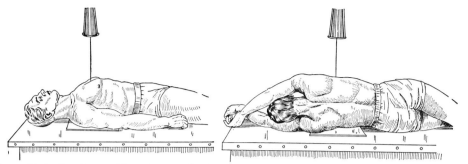

Figure 14-2 Routine positions for examination of the thoracic spine. *A*. A–P view. *B*. Lateral view.

ROUTINE POSITIONS
FOR EXAMINATION OF
THE LUMBAR SPINE (Figure 14–3)

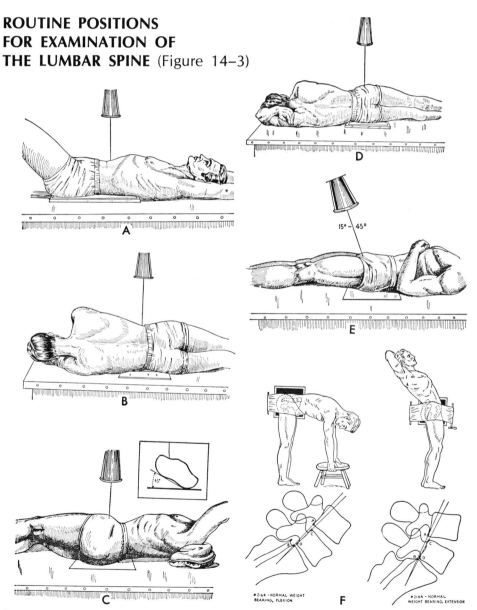

Figure 14-3 Routine positions for examination of the lumbar spine. *A*. A–P view. *B*. Lateral view. *C*. Oblique view. *D*. Special lateral view of sacrum and coccyx and lower-most lumbar segment. *E*. Distorted view of sacrum. *G*. Special views utilized for detecting degree of mobility of the lumbosacral spine in flexion and extension.

HOW TO ANALYZE SPINE FILMS AND WHAT TO LOOK FOR (Figures 14–4 through 14–21)

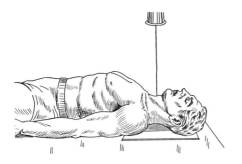

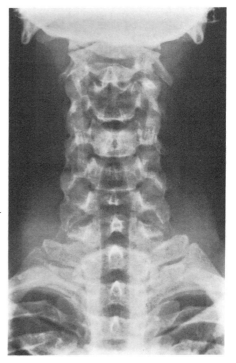

A

Figure 14–4 *A* and *B*. Antero-posterior views of cervical spine.

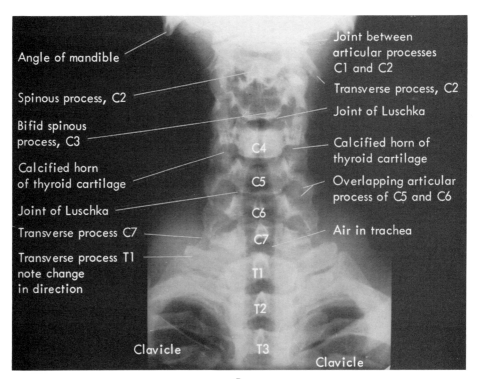

B

Figure 14–4 continued on opposite page.

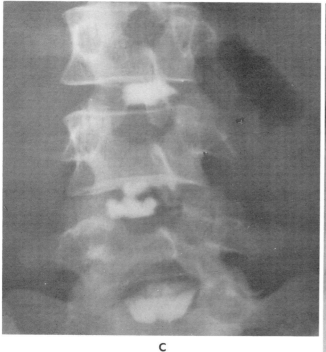

C

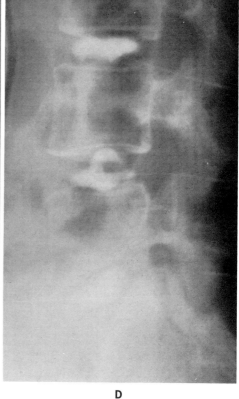

D

Figure 14-4 (*Continued*). *C.* Normal discogram in antero-posterior projection. *D.* Normal discogram of the lumbar region in lateral projection.

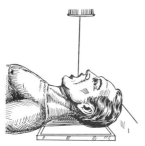

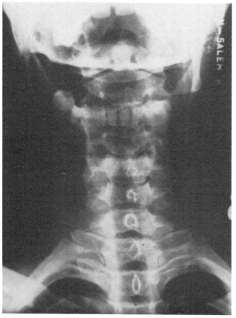

Figure 14-5 Antero-posterior view of the cervical spine obtained with a rhythmic motion of the lower jaw during the exposure. The head, of course, is rigidly immobilized to prevent movement of the cervical spine. When a view is obtained in this manner a concept of the upper two cervical segments may be obtained which otherwise is not possible in this projection, since these segments are invariably obscured by the shadow of the mandible (Ottonello method).

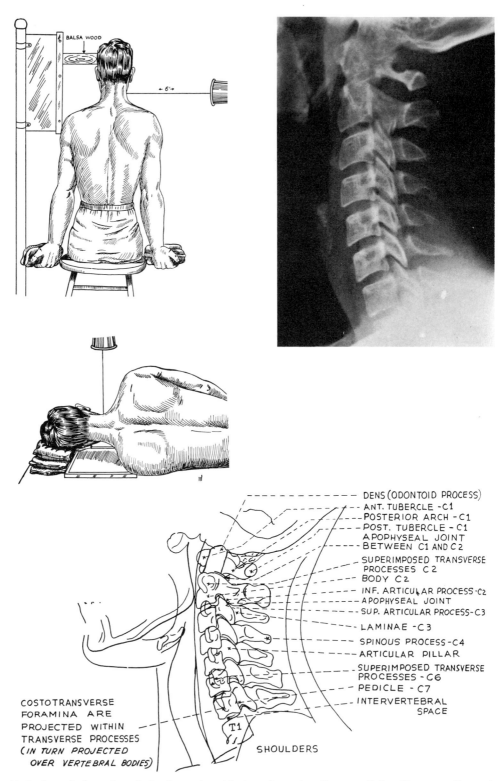

Figure 14–6 Lateral view of cervical spine and positioning of a patient for erect (6 foot film-target distance) and recumbent views. The erect view shown is the Grandy technique, described by C. C. Grandy in 1925 (Radiology 5:128–129, 1925).

NORMAL SAGITTAL MEASUREMENTS*

Region Evaluated	Normal Sagittal Measurements for Children 15 Years and Under (120 cases)		Normal Sagittal Measurements for Adults (480 cases)	
	AVERAGE (MM.)	RANGE (MM.)	AVERAGE (MM.)	RANGE (MM.)
Retropharyngeal space	3.5	2–7	3.4	1–7
Retrotracheal space	7.9	5–14	14.0	9–22
Cervical spinal canal:				
At first cervical vertebra	21.9	18–27	21.4	16–30
At second cervical vertebra	20.9	18–25	19.2	16–28
At third cervical vertebra	17.4	14–21	19.1	14–25
At fifth cervical vertebra	16.5	14–21	18.5	14–25
At seventh cervical vertebra	16.0	15–20	17.5	13–24

*From Wholey, M. H., et al.: Radiology, *71*:350, 1958.

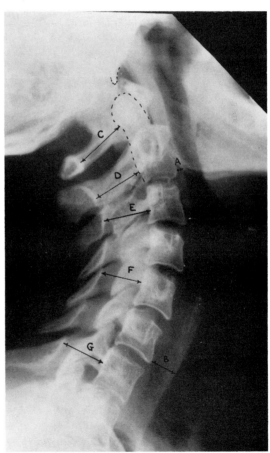

Figure 14–7 Normal lateral view of neck indicating regions evaluated. *A.* Retropharyngeal space, second cervical vertebra; *B.* retrotracheal space, sixth cervical vertebra; *C* to *G.* cervical spinal canal; *C,* first cervical vertebra; *D.* second cervical vertebra; *E.* third cervical vertebra; *F.* fifth cervical vertebra; *G.* seventh cervical vertebra (from Wholey, M. H., Brewer, A. J., and Baker, H. L., Jr.: Radiology *71*: 350, 1958).

CLASSIFICATION OF ABNORMALITIES OF THE SPINE FROM THE RADIOGRAPHIC STANDPOINT

The spine is analyzed in relation to the usual classification of radiographic pathology, namely, abnormalities of *size, shape, number* of the individual vertebral segments, *contour* of the spine generally, *density, architecture,* and *function* (study of the spine in motion).

In addition special consideration must be given to the following: *Joint abnormalities of the spine* — the intervertebral disks and true synovial joints are considered separately; and *special contrast studies* of the subarachnoid space (*myelography*).

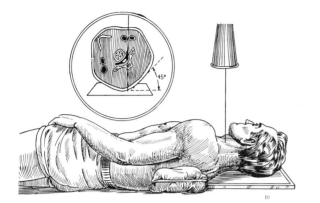

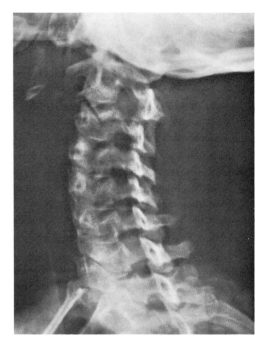

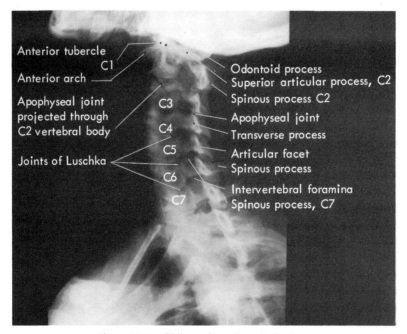

Anterior tubercle
C1
Anterior arch

Apophyseal joint
projected through
C2 vertebral body

Joints of Luschka

C3

C4

C5

C6

C7

Odontoid process
Superior articular process, C2
Spinous process C2

Apophyseal joint
Transverse process

Articular facet
Spinous process

Intervertebral foramina
Spinous process, C7

Figure 14–8 Oblique view of cervical spine.

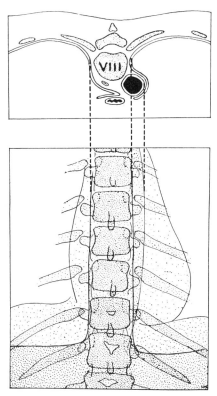

Figure 14–9   *Upper,* Cross section through the posterior mediastinum at the level of the eighth thoracic vertebra. *Lower,* Diagram taken from a roentgenogram depicting the posterior portions of the visceral and parietal pleura as lines along the vertebral column. Dotted lines indicate anatomical substrates of pleural lines and aortic lines in cross section. (From Lachman, E.: Anat. Rec. *83,* 1942.)

ABNORMALITIES IN NUMBER OF VERTEBRAL SEGMENTS

Failure of development.
Fusion of elements:
    1. Klippel-Feil deformity.
    2. Block vertebrae.
    3. The occipital vertebra.
    4. Atlantoaxial fusion.
    5. Lumbarization and sacralization.
Supernumerary elements.

Failure of Development of an Entire Vertebral Segment

This anomaly is frequently accompanied by other advanced congenital malformations (Giannini, Borrelli, and Greenberg).

The neural arch may itself persist while the rest of the vertebral segment is lacking (Reinhardt).

Total absence of the lumbar spine or sacrum (Frantz and Aitken; Alexander and Nashold).

(*Text continued on page 618*)

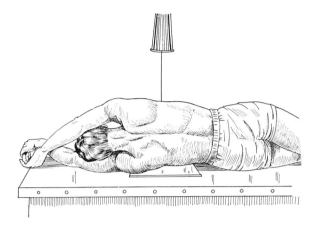

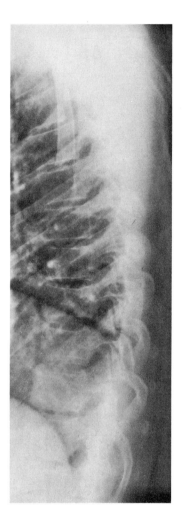

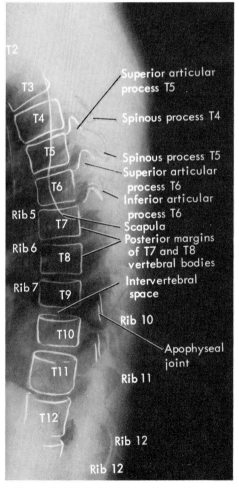

Figure 14–10   Lateral view of thoracic spine: positioning of patient, radiograph and labeled tracing.

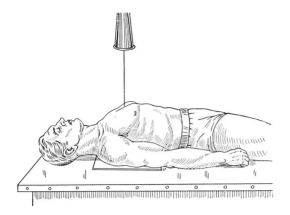

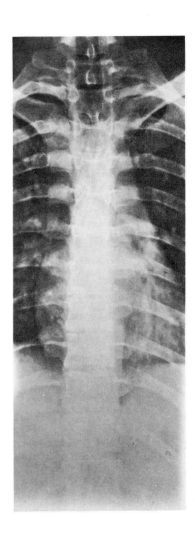

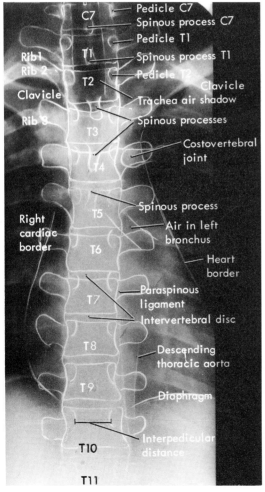

C7

Pedicle C7
Spinous process C7
Pedicle T1

Rib 1
Rib 2

T1

Spinous process T1

Pedicle T2

Clavicle

T2

Clavicle

Clavicle

Trachea air shadow

Rib 3

Spinous processes

T3

Costovertebral
joint

T4

Spinous process

T5

Air in left
bronchus

Right
cardiac
border

Heart
border

T6

Paraspinous
ligament

T7

Intervertebral disc

T8

Descending
thoracic aorta

T9

Diaphragm

Interpedicular
distance

T10

T11

Figure 14–11   Antero-posterior view of the thoracic spine: positioning of patient, radiograph and labeled tracing.

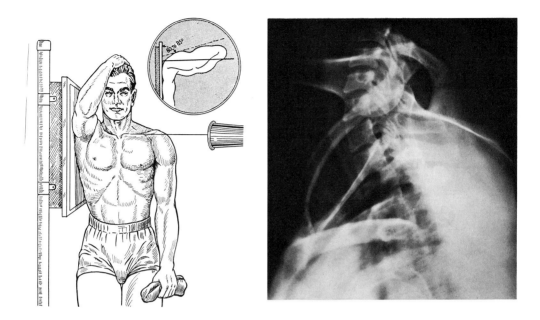

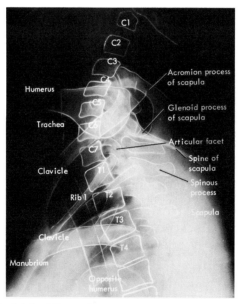

Figure 14–12   Lateral (slightly oblique) view of upper two thoracic segments (Twining position).

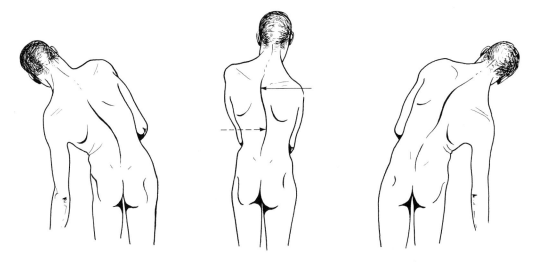

Primary curvature remains relatively constant (⟶).
Secondary curvature tends to correct itself (--⟶).

Figure 14–13   Method for positioning patient for study of scoliosis of the spine.

Figure 14–14   Method of measuring scoliosis.

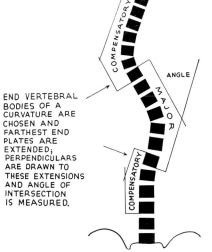

END VERTEBRAL
BODIES OF A
CURVATURE ARE
CHOSEN AND
FARTHEST END
PLATES ARE
EXTENDED;
PERPENDICULARS
ARE DRAWN TO
THESE EXTENSIONS
AND ANGLE OF
INTERSECTION
IS MEASURED.

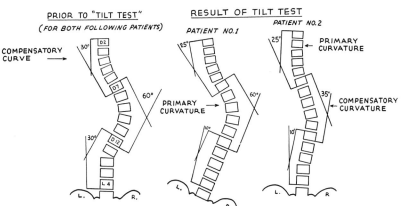

Figure 14–15   Determination of primary and secondary curvatures in dorsal scoliosis. (Modified from Ferguson, A. B.: *Roentgen Diagnosis of Extremities and Spine.* New York, Paul B. Hoeber, Inc., 1949.)

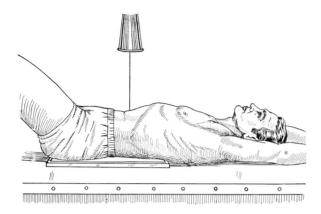

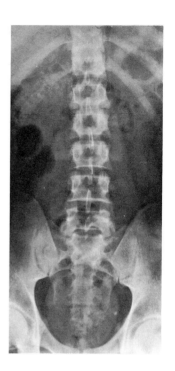

Figure 14–16 Antero-posterior view of lumbosacral spine: positioning of patient, radiograph and labeled tracing.

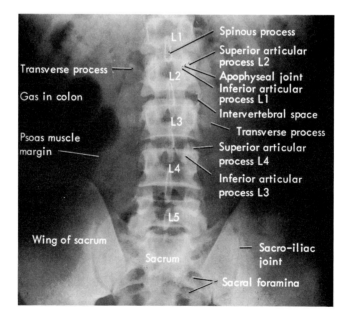

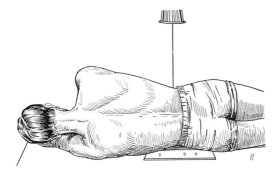

Figure 14–17 Lateral view of the lumbosacral spine.

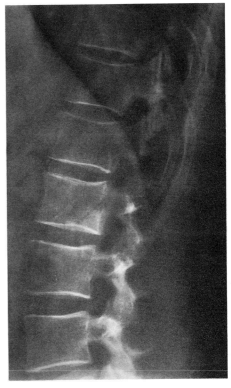

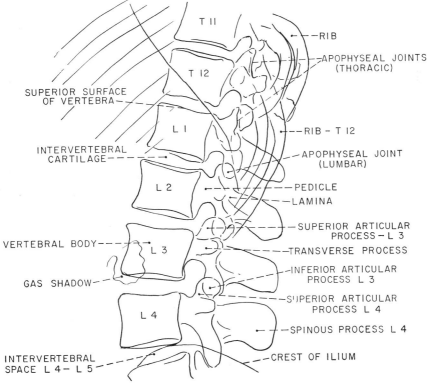

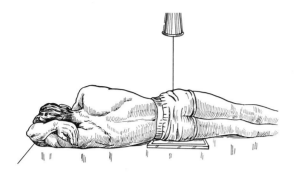

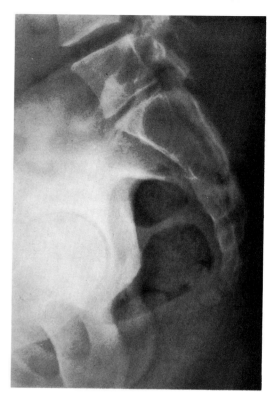

Figure 14–18 Special lateral view of sacrum and coccyx.

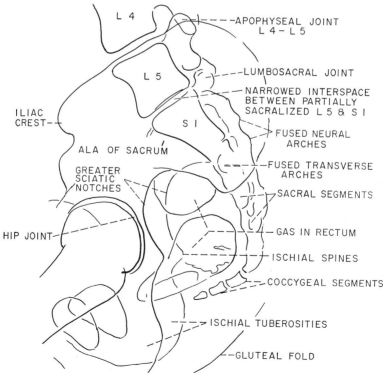

L 4

L 5

S I

ILIAC
CREST

ALA OF SACRUM

GREATER
SCIATIC
NOTCHES

HIP JOINT

APOPHYSEAL JOINT
L 4 - L 5

LUMBOSACRAL JOINT

NARROWED INTERSPACE
BETWEEN PARTIALLY
SACRALIZED L 5 & S I

FUSED NEURAL
ARCHES

FUSED TRANSVERSE
ARCHES

SACRAL SEGMENTS

GAS IN RECTUM

ISCHIAL SPINES

COCCYGEAL SEGMENTS

ISCHIAL TUBEROSITIES

GLUTEAL FOLD

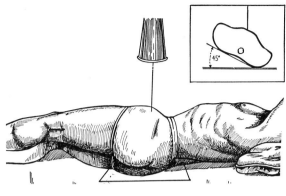

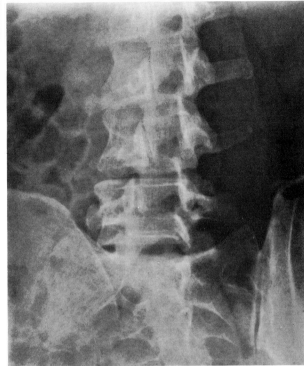

Figure 14–19   Oblique view of lumbosacral spine.

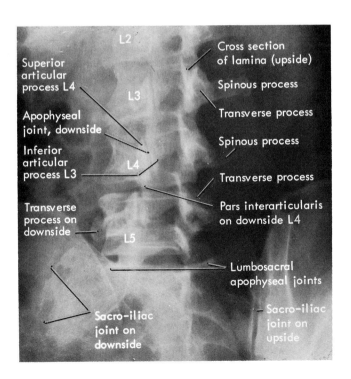

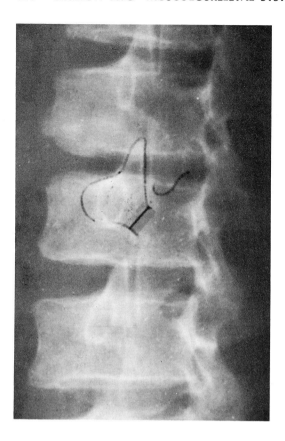

Figure 14–20 Oblique view of the lumbar spine demonstrating the "scotty dog" appearance of the transverse process, superior articular process and pars interarticularis. The collar on the "scotty dog" is the area of defective ossification most frequently encountered in association with spondylolisthesis.

Abnormalities of Number Due to Fusion of Elements

Klippel-Feil Deformity of the Cervical Spine (Figure 14–22)

This disorder is defined as a synostosis of two or more of the cervical segments with varying degrees of partial fusion and malformation giving rise to associated hemivertebrae and irregularities in the laminae and spinous processes.

There may be associated alteration in the upper ribs or cervico-occipital fusion. The involved portion of the spine is shortened and often kyphotic or scoliotic.

Infants with this disorder may have other severe malformations such as an encephalocele, facial and cranial asymmetry, a lowered nipple line, syndactylism, clubbed foot, and hypoplastic lumbar vertebrae. Sprengel's deformity may also coexist. Absence of the external auditory meatus, deafness, and mental deficiency may also be present.

Block Vertebra (Figure 14–23)

A fusion of two or more vertebrae is called a block vertebra. This fusion may involve the neural arches or ribs in the thoracic spine.

Usually, but not always, the total width of the block vertebra is equivalent to the width of two separate vertebrae plus the interspace between.

Differential Diagnosis

It must be distinguished from acquired block vertebrae which may follow trauma or infectious processes.

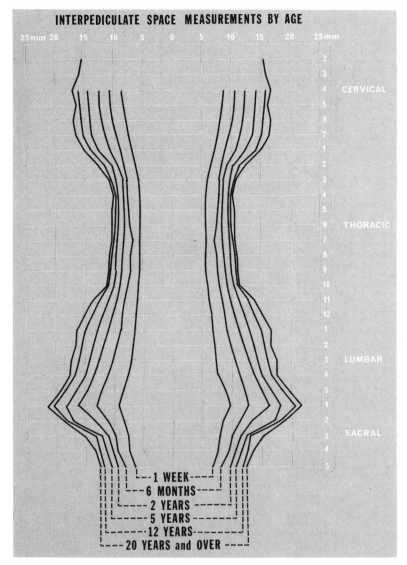

Figure 14–21   Chart for determination of interpedicular distances of the spine.

At times, patients with ankylosing spondylitis may present an appearance simulating synostosis of the vertebrae. Ordinarily, in the acquired forms of synostosis the disk margins, the persistence of interspaces, the evidence of bony overgrowth with paravertebral calcification, and the appearance of the neural arches help differentiate these conditions (Overton and Ghormley).

The Occipital Vertebrae

Anomalies of fusion of the occipital bone and C-1 may result in an extra partially fused vertebral segment between the formed occipital bone and the atlas. This has been called by some the "pro-atlas" (Epstein, 1969; Wollin).

Various deformations of the foramen magnum may occur as the result of the occipital vertebrae. There may be an anterior condyle or lateral paracondyloid and basilar processes. Various accessory bony elements may be fused with the rim of the foramen magnum.

A similar developmental abnormality is seen with achondroplasia.

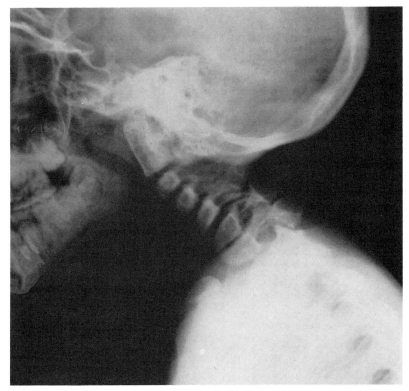

Figure 14–22   Lateral radiograph of the cervical spine in a patient with Klippel-Feil disease.

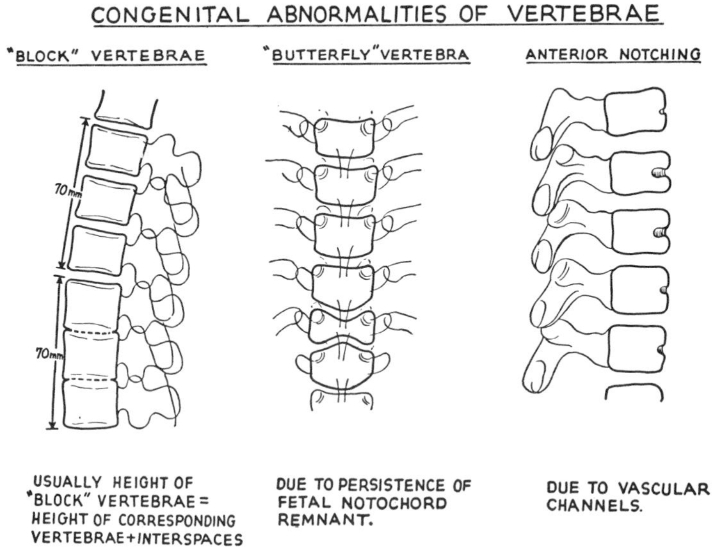

CONGENITAL ABNORMALITIES OF VERTEBRAE

"BLOCK" VERTEBRAE   "BUTTERFLY"VERTEBRA   ANTERIOR NOTCHING

USUALLY HEIGHT OF   DUE TO PERSISTENCE OF   DUE TO VASCULAR
"BLOCK" VERTEBRAE =   FETAL NOTOCHORD   CHANNELS.
HEIGHT OF CORRESPONDING   REMNANT.
VERTEBRAE+INTERSPACES

Figure 14–23   Congenital abnormalities of vertebrae including "block" vertebrae, "butterfly" vertebrae, and anterior notching due to vascular channels.

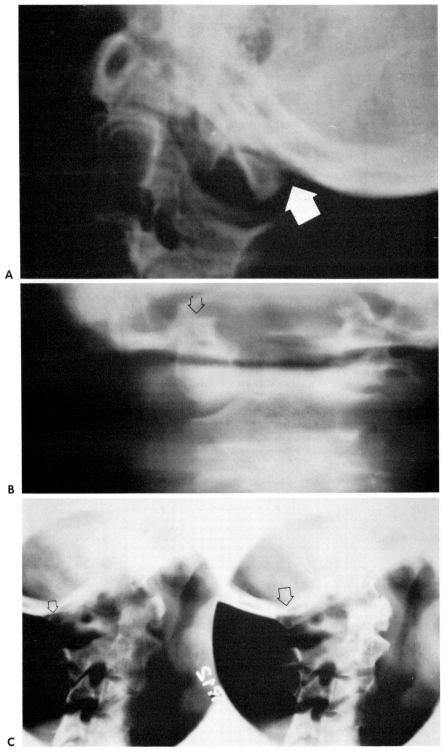

Figure 14–24 *A*. Occipitalization of the atlas in lateral projection. *B*. Tomogram of previous patient demonstrating occipitalization of the atlas by tomography. Note that the fusion is virtually complete on the right side (open arrow) but incomplete on the left side. *C*. Occipitalization of the spinous process of the atlas as demonstrated in the lateral projection.

Unless the space for the cord is compromised or mobility is limited because of articular alterations, such malformations are of little clinical importance.

Atlantoaxial Fusion (Figure 14–24)

In this condition there is an assimilation of the atlas and axis. There may be complete or partial circumferential union of the first cervical vertebrae with the foramen magnum. Instability of the atlas and axis or abnormal mobility of the dens may result.

Malformation of the foramen magnum may be associated with basilar invagination or impression.

The abnormal ranges of movement will require views in flexion and extension or cineradiographic studies for best demonstration. Atlantoaxial fusion may coexist with an occipital vertebra and may be very difficult to differentiate.

Congenital Fusions in the Cervical Spine

The most useful sign is the "wasp-waist" indentation at the site of the absent disk between the congenitally fused vertebral bodies.

Another valuable sign of congenital fusion is the absence of osteophyte formation at the uncovertebral joint (Brown).

Lumbarization and Sacralization (Figure 14–25)

Partial or complete fusion of the fifth lumbar segment with the sacrum may occur, and when partial fusion occurs it may only involve the transverse processes with the lateral masses of the sacrum on one or both sides.

When the fifth lumbar vertebra is completely assimilated in the sacrum it may be called "sacralization"; when the first sacral segment is integrated into the lumbar spine so that there are functionally six lumbar segments the condition is called "lumbarization."

Similar partial or complete fusion may occur at the junction of the sacrum and coccyx.

Supernumerary Ribs

A cervical rib can be identified by its association with the seventh cervical segment. The transverse process of C-7 is directed caudad while the transverse process of T-1 is directed cephalad.

It may be necessary to survey the entire spine to ascertain whether the abnormality is that of a supernumerary rib or a subnormal number of vertebral segments.

ABNORMALITIES OF SHAPE AND SIZE

1. Congenital absence of the dens.
2. Congenital absence of pedicles and articular facets.
3. Clefts in vertebrae
   a. The coronal cleft.
   b. The sagittal cleft.
   c. Cleft spinous processes
      —with meningocele or myelomeningocele.
      —failure of fusion of neural arches in cleidocranial dysostosis.

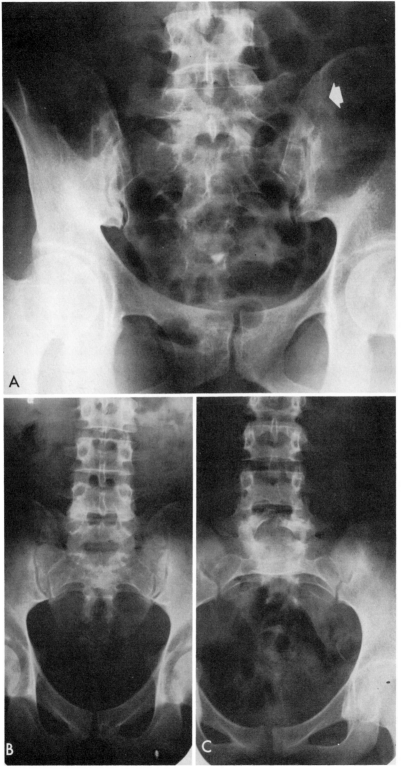

Figure 14–25 Sacralization of the fifth lumbar vertebra and lumbarization of the first sacral segment. *A.* Sacralization of the left lateral transverse process of L-5 vertebral body. *B.* Bilateral sacralization of the transverse process of L-5 vertebral body. *C.* Lumbarization of the first sacral segment, also demonstrating a spina bifida of this segment.

  4. Aberrations related to congenital, endocrine, or metabolic origin.
      a. Morquio's disease.
      b. Hurler's disease.
      c. Achondroplasia.
      d. Osteogenesis imperfecta.
      e. Marfan's syndrome.
      f. Down's syndrome.
      g. Turner's syndrome.
      h. Cushing's syndrome.
      i. Acromegaly.
      j. Hypothyroidism.
  5. Alterations in relation to contiguous vascular disorders
      a. Aortic aneurysm.
      b. Adjoining arterial malformations (vertebral artery erosion).

Abnormalities of Shape and Size

Congenital Absence of the Dens

In this rare anomaly, the odontoid process fails to develop while the lateral masses of the first cervical segment and the body of the second maintain a relatively normal position in respect to one another. Trauma may aggravate the situation and bring this condition to light when radiographs are obtained. Body section radiography may be necessary for final proof (Gwinn and Smith).

It must be differentiated from absence by a destructive process such as tuberculosis (Gwinn and Smith) or metastatic tumor.

Congenital Absence of Pedicles and Articular Facets of Cervical Vertebrae

In most cases the involved area presents an unusually large intervertebral foramen with no other evidence of adjacent bony destruction. There may be other associated anomalies in the adjoining bony structures (Wilson and Norrell).

Clefts in Vertebral Bodies

The Coronal Cleft. This may occur especially in the lower thoracic spine from failure of anterior and posterior ossification centers in the lower thoracic and upper lumbar vertebrae (Epstein, 1969) (Figure 14–26).

The Sagittal Cleft Vertebrae

It appears as a vertical bar in the body of the vertebra in the antero-posterior projection. There usually is concomitant upward or downward pointing of adjoining vertebrae.

The pedicles may be slightly increased in size and the interpedicular distance widened at the involved site.

The neural arch may also be malformed.

In the advanced form, this is referred to as a "butterfly" vertebra (Figure 14–27).

Cleft Spinous Processes

Failure of fusion of the spinous processes is very common, especially in the fifth lumbar and first sacral segments. It may, however, involve the entire length of the sacrum.

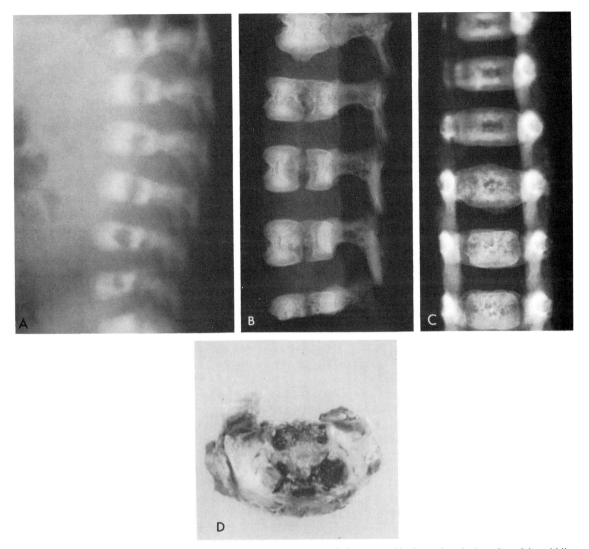

Figure 14–26   *A.* Coronal cleft vertebrae in a premature infant. The clefts are ovoid, situated at the junction of the middle and posterior thirds of the centra. *B.* Specimen roentgenogram, coronal cleft vertebrae, lateral. *C.* AP roentgenogram, same specimen. *D.* Craniad surface of horizontally cut vertebra. Cartilage extends from the coronal cleft to both sides. Centers of ossification are seen in front of and behind the cleft. (From Epstein, B. S.: *The Spine: A Radiologic Text and Atlas,* Philadelphia, Lea & Febiger, 1969.)

Most of these cleft spinous processes are in the midline but they may exist on either side of the midline.

The incidence is highly variable but has been estimated at approximately 16 to 18 per cent in the sacrum (Epstein).

Similar changes have been observed in the lower thoracic, upper lumbar, and in the cervical spinous processes. In the latter, the first, second, and seventh are most frequently involved.

Although usually these are asymptomatic, there may be an associated clue to a more serious neuroanatomic defect if there is a cutaneous manifestation of abnormality, such as a dimple or excessive hair growth. The possibilities may be either (a)

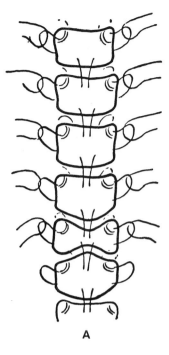

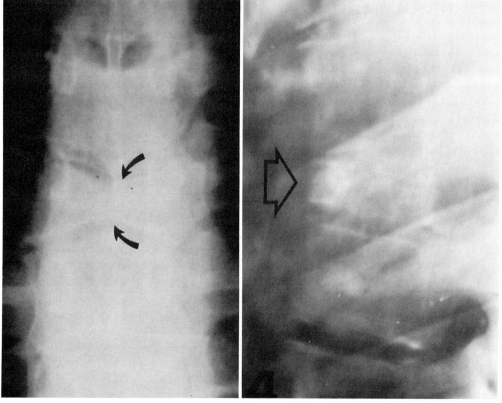

Figure 14-27   *A*. Tracing of a "butterfly vertebra" with compensatory overgrowth of adjoining vertebrae. *B*. Antero-posterior and lateral radiographs of "butterfly vertebra."

a tight filum terminale with a tethering of the conus medullaris, or (b) an associated lesion such as a fibrolipomatous mass or meningocele.

Lipomas of the Cauda Equina (Emery and Lendon).   In a study of one hundred spinal cords from children with neurospinal dysraphia, fibrofatty lesions were found in more than half. Lesions affecting the filum terminale were by far the most prominent. There were six types of fibrofatty masses identified.

It is important to make a clear distinction between a filum fibrolipoma, a dural fibrolipoma, or a leptomyelolipoma. In the first two conditions complete extirpation is practicable with good prognosis. In the third instance damage to the residual cord will probably ensue should extirpation be attempted.

The other rarer types of lipomas are diastematomyelia, hamartoma, heterotopia, and implantation fat. By far the greatest majority of cases involve the filum fibrolipoma which may be intrathecal, extrathecal, or both.

Myelography is usually necessary to demonstrate the latter entities (Figure 14–28).

The concurrence of additional defects with meningocele is quite frequent. These include: lacunar skull, hydrocephalus, the Arnold-Chiari syndrome, multiple congenital defects of the vertebral bodies, congenital dislocation of the hips, malformations of the viscera such as congenital anomaly of the kidneys, and malposition of portions of the gastrointestinal tract and lungs.

The meningocele is most frequent in the lumbosacral region and next most frequent in the region of the upper spine between the cervical spine and skull.

Other unusual varieties of meningocele include: (1) intrathoracic meningocele; (2) anterior sacral meningocele; (3) intrasacral meningoceles, often occult.

Failure of Fusion of the Neural Arches in Cleidocranial Dysostosis (Chapter 7)

In the spine there is often a failure of fusion of the neural arches. The bodies of the vertebrae may occasionally be wedged or biconvex in configuration. The thorax may be slender due to unusual mobility of the shoulders because of the clavicular deficiencies (Salmon).

Aberrations of Congenital, Endocrine, or Metabolic Origin

Spondyloepiphyseal Dysplasia Tarda (Weinfeld et al.).   Flattening of vertebral bodies may be universal in this condition.

Chondro-osteodystrophy (Morquio's disease or syndrome) (See Chapter 7)

Apart from the kyphosis, lumbodorsal beaking, and flattening and widening of the vertebral bodies, the odontoid process of C-2 is hypoplastic or may be absent and the posterior arch of C-1 indents the occipital bone, resulting in a deformity which may be regarded as a form of basilar impression.

The vertebral bodies assume, as growth proceeds, a rectangular shape but their borders retain their irregular curvilinear appearance. The disk spaces are disproportionately wide and the vertebral bodies flattened and rectangular with tonguelike protrusions from the anterior aspects of the vertebrae in the thoracolumbar region. The associated demonstration of corneal opacities, dental defects, and mucopolysaccharides in the urine help in accurate diagnosis. Langer and Carey (1966) have shown that this diagnosis has hitherto often been made inaccurately and may now be made on the basis of the appropriate chemistry in the urine.

Hurler's disease (Dysostosis multiplex; gargoylism) (Chapter 7)

Achondroplasia (Chondrodystrophia fetalis; micromelia) (Chapter 7)

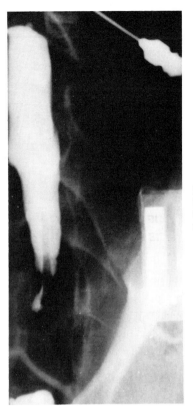

Figure 14–28 Myelograms demonstrating the tethered cord appearance. These may be associated with fibrolipomatous lesions or meningoceles.

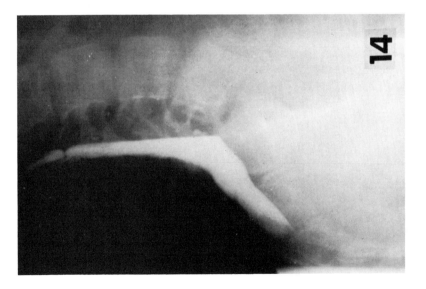

The changes in the spine are seen at birth with marked thinning of the vertebral bodies, wide intervertebral disks, and small linear, tonguelike projections from the anterior aspect of the vertebral bodies.

As growth proceeds, the lumbar lordotic curvature becomes much more marked and the sacrum assumes a horizontal position.

There is a marked diminution in size of the spinal canal with a diminution in interpedicular spaces progressing from lower thoracic to lower lumbar segments. The intervertebral foramina are elongated and narrow.

A kyphosis is usually present at the thoracolumbar junction and the fifth lumbar vertebra is wedged between the iliac bones. Decompressive laminectomies are usually required. The vertebrae at the apex of the kyphosis are wedge-shaped and above and below the kyphosis there is usually an elongated tonguelike projection from the vertebral body.

In *diastrophic dwarfism*, there is also a slight tendency to kyphoscoliosis and numerous osseous developmental anomalies. The vertebrae, however, maintain a fairly normal configuration and the interpedicular spaces and heights of the pedicles remain relatively normal for the most part (Langer). The skull also remains normal with no alteration at its base. This entity may thereby be differentiated from achondroplasia.

Osteogenesis Imperfecta (Chapter 7).   Because of marked softening the vertebrae become compressed and widened with a relative increase in size of the intervertebral disks. The vertebrae may become so compressed that they give the appearance of a thin biconcave lens. Each vertebra will vary in respect to the extent of compression.

Marfan's Syndrome (Arachnodactyly) (Mitoma; McKusick) (Chapter 7).

RADIOGRAPHIC MANIFESTATIONS IN THE SPINE.   The vertebral bodies are elongated and a tall appearance results. The pedicles are elongated also so that the width of the spinal canal is increased, although the interpedicular spaces are normal. The intervertebral disks appear narrowed and the opposing end-plates of the vertebrae appear irregular. Often other congenital defects are present (Nelson).

Down's Syndrome (Mongolism, Trisomy 21 Anomaly) (Chapter 7)

RADIOGRAPHIC MANIFESTATIONS

Spinal radiographic changes are minimal. Scoliosis may be present. A forward displacement of the atlanto-occipital joint together with an abnormally thin and small atlas has been noted (Spitzer et al.).

There is an increase in height of the vertebral bodies, a decrease in their anteroposterior diameters, and a broad concavity of the anterior margin (Rabinowitz and Mosely).

There may also be an increased mobility of the atlas in relation to a possible malformation or aplasia of the transverse ligament (Martel and Tishler).

Turner's Syndrome (Chapter 7)

RADIOGRAPHIC MANIFESTATIONS OF THE SPINE.   Scoliosis; irregularities in the opposing surfaces of the vertebral bodies, osteoporosis, and many associated minor congenital defects involving synostosis of cervical vertebrae; hypoplasia of C-1, and diminution in the size of the posterior arch of C-1 may be present.

The vertebral bodies appear "squared off." The intervertebral disks may be somewhat narrowed posteriorly. Sclerotic changes along the sacroiliac joints are often present (Keats and Burns; Finby and Archibald).

Cushing's Syndrome

GENERAL COMMENT.   This was originally thought by Cushing to be caused by basophilic adenomas of the pituitary gland (Cushing). More recently it has been found to have other causes including various adrenal cortical tumors, tumors of the ovary, the thymus, lungs, pancreas, breast, or thyroid (Eastridge, Hughes and Hamman; Sayle et al.; Hundler; Howland et al.).

PATHOPHYSIOLOGY. There is an abnormal corticosteroid function and the amount of osteoid present in all the bones is markedly diminished. There is an increased adrenal hormone which inhibits protein synthesis, diminishing the production of bone from osteoid.

RADIOGRAPHIC MANIFESTATIONS IN THE SPINE

Because of the severe osteoporosis there is a marked saucerlike indentation of both the superior and inferior end-plates of most of the vertebrae. The vertebrae may be affected variably depending upon pre-existing pressure. Nuclear intrusions into the vertebral bodies may be quite deep.

There is also a sclerotic zone at the end-plates of involved vertebrae representing compacted bony trabeculae in the depressed surfaces of the lumbar vertebrae. It appears that this compact sclerotic zone is related to prior trauma.

Acromegaly (Chapters 7 and 10)

RADIOGRAPHIC CHANGES IN THE SPINAL COLUMN (Erdheim; Waine et al.; Chester and Chester; Albright and Reifenstein; Lang and Bessler). The vertebral bodies tend to be increased in their antero-posterior dimensions with little increase in their height. The intervertebral disks retain their height. There may be prominent lateral and anterior spur formation on the vertebral bodies at the margins of the intervertebral disks.

Vertebral changes with acromegaly are relatively infrequent (Lang and Bessler; Epstein, 1969).

Hypothyroidism

DEFINITION. This condition is caused by a diminished or absent secretion of thyroid hormone.

RADIOGRAPHIC MANIFESTATIONS IN THE SPINE

In children the radiologic changes are caused by the delayed development of the skeletal structure. The vertebral bodies show osteoporosis and irregular ossifica-

DIFFERENCES IN VERTEBRAL EROSION BY:

1. Aneurysm of aorta ⎱ *most often thoracic*
2. Neurofibroma ⎰
3. Chordoma, *most often lumbosacral or at base of skull.*

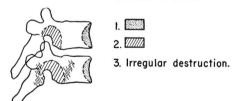

1. ▨
2. ▨
3. Irregular destruction.

Figure 14–29 Diagram demonstrating the differences between the vertebral erosion which occurs in association with tumors of nerve tissue origin and that erosion which occurs with aneurysms of the descending portion of the arch of the aorta or of the thoracic aorta.

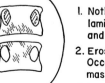

1. Nothing in body but laminated calcified clot and aneurysm are seen.
2. Erosion of pedicles Occasionally soft tissue mass — not calcified.
3. Irregular destruction.

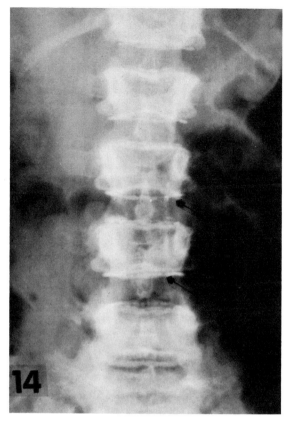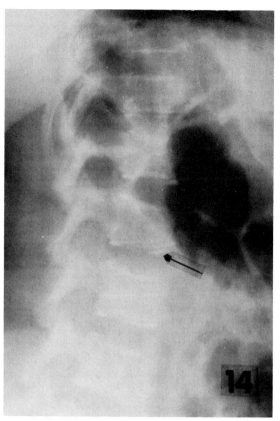

Figure 14–30   Antero-posterior and lateral views of the spine in a 33 year old cretin female with a bone age of 10. Note the fragmentation and dense sclerosis of the secondary ossification centers of the endplates of these vertebral bodies.

tion of the various centers within the vertebral bodies. Kyphosis at L-1 and L-2 similar to that noted in Hurler's disease may occur.

At times the involved vertebral bodies have a steplike wedging anteriorly and posteriorly (Caffey, 1967). At times a lumbar vertebral body may be hypoplastic, this in itself producing a kyphosis (cuneiform first lumbar).

Irregular ossification of the epiphyseal end-plates of the vertebral bodies is often present. Generally, the vertebrae tend to be flattened (platyspondyly) with increased intervertebral spaces (Figure 14–30). The secondary ossification centers appear fragmented and "stippled," and fuse very late, if at all, to the primary centers.

There may be dense zones at the upper and lower surfaces of the vertebral bodies.

There may also be partial absence of vertebral bodies causing hemivertebrae, abnormal segmentation of the ribs and abnormal rib-vertebral articulations (Lintermans and Seyhnaeve).

Alterations in Size and Shape of Vertebral Bodies in Relation to Contiguous Vascular Disorders

Aortic Aneurysms.   Aneurysms of the descending thoracic aorta produce erosive changes on the anterolateral aspects of the vertebrae, contiguous with the aneurysm because of the pulsatile and compressive trauma produced by the aneurysm (Figure 14–29). The intervertebral disks, being avascular, are resistant to these erosive changes.

Erosive Changes in the Vertebral Bodies or Arches from Adjoining Arterial Disease of Other Origin, for example, Vertebral Artery. Aneurysms of the vertebral artery can be of sufficient size to produce bone erosion. Usually this will require body section radiography for most accurate demonstration.

Abnormalities of Radiodensity and Architecture

1. Homogeneously lucent
    a. Osteogenesis imperfecta
    b. Hypophosphatasia
    c. Primary hyperparathyroidism
    d. Cushing's syndrome
    e. Osteoporosis
    f. Osteomalacia
    g. Rickets (hypovitaminosis D)
    h. Multiple myeloma
    i. Ewing's sarcoma (Occasionally, entire spine, but usually localized)
    j. Sickle cell anemia
    k. Thalassemia
2. Homogeneously sclerotic
    a. Osteopetrosis
    b. Ivory vertebrae
    c. Fluoride poisoning
    d. Myelosclerotic anemia
    e. Urticaria pigmentosa (mastocytosis)
    f. Idiopathic hypercalcemia of infancy
    g. Acquired hemolytic anemia
    h. Lymphoma
3. Spotted lucency
    a. Osteomyelitis
            Syphilitic
            Pyogenic
            Fungal
    b. Metastatic neoplasia and multiple myeloma
    c. Chordomas
    d. Sacrococcygeal teratoma
    e. Giant cell tumor
    f. Benign chondroblastoma
    g. Aneurysmal bone cyst
    h. Cystic angiomatosis
    i. Benign osteoblastoma (giant osteoid osteoma)
    j. Vertebral epiphysitis (Scheuermann's disease)
    k. Traumatic changes in the spine—Special considerations in each region of the spine.
    l. Spondylolysis; spondylolisthesis; pseudospondylolisthesis; reverse spondylolisthesis
    m. Reticuloendothelioses, such as eosinophilic granuloma.
4. Spotted sclerosis
    a. Osteopoikilosis
    b. Congenital stippled epiphysis

   c. Tuberous sclerosis
   d. Sclerotic bone islands
   e. Neoplastic metastatic disease
   f. Spinal lymphomas
   g. Osteoid osteoma
   h. Urticaria pigmentosa (mastocytosis)
5. Vertical irregular lucency and sclerosis
   a. Hemangioma
   b. Osteopathia striata (Voorhoeve's disease)
6. Boxlike sclerosis
   a. Paget's disease (osteitis deformans)
   b. Idiopathic hypercalcemia of infancy
7. Indiscriminate lucency and sclerosis
   a. Fibrous dysplasia
   b. Metastatic neoplasia:
        Malignant lymphomas
   c. Radiation effects on vertebrae
8. Spur formations with or without paraspinous ligamentous calcification
   a. Spondylosis deformans
   b. Syphilitic spondylitis
   c. Rheumatoid spondylitis
   d. Ankylosing spondylitis
   e. Ochronosis

Introduction.   Abnormalities of radiodensity and architecture may be further subdivided into the following eight groups (Figure 14–31):

1. Homogeneously lucent.
2. Homogeneously sclerotic.
3. Spotted radiolucency.
4. Spotted radiosclerosis.
5. A tendency to vertical or lacelike lucency or sclerosis.
6. A tendency to "picture framing" or boxlike sclerosis.
7. An indiscriminate alteration of the radiodensity or architecture.
8. The appearance of spurs with or without bony bridging or paraspinous ligament calcification.

When disease entities occur in each of these categories which have been described previously they will be mentioned by name only and occasionally illustrated. Specific abnormalities in relation to the spine will be described.

THE HOMOGENEOUSLY LUCENT ALTERATIONS

Osteogenesis Imperfecta (Chapter 7)

Hypophosphatasia (Chapter 7)

Radiographic Findings in the Vertebral Column.   The failure of ossification is paramount with delayed and irregular bone formation and occasionally dorsolumbar angulation (Currarino et al.)

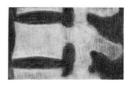

NORMAL

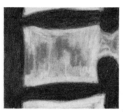

OSTEOPOROSIS WITHOUT
LOSS OF SHAPE

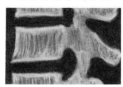

OSTEOPOROSIS WITH
BICONCAVE SHAPE,
OSTEOMALACIA,
HYPERPARATHYROIDISM,
CUSHING'S DISEASE

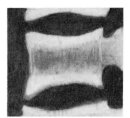

RUGGER JERSEY
APPEARANCE

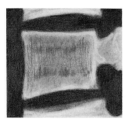

SPOTTED BLACK LYTIC
METASTASES FROM
CARCINOMA

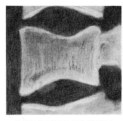

HEMANGIOMA VERTICAL
LUCENCY AND SCLEROSIS

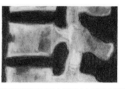

INDISCRIMINATE LUCENCY
AND SCLEROSIS, METASTASES

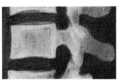

NORMAL

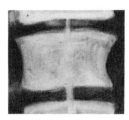

DIFFUSELY WHITE
OSTEOPETROSIS
(MARBLE BONE DISEASE)

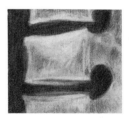

SPOTTED WHITE
(MALIGNANT LYMPHOMA)

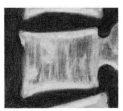

STREAKY WHITE AND
SPOTTED (METASTASIS
FROM CARCINOMA OF
PROSTATE)

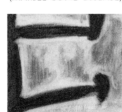

BOXLIKE SCLEROSIS
(PAGET'S DISEASE)

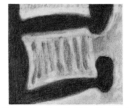

COARSENED TRABECULATION
AND SLIGHT EXPANSION
(FIBROUS DYSPLASIA)

Figure 14–31   General categories of roentgen changes in the architecture of vertebrae.

Figure 14–31 continued on opposite page.

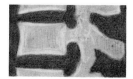

NORMAL

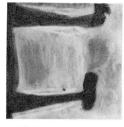

INCREASE HEIGHT
(ACROMEGALY)

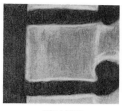

SQUARED
(TURNER'S SYNDROME)

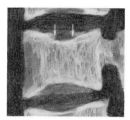

STEP-LIKE INDENTATION
END PLATES
(SICKLE CELL ANEMIA)

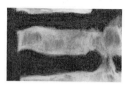

FLATTENED OSTEO-
CHONDRODYSTROPHY

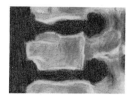

PERSISTANT EPIPHYSIS
INCREASED INTERSPACES
(CRETINISM
HYPOTHYROIDISM)

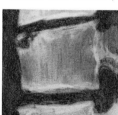

EPIPHYSITIS
SCHEUERMANN'S DISEASE

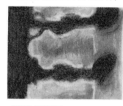

EPIPHYSITIS ADVANCED
WEDGED AND
UNDULATING END-PLATES
(ADVANCED
SCHEUERMANN'S DISEASE)

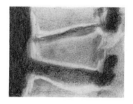

VERTEBRA PLANA
RETICULOENDOTHELIOSIS
EOSINOPHILIC GRANULOMA

Figure 14–31   (*Continued*).

Primary Hyperparathyroidism

Radiographic Changes in the Spine

Severe osteoporosis.

The vertebral bodies may collapse in a uniform fashion so that the normal height is reduced but the articular surfaces may be smooth.

There may be a biconcave appearance of the vertebral bodies due to protrusion of intervertebral disks into the vertebral bodies.

The vertebral body bony structure may have a reticular weblike alteration.

There may be marked decalcification of the sacrum adjoining the sacroiliac joints to the point of almost complete obliteration of these joints.

There may be some sclerotic foci within the osteoporotic vertebrae.

There may be erosion of the spinous and articular processes so that they appear to be more pointed than normal.

Osteosclerotic banded changes of the upper and lower aspects of the vertebral body have been reported (Crawford), but this also occurs in patients with uremia and secondary hypoparathyroidism of renal origin. This has been referred to as the "rugger jersey sign" (Figure 14–32). This also occurs in idiopathic hypercalcemia in infancy and osteopetrosis in adults.

Vertebral chondrocalcinosis may occur, especially in the cervical and lumbar regions in the vicinity of the synovial joints (Zitnan and Sit'aj).

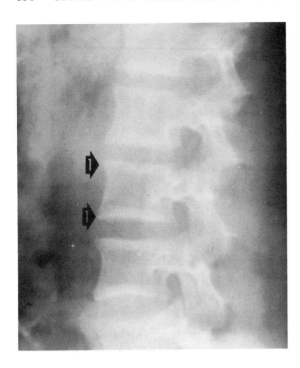

Figure 14-32 The "rugger jersey" pattern of the spine in a patient with Fanconi pancytopenia.

Cushing's Syndrome (has been previously described)

Osteoporosis

Radiographic Manifestations in the Spine.   The changes in the vertebral bodies may bear a close resemblance to those associated with hyperparathyroidism, osteomalacia, multiple myeloma, and other described radiolucent disorders.

Osteomalacia

Definition.   A disorder of bone in which there are abnormal amounts of osteoid with insufficient calcification produced by any condition which may deplete the body's calcium stores sufficiently. Albright and Reifenstein (1948) proposed four categories of the disorder: (1) with normal phosphatase; (2) with high phosphatase; (3) Milkman's syndrome; (4) advanced osteomalacia. The severity, therefore, depends on the relationship between serum phosphorus and serum calcium content.

Radiographic Manifestations in the Spine

Marked hyperlucency of the entire vertebral column, coupled with the formation of a heart-shaped pelvis and angulations under stress of the hips, ribs, and long bones.

Usually no callus formation is observed.

Pseudofractures or pathologic fractures are likely to occur (Milkman's syndrome).

As the disease progresses, biconcave vertebrae and markedly enlarged and biconvex intervertebral disks are noted.

Rickets (Vitamin D Deficiency) (Chapter 8)

Radiographic Manifestations in the Spine

Radiographic manifestations are similar to those observed in osteomalacia.

The softening of the bone may produce basilar impression and platybasia of the base of the skull (Hurwitz and Shepherd).

There may be an osteoid proliferation around areas of compression in the vertebral segments or neural arch.

Multiple Myeloma (Plasma Cell Myeloma) (Chapter 8)

Radiographic Manifestations in the Spine

The common change is that seen in osteoporosis.

Compression fractures are common, with wedging of the vertebrae in some instances and flattening in others, sometimes involving the pedicles and neural arches.

A paravertebral soft tissue mass may become apparent as the tumor grows outside the spine into the adjoining tissues.

There may be a single locus for some time in the sacrum and initially **in the sacrum this may appear as an expanding rarefied lesion with no specific marginal demarcation.**

Bone sclerosis as the predominating change is infrequent but does occur (Langley, Sabean, and Sorger).

Blockage of the spinal canal may occur as a result either of the plasma cell tumor per se or para-amyloid deposit.

Endothelioma of Bone (Ewing's Sarcoma) (Chapter 9)

Radiologic Aspects of Spinal Involvement

When the vertebrae are involved, the marrow space is extensively infiltrated and there is ordinarily extension of the tumor under the paraspinous ligaments and into the epidural space, giving rise to a paraspinal soft tissue mass.

Involvement may occur in one or more vertebrae or may involve virtually the entire spine and other bones of the body.

Basically, the lesion is destructive of bone most often in the long bones of the pelvis, but it can occur in any area in which marrow is found initially.

Sickle Cell Anemia

Radiographic Manifestations

Diffuse osteoporosis and slight widening of the intervertebral disks.

The vertebral bodies may become flattened and osteosclerotic foci may be visible interwoven with the zones of lucency, imparting a weblike or lacelike appearance.

The adjoining end-plates may take on a squared appearance at the sites where the nuclei pulposi protrude into the end-plates (Figure 14–33).

The changes in the vertebrae vary with the stages of the disease and the extent of reparative effort which has occurred. The vertebral bodies may assume a biconcave appearance together with patchy sclerotic areas.

The lucency surrounding the exit orifice of the anterior vertebral vein occasionally becomes very prominent because of loss of adjacent bone.

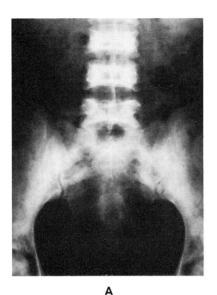 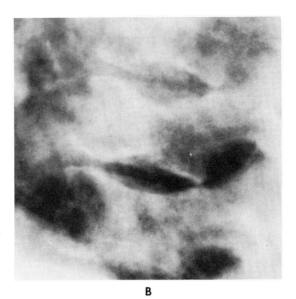

A   **B**

Figure 14–33 Spine in sickle cell anemia. *A*. Antero-posterior view of the lumbar spine and pelvis demonstrating the coarse trabecular pattern with interspersed lucency. *B*. Close-up view of the lower thoracic vertebrae in lateral projection demonstrating the squared indentations of the endplates often found in this condition. This is thought to be due to bone infarction at the site of indentations of the nucleus pulposus. It is not pathognomonic, however.

Thalassemia

Radiologic Changes in the Spine, Similar to Sickle Cell Anemia

HOMOGENEOUSLY SCLEROTIC

Osteopetrosis (Marble Bone Disease, Albers-Schonberg's Disease)

Radiographic Appearances of the Spine (Figure 14–34).

The configuration of the vertebrae is relatively normal except for a tendency to (a) rounding of the margins; (b) deepened indentations for the anterior and posterior veins.

The neural arch inclusive of spinous and transverse processes is also increased and densely sclerotic.

There is a marked tendency for the upper and lower end-plates to become densely sclerotic with a lesser zone of sclerosis or lucency between them, giving the vertebral bodies a "sandwiched" appearance.

At times the vertebral bodies become uniformly dense.

"Ivory Vertebrae"

Radiographic Manifestations. Dense, sclerotic vertebral body which may be isolated and separate from an otherwise relatively normal looking spine. This may resemble closely the findings in such diseases as Hodgkins' disease, Paget's disease, osteosclerotic metastases, and carcinomatous foci which have undergone treatment by chemotherapy or hormones (Ochsner and Moser).

Fluoride Poisoning

Radiographic Appearances. The vertebrae may be relatively normal in size and shape or slightly enlarged with considerable increase in density and calcification of the paraspinal ligaments, particularly the ligamenta flava, the intertransverse and the interspinous ligaments. Osteophytes are also observed in various muscle attach-

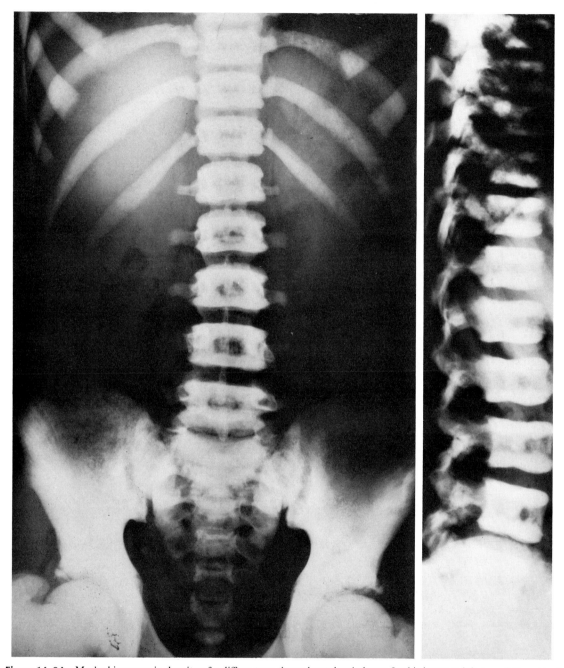

Figure 14–34   Marked increase in density of a diffuse type throughout the skeleton. In this instance it is especially evident in the lumbar spine and pelvis. The upper and lower thirds of the vertebral bodi s are especially sclerotic, imparting a striped appearance. In this instance there were stress fractures of the third and fourth lumbar neural arches that emphasized the fragile nature of this dense bone. Modeling abnormalities of the ribs are present. Neural arch fractures in this condition are not unusual. (Courtesy of Murray, R. O. and Jacobson, H. G.: *The Radiology of Skeletal Disorders.* Baltimore, Williams and Wilkins Co., 1971.)

ments. There is marked increase in density, thickened trabeculae, and narrowing of the marrow cavity.

Myelosclerotic Anemia

General Comments. This is an atypical form probably of myelogenous leukemia or a megakaryocytic leukemia in the bone marrow or other organs. It is characterized by generalized fibrosis of the bone marrow with excessive proliferation of endosteal bone (Epstein, 1969). There is usually a compensatory hyperplasia in the hematopoietic tissues outside the red marrow, such as that in the liver, spleen, and even in the ovaries, adrenals, mediastinum, and retroperitoneal regions (Lowman et al.).

Radiographic Appearances in the Spine

Confluent areas of increased density throughout the spongiosa of the thoracic and lumbar vertebrae, less frequently seen in cervical vertebrae.

The configuration of the vertebrae and the disks remains normal.

Sometimes the appearance is splotchy rather than diffuse.

Osteosclerosis in this condition must be differentiated from that which occurs with metastatic prostatic carcinoma, widespread metastases from carcinoma of the breast, or chronic myelogenous leukemia. It must especially be distinguished from the endosteal sclerosis which results after treatment by hormones or chemotherapy in metastatic disease.

Urticaria Pigmentosa (Mastocytosis)

Definition. This disease is a proliferative disorder of the mast cells affecting the reticuloendothelial system especially, but widely disseminated throughout the body, including the skin. The appearance suggests a mast-cell leukemia.

Radiographic Manifestations in the Spine

The bone lesions are characterized by resorption and proliferation intermixed.

The vertebrae retain their normal contours and configurations with thin cortical margins.

Although there are interspersed lytic lesions, the predominate manifestation is that of either a speckled sclerotic or diffusely sclerotic appearance.

Idiopathic Hypercalcemia of Infancy

Definition. In infancy, a state of abnormal sensitivity to vitamin D in the presence of a milk diet, resulting in excessive absorption of calcium from the gastrointestinal tract. This, in turn, is responsible for hypercalcemia, renal calcinosis, acidosis, and failure to thrive.

Radiologic Manifestations

Extensive osteosclerosis.

Defective ossification.

Widespread soft tissue calcifications.

The sclerotic changes in the long bones occur at their growing ends with "flaring" and osteosclerotic transverse lines. The bones are soft and bowed and the epiphyseal ends appear invaginated.

The vertebrae are also osteosclerotic but appear "framelike" with a relative central radiolucency. The vertebral bodies appear small.

Acquired Hemolytic Anemia (Chapter 8)

Lymphoma (Chapter 10)

SPOTTED RADIOLUCENCY

Osteomyelitis (spondylitis of infectious origin)

Classification.   There are many etiologic agents involved:
Pyogens.
Brucellosis.
Typhoid.
Tuberculosis.
Syphilis.
Fungus, protozoan, or parasitic infestation including blastomycosis, coccidioi-
domycosis, hydatid disease, and toxoplasmosis.
Radiologic Manifestations in the Spine (Figure 14–35).

RADIOLOGIC MANIFESTATIONS OF PYOGENIC AND TUBERCULOUS OSTEOMYELITIS OF THE SPINE

Nontuberculous	*Tuberculous*
1. Time lag: four to eight weeks	As much as six months
2. Earliest involvement: near end-plates	Same
3. Alteration in intervertebral disks: early	Same
4. Paravertebral soft tissue swelling: present	Present
5. Tendency to spread along soft tissue planes: absent	Present
6. Tendency to self-containment by zone of reaction: present	Absent
7. Collapse of involved vertebrae: present	Present
8. Destruction of intervertebral space: present	Present

9. Bony regeneration: rapid (four to six weeks)
    Typhoid   slow
    Syphilis   slow
	Delayed (many months)

10. Healing: dense sclerotic vertebrae are present	Not apt to form
11. Obliteration of intervertebral space: present	Present

Special Comment about Syphilitic Spondylitis (Freedman and Meschan).   Syphilis
of the spine is particularly apt to involve the lumbar and cervical regions. The bone is
destroyed and large bony bridges extend around the involved vertebrae. The foci of

DUE TO
<u>INFECTION</u>

1. TUBERCULOSIS

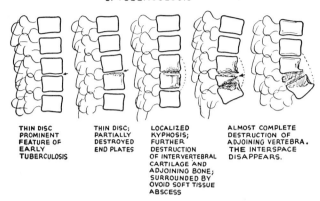

THIN DISC
PROMINENT
FEATURE OF
EARLY
TUBERCULOSIS

THIN DISC;
PARTIALLY
DESTROYED
END PLATES

LOCALIZED
KYPHOSIS;
FURTHER
DESTRUCTION
OF INTERVERTEBRAL
CARTILAGE AND
ADJOINING BONE;
SURROUNDED BY
OVOID SOFT TISSUE
ABSCESS

ALMOST COMPLETE
DESTRUCTION OF
ADJOINING VERTEBRA.
THE INTERSPACE
DISAPPEARS.

2. PYOGENIC

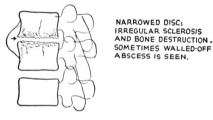

NARROWED DISC;
IRREGULAR SCLEROSIS
AND BONE DESTRUCTION.
SOMETIMES WALLED-OFF
ABSCESS IS SEEN.

<u>NEOPLASTIC</u>

IRREGULAR SCLEROSIS
AND OSTEOPOROSIS
(PARTICULARLY IN LYMPHOMAS)

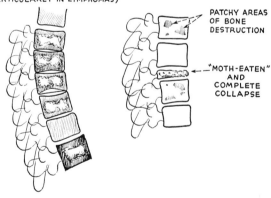

PATCHY AREAS
OF BONE
DESTRUCTION

"MOTH-EATEN"
AND
COMPLETE
COLLAPSE

<u>DUE TO METASTATIC NEOPLASM</u>

1. OBLITERATION OF VERTEBRAL STRUCTURAL DETAIL.

2. NO EXTENSION OF VERTEBRAL SUBSTANCE BEYOND
   COLUMN, BUT NEOPLASM MAY EXTEND.

3. DENSITY DECREASED - OCCASIONALLY SCLEROTIC.

4. NO DIVERGING SPINOUS PROCESS.

5. HOMOGENEOUS SCLEROSIS PARTICULARLY IN
   METASTATIC CARCINOMA OF PROSTATE.

A

Figure 14–35   *A*. The various types of wedged vertebral bodies.

Figure 14–35 continued on opposite page.

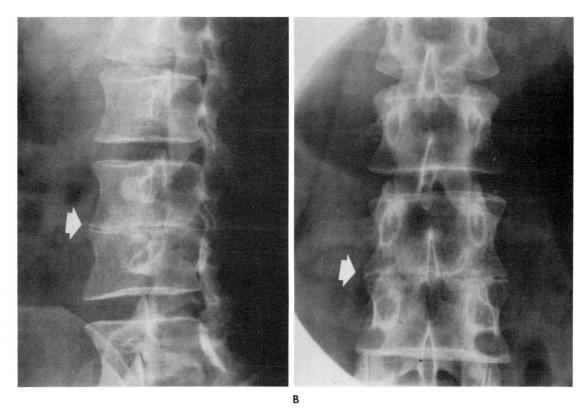

B

Figure 14–35 (*Continued*).   *B*. Paratyphoid spondylitis in a patient many years after the active disease process. *Left.* A-P projection. *Right.* Oblique projection. (Courtesy of Harold Landsman, M.D.)

DIFFERENTIATION BETWEEN PYOGENIC AND TUBERCULOUS SPONDYLITIS
AFFECTING VERTEBRAE

Tuberculous Spondylitis	Pyogenic Spondylitis
No osteoblastic response	Marked osteoblastic response
Large paravertebral abscess	Small or no paravertebral abscess
Marked rarefaction	Less rarefaction
Slow course	More rapid course
Marked destruction and collapse	Less destruction and collapse
	Arch involvement is more common in the nontuberculous group

C

Figure 14–35 (*Continued*).   *C*. Radiologic manifestations of tuberculous and pyogenic spondylitis. (From Richards, A. J.: J. Canad. Ass. Radiol., *11*:45–49, 1960.)

destruction tend, however, to be quite irregular, although greater resistance of the intervertebral disks has been noted. The process is apt to extend over all the lumbar vertebrae and many of the cervical vertebrae, producing a profound proliferation of spur formation and bony bridging. Calcification may involve the paraspinal ligaments. This process should be differentiated from the Charcot arthropathy which represents a true neuropathic process and not an involvement by an infectious agent such as the spirochete.

Metastatic Neoplastic Diseases and Multiple Myeloma

Multiple myeloma has been previously considered under the more homogeneous lucencies, but it may also have a spotted lucent appearance as well. Lucency and sclerosis may exist in the vertebral column simultaneously with metastatic neoplastic disease.

Common Sites of Origin are the breast, kidney, lung, thyroid, gastrointestinal tract, pancreas, and melanoma. (Sclerotic metastases are particularly apt to occur from prostatic carcinoma, lymphomas, and leukemias.)

Radiologic Manifestations

Small and large areas of bone destruction or interspersed foci of bony proliferation with no visible disturbance in the contour or size of the vertebra unless pathologic fracture supervenes. There is ordinarily no involvement of the intervertebral disks and no new bone formation across the interspace as in the case of the infectious spondylitides.

Vertebral metastases are frequently multiple and scattered with some vertebrae less involved or uninvolved.

Occasionally epidural metastases are encountered without associated bone destruction.

Great assistance in diagnosis is offered by spinal radioisotopic scans which may reveal (in 25 to 30 per cent of cases) bony metastases before they become manifest radiographically—recalling, however, that positive scans can also appear in other entities besides tumor metastases.

Chordomas

General Comment. These are tumors originating from remnants of the notochord and occurring mostly at the cephalic and caudal ends of the vertebral column, destroying the adjoining bone. The relative incidence in different areas varies in different series (Dahlin and MacCarty; Faust, Gilmore, and Mudgett).

Radiologic Manifestations

Predominantly bone destructive, although they may produce nerve pressure prior to detectable bone invasion and destruction.

Soft tissue swelling anteriorly into the nasopharynx occurs early.

Calcification is occasionally present in the soft tissue extravertebral tumor.

In the sacrum, expansion is often observed in the lateral projection. The sacrum, however, is slowly destroyed by the chordoma which extends to the adjoining soft tissues, producing a detectable mass. Remnants of calcification may be observed within the destroyed sacrum.

Sacrococcygeal Teratoma

General Comment. These are tumors appearing at birth as congenital malformations and usually arising from the dorsal aspect of the sacrum; they may become malignant. Congenital malformations elsewhere are frequently associated. The tumor is usually situated between the rectum and the sacrum, displacing these structures.

Radiographic Manifestations

The tumors are large, causing considerable displacement of the bladder and rectum with lesser destruction or none at all of the adjoining sacrum. The tumor is situated between the rectum and sacrum ordinarily, displacing the rectum markedly.

There may be calcification within the tumor, unlike other destructive lesions occurring in this region.

These tumors are manifest earlier in life than are chordomas. Eklöf (1965) has indicated that destruction of the sacrum and coccyx or aplasia of more than two distal sacral segments is unfavorable to the diagnosis of teratoma, a condition to be considered in the differential diagnosis.

Giant Cell Tumor, Benign Chondroblastoma, Aneurysmal Bone Cysts of the Vertebrae

Giant cell tumors, benign chondroblastomas, and aneurysmal bone cysts are different tumor entities that may produce rather similar radiographic changes within vertebral bodies and are difficult to distinguish without biopsy.

Radiographic Manifestations

These tumors may affect the vertebral bodies or the neural arches alone or in combination.

They are characterized by a rather sharply outlined area of bone destruction, an absence of adjacent bone reaction, and intact adjacent intervertebral disks usually.

In the presence of a collapsed vertebral body, however, a paravertebral swelling may occur which makes differentiation difficult.

Stippled calcific densities may be present within the benign chondroblastoma and strandlike appearances may occur with either the giant cell tumor or the aneurysmal bone cyst. The strandlike appearance may, on occasion, appear weblike.

Cystic Angiomatosis of Bone.   These are round or cystlike areas involving any bones but in the vertebrae they tend to occur without striations or honeycomb appearance and are ordinarily blood-filled or filled with a clear fluid (in which case they may be designated as lymphangiectases of bone).

Benign Osteoblastoma (Giant Osteoid Osteoma) (Figure 14–36)

General Comment.   This tumor resembles the osteoid osteoma histologically but is different radiologically. In the osteoblastoma, the so-called nidus is virtually the entire tumor, measuring up to one or two cm. in diameter. It is a vascular lesion producing resorptive changes in the bone.

Radiographic Appearances

Benign osteoblastomas have a predilection for the neural arches and pedicles of vertebrae and may cause extradural compression.

The tumor also occurs in the tubular bones, including those of the hands and feet where they may be eccentric in position.

A

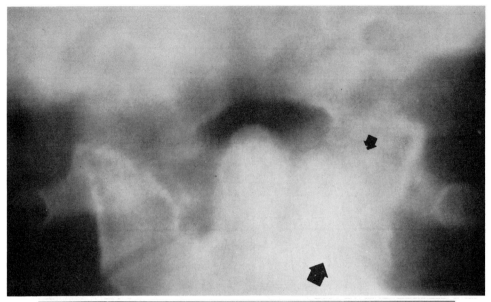

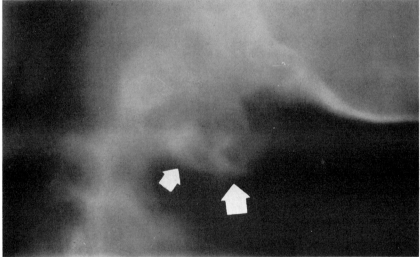

B

Figure 14–36 Giant osteoid osteoma. *A.* Tomogram in antero-posterior view showing the lateral mass of C-1 involved by the giant osteoid osteoma or osteoblastoma. *B.* Tomogram in the lateral view of this patient.

The nidus is ill-defined, expansile, and the lesion is predominantly lytic.

At times a stippled deposition of bone within the tumor is present, resembling an enchondroma.

Vertebral Epiphysitis (Juvenile Kyphosis Dorsalis; Scheuermann's Disease) (Figure 14–37)

General Comment. This is most likely caused by an inborn weakness or developmental error which produces fissures in the cartilaginous end-plates. There is, as a result, a prolapse of nuclear material into the spongiosa of the adjoining vertebral bodies. Defective growth follows (Beadle).

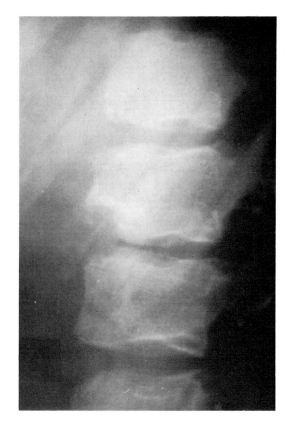

Figure 14–37 Vertebral epiphysitis. Lateral view demonstrating the fragmentation and steplike appearance of the secondary centers of ossification occasionally found in lower thoracic and lumbar vertebrae in this condition. This is thought to be a variation of Scheuermann's disease.

Radiological Appearance

In the early stage only a slight irregularity of the vertebral end-plates may be found or there may be a circumscribed zone of diminished density immediately beneath the anterior superior margin of the vertebral bodies (Figure 14–37 A).

As the disease progresses the marginal irregularity becomes greater and the adjoining vertebral body appears decalcified.

The intervertebral disks themselves become narrowed because of the nuclear extrusions into the involved vertebral bodies.

Late in the disease process, degenerative changes are superimposed with lipping and spur formation on involved vertebrae.

Although the posterior heights of the vertebral bodies are maintained, the anterior measurements become narrowed and kyphosis supervenes. Scoliosis may be observed more rarely.

Traumatic Changes in the Spine

Radiographic Appearances (Figure 14–38)

The fresh vertebral fracture is ordinarily recognized by either a loss of continuity in the substance of the neural arch or its processes, or a break in the trabecular continuity of a vertebral body. In the vertebral body, there may be a steplike appearance in silhouette on the anterior or lateral margin and an anterior or lateral narrowness (wedging).

There may be a compaction of the bone yielding a faint zone of sclerosis.

<u>DUE TO ISCHEMIC NECROSIS</u>

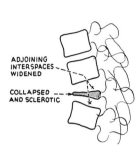

ADJOINING
INTERSPACES
WIDENED

COLLAPSED
AND SCLEROTIC

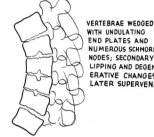

VERTEBRAE WEDGED
WITH UNDULATING
END PLATES AND
NUMEROUS SCHMORL'S
NODES; SECONDARY
LIPPING AND DEGEN-
ERATIVE CHANGES
LATER SUPERVENE

1. CALVE'S VERTEBRA PLANA.
AFFECTS PRIMARY OSSIFICATION
CENTER OF VERTEBRAL BODY
IN CHILDREN 2 TO 15 YEARS OF
AGE.

2. SCHEUERMANN'S DISEASE
(JUVENILE KYPHOSIS; KYPHOSIS
DORSALIS JUVENILIS;
OSTEOCHONDROSIS.)

<u>METABOLIC</u>

BICONCAVE APPEARANCE OF "FISH VERTEBRA"
*(OSTEOMALACIA; SENILE AND JUVENILE OSTEOPOROSIS; BLOOD
DYSCRASIAS; HYPERPARATHYROIDISM)*

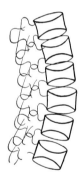

END PLATES OF VERTEBRAE
ARE BICONCAVE AND BODIES
ARE NARROWED IN MIDSECTION;
BONY TEXTURE RADIOLUCENT
WITH OCCASIONAL RELATIVE
SCLEROSIS OF PERIPHERY.

<u>CONGENITAL METABOLIC</u>
LIPOCHONDRODYSTROPHY

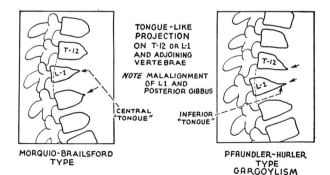

T-12

L-1

CENTRAL
"TONGUE"

TONGUE-LIKE
PROJECTION
ON T-12 OR L-1
AND ADJOINING
VERTEBRAE

NOTE MALALIGNMENT
OF L1 AND
POSTERIOR GIBBUS

T-12

L-1

INFERIOR
"TONGUE"

MORQUIO-BRAILSFORD
TYPE

PFAUNDLER-HURLER
TYPE
GARGOYLISM

Figure 14–38 The various types of wedged vertebral bodies.

Figure 14–38 continued on opposite page.

Shortly after initial injury, a resorption of bone along the fracture line occurs with a moderate amount of callus deposition.

The neural arches and processes tend to have more callus than the vertebral bodies themselves. A callus may give the fracture margin a very minimal sclerotic appearance.

Ultimately only the wedging or the deformity of the process remains as evidence of the injury.

Degenerative paraspinous ligamentous calcification surrounding the fracture site may also occur.

An injured intervertebral disk diminishes in height since it actually loses substance as a result of extrusion of the nucleus pulposus into the vertebral

CONGENITAL

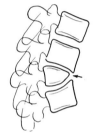
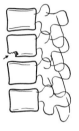

A. HEMIVERTEBRA

1. *ALL BONES APPEAR HEALTHY.*
2. *ANTERIOR HALF OF VERTEBRA IS ABSENT, NOT COMPRESSED.*
3. *ADJACENT VERTEBRAE ARE EXPANDED TO FIT DEFORMITY.*
4. *NO BULGING ANTERIORLY.*
5. *OTHER DEVELOPMENTAL ABNORMALITIES (RIB) MAY BE PRESENT.*
6. *INTERSPACES ARE WELL PRESERVED.*

B. DUE TO PERSISTENT ANTERIOR SCHMORL'S NODE (RARE)

1. *INFERIOR SURFACE AFFECTED USUALLY.*
2. *NO BULGING ANTERIORLY.*
3. *SHARPLY DEMARCATED END PLATE DEFECT.*
4. *INTERSPACES WELL PRESERVED.*

TRAUMATIC

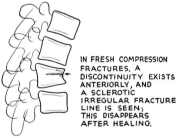
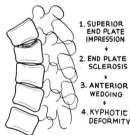

IN FRESH COMPRESSION FRACTURES, A DISCONTINUITY EXISTS ANTERIORLY, AND A SCLEROTIC IRREGULAR FRACTURE LINE IS SEEN; THIS DISAPPEARS AFTER HEALING.

1. SUPERIOR END PLATE IMPRESSION
↓
2. END PLATE SCLEROSIS
↓
3. ANTERIOR WEDGING
↓
4. KYPHOTIC DEFORMITY

A. COMPRESSION FRACTURE

1. *NONCONVULSIVE FRACTURES – LOCATIONS:*
   a. LOWER ½ OF CERVICAL SPINE.
   b. LOWER ½ OF THORACIC SPINE.
   c. ANYWHERE IN LUMBAR SPINE

2. *CONVULSIVE FRACTURES, USUALLY IN T3, T4, T5, T6.*

Figure 14–38 (*Continued*).   The various types of wedged vertebral bodies

Figure 14–38 continued on following page.

DUE TO
INFECTION

1. TUBERCULOSIS

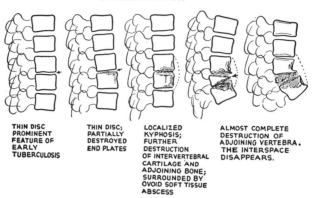

THIN DISC
PROMINENT
FEATURE OF
EARLY
TUBERCULOSIS

THIN DISC;
PARTIALLY
DESTROYED
END PLATES

LOCALIZED
KYPHOSIS;
FURTHER
DESTRUCTION
OF INTERVERTEBRAL
CARTILAGE AND
ADJOINING BONE;
SURROUNDED BY
OVOID SOFT TISSUE
ABSCESS

ALMOST COMPLETE
DESTRUCTION OF
ADJOINING VERTEBRA.
THE INTERSPACE
DISAPPEARS.

2. PYOGENIC

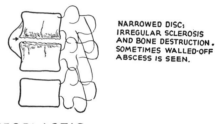

NARROWED DISC;
IRREGULAR SCLEROSIS
AND BONE DESTRUCTION.
SOMETIMES WALLED-OFF
ABSCESS IS SEEN.

NEOPLASTIC

IRREGULAR SCLEROSIS
AND OSTEOPOROSIS
(PARTICULARLY IN LYMPHOMAS)

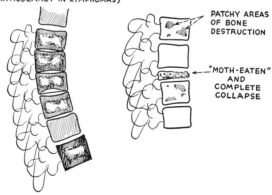

PATCHY AREAS
OF BONE
DESTRUCTION

"MOTH-EATEN"
AND
COMPLETE
COLLAPSE

DUE TO METASTATIC NEOPLASM

1. OBLITERATION OF VERTEBRAL STRUCTURAL DETAIL.

2. NO EXTENSION OF VERTEBRAL SUBSTANCE BEYOND
   COLUMN, BUT NEOPLASM MAY EXTEND.

3. DENSITY DECREASED - OCCASIONALLY SCLEROTIC.

4. NO DIVERGING SPINOUS PROCESS.

5. HOMOGENEOUS SCLEROSIS PARTICULARLY IN
   METASTATIC CARCINOMA OF PROSTATE.

Figure 14–38 (*Continued*).   The various types of wedged vertebral bodies.

body. The injured disk may undergo fibrosis or even calcification and associated paraspinous ligamentous calcification is also likely to occur.

Special Characteristics of Traumatic Disorders of the Spine in Specific Regions

CERVICAL SPINE.   The most frequent traumatic disorders of the cervical spine are (Whitley and Forsyth):

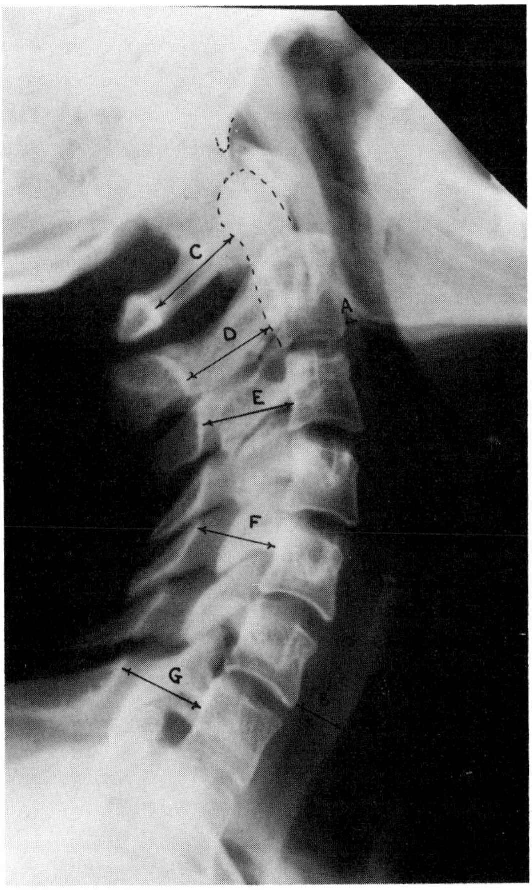

Figure 14–39   Normal lateral view of neck indicating regions evaluated. *A*. Retropharyngeal space, second cervical vertebra. *B*. Retrotracheal space, sixth cervical vertebra. *C* to *G*. Cervical spinal canal. *C*. First cervical vertebra. *D*. Second cervical vertebra. *E*. Third cervical vertebra. *F*. Fifth cervical vertebra. *G*. Seventh cervical vertebra. (From Wholey, M. H. et al.: Radiology, *71*:350, 1958.)

NORMAL SAGITTAL MEASUREMENTS*

Region Evaluated	Normal Sagittal Measurements for Children 15 Years and Under (120 cases)		Normal Sagittal Measurements for Adults (480 cases)	
	AVERAGE (MM.)	RANGE (MM.)	AVERAGE (MM.)	RANGE (MM.)
Retropharyngeal space	3.5	2–7	3.4	1–7
Retrotracheal space	7.9	5–14	14.0	9–22
Cervical spinal canal:				
At first cervical vertebra	21.9	18–27	21.4	16–30
At second cervical vertebra	20.9	18–25	19.2	16–28
At third cervical vertebra	17.4	14–21	19.1	14–25
At fifth cervical vertebra	16.5	14–21	18.5	14–25
At seventh cervical vertebra	16.0	15–20	17.5	13–24

*From Wholey, M. H., et al.: Radiology, *71*:350, 1958.

Figure 14–39   (*Continued*).

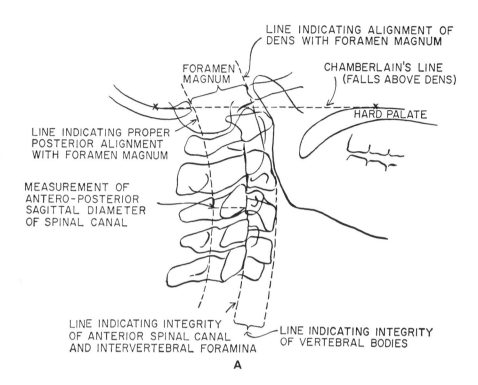

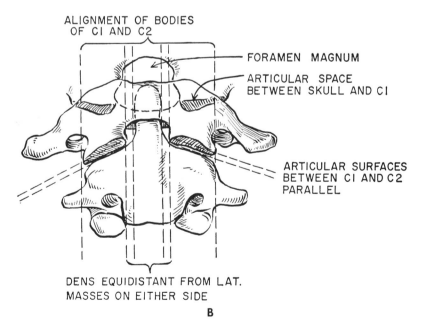

Figure 14–40 *A* and *B*. Alignment of cervical segments with respect to each other and the skull. *A*. Lateral projection. *B*. Odontoid projection. (From Wholey, M. H. et al.: Radiology, *71*:350, 1958.)

1. Fracture of the odontoid process, sometimes in association with a dislocation of the atlas.

2. Fracture of the atlas sometimes of an explosion or "Jeffersonian" variety.

3. Fractures of the neural arches.

4. Compression fractures, especially of the fifth or sixth cervical bodies.

5. Fractures of the spinous processes, especially of the seventh, with or without associated fractures of the upper dorsal regions.

A useful method of measuring the spinal canal and showing alignment of the cervical segments is shown in Figure 14–39.

"WHIPLASH INJURY"

Definition. Forcible flexion of the cervical spine following a sudden acceleration forward from a position of rest, and thereafter an elastic rebound of the head with consequent hyperextension of the spine. The automobile collision from behind is probably the most frequent cause. Injuries in and around the third to the fifth cervical segment and the fourth to the fifth lumbar segments are most responsible for symptoms. Although fractures are ordinarily not produced, careful search may reveal compression injuries of facets, particularly in oblique projections.

The fractures which are noted most frequently are avulsion fractures of the spinous processes, fractures of the articular facets, and dislocations of the vertebrae. Protrusion of a nucleus pulposus with herniation towards the spinal canal may also be produced.

UPPER THORACIC SEGMENT FRACTURES. These fractures, in association with convulsions, are most apt to occur in the upper thoracic spine and are particularly frequent in the third, fourth, and fifth dorsal segments (Figure 14–41). Other con-

Figure 14–41 Demonstration of the sequence of changes which occur in convulsive fractures of the upper spine. First there would appear to be a superior end plate indentation followed by wedging anteriorly. The kyphos deformity is usually slight in these cases. (Meschan, I., et al.: Radiology, *54*:180, 1950.)

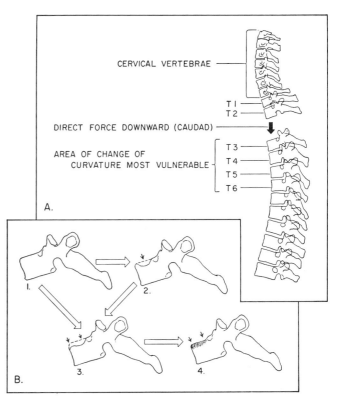

CERVICAL VERTEBRAE

T 1
T 2

DIRECT FORCE DOWNWARD (CAUDAD)

AREA OF CHANGE OF
CURVATURE MOST VULNERABLE

T 3
T 4
T 5
T 6

A.

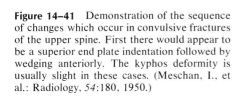

B.

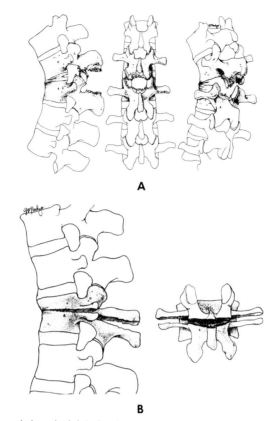

A

B

Figure 14–42 Characteristic spinal injuries in persons wearing seat belts in automobile collisions. Drawings show extensive ligament tearing (*A*), and composite of three cases of "chance fracture" (*B*). (Courtesy of Smith, W. S., and Kaufer, H.: Univ. Mich. Med. Center J., *33*:99–104, 1967.)

vulsive seizures such as those which occur with idiopathic epilepsy and with tetanus may produce similar involvement (Sujoy; Meschan et al.).

SEAT BELT FRACTURES OF THE SPINE (See later description) (Figure 14–42)

ILLUSTRATIONS OF SPECIAL FRACTURES (Figure 14–43)

Spondylolysis; Spondylolisthesis; Pseudospondylolisthesis; Reverse Spondylolisthesis

Definitions

SPONDYLOLYSIS: Defective ossification in the pars interarticularis of the neural arches, most commonly found in the fourth and fifth lumbar segments.

SPONDYLOLISTHESIS: A slippage forward of a vertebral body in respect to the vertebral body below it. This usually occurs in relation to a spondylolysis. Very seldom does it occur as the result of trauma to a neural arch. In true spondylolisthesis it is unknown what part trauma may play in this process.

PSEUDOSPONDYLOLISTHESIS (of Junghans): Displacement forward of a vertebral body anteriorly because of stretching and weakening of the apophyseal joints at their intervertebral articulations. The neural arch is intact and no spondylolysis is present.

REVERSE SPONDYLOLISTHESIS: A posterior displacement of the body of the lumbar vertebrae on the vertebrae beneath, usually resulting from an anatomic variation in the adjoining articular facets. The displacement is at the fourth or fifth lumbar interspaces almost invariably, and is only slight (Figure 14–44).

Degree of Slippage

Although the *degree of slipping* has been classified as slight, moderate, and severe, depending on the degree of angulation forward of the slipped vertebral body, even the most severe types of spondylolisthesis may be completely coincidental radiologic findings with no evidence of back pains. Also, there have been few proved demonstrations in which aggravation of the defect was demonstrated in the course of time, although this does occur.

SPOTTED SCLEROTIC LESIONS

Osteopoikilosis (See Chapter 7)

Congenital Stippled Epiphyses (Dysplasia Epiphysialis Punctata; Chondroangiopathia Calcificans Congenita) (See Chapter 7)

Tuberous Sclerosis

General Comment. This is a congenital hamartomatous disease affecting the central nervous system and many other organs. It is characterized by epilepsy, mental deficiency, adenoma sebaceum of the skin, and congenital tumors of the eye and many visceral organs.

Radiologic Changes in the Spine

The vertebrae may contain multiple sclerotic foci including the neural arches. This condition may resemble osteoblastic metastases or osteopoikilosis except that the most peripheral bones in the skeleton are not involved as in osteopoikilosis.

Sclerotic Bone Islands (Figure 14–45)

Neoplastic Metastatic Diseases characterized by osteoblastic metastases have been previously considered.

Spinal Lymphomas

Classification. Hodgkins's disease, lymphosarcoma, joint follicular lymphoma, and reticulum cell sarcoma.

Radiographic Manifestations in the Spine

Although usually the metastatic invasion of the vertebrae produces a lytic process, on occasion an osteoblastic or sclerotic reaction occurs (Hulten; Dresser and Spencer).

If the destruction proceeds sufficiently far, compression fractures and wedging of the vertebral bodies may result. Sclerosis similar to Cushing's disease may then be evident along the compressed margins of such involved vertebrae.

The intervertebral disks retain their integrity.

At times the bony appearance will, however, resemble a fine reticular network, especially in the vertebral processes.

Erosive changes occur especially along the anterior aspect of the vertebral bodies (Moseley).

Paravertebral swellings may occur by direct invasion of the paraspinous soft tissues or secondary to lymph node involvement. Extradural invasion of the spinal canal may occur, giving rise to neurological symptomatology. Myelography would be essential under these circumstances to establish the extent of the diagnosis.

Radiographic manifestations may be minimal even though extensive·involvement may be shown at autopsy.

Osteoid Osteoma

Definition.   Benign osteoblastic tumor composed principally of osteoid tissue and atypical bone.

Pathogenesis of Lesion.   The osteoid osteoma in spongy bone evokes a rim of sclerotic reaction, producing a pronounced sclerotic lesion. The nidus itself may not be demonstrable except by special body section radiography. At surgery the nidus may be seen as a bulging rubbery red nodule.

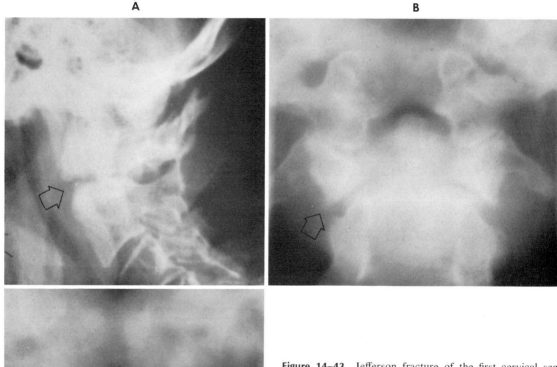

A

B

C

Figure 14–43 Jefferson fracture of the first cervical segment and fracture at the base of the odontoid process. *A.* Lateral view demonstrating the fracture of the odontoid process. The fracture of the neural arch of C-1 is also seen. *B.* Same patient demonstrating by tomogram the subluxation of the lateral mass of C-1 with respect to the occipital condyles and C-2. The fracture at the base of the odontoid is also shown. *C.* Another tomographic view, which demonstrates more clearly the subluxation of the articular mass of C-1 in respect to C-2 on the right (open arrow) and the fracture at the base of the odontoid (small open arrow).

Figure 14–43 continued on opposite page.

Radiographic Manifestations of the Spine

Involves chiefly the neural arches, particularly the isthmus and articular facets and the transverse processes (Walker; MacLellan and Wilson).

Lesions are usually small with a considerable sclerotic reaction. The nidus rarely exceeds 1 cm. in diameter. It appears as a central circular area of increased density surrounded by a radiolucent halo and this in turn is completely enveloped by sclerotic bone.

Mastocytosis (Urticaria Pigmentosa) (See Chapter 10 and earlier in this chapter also.)

VERTICAL IRREGULAR LUCENCY OR SCLEROSIS

Hemangioma

Radiographic Manifestations

Vertical wavy, striated, cancellous appearance of the bone (Figure 14–46). The horizontal trabeculae may appear somewhat thickened although diminished in number. The trabecular pattern may also be described as "weblike."

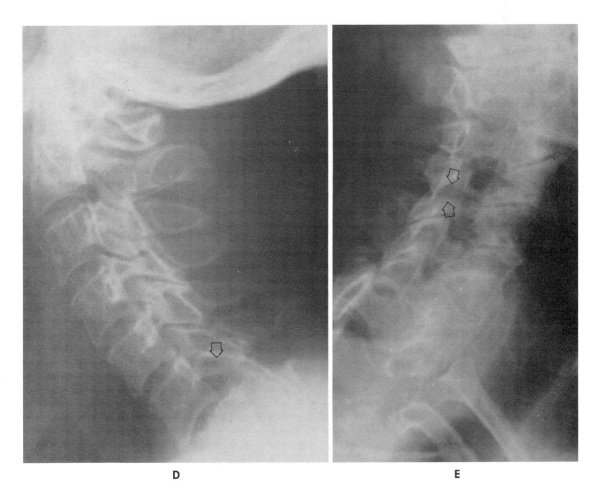

D   E

Figure 14–43 (*Continued*).   *D* and *E*. Horizontal fracture of the articular process of C-6. *D*. A lateral projection. *E*. An oblique projection demonstrating more clearly the horizontal type of fracture of this articular process. In the lateral view the subluxation of C-6 with respect to C-7 is just barely visible.

A RADIOGRAPHIC ANALYSIS OF SPONDYLOLISTHESIS

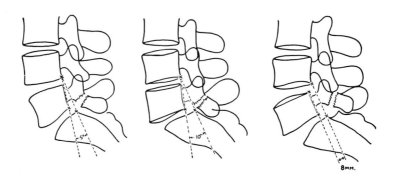

TRACINGS OF RADIOGRAPHS OF SUBJECTS WITH SPONDYLOLISTHESIS.
THE LINES EITHER INTERSECT ABOVE THE FIFTH LUMBAR VERTEBRA
AND FORM AN ANGLE EXCEEDING 2° (A and B) OR REMAIN PARALLEL,
BUT ARE MORE THAN 3 MM. APART (C).

[A]

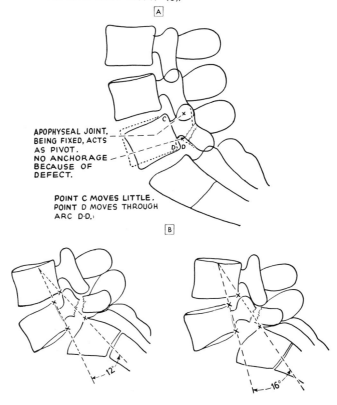

APOPHYSEAL JOINT,
BEING FIXED, ACTS
AS PIVOT.
NO ANCHORAGE
BECAUSE OF
DEFECT.

POINT C MOVES LITTLE.
POINT D MOVES THROUGH
ARC D·D.ı

[B]

SPONDYLOLISTHESIS AFFECTING THE FIFTH LUMBAR VERTEBRA. TRACINGS
OF RADIOGRAPHS TO DEMONSTRATE AN INSTABILITY OF 4° (16° MINUS 12°);
(A) WEIGHT-BEARING FLEXION – THE MINIMUM DEGREE OF SLIPPING IS
FREQUENTLY FOUND IN FLEXION.

(B) WEIGHT-BEARING EXTENSION – THE MAXIMUM DEGREE OF SLIPPING
IS FOUND IN EXTENSION.

[C]

Figure 14–44 *A.* Radiographic analysis of spondylolisthesis showing a method of lining and detection. *B.* Diagram illustrating the usual mechanism of spondylolisthesis. *C.* Tracings demonstrating method of measuring instability at the lumbosacral region in erect flexion and extension with spondylolisthesis.

Figure 14–44 continued on opposite page.

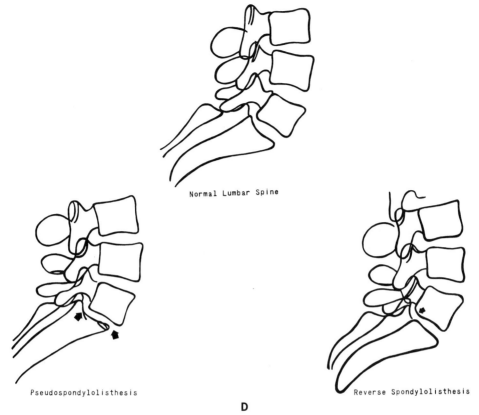

Normal Lumbar Spine

Pseudospondylolisthesis

Reverse Spondylolisthesis

D

Figure 14–44 (*Continued*).   *D.* Line diagram illustrating pseudospondylolisthesis and reverse spondylolisthesis.

The lesion may extend into the neural arch or may actually be responsible for some expansion of the vertebral bodies with pressure on the structures contained in the spinal canal at the level of the involved vertebrae.

The lesion may be single or multiple and is among the most frequent tumors affecting the spine (occurring in 10.7 per cent of cases according to Schmorl).

Osteopathia Striata (Voorhoeve's disease).

Definition.   Vertical striation of the skeleton, particularly the metaphyses of long bones but occasionally affecting vertebral bodies. It is related probably to osteopoikilosis, although this may not be accepted by all.

BOXLIKE SCLEROSIS OF THE VERTEBRAL BODIES

Paget's Disease (Osteitis Deformans)

Definition.   Mosiac-structured bone caused by rapid sequences of bone resorption and bone regeneration with secondary medullary fibrosis. There is a marked thickening of the cancellous tissue. The bone itself may appear to expand under the influence of the disease process. The disease may be monostotic or polyostotic.

Sites of Involvement.   In the spine, the lumbar spine and the sacrum are involved to the greatest extent, and the dorsal spine is next in frequency. The cervical spine is rarely involved.

Malignant degeneration of Paget's disease has been well documented (Summey and Pressley).

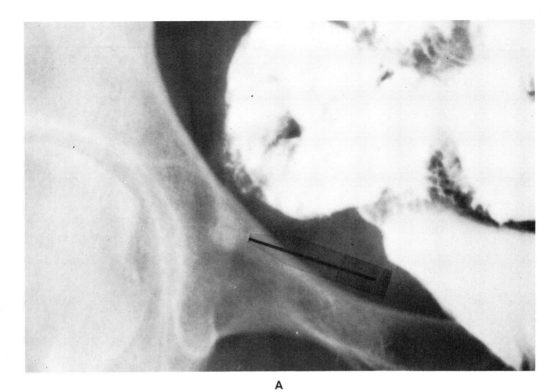

A

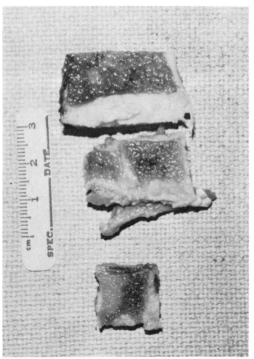

B

Figure 14–45   Sclerotic bone islands. *A*. In the superior ramus of the ischium. *B*. Gross appearance of vertebral bodies so affected at autopsy.

Radiographic Manifestations in the Spine

Early: slight diffuse increase in the density of the involved vertebrae with some tendency to coarsened and thickened trabecular pattern. This may be localized to a small portion of the vertebra or involve it entirely.

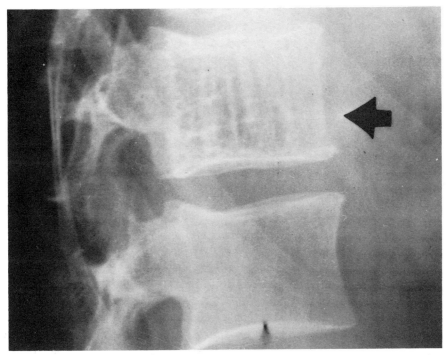

Figure 14–46   Hemangioma of the first lumbar vertebra showing typical striped trabeculation.

In well advanced cases there is a tendency to a boxlike coarsened configuration of the trabeculae with the central zone of the vertebrae being more lucent, yet still coarse, giving this boxlike appearance.

Occasionally, there is a diffuse increase in the density of the vertebral body with a cotton wool appearance like that which may occur more frequently in the flat bones such as the skull and pelvis.

The intervertebral disk is usually preserved.

Although Paget's involvement of the cervical spine is rare, the following features occur: (1) the involvement may be totally obscured by degenerative change; (2) there may be vertebral collapse simulating metastatic disease; (3) the entire neural arch, transverse process, and spinous process are involved (thus differing from hemangioma, which remains localized to the vertebral body); (4) the lumen of the intervertebral foramina and spinal canal may be encroached upon by the gradual overgrowth of the vertebral bodies and neural arch. (5) The collapse or overgrowth may interfere with the blood supply of the spinal cord (Feldman and Seaman).

Idiopathic Hypercalcemia at Infancy (Chapter 10)

INDISCRIMINATE LUCENCY AND SCLEROSIS

Fibrous Dysplasia

Definition.   Etiology is unknown. There is a gradual replacement of the skeletal tissues by an overgrowth of fibrous tissue, a proliferation on the outside of this fibrous tissue suggesting a regenerative process and producing the appearance of a "shell of bone." It may occur in association with certain endocrine dysfunctions, in which case the term "fibrous dysplasia with endocrine manifestations" has been used (also called Albright's disease) (Jaffe, 1958). The bone lesions tend to stabilize as the patient grows older and sexual precocity recedes.

Radiographic Manifestations of the Spine

Involvement of the vertebral column is relatively rare. Manifestations consist mainly of a thinning of the cortical bone, a loss of the trabecular markings, a widening of the intervertebral disk, and a tendency toward a shell of bone, which produces a zone of sclerosis along the outer margins of the lesion.

There may be numerous vertical striations traversing the medullary spaces.

The superior and inferior surfaces of the vertebrae assume a biconcave appearance.

The transverse processes may be re-directed and appear to be out of line in involved sites.

Neoplastic Metastatic Disease (Chapter 10) and previously described.

Malignant Lymphomas Involving Vertebrae have been previously considered.

Radiation Effects on Vertebrae

General Comment. Intensive x-ray irradiation over the vertebral column may produce spinal cord damage with doses in excess of 5000 rads in a period of approximately eight weeks. Boden has concluded that the limit of tolerance of the central nervous system is between 3500 and 4500 rads depending on the size of the field used in a matter of several weeks. Changes in bone may also occur (Spitz and Higgenbotham; Rubin et al., 1962).

Radiographic Manifestations

Horizontal transverse lines of increased density, parallel to the epiphyseal plate give the "bone within bone" appearance.

Gross contour abnormalities in the vertebral bodies suggest gross irregularity.

There is a reduction in size of the spinal canal and the interpedicular spaces are below normal.

Hypoplasia and underdevelopment of the sacrum occur.

Ingestion of radium may produce destructive changes in vertebrae, even before the destructive changes are noted in the mandible (Stevens).

Vertebral Sarcoidosis

This lesion produces a lytic focus in the vertebral body surrounded by reactive bone formation. If it is near the intervertebral disk, there is vertebral collapse with narrowing of the disk.

Lung findings: hilar adenopathy. Negative tuberculin tests are also associated (Berk and Brower).

SPUR FORMATION WITH OR WITHOUT PARASPINOUS LIGAMENTOUS CALCIFICATION

Spondylosis Deformans

Definition. Degenerative condition usually beginning in early middle age and characterized by spur formations along the margins of vertebral bodies with paraspinous ligamentous calcifications. Spurs may protrude into the spinal canal and the intervertebral foramina, producing pressure upon adjoining nerve structures.

Radiographic Appearances

The osteophytes tend to develop along the margins of the superior and inferior end-plates of the vertebrae, forming bone bridges and depositions sometimes over 1 cm. in thickness.

In the cervical spine, encroachment upon the spinal canal with diminution of the antero-posterior dimension to less than 13 mm. is considered significant from the standpoint of symptomatology.

There is an excellent correlation between the findings on lateral and oblique plain roentgenograms of the cervical spine and the findings on cervical myelography in respect to spurs. Transverse bars on myelography correlate almost perfectly with the posterior interbody spurs on plain roentgenograms. Encroachment upon the intervertebral foramina is also found to correlate well with the presence of significant posterior interbody spurs. The canal size must be judged by both its sagittal and transverse diameters. Both measurements should be correlated if possible, rather than one (Wilkinson et al.).

The cervical prevertebral fat stripe is of considerable assistance in detecting swelling which may arise from involvement of vertebrae or the intervertebral space. The prevertebral fat stripe tends to follow closely along the anterior margin of the vertebral bodies. This is not only of assistance in diagnosing cervical spondylosis but also in the detection of such processes as fractures, masses, inflammations, and other abnormalities related to the interface between the cervical spine and the prevertebral soft tissues (Whalen and Woodruff).

Herniated disks may coexist with spondylotic spurs. These also require myelography for demonstration.

Although spondylotic changes in the thoracic spine are frequent, they rarely affect the spinal cord since they are situated anteriorly and laterally for the most part. Occasionally they will encroach upon the intervertebral foramen. In the lumbar region association with herniated disks is frequent (Figure 14–47).

Syphilitic Spondylitis has been previously considered. An effort should be made to differentiate the appearance of typical syphilitic spondylitis from advanced deforming spondylosis since the two may resemble one another closely. In syphilitic spondylitis, however, there is evidence of some associated irregularity and destruction of the vertebral body, giving rise to irregular contours of the vertebral body. Generally the vertebral body is well preserved in deforming spondylosis.

Rheumatoid Spondylitis

Ankylosing Spondylitis, (Marie Strümpell's Disease, Ankylosing Spondylarthritis) (Figure 14–48)

Definition. Ankylosing spondylitis and rheumatoid arthritis resemble one another closely but have been separated from one another on the following differential points:

ROENTGENOLOGIC CRITERIA FOR RHEUMATOID ARTHRITIS OF THE CERVICAL SPINE

1. Atlantoaxial subluxation of 2.5 mm. or more.
2. Multiple subluxation of C-2 to C-3, C-3 to C-4, C-4 to C-5, C-5 to C-6.
3. Narrow disk spaces with little or no osteophytosis.

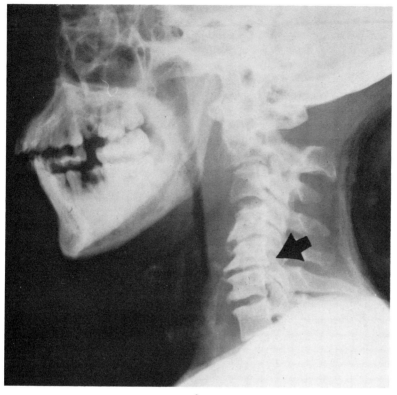

A

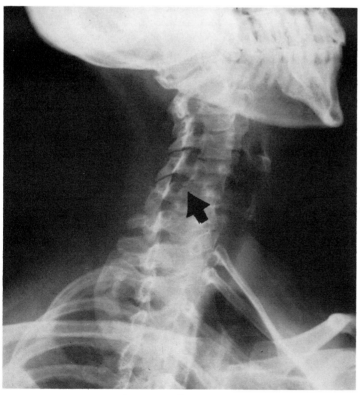

Figure 14–47 *A*. Lateral view of the cervical spine showing advanced degenerative changes in C-4, C-5 and C-6 vertebrae, with considerable narrowness of the interspaces and posterior spur formation extending in toward the spinal canal. This is very often associated with herniated disks. Note also the paraspinous ligamentous calcification and the loss of normal curvature in the spine. *B*. Oblique radiograph of the cervical spine demonstrating encroachment upon the intervertebral foramen.

B

Figure 14–47 continued on opposite page.

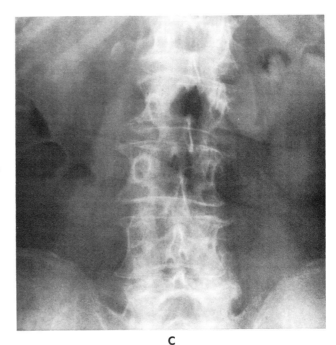

Figure 14–47 (*Continued*). *C*. Deforming spondylosis in the lumbar spine.

C

a. Pathognomonic at C-2 to C-3, C-3 to C-4.

b. Probable at C-4 to C-5 and C-5 to C-6.

4. Erosions of vertebrae, especially vertebral plates.

5. Odontoid small and pointed with eroded cortex.

6. Basilar impression.

7. Apophyseal joint erosion; blurred facets, narrow spaces; spinous process erosion.

8. Generalized osteoporosis.

9. A difference of 5 mm. or more between the posterior arch of the atlas and spinous process of the axis from flexion to extension.

10. Osteosclerosis, secondary, atlantoaxial occipital area (Bland et al.; Park and O'Brien).

1. There is a difference in incidence in males and females.

2. There is an absence of streptococcal and sheep red cell agglutinins in ankylosing spondylitis.

3. Subcutaneous nodules are absent in pure ankylosing spondylitis.

4. Severe osteoporotic changes in peripheral joints occur with rheumatoid arthritis, whereas this does not ordinarily occur with ankylosing spondylitis with peripheral joint involvement.

5. Calcification of the paraspinal ligaments is frequent in ankylosing spondylitis but is not present with rheumatoid arthritis.

6. Sacroiliac and spinal changes are predominant with ankylosing spondylitis while these are rare in rheumatoid arthritis. The cervical spine, however, is involved frequently with rheumatoid arthritis.

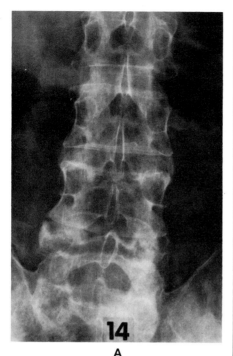

A

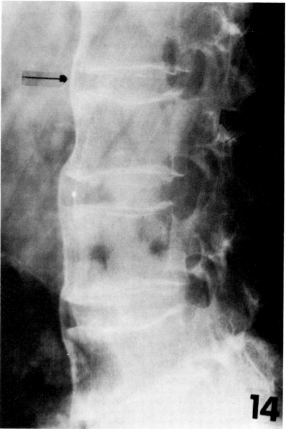

Figure 14–48   *A.* Moderate ankylosing spondylitis. The sacroiliac joints are fused as are the lumbar apophyseal joints. *B.* Lateral view. The extensive paraspinous ligamentous calcification is shown despite the fact that in the antero-posterior projection this does not appear to be nearly as extensive.

B

Figure 14–48 continued on opposite page.

Radiographic Manifestations

Usual sites of involvement in ankylosing spondylitis are the upper and lower corners of contiguous vertebrae beginning in the upper lumbar or lower thoracic spine and ascending and descending spine from the sites of origin. The paraspinous ligaments become thinly calcified and ultimately produce the so-called "bamboo" appearance.

Simultaneously there may also be involvement of the synovial joints between the intervertebral processes with a loss of the subarticular calcific zone first, and then gradual loss of definition of the subarticular bone to the point of complete obliteration of the intervertebral joint.

Peripheral joint manifestations are not uncommon in the early stages of ankylosing spondylitis as a transitory phenomenon.

The sacroiliac joints are involved very early in ankylosing spondylitis, perhaps in 98 per cent of cases (Forestier). There are stages of involvement of the sacroiliac joints: (1) cloudy opacities in the para-articular bones; (2) spotted osteoporosis of the subchondral bone; (3) ultimate blurred obliteration of the joint space itself with complete ankylosis.

It is said by some that the earliest manifestation of ankylosing spondylitis is actually in the apophyseal joints with rheumatoid-like changes therein (Epstein, 1969).

Ankylosing spondylitis is primarily a disease involving the synovial joints and intervertebral joints and affects the bones immediately adjoining these joint

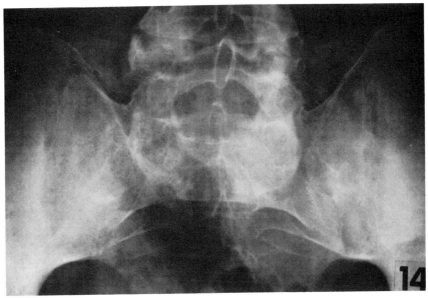

C

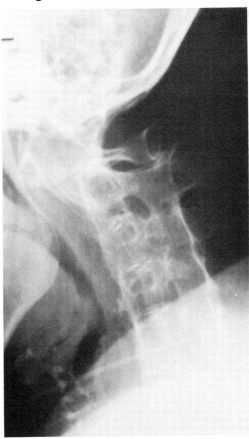

Figure 14–48 (*Continued*). *C.* More advanced case of ankylosing spondylitis with complete ankylosis also of the hip joints. *D.* Same case; very marked ankylosis of the cervical spine. C-1 is markedly subluxated forward with respect to C-2.

D

areas. Rheumatoid arthritis, on the other hand, may affect the bones of the vertebral bodies away from the joint.

The intervertebral disks may either appear wide or narrowed.

The joints between the ribs and the dorsal vertebrae are also involved, ultimately leading to a fixation of the thoracic cage and respiratory difficulties.

In true rheumatoid arthritis of the vertebrae, granulomatous nodules identical in appearance to the skin nodules make their appearance within the vertebral body itself (Baggenstass, Bickel, and Ward; Wholey, Pugh, and Bickel).

Atlantoaxial dislocation may occur with both rheumatoid arthritis and ankylosing spondylitis. The space involved by the atlantoaxial joints increases and the margins of the odontoid process become sharpened, resorbed, and the dens becomes pointed. Measurements for the atlantoaxial joints are given for both children and adults (see earlier discussion).

In early cases of juvenile rheumatoid arthritis no radiologic changes are ordinarily seen in the spine. Later, however, one finds radiologic changes similar to those of spondylitis with no calcification of the paraspinal ligaments. The vertebral bodies become osteoporotic and the lumbar lordotic curve may become straightened. The intervertebral disks may actually appear expanded. Complete ankylosis in juvenile rheumatoid arthritis may result (Saenger).

In the late stage in juvenile rheumatoid arthritis, the vertebral bodies may fuse to the point where they resemble block vertebrae.

Abnormalities of Contour and Alignment of the Spine as a Whole

1. Definition of Terms
    a. Scoliosis
        (1) Methods of measurement (Ferguson; Cobb)
    b. Lordosis
        (1) Methods of measurement
    c. Disease entities with kyphosis or scoliosis
        (1) Congenital torticollis
        (2) Morquio's disease
        (3) Hurler's disease
        (4) Arthrogryposis multiplex congenita
        (5) Mongolism
        (6) Turner's syndrome
        (7) Fractures and dislocation
        (8) Juvenile kyphosis (osteochondrosis; Scheuermann's disease)

2. Abnormalities of Alignment in Relation to the Skull
    a. Occipital vertebra
    b. Basilar invagination, impression, or platybasia
    c. Arnold-Chiari malformation
    d. Klippel-Feil deformity
    e. Chordoma
    f. Nasopharyngeal tumors

3. Abnormalities of Vertebral Alignment—One Vertebra with Another
    a. Hemivertebrae
    b. Atlantoaxial subluxation
    c. Trauma
    d. Spondylolisthesis
    e. Pseudospondylolisthesis
    f. Reverse spondylolisthesis

Abnormalities of Contour and Alignment
of the Spine as a Whole

The Normal Curvature of the Spine. These curves are illustrated in Figure 14–49. The major change with age occurs in the cervicothoracic junction when the child begins to lift its head and to assume the erect posture.

Definition of Terms

Scoliosis: lateral curvature and usually an associated rotation of several vertebrae in the longitudinal axis.

Lordosis: increased concavity in the spine on the posterior aspect.

Kyphosis: angulation of the spine on its posterior aspect.

Gibbus: a posterior hump or angulation similar to a kyphous deformity. As usually employed, there is no significant disturbance in the line of weight bearing. Each of these processes may be said to have a fulcrum around which the major curvature occurs.

Primary Curvature: one which cannot be changed significantly by bending the spine to one side or the other or by tilting the pelvis.

Secondary or Compensatory Curvature occurs when tilting the pelvis or bending the spine changes the curvature significantly.

Scoliosis

Measurement of Curvature in Dorsal Scoliosis (Figure 14–50)

Ferguson's original method of measuring scoliotic deformity (George and Rippstein):

1. Define the margin of the apical vertebra of a curvature as well as the vertebra which defines the ends of the curve at the upper and lowermost margins of the curve.

2. Place central points in each of these three vertebrae and connect them by lines forming an angle. This angle is called the angle of the curve, that is, the divergence from 180 degrees.

Cobb's method (introduced by Lippman). Define the end vertebra of a curvature and place a horizontal line on the uppermost margin of the upper vertebra and the lower end-plate of the lower vertebra. Extend these and draw perpendicular lines to the end-plates. The angle formed by these perpendiculars is the angle of scoliosis (Kittleson and Lim).

Orthopedists vary in their preferences for one method or another, but George

CHANGES IN SPINAL CURVATURE WITH AGE

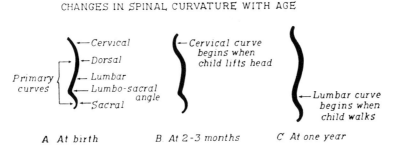

Figure 14–49   Changes in spinal curvature with age. (From Meschan, I., and Farrer-Meschan, R. M. F.: Radiology, *70:*637–648, 1958.)

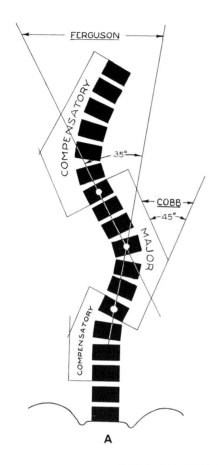

A

Figure 14–50 Methods of measuring dorsal spine scoliosis. *A.* Modified to show Cobb's method of measurement as well as Ferguson's. *B.* (Modified from Ferguson, A. B.: *Roentgen Diagnosis of Extremities and Spine.* New York, Paul B. Hoeber, Inc., 1949.) (See also George and Rippstein, Clark.)

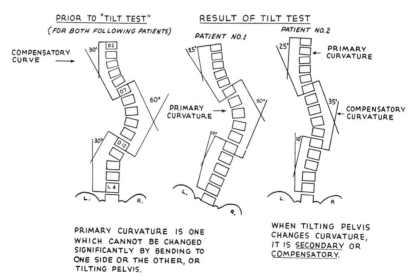

B

and Rippstein have indicated that the Ferguson method is more accurate. The merits of each method have been carefully studied by these authors.

Lordosis

Method of Measuring Lordosis of Lumbar Spine at Lumbosacral Angle

The relationship of the uppermost margin of the sacrum to the horizontal has been described as Ferguson's lumbosacral angle (Figure 14–51). Ferguson has indicated that when this angle exceeds approximately 34 degrees an unstable state is said to exist.

Another indication of instability with a lordotic lumbar spine is determined by extending the line of weight bearing of the dorsal spine — its longitudinal axis — to the level of the sacrum. If this line falls anterior to the sacrum, it may be concluded that there is inadequate spinal support and instability which, in turn, may cause muscle strain and back pain (Figure 14–51 *B*).

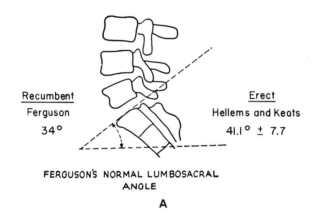

Recumbent
Ferguson
34°

Erect
Hellems and Keats
41.1° ± 7.7

FERGUSON'S NORMAL LUMBOSACRAL ANGLE

A

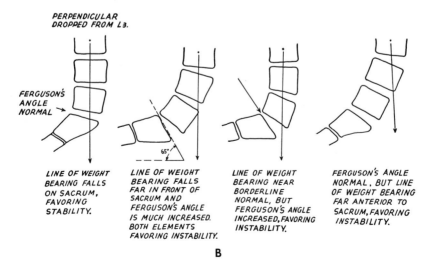

PERPENDICULAR DROPPED FROM L3.

FERGUSON'S ANGLE NORMAL →

LINE OF WEIGHT BEARING FALLS ON SACRUM, FAVORING STABILITY.

LINE OF WEIGHT BEARING FALLS FAR IN FRONT OF SACRUM AND FERGUSON'S ANGLE IS MUCH INCREASED. BOTH ELEMENTS FAVORING INSTABILITY.

LINE OF WEIGHT BEARING NEAR BORDERLINE NORMAL, BUT FERGUSON'S ANGLE INCREASED, FAVORING INSTABILITY.

FERGUSON'S ANGLE NORMAL, BUT LINE OF WEIGHT BEARING FAR ANTERIOR TO SACRUM, FAVORING INSTABILITY.

B

Figure 14–51 Analysis of two factors in lumbosacral instability. (Modified from Ferguson, A. B.: *Roentgen Diagnosis of Extremities and Spine*. New York, Paul B. Hoeber, Inc., 1949.)

Disease Entities Previously Described in Which Disorders of Alignment are Manifest (Figure 14–52)

Congenital Torticollis

Definition. Torticollis occurring at birth and not associated with a sterno-mastoid tumor. The latter occurs in about 20 per cent of the cases (Hulbert).

Radiographic Manifestations. Abnormality of cervical spinal curvature or muscle spasm.

Osteochondrodystrophy (Morquio-Brailsford's disease). Kyphosis usually manifest with elongation and flattening of the individual vertebral bodies.

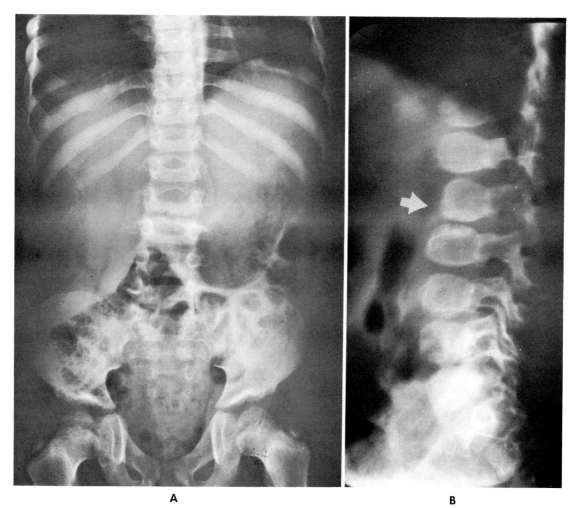

A   B

Figure 14–52 Some disorders of alignment of the spine in congenital or systemic diseases. *A*. Morquio-Brailsford disease (polytopic enchondral dysostosis). Film showing lower thorax, lumbar spine, pelvis, and hip. *B*. Lateral view of lumbar spine. Note that the ribs tend to be somewhat club-shaped; the vertebral bodies are broad from side to side and somewhat flattened in their appearance with a kyphos deformity in the upper lumbar spine, and with a tonguelike projection from the inferior aspect of L-2. There would appear to be a slight subluxation of L-2 with respect to L-1. Note also the characteristic appearance of the pelvis and hip as described in the text. In this instance the liver was also involved.

Figure 14–52 continued on opposite page.

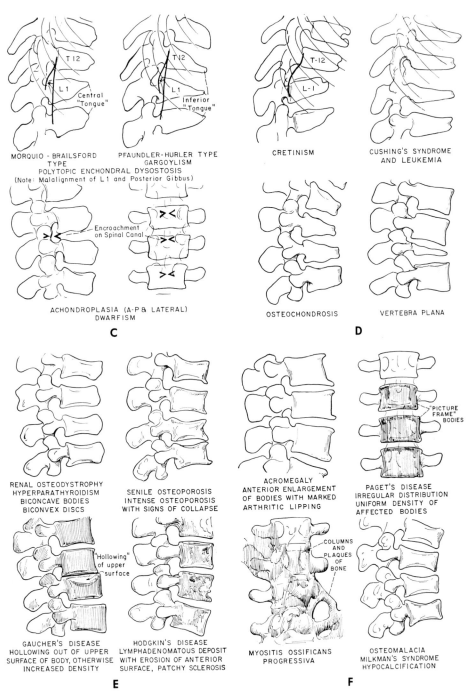

Figure 14–52 (*Continued*).

Figure 14–52 continued on following page.

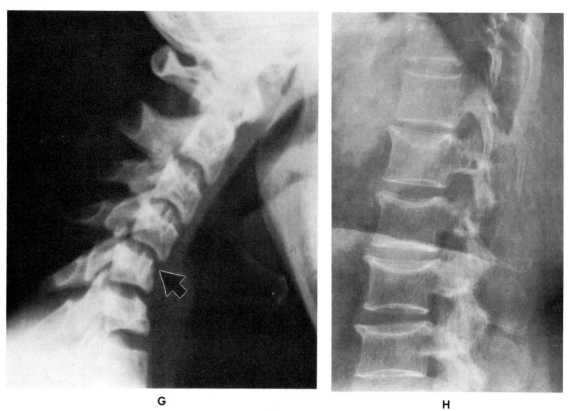

G   **H**

Figure 14–52 (*Continued*).   *G*. Subluxation of C-4 anteriorly. *H*. Osteomalacia involving the spine.

Hurler's Disease (gargoylism, dysostosis multiplex).   Kyphosis at the thoracolumbar junction with a rounded configuration of the individual vertebral segment.

Arthrogryposis Multiplex Congenita.   Lateral curvature of the muscle spine due to irregular muscle pull. The individual vertebrae may be narrow and somewhat elongated rarely.

Mongolism (Down's syndrome).   Subtle scoliosis. There is usually also a thin, small atlas, and forward displacement at the atlanto-occipital joint.

Turner's Syndrome.   Scoliosis, irregularities of opposing surfaces, and squared-off appearances of narrowed, intervertebral disks.

ROENTGENOLOGIC FINDINGS IN SYRINGOMYELIA AND HYDROMYELIA

1. Bone anomalies around foramen magnum.
2. Bone abnormalities of the cervical or thoracic spine.
3. Enlargement of the cervical or thoracic spinal canal either on the lateral, the antero-posterior projection or both.
4. Cervical or thoracic scoliosis either slight or definite (McRae and Standen).

Fractures and Dislocations with kyphosis, scoliosis, or displacement of vertebral segments.

Seat Belt Fractures (Smith and Kaufer):
1. Extensive ligament tearing with marked spreading of the posterior spinal elements. The synovial joint capsules may also tear along with the following: interlaminar ligament, ligamentum flavum, posterior longitudinal ligaments.
2. Thoracic paraplegia may result.
3. Radiographic findings
    a. Marked spreading of the posterior spinal elements.
    b. Occasionally, a horizontal fracture through the vertebral body continuing posteriorly through the pedicles, transverse processes, lamina, and spinous processes.

Dislocations (with or without fractures) in which the articular facets no longer articulate ("jump the track").

Juvenile Kyphosis Dorsalis (Scheuermann's disease; vertebral epiphysitis).

Abnormality of the Spine Alignment in Relation to the Skull

Occipital Vertebra.   This eminence, which distorts the periphery of the foramen magnum, has been previously described. It may appear anteriorly as a third condyle. Occasionally paracondyloid and basilar processes occur laterally. There may or may not be separate accessory bone elements fused with the rim of the foramen magnum.

Basilar Invagination, Basilar Impression, and Platybasia (Chapter 12)

Arnold-Chiari Malformation (Chapter 12)

Klippel-Feil Deformity (previously considered)

Chordomas

Nasopharyngeal Tumors.   These extend into the base of the skull, destroying the skull or invading the fissures of the base of the skull adjoining the malignant tumor.

Abnormality of Alignment of One Vertebral Segment with Respect to Another

Hemivertebrae

Definition.   Failure of development of a lateral half of a vertebral body resulting in a triangular wedge-shaped vertebral body from one side to the other or anteriorly. Usually the wedge is laterally situated but it may be anteriorly situated. A normal rib may project from the hemivertebrae.

Radiographic Manifestations.   The characteristic radiographic manifestations of the hemivertebra are illustrated in Figure 14–53.

Atlantoaxial Subluxation

Definition.   Displacement of the first cervical vertebral body in respect to the odontoid process of C-2. This may be related to one of several etiologies:

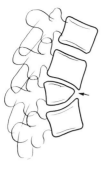

A. HEMIVERTEBRA

1. ALL BONES APPEAR HEALTHY.

2. ANTERIOR HALF OF VERTEBRA IS <u>ABSENT</u>, <u>NOT COMPRESSED</u>.

3. ADJACENT VERTEBRAE ARE EXPANDED TO FIT DEFORMITY.

4. NO BULGING ANTERIORLY.

5. OTHER DEVELOPMENTAL ABNORMALITIES (RIB) MAY BE PRESENT.

6. INTERSPACES ARE WELL PRESERVED.

A

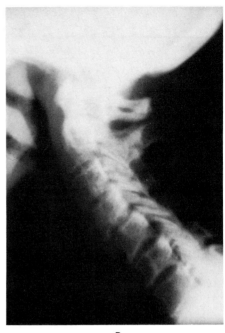

B

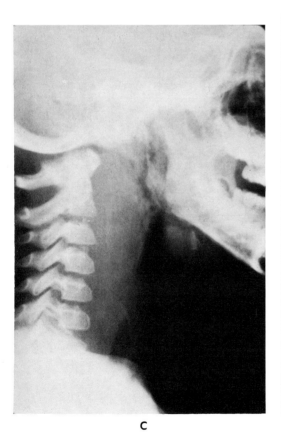

C

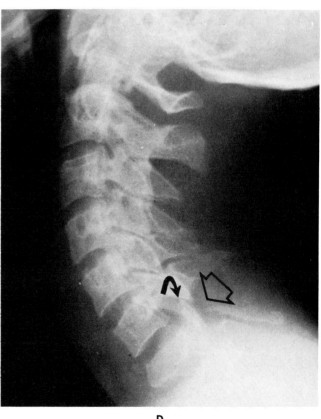

D

Figure 14–53 *A.* Hemivertebra. *B.* Rheumatoid arthritis involving the cervical spine with subluxation of C–4 in respect to C–5. *C.* Complete dislocation of the head with respect to the cervical spine with transection of the cord at this level. *D.* Facet dislocation of C–6 on C–7 with a fracture of the neural arch of C–6.

STRAIGHT BACK SYNDROME—RADIOGRAPHIC MANIFESTATIONS

1. Loss of normal kyphotic curvature of thoracic vertebrae on lateral views.
2. The normal distance between the vertebral column and sternum is diminished (diminished antero-posterior cardiothoracic ratio).
3. The heart assumes a pancake appearance in the postero-anterior projection, caused by compression between the sternum and the thoracic spine.
4. The heart may be displaced to the left with prominence of the pulmonary artery as in pectus excavatum.
5. The ratios of the antero-posterior transthoracic diameter are found to be uniformly below the mean normal for normal subjects.
6. Many of these patients also have functional cardiac murmurs (Twigg et al., 1967; Tampas and Lurie).

1. Developmental relaxation of ligaments surrounding the atlantoaxial joint.
2. Acquired relaxation of the ligaments such as occurs in mongolism or rheumatoid arthritis. Resorption of the odontoid process may also occur with rheumatoid arthritis of the cervical spine.
3. Ankylosis of the spinous process of C-1 with the occiput.
4. Trauma.
5. Neoplastic destruction of the odontoid process or neural arch of C-1. Subluxation with destruction of the atlantoaxial joint may also occur in association with lipoid dermatoarthritis (Martel, Abell, and Duff).

As a Result of Trauma various gradations of disorders of alignment may occur, ranging from fractures involving a single lamina or pedicle to complete dislocation of the pedicles with respect to one another. Severe trauma may cause the cephalad facets to dislocate over those which are caudad—"jumping the track." This type of trauma has been described especially with "laptype" seat belt injuries (see previous description).

Spondylolisthesis has been previously considered.

Pseudospondylolisthesis of Junghans has been previously considered.

Reverse Spondylolisthesis has been previously considered.

Joint Abnormalities of the Spine

1. Anatomical Considerations
2. Disease Entities
    a. Atlantoaxial fusion
    b. Alkaptonuria and ochronosis
    c. Ankylosing spondylitis
    d. Rheumatoid arthritis
        (1) Juvenile
        (2) Adult
        (3) Reiter's syndrome
    e. Ulcerative colitic arthritis
    f. Neuropathic arthropathy of the spine
    g. Paraplegic neuroarthropathy
    h. Traumatic arthropathy

     i. Intervertebral disk alterations
        (1) Injuries
        (2) Infections
        (3) Herniations
        (4) "Vacuum" phenomenon
    j. Hypervitaminosis A

JOINT ABNORMALITIES OF THE SPINE

Anatomical Considerations

The joints of the spine fall into two categories: (1) synovial joints or diarthroses, and (2) amphiarthroses.

The synovial joints may be found in the following sites:

1. Atlantoaxial joint.
2. Synovial joint between the occipital condyle and C-1.
3. Intervertebral joints between the articular processes of the vertebrae.
4. The costotransverse and costovertebral synovial joints: joints between the ribs and the transverse processes and vertebral bodies respectively.
5. The sacroiliac joints—synovial joints between the wings of the sacrum and the iliac bones.

The amphiarthrodial joints are the fibrocartilaginous junctions between the intervertebral disks and the vertebral endplates.

Disease Entities

Atlantoaxial Fusion

Definition. Assimilation of the atlas and axis resulting from maldevelopment of the occipital bone and first cervical segment. With complete fusion there is union of C-1 with the foramen magnum. With partial fusion there are varying degrees of segmental fixation of the first cervical segment with the foramen magnum. These anomalies may be associated with basilar impression.

RADIOLOGICAL ABNORMALITIES OF THE SACROILIAC JOINT IN ASSOCIATION WITH OTHER DISEASES

1. Ulcerative colitis, 18 per cent
2. Ulcerative colitis plus uveitis plus sacroiliac arthritis, 13 out of 25 cases.
3. Ulcerative colitis plus uveitis but no sacroiliac arthritis, 4 out of 119 cases.
4. Chronic prostatitis, 83 per cent (but same percentage with degenerative arthritis).
5. Reiter's syndrome, 20 out of 35 cases.

ATLAS-DENS INTERVAL (ADI) IN CHILDREN

1. At 40 inches target-to-film distance with patient supine and head neutral, all children have ADI 4 mm. or less.

2. At 72 inches target-to-film distance with patient erect, the maximum ADI was 5 mm. in a 13 year old boy.

3. Age and sex are not statistically significant factors. Position can, however, influence the measurements. Neutral position is recommended.

4. The mean difference in measurements between readers was 0.25 mm. in neutral position.

5. Other signs of atlantoaxial subluxation:

    a. Increased soft tissue anterior to cervical spine.

    b. Greater than 10 degree flexion between atlas and axis.

    c. Compensatory curve of the lower cervical spine.

    d. Narrowing of the atlantovertebral foramen (Locke et al.).

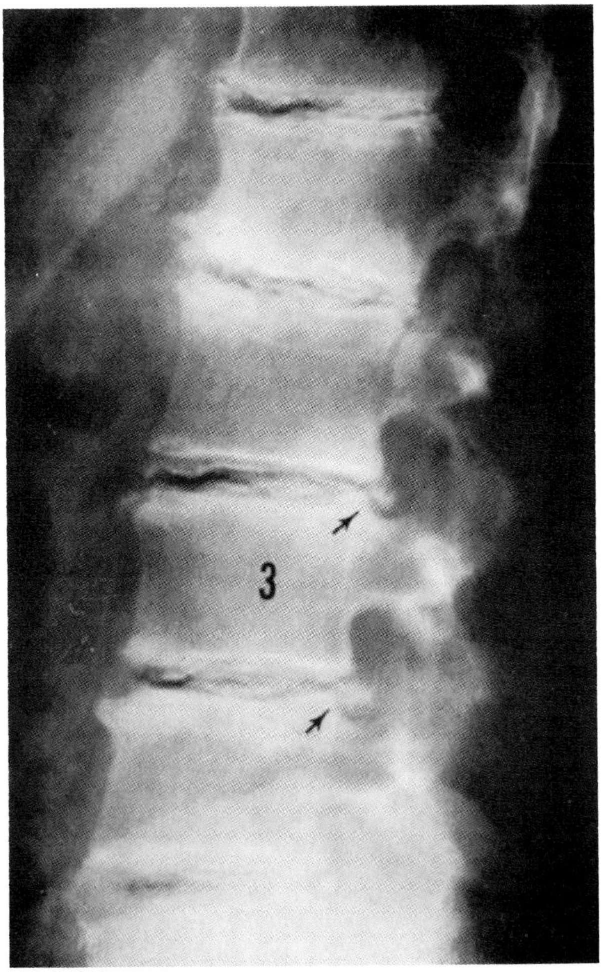

Figure 14–54 Ochronosis of the spine. Male, 69 years of age. Note the hypertrophic ankylosing changes with osteoporosis of the vertebral body. There is also a vertical and linear striation of the vertebral bodies, which are reduced in height. There is a diffuse calcification of practically all the intervertebral disks. In addition the degenerated intervertebral disks show a vacuum phenomenon. Some of the calcification in the disks protrudes posteriorly in toward the spinal canal. (From Hadley, L. A.: *Anatomico-roentgenographic Studies of the Spine.* Springfield, Ill., Charles C Thomas, 1964.)

Alkaptonuria and Ochronosis

Definition.   This disease is probably a hereditary metabolic disturbance characterized by the excretion of alkapton in the urine, rendering the urine dark after exposure to air. The excreted substance is homogentisic acid, an intermediary substance in the metabolism of phenylalanine.

Radiographic Manifestations in the Spine (Figure 14–54)

Dorsal kyphosis with loss of lumbar curve.
Hypertrophic ankylosing changes with osteoporosis of the vertebral bodies.
Vertical or linear striations of the vertebral bodies which may be reduced in height.
Diffuse calcification of practically all the intervertebral disks (Sacks).

Ankylosing Spondylitis has been previously considered.

Rheumatoid Arthritis has been previously considered.

Juvenile Rheumatoid Arthritis

Definition.   Rheumatoid arthritis in the very young. The joints most commonly affected are hand, wrist, feet, ankles, knee, and temperomandibular joints. The cervical spine, however, is involved in about 13 per cent of the cases (Epstein, 1969).

Radiographic Manifestations

Early: no radiologic changes are apparent in the spine.
Late: x-ray findings are similar to those previously described for ankylosing spondylarthritis. Decalcification of the vertebral body may take place. The intervertebral disks even appear to expand. Certain parts of vertebral bodies are especially prone to osteoporosis, especially at the atlantoaxial junction where subluxation may result.
Later in life, ankylosis of the apophyseal joints of the upper cervical vertebrae may occur. The antero-posterior diameter of the vertebrae may appear diminished and the entire process tends to simulate a block vertebra.

Reiter's Syndrome

Definition.   Disease of unknown etiology consisting of: (1) arthritis resembling rheumatoid arthritis; (2) conjunctivitis; (3) urethritis. (4) Involvement of the spine and sacroiliac joints is very infrequent (Hollander et al.). (5) In cases reported by Good (1962) Reiter's syndrome appeared to be closely associated with ankylosing spondylitis and clearly separable from rheumatoid arthritis involving the spine.

Ulcerative Colitis Arthropathy (Chapter 11)

Neuropathic Arthropathy of the Spine (Charcot's disease)

Definition and General Comment.   Changes which occur in the spine, usually secondary to central nervous system syphilis, but which may occur rarely with other neuropathic disorders such as diabetes, tumors of the caudaquina, spina bifida, traumatic paraplegia, transverse myelitis, and hematomyelia. This disease entity must not be confused with syphilitic spondylitis in which primary spirochetal infection of the spine is the cause of the disease process.

Radiographic Manifestations in the Spine

Marked bone atrophy, degenerative changes with extensive deposition of proliferating bone adjacent to the vertebral column and even some distance from it. There is usually accompanying calcification in the adjoining soft tissues.

The usual site is the lumbar spine but occasionally other vertebrae may be involved (Beetham et al.).

Paraplegic Neuroarthropathy

Definition and General Comment.   These are neuroarthropathic changes which occur especially in the lower extremities but which may occur in the spine following trauma and paraplegia resulting from this. The changes include intra-articular destructive and productive changes with large areas of extra-articular soft tissue ossification. Abramson and Kamberg noted these changes, especially when the trauma to the spine was above the level of L-1. Lesions below the first lumbar vertebra were not usually associated with alterations.

Traumatic Arthropathy (previously considered)

Intervertebral Disk Alterations

Disk Injuries.   Disk injury may produce degeneration, fragmentation, and ultimately protrusion or herniation of the injured disk.

RADIOGRAPHIC MANIFESTATIONS

Narrowness of the interspace.
Degenerate lipping of adjoining vertebral bodies and end-plates.
Undulation and irregularity of the end-plates of adjoining vertebral bodies.
Degenerative calcification of portions or all of the intervertebral disks.
Protrusion posteriorly toward the spinal canal, best demonstrated by myelography.

Disk Infections

In view of the fact that the intervertebral disk is avascular, direct infection of the intervertebral disk is rare. However, extension from an adjoining inflammatory process may occur. Thus, tuberculosis and other infectious processes may result in destructive changes in intervertebral disks. These have been previously described.

Intervertebral disk calcification, although very rare in children, has been reported by a number of investigators (Weens, Melnick, and Silverman). These calcifications may occur at any age, appear most frequently in the cervical spine, and do, on occasion, disappear over a period of several months.

Herniated Disks

Since herniation of a disk fragment toward the spinal canal is best demonstrated by myelography, it is outside the scope of this text and thus is best relegated to a special monograph dealing with this subject. Disk fragmentation and herniation can, however, occur in any direction with respect to the intervertebral space. Disk herniation is most prevalent in the lower lumbar region and is rare in the thoracic region, although it can occur.

It may also occur with somewhat greater frequency in the cervical region. The most common site for a cervical herniated disk is at the fifth and sixth interspaces (Spurling and Segerberg).

Protrusion of a disk anteriorly may also occur (Batts).

"Vacuum Phenomenon" in Intervertebral Disks

DEFINITION AND COMMENT.   Radiolucent streaks in the intervertebral space presumably representing gas or a vacuum phenomenon in the intervertebral disk region. This is usually, but not invariably, associated with interspace narrowness. No specific clinical significance is attributed to this change. It may be observed in multiple disks (Gershon-Cohen et al.).

Hypervitaminosis A

Hypervitaminosis A may produce changes in the spine virtually indistinguishable from those of ankylosing spondylitis (Gerber et al.).

Unlike the situation found in ankylosing spondylitis, there may be a retention of clarity in the bony margin of the sacroiliac joint, and other calcium depositions may occur such as in the insertions of the anterior tibial spine, the quadriceps tendon, the periphery of the hip joint, shoulder joint, and in the iliolumbar ligaments.

GENERAL COMMENTS CONCERNING MYELOGRAPHY

1. Indications
2. Method of distinguishing intramedullary, extramedullary, and intradural or extradural lesions
3. Some lesions which can be identified by myelography

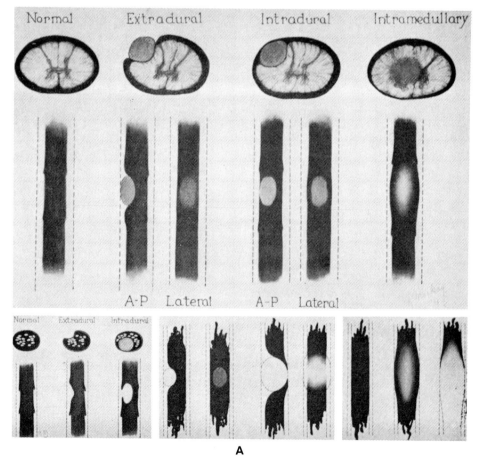

A

Figure 14–55   *A.* Methods of distinguishing intramedullary, extramedullary, and intradural or extradural lesions of the spinal canal. (Courtesy of John Camp, M.D.)

Figure 14–55 continued on opposite page.

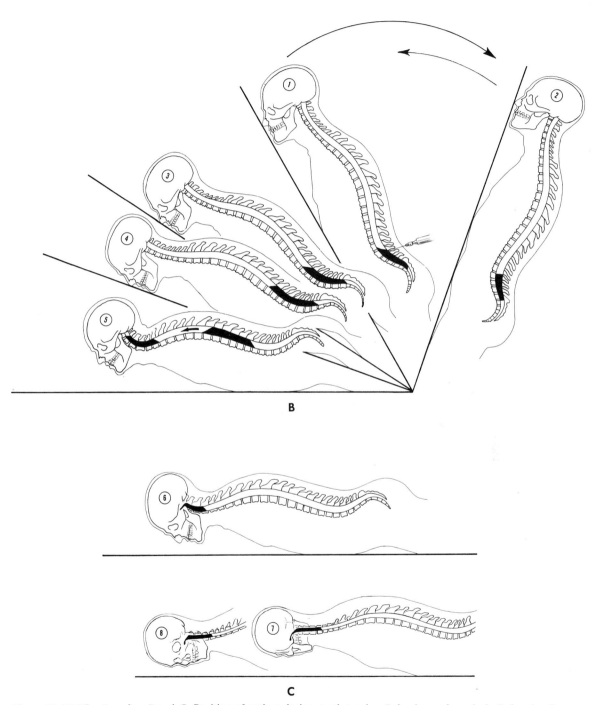

Figure 14–55 (*Continued*).   *B* and *C*. Position of patient during myelography: *B*. lumbar and cervical; *C*. for visualization of region of clivus and internal acoustic meati.

Figure 14–55 continued on following page.

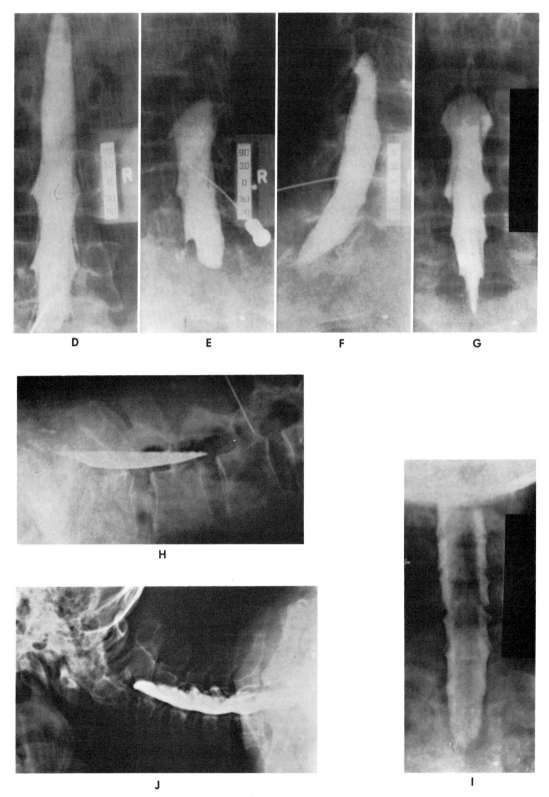

Figure 14–55 (*Continued*). *D* to *J*. Example radiographs of lumbar and cervical myelograms. *D* to *G*. Antero-posterior and oblique projections of lumbar myelograms; *H*. lateral horizontal beam study of lumbosacral myelogram; *I*. antero-posterior view of cervical myelogram; *J*. lateral horizontal beam study of cervical myelogram.

Figure 14–55 continued on opposite page.

Myelography (Shapiro; Epstein, 1969)

Definition.   Examination of the subarachnoid space of the spinal column by the injection of a suitable contrast material into this space. This contrast material may be gaseous or a positive contrast material such as Pantopaque.

Usual Procedure.   The usual procedure involves the injection of approximately 6 cc. or more of Pantopaque into the lumbar subarachnoid space. Pantopaque is usually removed following the procedure; if, however, small quantities do remain, they are slowly absorbed from the subarachnoid space over a period of approximately two years.

Indications.   This method of examination should be used only in accordance with the strictest care—depending upon when and where the technique has been completely mastered—and when sufficient experience has been accumulated in the interpretation of the results. It should be used only when surgical intervention following myelography is contemplated.

Myelography is Particularly Helpful in:

1. Demonstrating an operable lesion when the clinical and laboratory data are inconclusive.
2. Confirming or excluding an intraspinal lesion when all other methods have failed to establish a diagnosis.
3. Establishing the extent of a known lesion and possibly in giving some indication of its general pathologic nature.

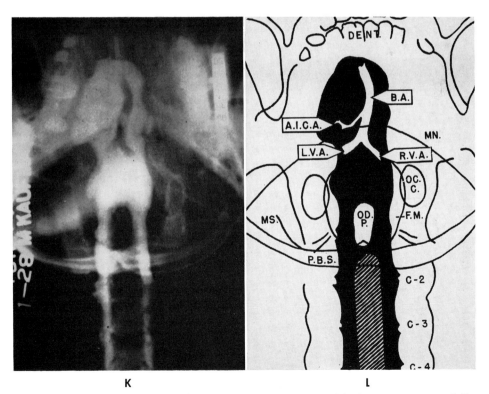

K   L

Figure 14–55 (*Continued*).   *K* and *L*. Normal antero-posterior views of the foramen magnum and clivus myelogram.

Figure 14–55 continued on following page.

4. Excluding multiple lesions, since approximately 4 per cent of spinal neoplasms are multiple.
5. Localizing the level of the lesion accurately prior to operation.
6. Determining the cause of recurrent symptoms in the patient with a previous laminectomy.
7. Medico-legal circumstances in which myelography may help to establish the presence or absence of a lesion, although a negative myelogram is not conclusive.

Methods of Distinguishing Intramedullary, Extramedullary, and Intradural or Extradural Lesions of the Spinal Canal (Figure 14–55).   These lesions include inflammatory lesions such as abscesses, hemorrhagic lesions such as hematoma, adhesions due to adhesive arachnoiditis, neoplasms, and herniated disks. It may not be possible on the basis of myelography alone to determine the exact nature of the lesion present. One may interpolate, however, by knowing whether the lesion is intramedullary, extramedullary but intradural, or extradural, especially when one relates this finding to the known incidence of disease processes in the spinal canal.

M

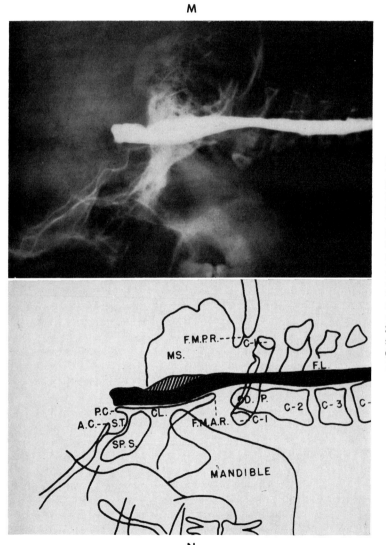

N

Figure 14–55 (*Continued*).   *M* and *N*. Normal cross-table (horizontal beam) lateral view in same position. B.A., basilar artery; A.I.C.A., anterior inferior cerebellar artery; L.V.A., left vertebral artery; R.V.A., right vertebral artery; OC. C., occipital condyle; OD. P., odontoid process; MS., mastoids; F.M., foramen magnum; P.B.S., posterior base of skull; F.M.P.R., foramen magnum posterior rim; F.M.A.R., foramen magnum anterior rim; CL, clivus; A.C., anterior clinoids; P.C., posterior clinoids; S.T., sella turcica; SP.S., sphenoid sinus; F.L., fluid level of Pantopaque. (From Malis, L. I.: Radiology *76*, 1958.)

Figure 14–55 continued on opposite page.

Subarachnoid myelography is employed most frequently to demonstrate herniated disks (Figure 14–56).

The performance of this procedure and the interpretation of findings are outside the scope of this text. Some other lesions which can be identified by this modality are:

1. Neurenteric cysts.
2. Diastematomyelia.
3. Meningoceles.
4. Traumatic avulsions of nerve roots.
5. Arachnoiditis.
6. Epidural adhesions.
7. Epidural and subdural infections.

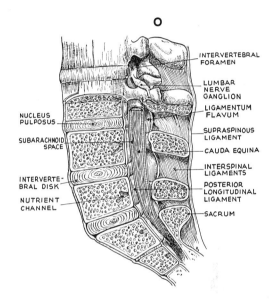

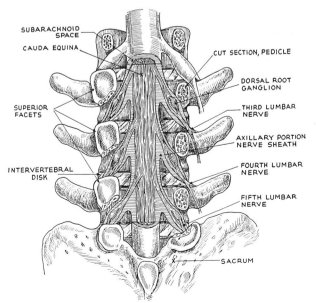

Figure 14–55 (*Continued*). *O*, Structure of intervertebral disk and its relationship to the subarachnoid space and adjoining ligamentous structures. *P*. Relationship of spinal nerve roots to axillary pouches of the subarachnoid space.

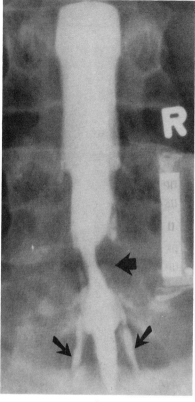

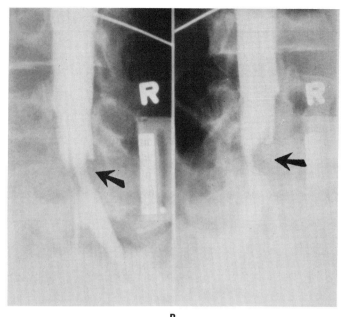

B

A

Figure 14–56   Myelogram demonstrating a herniated disk between L-4 and L-5 (*upper arrow*), producing an extradural type defect at this level and swollen nerve root sleeves (*lower arrows*). *A*. Frontal perspective. *B*. Oblique view.

8. Intraspinal dermoids, epidermoids, and dermal sinuses.
9. Intraspinal neoplasms.
10. Intraspinal lipomas.
11. Intraspinal meningeal tumor implants.
12. Archnoidal cysts.
13. Syringomyelia.
14. Intraspinal vascular malformations.
15. Spinal epidural hematomas.

Diagrammatic illustrations of some of these are shown in Figures 14–55 and 14–56.

Questions—Chapter 14

1. Indicate some of the abnormalities in number of vertebral segments.
2. Indicate several abnormalities in number of vertebral segments caused by faulty fusion of elements. Indicate five disease entities where this is primary.
3. What is meant by the term block vertebrae?
4. What is meant by the term occipital vertebra?
5. What is meant by the terms lumbarization and sacralization?
6. What is the clinical importance of congenital absence of the dens?
7. Name some of the "clefts in vertebrae" and indicate particularly how you would recognize a "butterfly" vertebra.

8. What is the clinical significance of cleft spinous processes?

9. What is the clinical significance of a meningocele and how would you recognize this radiologically? Where are meningoceles most frequently situated?

10. What type of abnormality of shape and size of vertebral segments is noted in Morquio's disease, Hurler's disease, achondroplasia, osteogenesis imperfecta, Marfan's syndrome, Cushing's syndrome, acromegaly, and hypothyroidism?

11. What alterations may be seen in vertebral bodies related to contiguous vascular structures?

12. What categories of abnormalities of radiodensity and architecture do we recognize?

13. In those diseases which produce homogeneous radiolucency of vertebrae, what differential features are there between sickle cell anemia and osteomalacia; osteoporosis and Cushing's syndrome; multiple myeloma and Ewing's sarcoma?

14. Name some of the disease entities which are responsible for the homogeneously sclerotic appearance of vertebrae.

15. Name some of the disease entities which are characterized by a spotted radiolucency of vertebrae.

16. Describe some of the differential features between tuberculous and nontuberculous involvement of vertebrae.

17. Describe some of the differential features of chordomas.

18. What is the general radiographic appearance of giant cell tumor, benign chondroblastoma, and aneurysmal bone cyst?

19. What are the most frequent sites of involvement of benign osteoblastoma? What is the most frequent radiographic appearance?

20. Define "vertebral epiphysitis." Is this truly an inflammatory process? What is the pathogenesis of lesions and what is their ultimate radiographic appearance?

21. Describe some of the traumatic changes in the spine. What are the most frequent appearances in the cervical region; the thoracic region, and the lumbosacral region?

22. Define the following terms: spondylolysis; spondylolisthesis; pseudospondylolisthesis; reverse spondylolisthesis?

23. Indicate five or six disease entities characterized by spotted osteosclerosis of vertebrae.

24. What are some of the clinical and radiologic features of tuberous sclerosis?

25. Describe some of the radiologic features of spinal lymphomas.

26. What is the radiographic appearance of an osteoid osteoma as it affects the spine?

27. Describe some of the radiographic appearances of urticaria pigmentosa as it affects the spine.

28. What is the most frequent lesion of vertebral bodies which is characterized by vertical irregular radiolucency and sclerosis?

29. What is the most frequent disease affecting vertebrae which is characterized by box-like sclerosis or a "picture frame" appearance? Is there a disease entity in infants which also produces this appearance?

30. What is the radiographic appearance in fibrous dysplasia as it affects the spine?

31. What differential features in respect to spur formation can you enumerate in respect to the following: spondylosis deformans; syphilitic spondylitis; ankylosing spondylitis; rheumatoid spondylitis?

32. Define the following terms: (1) scoliosis; (2) lordosis; (3) kyphosis; (4) gibbus; (5) primary curvature in scoliosis; (6) secondary curvature in scoliosis.

33. Describe two methods of measurement in scoliosis of the spine.

34. Describe two methods of recording and/or measuring lordosis of the lumbosacral region.

35. Name five diseases characterized by kyphosis and/or scoliosis which have a systemic origin.

36. What is characteristic of a "seat belt" fracture?

37. What is characteristic of a "whiplash spine injury"?

38. What is meant by occipital vertebra?

39. Define platybasia.

40. How does Arnold-Chiari malformation affect the spine?

41. Describe the deformity in Klippel-Feil deformity.

42. What is meant by "hemivertebrae"?

43. What is meant by atlantoaxial subluxation and what are some of its causes?

44. What types of joints are found in the spine? Which of these are synovial joints?

45. Describe the radiologic findings in ochronosis.

46. Describe the differences which are generally recognized between ankylosing spondylitis and rheumatoid arthritis as it affects the spine in both the juvenile and adult.

47. What is neuropathic arthropathy of the spine?

48. What is characteristic of paraplegic neuroarthropathy as it affects the spine?

49. What is the radiographic appearance when the intervertebral disk is injured?

50. What is the radiographic appearance when infection involves the intervertebral disk? Name some agents which are responsible for this.

51. What is meant by the term "herniated disks"? Where is it found most frequently? How is it best demonstrated radiologically?

52. Define "vacuum phenomenon" as it affects the intervertebral disks.

53. What is the spine manifestation of hypervitaminosis A?

54. Relate some of the indications for myelography.

55. How would you distinguish between intramedullary, extramedullary, and intradural or extradural lesions of the spine?

56. List some lesions (approximately ten) which can be identified by myelography.

References

Abramson, D. J., and Kamberg, S.: Spondylitis, pathological ossification and calcification associated with spinal cord injury. J. Bone Joint Surg., 31-A:275–283, 1949.

Ackermann, W., and Schwarz, G. S.: Non-neoplastic sclerosis in vertebral bodies. Cancer, 11:703–798, 1958.

Albright, F.: Osteoporosis. Ann. Intern Med., 27:861–882, 1947.

Albright, F., and Reifenstein, E. C. Jr.: Parathyroid Glands and Metabolic Bone Disease. Baltimore, Williams and Wilkins Co., 1948.

Albright, F., Bennett, C. H., Parson, W., Reifenstein, E. C. Jr., and Roos, A.: Osteomalacia and late rickets. Medicine 25:399–479, 1946.

Albright, F., Butler, A. M., Hampton, A. O., and Smith, P.: Syndrome characterized by osteitis fibrosa disseminata. New Eng. J. Med., 216, 727–746, 1937.

Alexander, E., Jr., and Nashold, B. S. Jr.: Agenesis of the sacrococcygeal region. J. Neurosurg., 13:507–513, 1956.

Baggenstass, A. H., Bickel, W. H., and Ward, L. E.: Rheumatoid granulomatous nodules as destructive lesions of vertebrae. J. Bone Joint Surg., 34-A:601–609, 1952.

Bailey, D. K.: The normal cervical spine in infants and children. Radiology, 59:712–719, 1952.

Barer, M., Peterson, L. F. A., Dahlin, W. H., Winkelman, P. K., and Stewart, J. R.: Mastocytosis with osseous lesions resembling metastatic malignant lesions in bone. J. Bone Joint Surg., 50-A:142–152, 1968.

Barton, C. J., and Cockshott, W. P.: Bone changes in hemoglobin S-C disease. Amer. J. Roentgenol., 88:523–532, 1962.

Batts, M. Jr.: Rupture of the nucleus pulposus. J. Bone Joint Surg., 21:121–126, 1939.

Beadle, O. A.: The intervertebral disks: Observations of their normal and morbid anatomy in relation to certain spinal deformities. Med. Res. Council, 161:1, 1931.

Becker, J. A.: Hemoglobin S-C disease. Amer. J. Roentgenol., 88:503–511, 1962.

Beetham, W. P. Jr., Kaye, R. L., and Polley, H. F.: Charcot's joints. Ann. Intern. Med., 58:1002–1012, 1963.

Begg, A. C., and Falconer, M. A.: Plain radiography in intraspinal protrusion of lumbar intervertebral disks. Correlation with operative findings. Radiology, 53:898, 1949.

Berggard, I., and Bearn, A. G.: The Hurler syndrome: A biochemical and clinical study. Amer. J. Med., 39:221–229, 1965.

Berk, R. N., and Brower, T. D.: Vertebral sarcoidosis. Radiology, 82:660–663, 1964.

Beveridge, B., Vaughan, B. F., and Walters, M. N. I.: Primary hyperparathyroidism and secondary renal failure with osteosclerosis. Fac. Radiol., 10:197–200, 1959.

Birkett, A. N.: Injuries and derangements of the spinal column. In Platt, G. H., ed.: Modern Trends in Orthopedics. New York, Paul B. Hoeber, 1950.

Biwaters, E. G. L., Dickson, A. St. J., and Scott, J. T.: Joint lesions of hyperparathyroidism. Ann. Rheum. Dis., 22:171–187, 1963.

Bland, J. H., Van Buskirk, F. W., Tampas, J. P., Brown, E., and Clayton, R.: A study of roentgenologic criteria for rheumatoid arthritis of the cervical spine. Amer. J. Roentgenol., 95:949–954, 1965.

Bland, J. H., Davis, P. H., London, M. G.,

Van Buskirk, F. W., and Duarte, C. G.: Rheumatoid arthritis of the cervical spine. Arch. Intern. Med., *112*:892–898, 1963.

Bligh, A. S.: Diastematomyelia. Clin. Radiol., *12*:58–63, 1961.

Boden, G.: Radiation myelitis of the brain stem. Fac. Radiol., *2*:79–94, 1950.

Boden, G.: Radiation myelitis of the cervical spinal cord. Brit. J. Radiol., *21*:464–469, 1948.

Boreadis, A. G., and Gershon-Cohen, J.: Luschka joints of the cervical spine. Radiology, *66*:181–187, 1956.

Brain, R.: Some aspects of the neurology of the cervical spine. J. Fac. Radiol., *8*:74–91, 1956.

Brown, M. W., Templeton, A. W., and Hodges, F. J. III: The incidence of acquired and congenital fusions in the cervical spine. Amer. J. Roentgenol., *92*:1255–1259, 1964.

Brunner, R.: Lateral intrathoracic meningocele. Acta Radiol., *51*:1–9, 1959.

Burkhart, J. M., Burke, E. C., and Kelly, P. J.: The chondrodystrophies. Proc. Mayo Clin. Bull., *40*:481–499, 1965.

Caffey, J.: Achondroplasia of the pelvis and lumbosacral spine. Amer. J. Roentgenol., *80*:449–457, 1968.

Caffey, J.: Cooley's anemia: a review of the roentgenographic findings in the skeleton. Amer. J. Roentgenol., *78*:381–391, 1957.

Caffey, J.: Gargoylism (Hunter-Hurler disease, dysostosis multiple lipochondrodystrophy). Amer. J. Roentgenol., *67*:715–731, 1952.

Caffey, J.: Pediatric X-ray Diagnosis. Fifth Edition. Chicago, Year Book Medical Publishers, 1967.

Caldicott, W. J. H.: Diagnosis of spinal osteoid osteoma. Radiology, *92*:1192–1195, 1969.

Calenoff, L.: Osteosclerosis from intentional ingestion of hydrofluoric acid. Amer. J. Roentgenol., *87*:1112–1115, 1962.

Calhoun, J. D., and Thompson, S. B.: Vertebra plana in children produced by xanthomatous disease. Amer. J. Roentgenol., *82*:482–489, 1959.

Camp. J. D.: Contrast myelography, past and present. Radiology, *54*:477–506, 1950.

Camp, J. D., and McCullough, J. A. L.: Pseudofractures in diseases affecting the skeletal system. Radiology, *36*:651–663, 1941.

Castro, A. F.: Presacral tumors. South. Med. J., *54*:969–977, 1961.

Cave, P.: Butterfly vertebrae. Brit. J. Radiology, *31*:503–506, 1958.

Cervenansky, J., Sitaj, S., and Urbanek, T.: Alkaptonuria and ochronosis. J. Bone Joint Surg. (Amer.), *41-A*:1169–1182, 1959.

Chester, W., and Chester, E. M.: Vertebral column in acromegaly. Amer. J. Roentgenol., *44*:552–557, 1940.

Child, A. E., and Tucker, F. R.: Spondylarthritis in infants and children. J. Canad. Ass. Radiol., *12*:47–51, 1961.

Cimmino, C. V., and Painter, J. W.: Iniencephaly. Radiology, *79*:942–944, 1962.

Clarke, E.: Spinal cord involvement in multiple myelomatosis. Brain, *79*:332–338, 1956.

Clark, H. O.: Scoliosis. In Platt, G. H., ed.: Modern Trends in Orthopedics. New York, Paul B. Hoeber, Inc., 1950.

Clifton, E. E., and Rydell, J. R.: Congenital dermal (pilonidal) sinus with dural connection. J. Neurosurg., *4*:276–282, 1947.

Cloward, R. B., and Buzaid, L. L.: Discography: technique, indications and evaluation of the normal and abnormal intervertebral disc. Amer. J. Roentgenol., *68*:552–564, 1952.

Cobb, J. R.: Outline for study of scoliosis. Instructional course Lecture. Amer. Acad. Orthoped. Surg., *5*:261–275, Ann Arbor, J. W. Edwards, 1948.

Cohen, J., Currarino, G., Neuhauser, E. B. D.: A significant variant in the ossification centers of the vertebral bodies. Amer. J. Roentgenol., *76*:469–475, 1956.

Craig, W. M., Svien, H. J., Dodge, H. W., and Camp, J. D.: Intraspinal lesions masquerading as protruded lumbar intervertebral discs. Radiology, *60*:464, 1953.

Crandall, P. H., and Batzdorf, U.: Cervical spondylotic myelopathy. J. Neurosurg., *25*:57–66, 1966.

Crawford, T., Dent, C. E., Lucas, P., Martin, N. H., and Nassim, J. R.: Osteosclerosis associated with renal failure. Lancet, *2*:981–988, 1954.

Cronqvist, S., and Fuchs, W.: Lumbar myelography in complete obstruction of the spinal canal. Acta Radiol. (Diagnosis) *2*:145–152, 1964.

Currarino, G., and Erlandson, M. E.: Premature fusion of epiphyses in Cooley's anemia. Radiology, *83*:656–664, 1964.

Currarino, G., Neuhauser, E. B. D., Reyersbach, G. C., Sobel, E. H.: Hypophosphatasia. Amer. J. Roentgenol., *78*:392–419, 1957.

Cushing, H.: Intracranial tumors. Notes upon a series of 2,000 verified cases with surgical mortality percentages pertaining thereto. Springfield, Charles C Thomas, 1932.

Dahlin, D. C., and MacCarty, C. S.: Chordoma. Cancer, *5*:1170–1178, 1952.

Dalton, C. J., and Schwartz, S. S.: Evaluation of the paraspinal line in roentgen examination of the thorax. Radiology, *66*:195–200, 1956.

Dassel, P. M.: Agenesis of the sacrum and coccyx. Amer. J. Roentgenol., *85*:697–700, 1961.

Daum, H. F., Smith, A. B., Walker, J. W., Chapman, S. B., and Eversman, G. H.: Protrusions of the lumbar disk: A correlation of the radiographic diagnosis and surgical findings. South. Med. J., *52*:1479–1484, 1959.

Daves, M. L., and Yardley, J. H.: Fibrous dysplasia of bone. Amer. J. Med. Sci., *234*:590–606, 1957.

Derry, D. E.: The influence of sex on the position and composition of the human sacrum. J. Anat. and Physiol. London, *46*:184–192, 1911–12.

Dickson, D. D., Camp, J. D., and Ghormley, R. K.: Osteitis deformans. Radiology, *44*:449–470, 1945.

Djindjian, R.: Arteriography of the spinal cord. Amer. J. Roentgenol., *107*:461–478, 1969.

Dorfman, A.: Heritable diseases of connective

tissue: The Hurler syndrome. In Stanbury, J. B., Wyngaarden, J. B., and Fredrickson, D. S., eds., The Metabolic Basis of Inherited Disease. Second Edition. New York, McGraw Hill, 1966. pp. 963–994.

Dresser, R., and Spencer, J.: Hodgkin's disease and allied conditions of bone. Amer. J. Roentgenol., 36:809–815, 1936.

Dugger, G. I., and Vandiver, R. W.: Spinal cord compression caused by vitamin D resistant rickets. J. Neurosurg., 25:300–303, 1966.

Dunlap, J. P., Morris, M., and Thompson, R. G.: Cervical spine injuries in children. J. Bone Joint Surg. (Amer.), 40-A:681–686, 1958.

Eastridge, C. E., Hughes, F. A. Jr., Hamman, J. L.: Cushing's syndrome in association with carcinoma of the respiratory tract. Ann. Thoracic Surg., 1:151–158, 1965.

Eban, R.: Idiopathic hypercalcemia of infancy. Clin. Radiol., 12:31–40, 1961.

Eklöf, O.: Roentgenologic findings in sacrococcygeal teratoma. Acta Radiol. (Diagnosis), 3:41–48, 1965.

Emery, J. L., and Lendon, R. G.: Lipomas of the cauda equina and other fatty tumors related to neurospinal dysraphism. Develop. Med. Child Neurol. (Suppl.) 20:62–70, 1969.

Engles, E. P., Smith, R. C., and Krantz, S.: Bone sclerosis in multiple myeloma. Radiology, 75:242–247, 1960.

Epstein, B. S., and Epstein, J. A.: Osteoarthritis and spondylosis of the spine. Rheum. 13: 82–87, 1957.

Epstein, B. S.: The Spine: A Radiologic Text and Atlas. Third Edition. Philadelphia, Lea and Febiger, 1969.

Erdheim, J.: Über Wirbelsaüleveranderungen bei Akromegalie. Virchow's Arch. f. Path. Anat., 281:197, 1931.

Erf, L. A., and Herbut, P. A.: Primary and secondary myelofibrosis. Ann. Intern. Med., 21: 863–889, 1944.

Evans, P. R.: Deformity of the vertebral bodies in cretinism. J. Pediat., 41:706–712, 1952.

Evison, G., and Evans, K. T.: Bone sclerosis in multiple myeloma. Brit. J. Radiol., 40:81–89, 1967.

Ewing, J. E.: Neoplastic Disease. Fourth Edition. Philadelphia, W. B. Saunders Co., 1940.

Fairbank, H. A. T.: Achondroplasia. J. Bone Joint Surg., 31-B:600–607, 1949.

Fairbank, H. A. T.: Chondro-osteodystrophy, Morquio-Brailsford type. J. Bone Joint Surg., 31-B:291–301, 1949.

Fairbank, H. A. T.: Osteopathia Striata. J. Bone Joint Surg., 32-B:117–125, 1950.

Faust, D. B., Gilmore, H. R. Jr., and Mudgett, C. S.: Chordomata. Ann. Intern. Med., 21: 678–698, 1944.

Feldman, F., and Seaman, W. B.: The neurologic complications of Paget's disease in the cervical spine. Amer. J. Roentgenol., 105: 375–382, 1969.

Ferguson, A. B.: The plane of the lumbosacral facets in relation to stability. In Roentgen Diagnosis of the Extremities and Spine. Second Edition. New York, Paul B. Hoeber, 1949.

Fiebelkorn, H. J.: Über Aufhellungsstreifen

(sog. Vakuum-Phänomen) in den lumbalen zwischen Wirbelscheiben. Fortschr. a. d. Geb. d. Roentgenstr., 81:601–605, 1954.

Fielding, J.: Cineroentgenography of the normal cervical spine. J. Bone Joint Surg. (Amer.), 39-A:1280–1288, 1957.

Finby, N., and Archibald, R. M.: Skeletal abnormality associated with gonadal dysgenesis. Amer. J. Roentgenol., 89:1222–1235, 1963.

Follmer, B.: Wirbelfrakturen bei Tetanuser Krankung (Spinal fractures in tetanus). Zbl. Chir., 77:411–416, 1952.

Forestier, J.: Sacroiliac changes in early diagnosis of ankylosing spondylosis. Radiology, 33: 389–402, 1939.

Frantz, C. H. and Aitken, G. T.: Complete absence of the lumbar spine and sacrum. J. Bone Joint Surg., 49-A:1531–1540, 1967.

Fraser, R.: The problem of osteoporosis. J. Bone Joint Surg., 44-B:485–495, 1962.

Freedman, E., and Meschan, I.: Syphilitic spondylitis. Amer. J. Roentgenol., 49:756–765, 1943.

Freiberger, R. H.: Osteoid osteoma of the spine: Cause of backache and scoliosis in children and young adults. Radiology, 75: 232–236, 1960.

George, K., and Rippstein, J.: Comparative study of two popular methods of measuring scoliotic deformity of the spine. J. Bone Joint Surg. (Amer.), 43-A:809–818, 1961.

Gerber, A., Raab, A. P., and Sobel, A. E.: Vitamin A poisoning in adults. Amer. J. Med., 16:729–745, 1954.

Gershon-Cohen, J., Schraer, H., Sklaroff, D. M., and Blumberg, N.: Dissolution of the intervertebral disk in the aged normal. The phantom nucleus pulposus. Radiology, 62:383–387, 1954.

Giannini, M. J., Borrelli, F. J., and Greenberg, W. H.: Agenesis of the vertebral bodies, a cause of dwarfism. Amer. J. Roentgenol., 59:705–711, 1948.

Giraudi, G.: Contributo anatomico e radiologico alla conoscenza delle "articolazioni sacro-iliache accessorie" (Diartrosi sacro-iliache dorsali). Radiol. Med., 23:987–994, 1936.

Glay, A., and Rona, G.: Nodular rheumatoid vertebral lesions versus ankylosing spondylitis. Amer. J. Roentgenol., 94:631–638, 1965.

Goff, C. W., and Aldes, J. H.: Fractures and dislocations of the neck. Med. Sci., 15:45–50, 1964.

Good, A. E.: Involvement of the back in Reiter's syndrome. Ann. Intern. Med., 57:44–59, 1962.

Griffith, G. C., Nichols, G. Jr., Asher, J. D., and Flanagan, B.: Heparin osteoporosis. J.A.M.A., 193:91–94, 1965.

Gwinn, J. L., and Smith, J. L.: Acquired and congenital absence of odontoid process. Amer. J. Roentgenol., 88:424–431, 1962.

Hadley, L. A.: Accessory sacroiliac articulations with arthritic changes. Personal communication.

Hadley, L. A.: Anatomico-Roentgenographic Studies of the Spine. Springfield, Charles C Thomas, 1964.

Hadley, L. A.: The covertebral articulations and

cervical foramen encroachment. J. Bone Joint Surg. (Amer.), *39-A*:910–920, 1957.

Hadley, L. A.: Value of routine plain roentgenograms in the diagnosis of sacral perineurial cysts. Amer. J. Roentgenol., *84*:119–124, 1960.

Hadley, L. A.: Congenital absence of a pedicle from cervical vertebrae. Amer. J. Roentgenol., *55*:193–197, 1946.

Halaby, F. A., Peterson, R. B., and Leaver, R. C.: Spinal lipoma Amer. J. Roentgenol., *92*:1293–1297, 1964 (16 ref.).

Hamburg, A. E.: Skeletal changes in sickle cell anemia. J. Bone Joint Surg., *32-A*:893–900, 1950.

Harris, W. H., Dudley, H. R. Jr., and Barry, R. J.: A natural history of fibrous dysplasia. J. Bone Joint Surg., *44-A*:207–233, 1962.

Heinbecker, P.: Cushing syndrome. Ann. Surg., *124*:252–261, 1946.

Hinck, V. C., Clark, W. M. Jr., and Hopkins, C. E. Normal interpediculate distance; minimum and maximum in children and adults. Amer. J. Roentgenol., *97*:141–153, 1966.

Hinck, V. C.: Cervical fracture dislocation in rheumatoid spondylitis. Amer. J. Roentgenol., *82*:257, 1959.

Hinck, V. C., and Hopkins, C. E.: Measurement of the atlanto-dental interval in the adult. Amer. J. Roentgenol., *84*:945–951, 1960.

Hinck, V. C., Hopkins, C. E., and Savara, B. S.: The sagittal diameter of the cervical spinal canal in children. Radiology, *79*:97–108, 1962 (14 ref.).

Hodges, P. C., Phemister, D. B., and Brunschwig, A.: Charcot's neuropathic lesion of the spine. New York, Thomas Nelson and Sons, 1941.

Holland, H. W.: Charcot's arthropathy of the spine. Brit. J. Radiology, *25*:267–269, 1952.

Hollander, J. L., Fogarty, C. W. Jr., Abrams, N. R., and Kydd, D. M.: Arthritis resembling Reiter's syndrome. J.A.M.A., *129*:593–595, 1945.

Horrigan, W. D., and Baker, D. H.: Gargoylism: a review of the roentgen skull changes with a description of a new finding. Amer. J. Roentgenol., *86*:473–477, 1961.

Howland, W. J. Jr., Pugh, D. G., and Sprague, R. G.: Roentgenologic changes in the skeletal system in Cushing syndrome. Radiology, *71*: 69–78, 1958.

Hulbert, K. F.: Congenital torticollis. J. Bone Joint Surg., *32-B*:50–59, 1950.

Hulten, O.: Ein Fall von "Elfenbeinwirbel" bei lymphogranulomatose. Acta Radiol., *8*:245, 1927.

Hundler, G. G.: Pathogenesis of Cushing's disease. Proc. Mayo Clin., *41*:29–39, 1966.

Hurwitz, L. J., and Shepherd, W. H. T.: Basilar impression and disordered metabolism of bone. Brain, *89*:223–234, 1966.

Ivie, J. M.: Congenital absence of the odontoid process. Radiology, *46*:268–269, 1946.

Jacobson, G., and Adler, D. C.: An evaluation of lateral atlanto-axial displacement in injuries of the cervical spine. Radiology, *61*:355–362, 1953.

Jacobson, G., and Bleecker, H. H.: Pseudo sub-

luxation of the axis in children. Amer. J. Roentgenol., *82*:472–481, 1959.

Jacobson, H. G., Poppel, M. H., Shapiro, J. H., and Grossberger, S.: The vertebral pedicle sign: A roentgen finding to differentiate metastatic carcinoma from multiple myeloma. Amer. J. Roentgenol., *80*:817–821, 1958.

Jaffe, H. L.: Tumors and Tumorous Conditions of the Bones and Joints. Philadelphia, Lea and Febiger, 1958.

Jaffe, M. D., and Willis, P. W. III: Multiple fractures associated with long term sodium heparin therapy. J. A. M. A., *193*:158–160, 1965.

James, W., and Moule, B.: Hypophosphatasia. Clin. Radiol., *17*:368–376, 1966.

Jones, M. D.: Cervical spine cineradiography after traffic accidents. Arch. Surg., *85*:974–981, 1962.

Katz, I., Rabinowitcz, J. G., and Dziadiw, R.: Early changes in Charcot's joints. Amer. J. Roentgenol., *86*:965–974, 1961.

Keats, T. E., and Burns, T. W.: Radiographic manifestations of gonadal dysgenesis. Radiol. Clin. N. Amer., *2*:297–313, 1964.

Key, J. A.: Intervertebral-disc lesions in children and adolescents. J. Bone Joint Surg., *32–A:* 97–102, 1950.

Khilnani, M. T., and Wolf, B. S.: Transverse diameter of the cervical spinal cord in pantopaque myelography. J. Neurosurg., *20*:660–664, 1963.

Kieffer, S. A., Nesbit, M. E., and D'Angio, G. J.: Vertebra plana due to histiocytosis X: serial studies. Acta Radiol. (Diagnosis) *8*:241–251, 1969.

Kittleson, A. C., and Lim, L. W.: Measurement of scoliosis. Amer. J. Roentgenol., *108*:775–777, 1970.

Knutsson, F.: Vacuum phenomenon in intervertebral disks. Acta Radiol., *23*:173–179, 1942.

Knutsson, F.: Vertebral genesis of idiopathic scoliosis in children. Acta Radiol. (Diagnosis) *4*:395–402, 1966.

Lang, E. K., and Bessler, W. T.: The roentgenologic features of acromegaly. Amer. J. Roentgenol., *86*:321–328, 1961.

Langer, L. O.: Diastrophic dwarfism in early infancy. Amer. J. Roentgenol., *93*:399–404, 1965.

Langer, L. O., and Carey, L. S.: The roentgenographic features of KS mucopolysaccharidosis of Morquio (Morquio-Brailsford disease). Amer. J. Roentgenol., *97*:1–20, 1966.

Langley, G. R., Sabean, H. B., and Sorger, K.: Sclerotic lesions of bone in myeloma. Canad. Med. Ass. J., *94*:940–946, 1966.

Lasorte, A. F., and Brown, N.: Ruptured anterior nucleus pulposus between T-1 and T-2 causing a discrete esophageal defect and minimal dysphagia. Amer. J. Surg., *98*:631–634, 1959.

Legre, J., and Serratrice, G.: Radiological aspects of primary tumors of the spine and their treatment (apropos of cases). J. de Radiol. Electrol., *41*:217–229, 1960. Quoted from Abstracts of radiological literature. Amer. J. Roentgenol., *85*:388–389, 1961.

Leigh, T. F., Corely, C. C. Jr., Huguley, C. M.

Jr., and Rogers, J. V. Jr.: Myelofibrosis: the general and radiologic findings in 25 proved cases. Amer. J. Roentgenol., *82*:183–193, 1959.

Leigh, T. H., and Rogers, J. V. Jr.: Anterior sacral meningocele. Amer. J. Roentgenol., *71*:808–812, 1954.

Lemmen, L. J., and Laing, P. G.: Fracture of the cervical spine in patients with rheumatoid arthritis. J. Neurosurg., *16*:542–550, 1959.

Lewis, S. M., Szur, L.: Malignant myelosclerosis. Brit. Med. J., *2*:472–477, 1963.

Liberson, M.: Soft tissue calcification in cord lesions. J. A. M. A., *152*:1010–1013, 1953.

Lintermans, J. P., and Seyhnaeve, V.: Hypothyroidism and vertebral anomalies: a new syndrome? Amer. J. Roentgenol., *109*:294–298, 1970.

Lipow, E. G.: Whiplash injuries. South. Med. J., *48*:1305–1311, 1955.

Locke, G. R., Gardner, J. I., and VanEpps, E. F.: Atlas-dens interval (ADI) in children. A survey based on 200 normal cervical spines. Amer. J. Roentgenol., *97*:135–140, 1966.

Lombardi, G., and Passerini, A.: Spinal cord tumors. Radiology, *76*:381–392, 1961.

Lott, G., and Klein, E.: Osteoporosis. Amer. J. Roentgenol., *94*:616–620, 1965.

Lowman, R. M., Bloor, C. M., and Newcomb, A. W.: Roentgen manifestations of thoracic extramedullary hematopoiesis. Dis. Chest., *44*:154–162, 1963.

MacCarty, W. C., and Lane, F. W., Jr.: Pitfalls of myelography. Radiology, *65*:663–670, 1955.

MacLellan, D. I., and Wilson, F. C.: Osteoid osteoma of the spine. J. Bone Joint Surg., *49–A*:111–121, 1967.

Maroteaux, P., and Lamey, M.: Hurler's disease, Morquio's disease and related mucopolysaccharidosis. J. Pediat., *67*:312–323, 1965.

Martel, W.: The occipito-atlanto-axial joints in rheumatoid arthritis and ankylosing spondylitis. Amer. J. Roentgenol., *86*:223–240, 1961.

Martel, W., Abell, M. R., and Duff, I. F.: Cervical spine involvement in lipoid dermatoarthritis. Radiology, *77*:613–617, 1961.

Martel, W., and Page, J. W.: Cervical vertebral erosions and subluxations in rheumatoid arthritis and ankylosing spondylitis. Arthritis, *3*:546–556, 1960.

Martel, W., Tishler, J. M.: Observations on the spine in mongoloidism. Amer. J. Roentgenol., *97*:630–638, 1966.

Matson, D. D., and Jerva, M. J.: Recurrent meningitis association with congenital lumbosacral dermal sinus tract. J. Neurosurg., *25*:288–297, 1966.

McCollum, D. E., and Odom, G. L.: Alkaptonuria, ochronosis and low back pain. J. Bone Joint Surg., *47–A*:1389–1392, 1965.

McCormack, L. J., Dockerty, M. B., and Ghormley, R. K.: Ewing's sarcoma. Cancer, *5*:85–99, 1952.

McKusick, V. A.: Heritable Disorders of Connective Tissue. Second Edition. St. Louis, C. V. Mosby Co., 1960.

McKusick, V. A.: Heritable disorders of connective tissue: the Hurler syndrome. J. Chronic Dis., *3*:360–389, 1956.

McRae, D. L.: The significance of abnormalities of the cervical spine. Amer. J. Roentgenol., *84*:3–25, 1960 (8 ref.).

McRae, D. L., and Barnum, A. S.: Occipitalization of the atlas. Amer. J. Roentgenol., *70*:23–46, 1953.

McRae, D. L., and Standen, J.: Roentgenologic findings in syringomyelia and hydromyelia. Amer. J. Roentgenol., *98*:695–703, 1966.

Melamed, A., and Ansfield, D. J.: Posterior displacement of lumbar vertebrae; classification and criteria for diagnosis of true retrodisplacement of lumbar vertebrae. Amer. J. Roentgenol., *58*:307–328, 1947.

Melnick, J. C., and Silverman, F. N.: Intervertebral disk calcification in childhood. Radiology, *80*:399–408, 1963.

Meschan, I.: A radiographic analysis of spondylolisthesis. Med. J. Aust., *1*:465–469, 1946.

Meschan, I.: Radiographic study of spondylolisthesis with special reference to stability determination. Radiology, *47*:249–262, 1946.

Meschan, I.: Spondylolisthesis: commentary on etiology and improved method of roentgenographic mensuration and detection of instability. Amer. J. Roentgenol., *53*:230–243, 1945.

Meschan, I., Scruggs, J. G. Jr., and Calhoun, J. D.: Convulsive fractures of dorsal spine following electro-shock therapy. Radiology, *43*:180, 1950.

Milkman, L. A.: Multiple spontaneous idiopathic symmetrical fractures. Amer. J. Roentgenol., *32*:622–634, 1934.

Miller, G. A., Ridley, M., and Medd, W. E.: Typhoid osteomyelitis of the spine. Brit. Med. J., *1*:1068–1069, 1963.

Mitoma, C. et al.: Improvement in methods of measuring hydroxylproline. J. Lab. Clin. Med., *53*:970–976, 1959.

Möes, C. A. F.: Spondylarthritis in childhood. Amer. J. Roentgenol., *91*:578–587, 1964.

Moore, J. E.: Spina bifida with report of 384 cases treated by excision. Surg. Gynec. Obst., *1*:137–140, 1905.

Moseley, J. E.: Patterns of bone changes in the malignant lymphomas. J. Mt. Sinai Hosp., *29*:463–503, 1962.

Moseley, J. E.: Patterns of bone changes in the sickle cell states. J. Mt. Sinai Hosp., *26*:424–439, 1959.

Mulcahy, F.: Bone changes in myelosclerosis. Proc. Royal Soc. Med., *50*:100–103, 1957.

Munk, J., Peyser, E., and Gellei, B.: Osteoid osteoma of the frontal bone. Brit. J. Radiol. *33*:328–330, 1960.

Murray, R. O., and Jacobson, H. G.: The Radiology of Skeletal Disorders. Baltimore, Williams and Wilkins Co., 1971.

Nathan, H.: Osteophytes of the vertebral column. J. Bone Joint Surg., *44–A*:243–268, 1962.

Nelson, J. D.: The Marfan syndrome with special reference to congenital enlargement of the spinal canal. Brit. J. Radiol., *31*:561–564, 1958.

Neuhauser, E. B. D., Wittenborg, M. H., and Dehlinger, K.: Diastematomyelia. Transfixation of cord or cauda equina with congenital anomalies of the spine. Radiology, *54*:659–664, 1950.

Nicholas, J. A., Wilson, P. D., and Frieberger,

R.: Pathological fractures of spine: etiology and diagnosis. J. Bone Joint Surg., *42–A*:127–137, 1960.

Norman, A., and Kambolis, C. P.: Tumors of the spine and their relationship to the intervertebral disk. Amer. J. Roentgenol., *92*:1270–1274, 1964.

Ochsner, H. C., and Moser, R. H.: "Ivory vertebrae." Amer. J. Roentgenol., *29*:635–637, 1933.

Oppenheimer, A.: Rickets of spinal column. Radiol. Clin. N. Amer., *8*:332, 1939.

Overton, L. M., and Ghormely, R. K.: Congenital fusion of the spine. J. Bone Joint Surg., *16*:929–934, 1934.

Overton, L. M., and Grossman, J. W.: Anatomical variations in the articulations between the second and third cervical vertebrae. J. Bone Joint Surg. (Amer.), *34–A*:155–161, 1952.

Park, W. M., and O'Brien, W.: Computer-assisted analysis of radiographically diagnosed neck lesions in chronic rheumatoid arthritis. Acta Radiol. (Diagnosis), *8*:529–535, 1969.

Patterson, H. A., and Byerly, G.: Esophageal obstruction due to lesions of the cervical spine. Ann. Surg., *147*:863–867, 1958.

Perman, E.: Hemangiomata in the spinal column. Acta Chir. Scand., *61*:91–105, 1926.

Pirkey, E. L., and Purcell, J. H.: Agenesis of lumbosacral vertebrae. Radiology, *69*:726–729, 1957.

Poker, N., Finby, N., Archibald, R. M.: Spondylo-epiphyseal dysplasia tarda: four cases in childhood and adolescence, and some consideration regarding platyspondyly. Radiology, *85*:474–480, 1965.

Poppel, M. H., Gruber, W. F., Silber, R., Holder, A. K., and Christman, R. O.: Roentgen manifestations of urticaria pigmentosa (mastocytosis). Amer. J. Roentgenol., *82*:239–249, 1959.

Porretta, C. A., Dahlin, D. C., and Janes, J. M.: Sarcoma in Paget's disease of bone. J. Bone Joint Surg., *39–A*:1314–1329, 1957.

Rabinowitz, J. G., and Moseley, J. E.: The lateral lumbar spine in Down's syndrome. Radiology, *83*:74–79, 1964.

Ravitch, M. M., and Smith, E. I.: Sacrococcygeal teratoma in infants and children. Surgery, *30*:733–762, 1951.

Reed, R. J.: Fibrous dysplasia of bone. Arch. Path., *75*:480–495, 1963.

Reinhardt, K.: Asoma an der lendenwirbelsaule. Fortschr. Roentgenstr., *99*:197–203, 1963.

Reynolds, J.: A re-evaluation of "fish vertebrae" sign in sickle cell hemoglobinopathy. Amer. J. Roentgenol., *97*:693–707, 1966.

Richards, A. J.: Non-tuberculous pyogenic osteomyelitis of the spine. J. Canad. Ass. Radiol., *11*:45–49, 1960.

Robins, M. M., Stevens, H. F., and Linker, A.: Morquio's disease: an abnormality of mucopolysaccharide metabolism. J. Pediat., *62*:881–889, 1963.

Rodman, T., Funderburk, E. E., Jr., and Myerson, R. M.: Sarcoidosis with vertebral involvement. Ann. Intern. Med., *50*:213–218, 1959.

Rose, G. A.: Radiological diagnosis of osteoporosis, osteomalacia, and hyperparathyroidism. Clin. Radiol., *15*:75–83, 1964.

Rosendahl-Jenson, S.: Fibrous dysplasia of the vertebral column. Acta Chir. Scand., *111*:490–494, 1956.

Rowlands, B. C.: Anterior sacral meningocele. Brit. J. Surg., *43*:301–304, 1955.

Rowley, K. A.: Coronal cleft vertebrae. J. Fac. Radiol., *6*:267–274, 1955.

Rubin, P., Duthie, R. B., and Young, L. W.: The significance of scoliosis in post-irradiated Wilms' tumor and neuroblastoma. Radiology, *79*:539–559, 1962.

Rubin, S., and Stratemeier, E. H.: Intrathoracic meningocele. Radiology, *58*:552–555, 1952.

Sacks, S.: Alkaptonuric arthritis: Report of a case. J. Bone Joint Surg. (Brit), *33–B*:407–414, 1951.

Saenger, E. L.: Spondylarthritis in children. Amer. J. Roentgenol., *64*:20–31, 1950.

Salmon, D. D.: Hereditary cleidocranial dysostosis. Radiology, *42*:391–395, 1944.

Sanfillipo, S. J., Podosin, R., Langer, L., and Good, R. A.: Mental retardation associated with acid mucopolysacchariduria (heparin sulfate type). J. Pediat., *63*:837–838, 1963.

Sayle, B. A., Lange, P. A., Green, W. O. Jr., Bosworth, W. C., and Gregory, R.: Cushing's syndrome due to islet cell carcinoma of pancreas. Ann. Intern. Med., *63*:58–68, 1965.

Schmorl, G.: Osteitis deformans of Paget. Virchow's Arch. Path. AMAT *283*:694–751, 1932 (Über Osteitis deformans Paget).

Schmorl, G., and Junghans, H.: Die Gesunde und Kranke Wirbelsaule in Röntgenbild und Klinik. Second Edition. Stuttgart, Georg Thieme Verlag, 1951.

Schmorl, G., and Junghans, H.: The radiographic picture of the spine in health and disease. Die Gesunde und die Kranke Wirbelsaule in Röntgenbild und Klinik. Stuttgart, Georg Thieme Verlag, 1957. Translated and edited by Wilk, S. P., and Goin, L. S. New York, Grune and Stratton, 1959.

Schreiber, M. H., and Richardson, G. A.: Paget's disease confined to one lumbar vertebra. Amer. J. Roentgenol., *90*:1271–1276, 1963.

Schorr, S., Frankel, M., and Adler, E.: Right unilateral thoracic spondylosis. J. Fac. Radiol., *8*:59–65, 1956.

Schultz, E. H., Jr., Levy, R. W., and Russo, R. E.: Agenesis of the odontoid process. Radiology, *67*:102–105, 1956.

Schurr, P. H.: Sacro-extradural cyst. J. Bone Joint Surg., *37–B*:601–605, 1955.

Schwartz, D. T., and Alpert, M.: The malignant transformation of fibrous dysplasia. Amer. J. Med. Sci., *247*:1–20, 1964.

Seaman, W. B., and Wells, J.: Destructive lesions of the vertebral bodies in rheumatoid disease. Amer. J. Roentgenol., *86*:241–250, 1961 (25 ref.).

Shapiro, R.: Myelography. Chicago, Year Book Publishers, 1962.

Sharp, J., and Purser, D. W.: Spontaneous atlanto-axial dislocation in ankylosing spondylitis and rheumatoid arthritis. Ann. Rheum. Dis., *20*:47–77, 1961.

Sherman, R. S., and Wilner, D.: The roentgen diagnosis of hemangioma of bone. Amer. J. Roentgenol., *86*:1146–1159, 1961 (60 ref.).

Shiers, J. A., Neuhauser, E. B. D., and Bowman,

J. R.: Idiopathic hypercalcemia. Amer. J. Roentgenol., *78*:19–29, 1957.

Singh, H. A., Dass, R., Hayredh, S. S., and Jolly, S. S.: Skeletal changes in endemic fluorosis. J. Bone Joint Surg., *44–B*:806–815, 1962.

Singleton, E. B.: The radiographic features of severe idiopathic hypercalcemia of infancy. Radiology, *68*:721–726, 1957.

Sissons, H. A.: The osteoporosis of Cushing syndrome. J. Bone Joint Surg., *38–B*:418–433, 1956.

Smith, C. F., Pugh, D. G., and Polley, H. F.: Physiologic vertebral ligamentous calcification: An aging process. Amer. J. Roentgenol., *74*:1049–1058, 1955.

Smith, R. W. Jr., Eyler, W. R., and Mellinger, R. C.: On the incidence of senile osteoporosis. Ann. Intern. Med., *52*:773–781, 1960.

Smith, W. S., and Kaufer, H.: New pattern of spine injury associated with lap-type seat belts: preliminary report. Univ. Mich. Med. Center. J., *33*:99–104, 1967.

Snure, H., and Maner, G. D.: Metastatic malignancy in bone. Radiology, *28*:172–177, 1937.

Sole-Llenas, J., Rotes-Querol, J., Dalmau-Ciria, M.: Radiologic aspects of spinal brucellosis. Acta Radiol. (Diagnosis), *5*:1132–1139, 1966.

Solovay, J., and Solovay, H. U.: Paraplegic neuroarthropathy. Amer. J. Roentgenol., *61*:475–481, 1949.

Spillane, J. D.: Achondroplasia. J. Neurol. Neurosurg. Psychiat., *15*:246–252, 1952.

Spitz, S., and Higginbotham, N. L.: Osteogenic sarcoma following prophylactic roentgen ray therapy. Cancer, *4*:1107–1112, 1951.

Spitzer, R., Rabinowitch, J. Y., and Wybar, K. C.: A study of the abnormalities of the skull, teeth and lenses in mongolism. Canad. Med. Ass. J., *84*:567–572, 1961.

Spurling, R. G., and Segerberg, L. H.: Lateral intervertebral disk lesions in the lower cervical region. Radiology, *61*:853, 1953.

Stein, F., Block, H., and Kenin, A.: Nontraumatic subluxation of the atlanto-axial articulation: Report of a case. J. A. M. A., *152*:131–132, 1953.

Steinbach, H. L., Gordon, G. S., Eisenberg, E., Crane, J. T., Silverman, S., and Goldman, L.: Primary hyperparathyroidism: a correlation of roentgen, clinical and pathologic features. Amer. J. Roentgenol., *86*:329–343, 1961.

Steinbach, H. L., and Noetzli, M.: Roentgen appearances of the skeleton in osteomalacia and rickets. Amer. J. Roentgenol., *91*:955–972, 1964.

Stevens, R. H.: Radium poisoning. Radiology, *39*:39–47, 1942.

Sujoy, E.: Spinal lesions in tetanus in children. Pediatrics, *29*:629–635, 1962.

Summey, T. J., and Pressley, C. L.: Sarcoma complicating Paget's disease of bone. Ann. Surg., *123*:135–153, 1946.

Swedberg, M.: Meningocele and myelomeningocele studied by gas myelography. Acta Radiol., *1*:796–805, 1963.

Swenson, P. C., Teplick, J. G.: Ewing's sarcoma. Radiology, *45*:594–598, 1945.

Tampas, J. P., and Lurie, P. R.: The roentgeno-graphic appearance of the chest in children with functional murmurs. Amer. J. Roentgenol., *103*:78–86, 1968.

Tanz, J. S.: To-and-fro motion range at the 4th and 5th lumbar interspaces. J. Mount Sinai Hosp., *16*:303–307, 1950.

Taybi, H.: Diastrophic dwarfism. Radiology, *80*:1–10, 1963.

Templeton, A. W., Jaconette, J. R., and Ormond, R. S.: Localized osteosclerosis and hyperparathyroidism. Radiology, *78*:955–957, 1962.

Teng, P., and Papatheodorou, C.: Combined cervical and lumbar spondylosis. Arch. Neurol., *10*:298–307, 1964.

Thoms, J.: Cleidocranial dysostosis. Acta Radiol., *50*:514–520, 1958.

Townsend, E. H., Jr., and Rowe, M.: Mobility of the upper cervical spine in health and disease. Pediatrics, *10*:567–573, 1952.

Treasure, E. R.: Benign chondroblastoma of bone. J. Bone Joint Surg., *37–B*:462–465, 1955.

Trotter, M.: Common anatomical variations in the sacroiliac regions. J. Bone Joint Surg., *22*:293–299, 1940.

Twigg, H. L., de Leon, A. C., Perloff, J. K., and Majd, M.: Straight back syndrome. Radiographic manifestations. Radiology, *88*:274–277, 1967.

Twigg, H. L., Zvaifler, N. J., and Nelson, C. W.: Chondrocalcinosis. Radiology, *82*:655–659, 1964.

Vaughan, B. F., and Walters, M. N. I.: Sclerotic banded vertebrae (Rugger-jersey sign). J. Coll. Radiol. Austr., *7*:87–92, 1963.

Verbiest, H.: Giant cell tumors and aneurysmal bone cysts of the spine. J. Bone Joint Surg., *47–B*:699, 1965.

Vestermark, S.: Osteochondrodystrophia deformans with mucopolysaccharidosis. Arch. Dis. Child., *40*:106–110, 1965.

Waine, H., Bennett, G. A., and Bauer, W.: Joint disease associaed with acromegaly. Amer. J. Med. Sci., *209*:671–687, 1945.

Walker, J. W.: Benign bone tumors in pediatric practice. Radiology, *58*:662–673, 1952.

Weens, H. S.: Calcification of intervertebral disks in children. J. Pediat., *26*:178–188, 1945.

Weinfeld, A., Ross, M. W., Sarasohn, S. H.: Spondylo-epiphyseal dysplasia tarda. Amer. J. Roentgenol., *101*:851–859, 1967.

Weston, W. J., and Goodson, G. M.: Vertebra plana (Calvé). J. Bone Joint Surg. (Brit.) *41–B*:477–485, 1959.

Whalen, J. P., and Woodruff, C. L.: Cervical prevertebral fat stripe: a new aid in evaluating the cervical prevertebral soft tissue space. Amer. J. Roentgenol., *109*:445–451, 1970.

Whitaker, P. H.: Radiological manifestations of tuberous sclerosis. Brit. J. Radiol., *32*:152–156, 1959.

Whitley, J. E., and Forsyth, H. F.: The classification of cervical spine injuries. Amer. J. Roentgenol., *83*:633–644, 1960.

Wholey, M. H., Bruwer, A. J., and Baker, H. L., Jr.: Lateral roentgenogram of neck; with comments on atlanto-odontoid-basion relationship. Radiology, *71*:350–356, 1958.

Wholey, M. H., Pugh, D. G., and Bickel, W. H.: Localized destructive lesions in rheumatoid spondylitis, Radiology, 74:54–56, 1960.

Wilkinson, H. A., LeMay, M. L., and Ferris, E. J.: Roentgenographic correlation in cervical spondylosis. Amer. J. Roentgenol., 105:370–374, 1969.

Williams, H. J., and Pugh, D. G.: Vertebral epiphysitis: a comparison of the clinical and roentgenologic findings. Amer. J. Roentgenol., 90:1236–1247, 1963.

Wilner, H. I., and Finby, N.: Skeletal manifestations in the Marfan syndrome. J. A. M. A., 187:490–495, 1964.

Wilson, C. B., and Norrell, H. A., Jr.: Congenital absence of a pedicle in the cervical spine. Amer. J. Roentgenol., 97:639–647, 1966.

Wolf, B. S., Khilnani, M., and Malis, L.: Sagittal diameter of the bony cervical spinal canal and its significance in cervical spondylosis. J. Mount Sinai Hosp., 23:283–292, 1956.

Wollin, D. G.: The os odontoideum. J. Bone Joint Surg., 45–A:1459–1471, 1963.

Woodruff, F. P., and Dewing, S. B.: Fracture of the cervical spine in patients with ankylosing spondylitis. Radiology, 80:17–21, 1963.

YaDeau, R. E., Clagett, O. T., and Divertie, M. B.: Intrathoracic meningocele. J. Thoracic Cardiovasc. Surg., 49:202–209, 1965.

Yentis, I.: Radiological aspects of myelomatosis. Clin. Radiol., 12:1–7, 1961.

Zatz, L. M., Burgess, P. W., and Hanberry, J. W.: Agenesis of a pedicle in the cervical spine. J. Neurosurg., 20:564–569, 1963.

Zellweger, H., Ponsetti, I. V., Pedrini, V., Stamler, F. S., VonNoorden, G. K.: Morquio-Ullrich's disease. J. Pediat., 59:549–561, 1961.

Zitnan, D., and Sit'aj, S.: Chondrocalcinosis articularis. Ann. Rheum. Dis., 22:142–152, 1963.

Zucker, G., and Marder, M. J.: Charcot's spine due to diabetic neuropathy. Amer. J. Med., 12:118–124, 1952.

INDEX

Note: numbers in *italics* indicate pages containing illustrations.

Syndromes and signs are listed alphabetically under *Syndrome* and *Sign* as well as under their adjectival and eponymic names.

Abdomen
   abscesses within, recognized on plain films, *1226*
   calcification 1279, *1280, 1281, 1282*, 1283, *1284*, 1288
      in infancy and early childhood, 1287
   contents of, displacement with subdiaphragmatic abscess, 759
   displacement of organs outside, *757*
   extraluminal gas patterns, *1276, 1277*
      classification of, 1271
      caused by trauma, *1275*
      in abscess pockets, 1274
      in biliary tree, *1272*
      in cystitis emphysematosis of urinary bladder and gallbladder, 1278
      in portal venous system, 1277
      in vaginitis emphysematosa, 1279
      projected over liver, 1274
   flank area
      anatomy of, *1220*, 1221
      and abdominal wall, 1225
   fluid levels within, *1222*
      appearance separating loops of bowel, *1227*
   free air beneath diaphragm, *1223*
   gastrointestinal loops, displacement by ovarian cyst, *1230*
   gastrointestinal tract, rotation of bowel, *1259*
   hematoma (retroperitoneal), *1227*
   hernia, *1253*
   increased pressure in, shown by Valsalva and Mueller tests, 755
   intestine(s). See also *Intestine, small,* and *Colon.*
      as sign in peritonitis, 1232–1233
      large
         differentiation from small intestine, *1222*
         haustrations of, *1222*
         isolated distention of small portions, 1257
         volvulus of, 1257
      small
         coiled spring appearance, *1229*
         differentiation from large intestine, *1222*
         malrotation, 1263
         nonrotation of, 1263
         reverse rotation, 1263
         valvulae conniventes, *1222*, 1241
         volvulus of, 1255

Abdomen (*Continued*)
   kidneys, abnormalities on plain film, 1223
   masses in
      associated with elevation of diaphragm, 750
      identification of, 1288
      in children, 1290–1292
   median section of, *1702*
   plain film study, 1223, *1224*, 1225, *1226*, 1246
   psoas shadows on plain films, 1225
   roentgen signs of abnormality, 1222, 1251
   routine films, 1217–1219, *1219*
   trauma
      and sequelae, *1226*
      roentgenologic signs of, *1230*
   urinary tract abnormalities on plain films, *1224*
   vascular disease, on plain film, 1246, 1248
   vasculature changes in position of abdominal aorta, 1289
   "vector principle"
      in diagnosis of abdominal masses, 1265
      in relation to displacement of intra-abdominal organs, *1264*
   wall
      abnormalities of, 1222, 1304
      anatomy of, *1220,* 1221
      and flank area, 1225
Abdomen, and urinary tract (radiologic study of abdomen without added contrast media), 1217–1309
Abdominal disease
   associated with changes in mediastinum, 1030
Abscess
   amebic, of liver, 1297
   and colon, 1790
   and regional enteritis, 1717
   Brodie's, 66, *285, 287, 288, 289, 354, 356*
   "cold," of tuberculosis, 403
   granulomatous, of bone, 66
   intra-abdominal, *1229*
      Crohn's disease, 1717
      demonstrating extraluminal gas, 1274
      differentiation from fecal material, 1269
      in sac of lesser omentum, *1704*
      perisigmoidal, *1268*
      with speckled gas appearance, 1267, *1273*
   intracranial, 580, 585
   of appendix, *1848*
   of kidney, 1353, 1454, 1455

Abdomen (*Continued*)
  of lung, 857, 894, 895, 896, 897, 920
    connecting with pleura, 895
    with aspiration pneumonia, 857
    with pneumatocele, 874
  of psoas muscle, *1404*
  paraspinous, *1012*
    simulating mediastinal tumor, 1057
  periapical, *548*
    in hyperparathyroidism, *240*
  perirenal, 1454
  perisigmoidal, *1226*
  peritoneal, in neonate, *1761*
  psoas, *1284*
    in tuberculosis, 403
  pulmonary, and cavitation, *1004*
  retroperitoneal, *1226*, 1228
  splenic, roentgenographic diagnosis of, 1300
  subhepatic, *1226, 1273*
  subphrenic, *1226*
Accessory diaphragm, 758
Acetabular angle, *213*, 213 (table)
Acetabular dysplasia, 147
Acetone, as cause of pneumoconiosis, 929
Achalasia
  and tracheal displacement, 794
  of esophagus, *1554*
Achondrogenesis, 204
Achondroplasia, 94, 201, 202, 627, 774, 1873
  and changes of thoracic cage, 770
    roentgenologic signs of, 775
  and spinal malalignment, *673*
Acid fumes, secondary effects of, on lung, 877
Acid phosphatase, elevation in carcinoma of
    prostate, 368
Acoustic neuroma, 568, *571, 572, 593*
  and destruction of temporal bone, 568
Acrocephalosyndactylia, *210*
Acrolein, as cause of pneumoconiosis, 929
Acromegaly, 59, *359, 360, 365, 538, 539,*
    630, *635*
  and spinal malalignment, *673*
  phalangeal changes in, *62, 364*
Acro-osteolysis, 315
  idiopathic
    familial, *284*
    nonfamilial, 282
Actinomycosis
  as cause of colon constriction, 1824
  of bone, 305, 344
  of colon, 1837
  of jaw, 338, *548*
  of lung, 844, 845
  of skull, 494
Adamantinoma, 549, *550*
Addison's disease, 1428, 1431
  and calcification of adrenal gland, 1428
Adenoid hypertrophy, 702
Adenoma
  adenomatosis, multiple endocrine, 1841
  adenomyosis, of uterus, 1897, 1899
  of adrenal gland, 1433
  of bronchus, 897
  of colon, *1798*, 1840
    compared with colitis cystica profunda, 1845
  of gallbladder, *1495, 1496, 1497*
  of hypophysis, 526, 532, *587*
  of lung, *891*
  of parathyroid
    and indentation of esophagus, *237, 238*
    and osteosclerosis, 345, 346

Adenoma (*Continued*)
  of pituitary gland, with calcification, *467*
  of renal cortex, *1366*
  of stomach, 1647
  of suprarenal gland, *1428*
  parathyroid
    and hyperparathyroidism, *237*
    and osteosclerosis, 350
    changes in skull, 509
Adenomatosis
  pulmonary, 980
Adenomyomatosis
  of gallbladder, *1494*
Adhesions, with pneumothorax, *762*
Adrenal disease, as cause of respiratory
    obstruction, 786
Adrenal gland
  adenoma of, 1433
  carcinoma of, 1433
  changes in Cushing's syndrome, 236
  primary aldosteronism, 1433
  visualization by retroperitoneal pneumography,
    1334
Aeroesophagography, 1549
Agammaglobulinemia, 1030
  and thymic pathology, 1034
Agnogenic myeloid metaplasia, and
    osteosclerosis, 332
Air, in mediastinum, 1046
  with ruptured uterus, 1883
Air passages, obstruction of, 786–788
  upper, 701, 786–795
    classification of roentgen signs of, 789
Air space, oropharynx, 1523
Alban-Koehler's disease, *277*
Albers-Schönberg disease. See *Marble bone
    disease.*
  producing sclerotic changes of bone, 325
Alimentary tract, 1479, 1521
  upper (including oropharynx, laryngopharynx,
    and esophagus), 1522–1581
Alpha-1 antitrypsin deficiency, 1005
Altitude, and pulmonary edema, 866
Aluminum, as cause of pneumoconiosis, 929
Alveolar proteinosis, *803*, 864, 869, *870, 871*
  clinical aspects of, 869
Amebiasis
  of appendix, 1850
  of colon, 1836
  of lung, *802*
Amebic hepatic abscess, 1297
Ammonia, as cause of pneumoconiosis, 929
Amniography, 1879
Amyloidosis
  associated with myocardiopathy, 1158
  bone and joint lesions of, 417
  of colon, 1844, 1845
  of small intestine, 1707, 1735, 1737, 1738
  of lung, 921
Anemia
  aplastic, 255
  hemolytic
    causing sclerotic lesions of spine, 632
    changes in bones, 253
    changes in skull, *482*
    classification, 253
    congenital, in infancy, 484
  iron deficiency, bony changes in, 255
    changes in skull, *482*
  myelophthisic, 255
  myelosclerotic, 632, 640

Anemia (*Continued*)
  producing osteosclerosis of bone, *325*
  radiographic bony changes in, *331, 338*
  sickle cell, 254, 256, 632, 635, 637, 638
    appearance of vertebra, *635*
    radiographic changes in spine, 637
Anencephaly, 1873, 1876
Aneurysm
  causing esophageal displacement, *1562*
  causing vertebral erosion, 632
  in Marfan's syndrome, 191
  intracranial calcification and, 586
  laminated calcification and, 1028
  of aorta, 1117
    abdominal, 1288, *1289*
    descending, 631, *1012, 1058*
  of carotid artery, calcification of, *467, 587*
  of heart, 1013, *1152*
  of renal artery, 1288, 1366, *1394*
  of sinus of Valsalva, 1117
  of vein of Galen, 586
  pulmonary arteriovenous, 894, *1142*
  relationship to mediastinal compartments, *1012*
Angiocardiograms, 729, 736
Angiocardiography, in evaluation of mitral stenosis, 1111
Angiofibroma, nasopharyngeal, *792,* 795
Angiogram, associated with hydrocephalus, 471
  cerebral, 518
  of kidney, 1321, 1358
  of skull, 498, 579
Angiography
  as aid in diagnosis of solitary pulmonary varix, 961
  biliary, 1515
  mediastinal lesions, identification of, 1026, 1028
  of hepatic vein, 1294
  of lung, 833
  of pancreas, 1675
  pulmonary agenesis, diagnosis of, 771
  pulmonary hypertension, demonstration of, 952
  pulmonary hypoplasia, demonstration of, 771
  pulmonary thromboembolism, localization of, 830
Angioma, of pleura, 768
  of skull, 585
Angiomatosis, of bone, 260, 282, 632, 645
Angiomyolipoma, of kidney, 1363, *1364*
Angioneurotic edema, 1737
Angle
  acetabular, *427*
  arteriovenous, with bronchogenic carcinoma, 901
  Boogaard's, 449, 488, 490, *490*
  cardiophrenic, 718
    relation to pericardial cyst, *1041*
  costophrenic, 718, *731, 1014*
    blunting, with bilateral low position of diaphragm, *753*
      with varicella pneumonia, 876
    lobar pneumonia, appearance with, 829
    obliteration of, *764*
    pneumonia and effusion, appearance contrasted with, *764*
    relationship to azygos venous system, *943*
    right, *1023*
    subdiaphragmatic abscess, appearance with, 759
  facial, *449*

Angle (*Continued*)
  iliac, *427*
  nasopineal, *449*
  sphenoid, *449*
Ankylosing spondylitis, *409*
Ankylosis, diseases associated with, 386
Anoxia, as cause of respiratory obstruction, 786
Antero-posterior view, definition of, 39
Anus
  ectopic, *1816*
  imperforate, 1814, 1815
    classification of, *1816,* 1817
      by pubococcygeal line, *1817*
Aorta, *709, 710, 732, 733,* 1024, 1025
  abdominal, aneurysm of, *1228, 1285*
    calcification of, 1288
    changes in position, 1289
    connection with anomalous arterial supply to right lower lobe, 961
  aneurysm, formation of, 1013, 1117, *1125*
    associated with aortitis syndrome, 1158
    effects on spine, 631
    of arch, 1120, *1120*
    of ascending, *1119*
    of descending, and mediastinal compartments, *1012*
    of sinus of Valsalva, 1013
    vertebral erosion by, *1052*
  angiography in relation to, 1026
  aortitis syndrome, 1158
  arch of, 731, *942, 948, 1015, 1018, 1021*
    calcification in, *1127*
    relationship to superior mediastinum, 1020
    relationship to thoracic spine, 1016
    vascular anomalies of, 1206, *1561*
  ascending, *942, 1012, 1022*
  atresia of, *1203*
  classification of roentgen signs, 1089
  contour, changes in, *1117*
  coarctation of, 1018, 1195, 1202, 1203
    rib notching and, 775, 780
    Turner's syndrome and, 221
  constriction, by mediastinal fibrosis, 1047
  descending thoracic, *735, 948, 1015,* 1018, *1022, 1023*
    aneurysm formation in, 1057, 1058, 1121
    azygos venous system, relationship to, *943*
    bronchi, relationship to, *941*
    mediastinal lymph nodes, relationship to, 1026
    thoracic spine, relationship to, 1016
  dissecting aneurysm of, *1122,* 1125, 1126, 1127
  dissection of, *1054*
    nontraumatic, *1055*
  indentation on trachea, 1025
  knob of, in hypertensive heart disease, *1154*
    double contour appearance, with bronchogenic carcinoma, 911
    shadow of, in nonpenetrating chest injuries, 1053
  measurements of, *1080, 1084*
  nonpenetrating injuries to, 1052
  poststenotic dilatation of, 1105
  pseudocoarctation, *1118,* 1120, 1201
  pulmonary window of, 956
  right sided, causing impression on esophagus, *1560*
  roentgen signs of abnormality, 1089, 1117
  thoracic, relationship to esophagus, *1537*

Aorta (*Continued*)
  window of, *709, 733, 1015*
    detection in cardiac fluoroscopy and, 1072
    in lateral views of chest, *948, 1018*
Aortography, 1329
  distinction between mediastinal tumors and
    aneurysm, 1051
  in visualization of kidney, 1329
Aplasia, 221
Appendage, auricular, *731, 735*
Appendices epiploicae, 1754
  calcification of, 1831
Appendicitis. See *Appendix, inflammation of.*
Appendix
  coproliths of, 1287, 1848
  appendicitis and, *1849*
  deformities following surgery, 1849
  fecaliths of, 1850
    calcification of, 1831
  in regional enteritis, 1850
  inflammation of, roentgen findings in, 1848
    roentgen sign of gangrenous, 1849
  perforation, as cause of subdiaphragmatic
    abscess, 759
  position, variations in, 1848
  vermiform, 1754, 1848
Arachnodactylia, *190,* 360
Arachnoidal granulations, *502, 503*
Arc welder's disease, 877
Argyrosiderosis, 929
Arnold-Chiari malformation
  foramen magnum, measurements of, *471* (table)
  radiograph and line diagram, *472*
  skull, posterior fossa of, 595
    abnormality of alignment with, 668
    and upper cervical spine abnormalities, 469
Artefacts
  definition of, 40
Arteriography
  of colon, 1778
  of kidney, 1321, *1329*
    differentiation between cyst and neoplasm,
      1327
  percutaneous transfemoral renal, 1329
Arteriosclerosis
  of kidney, 1464
  of peripheral lung vessels secondary to
    congenital heart lesions, 951
Arteritis, Wegener's necrotizing granuloma, 988
Artery(ies)
  aneurysm, and bone destruction, 1028
  aorta, abdominal, and aneurysm, 1288
    calcification of, 1288
  brachiocephalic, *948*
  carotid, aneurysm of, *532*
    common, *1024*
    internal, aneurysm of, *532*
      calcification of, *467*
    left common, *1014, 1020*
  celiac, *1024*
  coronary, *1022, 1132, 1133*
    calcification in, *1128*
  innominate, *1020*
    aneurysm of, 1057, *1060, 1124,* 1127
  intercostal, azygos venous system and, *943*
    coarctation of aorta and, 779
  mammary, coarctation of aorta, 779
    internal, identification of, 1026
  mesenteric, superior, *1024*
    thrombosis of, *1240*
    vascular occlusion of, 1712, 1807, 1819

Artery(ies) (*Continued*)
  nutrient of bone, 51, 54
  of pleura, associated with aneurysms, 960
  of skull, calcification in, 585
  phrenic, *1024*
  pulmonary, *734,* 1015, *1015, 1018, 1022*
    aneurysm of, with pulmonary meniscus sign,
      912
    classification of roentgen signs of
      abnormality, 1128, 1132
    coarctations, classification of, *1183*
    constriction, in mediastinal fibrosis, 1047
    conditions accompanied by dilatation,
      classification of, 1139
    dilatation, most frequent causes of, 1135
    diminution in size, classification of, 1137
    enlargement with associated low position
      of diaphragm, *753*
    identification of, 1026
    measurements of, 1133
    pulmonary infarction, 831
    roentgen abnormalities of (classification),
      1128, 1132
    thrombosis, changes with, *1140*
  renal, *1024,* 1348
    aneurysm of, *1394*
    calcification of, 1288
    fibromuscular defects of, *1397*
    fibromuscular hyperplasia of, *1463,* 1464
    thrombosis, site of, 1389
  sinuses of Valsalva, aneurysm of, 1127
  splenic, calcification of, 1288, 1299
  subclavian, *1020,* 1024
    aneurysm of, 1127
    left, *1014*
    right, causing displacement of esophagus,
      1559
  to kidney, *1349*
  vertebral, *1024*
Arthritis, degenerative. See *Arthritis,*
    hypertrophic.
  hemophilic, 386
    pathology and radiographic findings, *398*
    sites of occurrence, *398*
  hypertrophic, 386, 393, *394, 395,* 397
  in collagen disease, 413
  neurotrophic, 421
  ochronosis and, 425
  psoriatic, roentgenologic features, 411
  pyogenic, 386, 387, *389,* 390, *390, 391*
  rheumatoid, 386, 403, *404, 405, 406*
    ankylosing spondylitis, differentiation from,
      408
    hands, radiographic changes in, *403*
    juvenile forms of, 406, 407
    of spine, 408, *410*
    rheumatic fever, differentiation from, 407
    secondary to, 391
  traumatic, 386, 393, *394,* 421
  tuberculous, 386, *401, 402,* 403
  with ulcerative colitis, 412, 1833
Arthrogryposis, *63*
Arthrogryposis multiplex congenita, 210, 425, 674
  with spinal curvature, 668
Arthrokatadysis, 1894
Arthropathy
  neurogenic, *399, 400*
  neurotrophic, 386, 387
  steroid therapy and, 413, *414, 415*
  traumatic, 387, 394
Arthrosis, periarticular, *392*

Aryepiglottic folds, 790
Asbestosis, 927, 929, 970, 976, 977
    with pleural calcification, 921
    with rheumatoid arthritis, 927
Ascariasis infestation
    of abdomen, 1271, *1272*
    of small intestine, *1706*
Ascites, 1231, 1263
    associated with diaphragmatic elevation, 750
Aspergillosis
    of lung, 848, 850, 988, 1000
Asthma
    mucoid impactions causing accentuation of
        bronchial pattern, 961
    increased radiolucency of 987
    respiratory tract obstruction, 788
Astrocytoma
    calcification in, *467, 589, 590*
        intracranial, *587*
Atelectasis, 744, *802,* 814–825
    acute exanthemas of childhood and, 871
    alveolar proteinosis and, 869, 871
    as cause of linear markings of parenchyma,
        939, 975
    bronchial adenoma and 824, 897
    bronchiectasis and, 961, 966
    bronchogenic carcinoma and, 901, 911
    bronchopulmonary dysplasia and, 880
    carcinoma of lung and, *899*
    chronic aspiration pneumonia with, 857
    classification of, 814, 971
    diaphragm, elevation of, *749,* 814
    emphysema and, *826*
    histopathology of, *804*
    Hodgkin's disease and, 1036
    interspaces, appearance of, *764*
    lobar, and lobar emphysema, distinction
        between, *817*
    lung abscess, associated with, *896*
    lung parenchyma, as cause of line shadows in,
        939, 970, 971, 975
    lung vessels associated with, 820
    lupus erythematosus, changes with, 858
    massive pleural effusion and lobar pneumonia,
        differentiation from, *816*
    mediastinum, displacement of, 814
    new-born and, *818*
    platelike, 814, *817, 939*
    pneumothorax and, *821*
    psittacosis and, 877
    pulmonary infarction and, 833
    pulmonary thromboembolism and, 830
    thorax, changes in shape of, *771*
    Wegener's granulomatosis, 920
Atlantoaxial dislocation, in rheumatoid arthritis
    and ankylosing spondylitis, 668
Atlantoaxial fusion, 622, 678
Atlantoaxial subluxation, 679
    associated with abnormalities of vertebral
        alignment, 668
    classification of causes, 675, 677
Atlas, occipitalization of, *621*
Atlas-dens interval, measurement of, 679
Atrium
    auricle of, *1022*
    changes in, 1095, *1098*
    relationship of left, to esophagus, *1537*
Auricular appendage, *942*
Autoimmunologic disease, in lung, 921, 970
    interstitial pneumonia, cause of, 977

Axillary fold, *787*
Azygos knob, *942*

Bacterioides, *803*
Bagassosis, as cause of pneumoconiosis, 929
Banana oil, as cause of pneumoconiosis, 929
Baritosis, as cause of pneumoconiosis, 929
Barium, 929
    involving lung, 923, 929
Barium column, radiographic changes of,
        1804, *1806*
Barium enema
    barium-air double contrast study, *1776*
    cathartic colon, appearance of, *1813*
    complications of, *1777,* 1778
    examination, barium-air double contrast, 1775
        obstruction to flow, *1783,* 1796, 1799
        routine, 1767, 1773, 1774
    filling defects (feces), *1813*
    following surgery for carcinoma, 1847
    glands of Lieberkühn, *1765*
    implications of, 1776
Barium meal, accelerated, 1692–1693
Barrel chest, 770
Basilar impression, *447*
    roentgen criteria for, *488*
Bechet's disease, 1535
Benign osteoblastoma. See *Osteoma, giant
    osteoid.*
Berteil's projection, *575*
Berylliosis, 980
    of lung, *928, 933*
Beryllium, 929
    interstitial pneumonia, cause of, 977
    poisoning, changes in lung, 970, 977
Bezoar, of stomach, *1629*
Bile duct, common, 1506
    abnormalities, of architecture, 1507
        of size, 1506
        of contour, 1507
    carcinoma, anatomic sites of, 1512
    carcinoma and stone, distinction between,
        1510
    contrast agent, comparison of, *1510* (table)
    cystic dilatation of, 1509
    diverticulum of, *1509*
    filling defects, 1508
    intramural portion of, (duodenum), *1509*
    sphincter of Oddi, alterations in, 1508
Biliary sclerosis, 980
Biliary system, anatomic studies of, 1482,
        1484, 1485
    methods of study, 1479
Biliary tract, abnormality in KUB films, 1480
Birdheaded dwarf of Seckel, 222
Bismuth poisoning, *334*
Bladder, urinary
    achalasia of, 1411
    alterations, in architecture, 1420
        in size and contour, *1413*
    "bladder ears," *1413*
    calcification of, 1410, 1421
    calculi of, 1410
    classification of roentgen signs of abnormality,
        1410
    cystitis emphysematosa, 1410, 1420
    cystitis granularis, 1420
    diverticulum of, 1421

Bladder (*Continued*)
  exstrophy, 1304, 1410, 1411, *1412*
  filling defect, *1414*
  neurogenic, *1413*, 1415, *1416*
  tuberculosis of, *1406*
Blastomycosis
  finely granular shadows, associated with, 933
  of bone, 250, *252*, 306, 345
  of lung, 844, 845
Blebs, pulmonary, 988
Blineau's projection, *575*
Body section radiography
  in analysis of nodular lung lesions, 894
  in examination of mediastinum, 1026
  in study of Pancoast tumor, 909
Body surface area, nomogram for determination
    of, *1082, 1083*
Boehler, critical angle of, *162*
Bone(s). See also names of specific bones.
  aberrations, chromosomal, 215
  actinomycosis of, 305
  architecture of, *66*
  biochemistry and roentgen appearance, 95, 96
  blood supply of, 51, 54, 55
  changes due to adjoining pathology, 105 (table)
  composition of, 55
  congenital diseases, related to extrinsic disease,
    213
  contour change and disease process, 98
  cortex, involvement in bone pathology,
      59 (table)
    normal appearance, *61*
  Cushing's syndrome and, 236
  density, diminished, 100, 101
    increased, 102, 103
  development of, classification of pathologic
      conditions, 184
    maldevelopment of, 198, 222
    overdevelopment of, 190, 222
    underdevelopment of, 185, 221
  diabetes, changes in, 282
  eburnation of, 40
  endocrine abnormalities associated,
    375 (table)
  eosinophilic granuloma of, 305
  erosion, differentiation between kinds, *1052*
  extremities, diseases of, 323–379
  formation of, 49, 55, 56 (table)
  fungus infections of, 305
  hemangioma of, *287*
  hypertrophic disease of, *324*
  lesions causing destruction of, 1028
  lipoatrophic diabetes mellitus and, 332
  lymphangiomatosis of, 260
  metastatic carcinomatous spread, association
    with, 921
  necrosis of, focal aseptic, 274. See also
      Osteochondroses.
  neoplasms of, *67, 320*
  neuroblastoma of, 314
  neurofibromatosis, involvement of, 241
  ossification and growth of, *50, 51, 52*
  osteolysis, progressive, 315
  osteomalacia, 59. See also *Osteomalacia.*
  osteomyelitis (acute and chronic), *301*
  osteoporosis, 59. See also *Osteoporosis.*
  osteosclerosis, 59. See also *Osteosclerosis.*
    affecting several extremities, 323
  overgrowth or outgrowth, diseases producing,
    358

Bone(s) (*Continued*)
  pathology, radiographic, 59 (table), *231*
    site of, 106–107 (tables)
  pathophysiology and biochemistry of, 55
  periosteum of, 59. See also *Periosteum.*
  pulmonary parenchyma and, 1110
  radiolucency
    diseases of a single extremity, 274–322
    diseases of multiple extremities, 230–273
      classification, 230, 231, 232
    lesions of, analysis by marginal appearance,
      287
    multiple areas of diseases causing, 241
    osteosclerosis and, mixed, 104
  regional maldevelopment, 197
    remodeling of, *53*
  roentgen analysis of, 65, *65*
  sarcoma of, appearance of pulmonary
    metastases, *922*
  sclerosis of, 40, *325*
    marginal, associated with radiolucent bone
      disease, *275*
    normal bone islands, 345
    sclerotic bone islands, *346, 347*
    tuberous, 260
  structure of, *59*
  trabeculae of medulla, 59
  trabecular patterns of, 104, *254, 371*
  trabeculation, cause of, in sickle cell anemia,
    254
    course of, in leukemia, *258, 259*
  tuberculosis of, periosteal reaction, *374*
  tumors, classification of, 366, 367
    statistics of, 371
  urologic diagnosis, *1422*
  yeast and fungus infections of, 241
Bone age. See also *Skeletal Maturation.*
  data, general rules for use, 89
  sampling method, *111*
  versus chronological age, *88*
Bones and joints, basic concepts in
  radiographic study of, 49–115
Brachiocephalic vessels, in left lateral view of
  chest, *1018*
Brachydactyly, 221
Breast, *787*
  identification of, 738
  malignancy of, in lung, *900, 922*
Bronchiectasis, 744, *803*, 852, *897*, 965, 999
  atelectasis and, 961
  cavities associated with, 896, *1004*
  characteristics of, 965, 966
  histopathology of, *811*
  pneumonitis and, 961
  pulmonary hypoplasia and, 771
  saccular or cystic, identified by
    bronchography, 966
  scimitar syndrome and, 961
  tumorlet of lung, similarity to, 909
  varicose, identification by bronchography, 966
  web formation and honeycombing, associated
    with, 976
Bronchiolectasis, with muscular hyperplasia, 981
Bronchioles, *799*, 993
Bronchiolitis, associated with silo filler's disease,
  962
Bronchiolitis fibrosa obliterans, 932, 933, 962,
  977, 999
Bronchitis, chronic, 991
Bronchogenic carcinoma, 894, *897*, 907, 1004

Bronchogenic carcinoma (*Continued*)
  obstruction of bronchus with, *907*
  "rat-tail narrowness" with, 901
  thumbprint indentation with, 901
Bronchogenic cyst, 987, 1043, 1045
  involving mediastinum, *1044*
  pathological specimen of, *1045*
Bronchogram, roentgenographic appearance of, *963, 964, 965*
Bronchography, 729
  air bronchogram, with pseudomonas aeruginosa pneumonia, 874
  bronchiectasis, cylindrical and saccular, *967*
  classification of, 966
  emphysema, changes in, 993, *994*
  mediastinal lesions and, 1027
  idiopathic unilateral hyperlucent lung, appearances in, *998, 999*
  muscular sclerosis of lung, diagnosis of, 981
  pulmonary agenesis, diagnosis of, 771
  pulmonary hypoplasia, 771
  tracheobronchiomegaly, diagnosis of, 794
Bronchopneumonias
  acute exanthemas of childhood and, *872*
  arteries, pulmonary (dilatation of), 951
  bronchogenic carcinoma, relation to, 911
  carcinoma, relation to, 901
  coccidioidomycosis and, 848
  collagen disease of lung, association with, 858
  Echinococcus granulosis, associated with, 836
  hypostatic, 853
  Loeffler's, 858
  parasitic round worms (nematodes) and, 836
  pork tapeworm and, 836
  tularemia, 872
Bronchopulmonary dysplasia, 803, 877, 880, 970, 976, *978*
Bronchus(i), 702, *731, 734, 799, 1022*
  abnormal architecture of, 789
  adenoma of, 824, 897
    atelectasis and, *827*
    clinical manifestations of, 824
    elevated hemidiaphragm, association with, *827*
    roentgenologic appearance of, 824, *826*
    segmental atelectasis with, *827*
  anatomy of, 705
  check valve obstruction, *754*
  depression of left main stem with nonpenetrating chest injuries, 1053
  displacement of, 789, 1052
  esophagus, relationship to, *1537, 1538*
  lateral views of chest, *1015, 1018*
  mediastinum, *1014*
  narrowing of lumen, secondary to carcinoma of bronchus, 901
  neoplasms of, 883
  size, variations in, 789
  "spidering," accompanying pulmonary emphysema, 991
  transection of, 763
Build, asthenic, 750
Bullae, 988
Bursa, diseases of, 423
Bursitis, traumatic, and elbow injury, *131*
Busulfan therapy, and pulmonary fibrosis, 980
Byssinosis, 929

Cadmium, fumes, 929
  interstitial pneumonia, as cause of, 977
Caisson disease, infarction of bone, *354*

Calcaneus, 161
  talus, aligned with, *385*
  tuber angle of, *162*
Calcification
  abdominal, *1228, 1279, 1280, 1281, 1282, 1283, 1284, 1285, 1287,* 1288, *1289,* 1289
    in infancy and early childhood, 1287
    mucinous adenocarcinoma of stomach, *1651,* 1660
  aortic sinus of Valsalva, 1072
  appendiceal fecalith, 1831, 1850
  appendices epiploicae, 1831
  cysts of liver, 738, 1295
  deficiency of deposition, 232
  dystrophic, 1377 (table)
  ectopic, 57
  eggshell type, 925, *927*
  enterolithiasis, 1744
  gallbladder, wall of, *1500*
  gallstone, in bowel, 1744
  habenular, *452*
  hemangiomas, of gastrointestinal tract, 1743, 1831
    of tissues, *317*
  heart, *1073, 1074, 1075,* 1078, 1095, *1126, 1129, 1130, 1131*
    aortic, 1052, *1122,* 1157
      aneurysm of *1125*
      arch, 1117, *1123, 1127*
      stenosis of valve, *1191*
    cardiac valves, 1072
    coronary vessels, 1072, *1128, 1136*
    disease
      hypertensive, 1153
      rheumatic, 923
      valvular, 1110
    inferior vena caval, 1287
    mitral ring, *1136*
    mitral stenosis, chronic, and, 923
    myocardial, 1072
    paraventricular, 585
    pericardial, 1072, *1137, 1146*
    sites of occurrence, 1072
  in adenocarcinoma of bowel, 1832
  adrenal cyst, *1285*
  in capsular fibrositis, 387
  in chondromyxoid fibroma, *285*
  in clivus, 497
  in colon, wall of, 1805
  in common bile duct, *1510*
  in coprolith of appendix, 1848
  in dermoid cyst, *1269, 1270*
  in enchondroma, *290*
  in fallopian tube, 1885
  in gallbladder, *1490, 1491,* 1499
  in intrathoracic goiter, 1032
  in neuroblastoma, 1287
  in papillary muscles, 1072
  in pelvic extrauterine masses, *1884*
  in seminal vesicles, *1370*
  in thyroid gland, 795
  in vas deferens, *1370*
  intracranial, *466, 467,* 581, *583, 584*
    abnormal deposits in, classification of, 585, 586, 587, 588, 589, 590, 591, 592
    craniopharyngioma, 532
    hydrocephalus and, 468
    meningioma, *594*
    parasellar or intrasellar, 532
    pituitary adenomas, 527
    sella turcica, *532*

Calcification (*Continued*)
  intracranial pressure and, *580*, 581
  intraorbital, classification of, 577
  leiomyoma of stomach, 1659
  leiomyosarcoma of bowel, 1832
  lung, 892, *893*, 895, 923
    anonymous mycobacteria of, 841
    barium or tin inhalation, resemblance to, 923
    classification of, 921
    hamartoma of, 911, 923
    histoplasmosis of, 845, 846, *847*, 933
    hydatid cysts, 923
    hypo- or hyperparathyroidism, 923
    in arrested mycoses, 933
    in mass shadows, 892
    in pulmonary pathology, 917
    infectious granulomas and, 921
    microlithiasis and, 921
    nodular lesions of lung parenchyma, 919
    pleural, 921, 925
      asbestosis and, 921, 927
    pneumoconiosis and, 921
    "popcorn" type, 923
    rheumatic heart disease and, 923
    tumors, *910*
    with aspergillosis, 850
    with chronic granulomatous disease of
      childhood, 846
  mediastinal, 1026, 1028, *1029*
  metabolism, factors governing, *56*
  mica inhalation and, 921
  of basal ganglia, 581
  of blood vessels, *252*
  of carotid arteries, 532
  of epiphyses, 193
  of petroclinoid ligament, 532
  of urinary bladder, *1370*, 1410, 1421
  pancreatic, 1670
  placental, 1287
  "popcornlike," 362, 892, 923, 1028
  primary myeloid metaplasia and, 923
  prostatic, *1370*
  psammomatous type, 795
  renal, 1288, 1365, *1366*, 1367, 1371, 1374,
      1375, 1376, 1391
    in childhood, 1378
    in renal tuberculosis, *1406*
    of renal pyramids, with parathyroid
      adenoma, *237*
    of suprarenal gland, 1428, 1429, *1431*
  silicosis, 921
  splenic, 1298
    splenic artery, 1288
  subperiosteal, in osteomyelitis of Garré, 352
  talc inhalation and, 921
  thymoma, 1034
  "tramline," 1366
    of kidney, 1450
  urinary, *1370*, 1407
  vascular, within abdomen, 1288
  Wilms' tumor, 1287
Calcitonin, 56
Calculus(i)
  biliary, 1499
  in common bile duct, differentiation from
    stone, *1510*
  fallopian tube, 1885
  in kidney, *1369*, *1372*
  staghorn, *1367*, 1374

Calculus(i) (*Continued*)
  urinary bladder, 1421
  urinary tract, *1370*
  vesical, *1370*
Caldwell's view, and acoustic neuroma, *572*
Caliectasis, in sickle cell disease, 255
Calvé's disease, *277*
Calyx, pyelocaliectasis, *1379*
Canal
  cervical spinal, sagittal measurements of, 607
    (table)
  external auditory, atresia of, 555
  optic, pathologic states of, 574
    erosion of, parasellar, 576
  spinal, measurements of, 651 (table)
Capitate, fractures of, 135
Capsule,
  joint, diseases of, 423
    fibrositis of, 387
    idiopathic capsulitis, 386, *388*
    rheumatic fever, changes in, *392*
  "radiologic," in abscess of bone, 66
    in Brodie's abscess, *66*
    in fibroma (chondromyxoid), *66*
    in fibrous dysplasia, *66*
    in radiolucent disease of bone, *287*
Carbon tetrachloride, 877, 929
Carcinoid, 1030
  in appendix, 1842, 1850
  in cecum, 1799
  in colon, 1842
  in stomach and duodenum, 1647, 1650
Carcinoid tumor, gastrointestinal, classification
    of, 1648
  small intestine, 1719, 1743
Carcinoma, 744
  bronchogenic, *897*, 907, 1004
  clear cell type, *922*
  metastatic, of small intestine, 1737
  of common bile duct, distinction from
    stone, *1510*
  of lung, 740, 768, *891*, 894, 921
    "golfball" type, 925
  of tongue, *1527*
Cardiac pacemakers, 1149, 1150, *1150*
Carina, *735*
Cartilage, zone of development in epiphyseal
    plate, *52*
Cavity, involving lung, *920*, *1004*
  mycotic, 895
Cecum, abnormalities of position, 1762
  hyperrotation of, 1755
  incomplete rotation of, 1755
  roentgen signs of lesions, 1838
  with volvulus, 1257
Cementoma, *548*
Cephalohematoma, *484*, 486
Cephalopelvic disproportion, 1885, 1887, *1893*
Cerebral aqueduct, perimeter ratio, *478*
  stenosis of, 473, *476*, *478*
Cervix
  canal, 1901, *1904*
  carcinoma of, *1902*
  funnel, *1903*
  inflammation of (cervicitis), *1902*
Chalasia, of esophagus, 1555, *1556*
Chamberlain's line, 449
Chassard-Lapiné view, of rectum and sigmoid
    colon, *1772*, *1773*

Chaussé III position, 551, *554, 555*
Check valve mechanism, associated with
    pneumothorax, 761
Chemodectoma, 498, 1013, 1030
    of head and neck, 571
    of mediastinum, 1013
Cherubism, *552*
Chest
    abdominal contents in, 755, *757*
    air column relationships, 948
    anatomy of, 701–729
        features responsible for linear or reticular
            markings of lung, 939
        sagittal, *1019*
    apical lordotic view, *735, 906, 909*
    arteries, veins, and bronchi, diagram of, *942*
    body section radiography of, 729, 730
    Bucky films of, 729
    deformities of, affecting cardiac position, 1089
    disease of, localization of, 736
    esophagrams of, 729
    flail, *773*
    fluoroscopy of, 730
    hourglass, *773*
    lymphadenopathy, identification of, 739
    measurements, and head measurements in
        American children, *443* (table)
    positions for examination of, 730
    radiologic methods of examination of, 730–739
    roentgen signs of, 745
    roentgenologic analysis, introduction to, 712–
        747
    shadows of, differentiation of, *764*
    size, decrease of, with small hemithorax, 750
        narrowing of, *771*
        widening of, *771*
        variation in, with elevation of diaphragm,
            749
    soft tissue structures, identification of, *737*
    superimposition of liver or pancreas over, 755
    thoracic cage in congenital heart disease, 1195
    views of,
        anterior oblique, *709, 710*
        lateral, *709, 732, 948, 949, 957, 958, 959,
            1018*
            advantages of, 739
            decubitus films of, 729
        posteroanterior, *708, 731, 942*
        posteroanterior oblique, *733, 734*
China clay, 929
Cinebronchographic studies, 993
Chlorine compound fumes, 929
Choanae, atresia of, *537*
Cholangiography
    abnormalities of function, 1509
    direct, complications of, 1514
    evaluation with gallbladder intact, 1510
    evaluation in postcholecystectomy, *1507,
        1508,* 1511
    hazards of use, 1511
    indications for use, 1511
    intravenous, 1503
        indications for, 1504
        radiographic signs of abnormality, 1505,
            1506
        technique of examination, 1505
    operative, 1513
    percutaneous, 1511
        evaluation of, 1513
        procedure, 1511
        related to pancreatic disease, 1671

Cholangiography (*Continued*)
    percutaneous, roentgen signs of abnormality,
        1512
    postoperative, 1513
    radiographic signs of abnormality, 1506
    selection of patients, 1516
    T-tube, 1513
    value of, 1515
Cholecystography
    abnormalities of density, 1492
    biliary tract, changes in, *1507*
    compounds used, comparison of, 1481 (table)
    film and fluoroscopic technique, *1486*
    oral
        complications of, 1503
        evaluation of, 1502
        major compounds used, 1480
        technical aspects of, 1483
    pancreatic disease and, 1671
    radiographic study, *1486*
    rectal, 1503
    roentgen signs of abnormality, 1480
    selection of patients, 1516
Cholecystitis, chronic, with calcified plaques,
    1499
    emphysematous, 1497, *1498*
Cholecystoses, hyperplastic, classification of,
    1496
Cholesteatoma, bone absorption of periantral
    area, *570*
    destruction of temporal bone and, 568
    radiographic appearance of, 569, *570*
Chondroangiopathia calcificans congenita, *194,
    195*
Chondroblastoma, 281
    of epiphysis, *276*
    of femoral head, *281*
    of vertebra, 645
Chondrocalcinosis, 421–423. See also
    Chondromatosis.
Chondrodysplasia, 199
    detectable at birth, 204, 205
Chondrodysplasia punctata, 204
Chondrodystrophy, 201
Chondroectodermal dysplasia, 204, 209
Chondroma, of lung, *910*
    of pleura, 768
    "popcorn-like" calcification in, 1028
Chondroma leiomyoma, *910*
Chondromatosis, of joints, 386
Chondromatosis with synovial chondrometa-
    plasia. See *Chondrocalcinosis.*
Chondromyxoid fibroma, *285, 287, 288, 292*
Chondromyxosarcoma, *286, 288,* 300
Chondro-osteodystrophy, 627
Chondrosarcoma, 358, 359, 362, *362,* 420
    comparison with osteosarcoma, *363*
Chordoma, 498, *532,* 644
    abnormalities of alignment in relation to
        skull, 668
    calcification of, *467,* 587
    of sacrum and coccyx, *1829*
    spotted lucency of spine and, 632
    vertebral erosion and, 1052
Chorioepithelioma, of mediastinum, 1031
    with pulmonary involvement of, *922*
Choroid plexuses, calcification of, *582, 583*
    displacement with increased intracranial
        pressure, 581
Chromosomal aberrations, with skeletal ab-
    normalities, classification of, 515

Cineradiography
  oropharynx, study of, 1531
  stomach-duodenum, examination of, 1596
  swallowing function, study of, 1524, 1542, 1544
  urinary tract and, 1334
Cisterna chyli, *1024, 1025*
Cisternomyelogram, intracranial space-occupying lesion, identification of, 579
Clavicle, *942, 1015*
  articulation with coracoid process, 781
  congenital defect of, 781
  fractures of, *123*
  in cleidocranial dysostosis, *186,* 781, *782*
  in infantile cortical hyperostosis, *783*
  in lateral view of chest, *948*
  resorption, in rheumatoid arthritis, 781, *783, 784*
    of acromioclavicular junction, 781
  rhomboid fossae of, 781
  supernumerary, 781
  thickening of inferior margin in rheumatoid arthritis, 781
Cleidocranial dysostosis, 185, *186, 187, 188, 189, 491,* 781, *782*
  fusion of neural arches, failure of, 622, 627
  skull, changes in, 488, *490*
Clivus, chordoma of, 497
Clubbing of fingers, with Kartagener's syndrome, 968
Coccidioidomycosis, *847*
  in bone, 344
  in lung, 844
  with cavitation, *1000*
Coccyx, interference in parturition, 1894
  variations of, *1892*
Codman's triangle, *275*
  in fibrosarcoma of bone, *319*
  in osteosarcoma of bone, *309*
Colitis cystica profunda, 1845
Colitis, ischemic, 1819
Collagen diseases, 859
  arthritis and, 413
  involving bone, 345
  involving lung, *802,* 810, 864
    fibrotic disease of parenchyma, 977
    finely granular shadows of parenchyma, 932
    linear changes, 970
  lupus erythematosus, 867
  pharyngeal pathology, 1535
  radiographic manifestations of, 867
  rheumatic fever, 864
  scleroderma, *859*
  Wegener's granulomatosis, 864
Collapse of lung, producing linear markings, 939, 970
Colon
  abnormalities, of architecture, 1832
    internal, 1799
    of contour, *1760,* 1825
    of density, 1830
    of function, 1847
    of position, 1827
    of rotation, 1790
    of rotation and descent, 1828
    of size, diffuse increase in, 1807
      narrowness of lumen, 1823
      narrowness, segmental, 1823
      segmental or localized, 1807

Colon (*Continued*)
  actinomycosis of, 1837
  adenoma of, villous, *1798*
  amyloidosis of, 1844
  anatomy of, 1754
  appendices epiploicae, 1754
  arteriography of, 1778
  blood supply of, 1755
  calcification in wall of, 1805
  carcinoid of. See *Carcinoid.*
  carcinoma of, *1788*
    calcification in, *1832*
    distribution of, *1843*
    perforation as cause of subdiaphragmatic abscess, 759
    roentgenologic findings, 1843
    with ulcerative colitis, 1834
  cathartic colon, *1779,* 1808, *1813*
  cecum. See *Cecum.*
  congenital abnormalities of
    Hirschsprung's disease, *1781, 1782*
    megacolon, *1780*
    microcolon, 1825
    stricture or atresia, 1825
  contracture, of transverse colon, *1763*
    sites of, *1763*
  contrast studies, 1780
  displacement of, 1790, *1795,* 1830
  diverticula of, *1793,* 1825
  diverticulosis of, 759
  examination, following barium meal, 1777
    through colostomy, 1774
  foramen of Morgagni, appearance in, 758
  gastric resection, changes following, 1847
  haustral sacculations, 1754
  herniation of, 1794, *1795,* 1830
  ileac, *1771*
  ileocecal junction, *1759*
  inflammation of, rupture following barium enema, 1776
  interposition of, 1234, *1796,* 1828
    beneath right hemidiaphragm, *751*
    with unilateral elevation of diaphragm, 750
  intussusception, enterocolic, *1798*
  irritable, 1766
  ischemic colitis, 1819
  leiomyosarcoma of, 1832
  lymphosarcoma of, 1843
  mucoviscidosis, involvement with, *1809*
  noninfectious enterocolitis, as cause of respiratory obstruction, 786
  normal appearance of, *1756, 1757*
  obstruction of, disease entities producing, 1818
  organoaxial rotation of stomach, changes with, *1797*
  pelvic, *1771*
  physiology of, 1766
  polypoid defects of, 1799, 1840
  polyposis, familial, 1841
  pseudovolvulus of, 1823
  radiologic examination of, *1767, 1768,* 1769
  radiology of, 1734–1859
  rectosigmoid junction, *1764, 1770*
  rectum, Chassard-Lapiné view, *1772, 1773*
  roentgen signs of, *1778, 1779,* 1807
  scleroderma of, *1793*
  segmental narrowness, 1788
  sigmoid, Chassard-Lapiné view, *1772, 1773*
  spasm of, 1766

Colon (*Continued*)
  splenic flexure, annular constriction of, *1762*
  surgical resection of, *1784*
  taeniae coli, 1754
  toxic dilatation of, 1807, 1823
  toxic enterocolitis, *1791*
  tuberculosis of, *1792*, 1837
  tumor, benign, 1842
  "unused colon," *1761*
  variations of normal, 1755
  volvulus of, *1786, 1807*, 1818
    of cecum, *1787*
Colostomy, examination of colon through, 1774
Common mesentery deformity, *1704, 1794*
Congenital and hereditary abnormalities of
    skeletal system, 182–229
Congenital heart disease
  anatomic classification of, 1167, 1168
  aorta
    arch of, abnormalities, *1196*, 1206
    atresia of, *1203*
    coarctation of, 1195, *1202, 1203*
    right-sided, anomalies of, *1197*
    stenosis, 1185
  as cause of respiratory obstruction, 786
  atrial septal defect, 1175, *1176*
  blood vessels, transposition of, 1184–1185,
    1186
  classification of, 1165, 1166
  contour, changes in, *1170*
  cor triatriatum associated with pulmonary
    hypertension, 952
  dextrocardia, mirror image, 1206
  dextroversion, *1200, 1204*, 1206
  Ebstein's disease, 1189, *1193*
  endocardial fibroelastosis, 1187, *1192*, 1204
  frequency of, 1210 (table)
  increased radiolucency of chest, 988
  interatrial septal defect, *1205*
  interventricular septal defect, *1205*
  Kartagener's triad, 1206
  levocardia, 1206
  levoversion, *1200, 1204*, 1206
  patent ductus arteriosus, 1178, *1179*
  patent foramen ovale, *1193*
  patent interatrial septum, *1176*
  patent interventricular septum, *1177*
  pericardium, absence of, 1210
  positional abnormalities, 1206
  pulmonary artery, coarctations of, classifica-
    tion, *1183*
    ectopia of left, 1207, 1209
  pulmonary vasculature, changes in, 1170, *1170*,
    1171–1174, 1201, 1204
  pulmonic stenosis, *1181*, 1182
  routine of analysis of films, 1167
  situs inversus, *1200, 1204*
  situs solitis, *1200, 1204*, 1206
  tetralogy of Fallot, 1182, 1184, *1184*
  tricuspid atresia, 1178, *1180*
  truncus arteriosus, communis, *1188*
    persistent, 1185, *1189, 1190*
    pseudocommunis, *1188*
  ventricular septal defect, 1175, *1177*
Congenital insensitivity to pain, complicated by
    fractures, *175*
Contraceptive devices, complications of in-
    sertion, 1895
  radiographic appearance in uterus, 1894
  types, *1895*
Contrast media, 16–17
  barium sulphate, 16
  carbon dioxide for fetal localization, 1880
  double contrast air in barium, in examina-
    tion of stomach-duodenum, 1596
    with duodenal ulcer, *1619*
  gases, 17
  iodides, 16
  in cholecystography, 1480, 1482
  in hysterosalpingography, 1896
  nitrous oxide in pelvic pneumography, 1908
  reactions to, 1337, 1338
  water soluble, in study of gastrointestinal tract,
    1597
    iodinated, in study of small intestine, 1695
  water test for hiatal hernia, 1594
Convolutional impression, 580
Coracoclavicular joint, 781
Cor pulmonale, 830
  changes in lung and heart, 1155, *1156*
  disease responsible for entity, 1155
  fibrotic changes in lung, 977
  with emphysema, 993
  with Goodpasture's syndrome, 879
Cranial indices, *446*
Cranial lacunar osteoagenesis (luckenschädel),
    505
Craniocarpotarsal dystrophy, 222
Craniofacial dysostosis, 211
Craniolacunia, 1873, 1876
Craniometaphyseal dysplasia. See *Metaphyseal
    dysplasia.*
Craniopharyngioma, *532*
  calcification of, 467, *587*
  sella turcica, changes in, 528
Cranium
  neoplastic tumors of, with calcification,
    588–592
  radiological evidence of intracranial space-
    occupying lesion, 579, 580
Cretinism, 233
  metaphyseal changes with, *332*, 333
  radiographic findings, 336
  skeletal changes with, *335*
  with spinal malalignment, *673*
Crohn's disease (granulomatous colitis), 1799,
    1802, 1808, 1834, 1835
Crosby capsules, use in intestinal biopsy, 1696
Cross-sectional anatomy, at level of fifth thoracic
    vertebra, *1022*
  at level of manubrium, *1020*
  at level of fourth thoracic vertebra, *1021*
  at level of T-7 and T-8, *1022*
Croup, 790
  radiographic appearances of, *789,* 790
  with upper respiratory tract obstruction, 788
Crouzon's disease, 211, *463*
Cryptococcosis (torulosis), of lung, 844
Cuboid bone, 162
Cuneiform bone, 162
Cushing's syndrome, 1429
  causing calcification of kidney, *1367*
  with mediastinal changes, 1030
Cyst
  adrenal, calcification in, *1285*
  aneurysmal bone, *66, 286, 287, 288, 298*
    of vertebra, 645
  arachnoid, of skull, simulating Dandy-
    Walker syndrome, *475*
  bone, *66, 287*

Cyst (*Continued*)
  bronchogenic, 1013, 1043, *1043,* 1045
    classification of, 1045
    of mediastinum, *1012, 1044*
    pathological specimen of, *1045*
  choledochal, 1290
  congenital mediastinal, 1606
  Dandy-Walker, *448*
  dental root, *548*
  dentigerous, *542*
  dermoid, of mediastinum, 1030
    of nose, 549
    of pelvis, *1269, 1270*
    of skull (teratoma), 497
  echinococcus, intracranial calcification, *587*
  enteric, 1013
  enterogenous, 1699
  fissural, 549
  gas, in pneumatosis cystoides intestinalis, *1812*
  gastrogenic, 1606
  hydatid, 988
    calcification in, *467*
    intracranial calcification, *587*
  leptomeningeal, 492
  lipomatous, of os calcis, *293*
  mediastinal, 1028, 1031
  mycosis, as cause of, *920*
  neurenteric, *1012*
  neurenteric canal, 1013
  of carpus in Wilson's disease, 266
  of kidney, *1321,* 1358, 1362
    classification of, 1434
    differentiation, from carcinoma, 1445
      from neoplasm, 1327
    radiographic features of, *1380,* 1435
  of suprarenal gland, 1433
  of thoracic duct, 1013
  of thyroglossal duct, with respiratory tract
    obstruction, 788
  osteitis fibrosa cystica, 66
  ovarian, 1885
  pancreas, in relation to, *1674*
  pancreatic pseudocyst, in mediastinum, 1013
  paracytic, 1031
  periapical, *542*
  pericardial, 1013, *1040,* 1141
    celomic, *1012,* 1031, 1036
    differentiation from mediastinal lesion, 1030
    inflammatory, 1031
  pulmonary, 894, 895, *920,* 988
    classification, 999, 1003
  solitary bone, 288, *293, 294*
  thymic, *1012,* 1032
Cystic disease, pulmonary, *897, 1004*
Cysticercosis, with intracranial calcification, 585
Cystitis emphysematosa, *1408,* 1410
Cystocele, investigation by chain cystourethrography, *1328*
Cystography, 1316, 1323, *1415*
  air cystogram, 1325
  delayed, in children, 1326
  polycystogram, 1325
  postvoiding study, 1324
  simple retrograde, 1324
  superimposition, 1325
  triple voiding, 1326
Cystourethrography, 1316, *1318,* 1323, 1341,
    1417, 1418
  chain type, 1327, 1328, 1421
  posterior urethral valves, *1418*

Cystourethrography (*Continued*)
  retrograde, 1326
  voiding, 1316, 1326
    expression cystourethrography, 1326
    technique of, *1318*
Cytomegalic inclusion disease, with intracranial
  calcification, *586*
Cytomegalovirus, *803*

Decalcification, of foramen rotundum, with angiofibroma of the nasopharynx, 795
Decubitus films, definition of, 40
Deforming spondylosis, 665
Dens, congenital absence of, 622, 624
Density, decreased, definition of, 39
  increased, definition of, 39
Dermatomyositis, in lung, 877, 970
  phalangeal changes, *62*
Dermoid, of mediastinum, *1033*
  of skull, *497*
Dermoid cyst, 1030
  of abdomen, *1269*
Diabetes
  gastric atrophy and, *1638*
  lipoatrophic diabetes mellitus, 332
  mucormycosis and, 549
  osteopathy, 282
Diaphragm, 723, 1014, 1018
  abnormalities, in density, 758
    in function, classification of, 748
    in number, 758
    in position, 750
      bilateral low position, 750, *753*
      unilateral low position, 753, *754*
      with pulmonary emphysema, 750
    in size and integrity, classification of, 755
  acute bronchiolitis, with, *989*
  air under, 738, *749, 1223*
  alpha-1 antitrypsin deficiency, appearance with,
    1005
  attachments of, 729
  contour of, changes in (classification), 755
  costal attachments, with emphysema, 993
  delineation by pneumoperitoneum, 766
  diaphyseal sclerosis of, 222
  elevation of, 723, 749
    secondary to left heart failure, 960
    secondary to pulmonary hypertension, 956
    secondary to pulmonary thromboembolism,
      830
    unilateral
      causes associated with, 750
      radiographic appearance with, *750*
      with abscess formation, 750
      with accessory diaphragm, 758
      with fluid, 750
      with gas-containing loops of bowel, *751*
      with inflammation, 750
      with infrapulmonary effusion, 766
      with massive atelectasis, *764*
      with splenic enlargement, 750
    with ascites, *749*
    with atelectasis, *816*
    with bronchogenic carcinoma, 901, *905,* 911
    with chronic passive hyperemia of chest, *958*
    with lupus erythematosus, 858
    with subdiaphragmatic abscess, 759

Diaphragm (*Continued*)
emphysema, appearance with, 995
flattening, with bronchogenic carcinoma, *898*
with emphysema, 993
foramina, of Bochdalek, 729
of Morgagni, *729*
hepatodiaphragmatic interposition, 1263
herniation through, *729*, 755, *1564*
of greater omentum through, 1796
of stomach through, *1610*
widening of thoracic cage and, *771*
in Hodgkin's disease, 1035, 1036
increased linear markings of lung parenchyma, appearance with, *938*
infrapulmonary effusion simulating tumor and, 752
interposition of colon beneath, *1223, 1796*
leiomyoma of, *752*
linear shadow associated with pleural adhesion, *768, 973*
methods of study of, 748
movement of, 759
paradoxical, 750
Potter-Bucky, as accessory for recording of x-ray image, 8
in production of x-rays, *10*
pulmonary agenesis of, changes with, 771
radiologic examination of, 728
radiology of, 748–761
relationship, of right dome to left, 723
to congested liver as seen with passive hyperemia of lung, *958*
to esophagus, *1537*
to pleura, 971
to ribs, 723, *749*
scalloping of, *728, 729*, 731
stomach, distance from, 738
structures penetrating, 729
subdiaphragmatic abscess, 759, *759*
subdiaphragmatic gas (air fluid level), 759
tenting of, *728, 729, 757*
tumor of, with unilateral elevation, 750
venous drainage of, *943, 1023*
x-ray, adjustable, for delimiting beam, *11*
Diaphragma sellae, 524
Diaphyseal aclasis. See *Exostoses, hereditary multiple cartilaginous.*
Diaphysis, aneurysmal bone cyst, appearance in, 298
corticoperiosteal radiolucent lesions, *311*
Engelmann's disease, involvement in, 327
osteomyelitis, appearance in, 249
radiolucent lesions of, corticoperiosteal changes, 310
thyroid acropachy, changes in, 341
tuberculosis of, 304
Diastrophic dwarfism, 201, 205
Diatomite, 929
Diploë, venous, *504*
Dissection, air, in bowel wall, *1810*
Distortion, in estimation of cephalopelvic disproportion, 1885
Diverticulitis, as cause of colon constriction, 1824
Diverticulosis, of colon, 1790, 1793, 1827
of esophagus, 1566
of fallopian tube, 1901
of sigmoid, *1826*
of small intestine, *1713*
simulation by normal glands of Lieberkühn, *1765*

Diverticulum(a)
epiphrenic, in mediastinal compartment, *1012*
of esophagus, 1030, 1032, 1053, 1565, *1566*
inflammation of. See *Diverticulitis.*
involving mediastinum, 1031
of colon, 1825
of common bile duct, *1509*
of duodenum, *1632*, 1633
of gallbladder, *1494*
of jejunum, *1633*
of kidney calyx, *1369*
Meckel's, 1287, 1712, *1714*
as cause of intussusception, 1821
of pericardium, 1036
of small intestine, 1712
of sigmoid, *1826*
of stomach, *1630*, 1631
pharyngeal, 1534
of esophagus, 1565
pulsion, *1533*, 1565
traction, of esophagus, 1565
Down's syndrome, spinal changes, 629
Ducts, alveolar, 799
thoracic, anatomic relationships of, *1024*
Dunham's fan, 895
Duodenum
anatomic relationships of, *1603*
carcinoma of, *1673, 1724*
congenital anomalies of, *1605*
dilatation in nontropical sprue, *1709*
diverticula of, *1633, 1714*
intraluminal, 1631, *1633*
postbulbar, *1632*
duodenography, hypotonic, 1674, 1676, 1677
hematoma, intramural, 1659, *1659*
inflammation of (duodenitis), *1604*
inversion of, 1616
megaduodenum, 1603
normal measurements of, 1602
normal rugal pattern of, *1583*
obstruction, chronic, *1604*
position, changes in, 1613
pseudodiverticula of, 1631, *1631*
roentgenologic appearance, normal, *1623*
pathological, *1604*
reduplication of, 1606
retroperitoneal rupture of, 1659
scarring of duodenal bulb, 1621
tumors of, benign, 1656, *1657*
malignant, 1658
ulceration of, *1618, 1619*, 1620
diseases associated with, 1646
perforation as cause of subdiaphragmatic abscess, 759
umbilication of duodenal bulb, *1625*
Dysphagia lusoria, 1559
Dysgammaglobulinemia, in small intestine, 1738, 1739

Ear. See also *Temporal bone* and *Mastoid.*
middle ear, tomogram, *565*
Echinococcosis, intracranial calcification and, 585
Echinococcus granulosis, bronchopneumonia and, 835
Ectopia, crossed, *1354*
of pelvis, *1354*

Effusion
  alveolar cell carcinoma of lung and, 908
  chilus, of pleura, 766
  cirrhous, of pleura, 766
  esophageal rupture and, 1566
  hemorrhagic, of pleura, 766
  infrapulmonary, *754*, 766
  interlobar, *765*, 766
    major fissure, *765*
  of joints (knee), 387
  pericardial, 802, 1143, *1144*
    autoimmune disease and, 921
    Hodgkins disease and, 1036
    rheumatic heart disease and, 1153
    special methods for examination of, 1067
  pleural, 763, *764*, 766, *802*
    pneumonia and, *816*, 835, 871, 874
      of atypical measles, 871
      pseudomonas aeruginosa, 874
      staphylococcal, vs. atelectasis, *816*, 874
    pulmonary thromboembolism as cause of, 830
    with Hodgkins disease, 1036
    with hydrocarbon ingestion, 995
    with left heart failure, 960
    with mediastinal disease, 1030
    with nonpenetrating chest injuries, 1053
    with pleural mesothelioma, 769
    with pulmonary infarction, 833
  pulmonary edema and, 867
  Q fever pneumonia and, 857
  tuberculosis of lung and, *838*
Elbow, changes in fat plane with fracture, *131*
  fractures and dislocations of, 127, *128, 129, 130*
    tear of orbicular ligament of radius and, 132
  Monteggia fractures of, *130*, 132
  traumatic bursitis, and changes in fat pad
    contour, *131*
Ellis-Van Creveld disease, 204, 209
Emphysema, *967*, *990–999, 996*
  atelectasis and, *817, 826*
  barrel-shaped chest and, 775
  bronchiectasis and, 966
  bronchitis and, 965
  bronchogenic carcinoma and, *898, 901*, 911
  bronchographic appearance of, *967, 993*
  bronchopulmonary dysplasia and, 880
  bullous type, *1003*
    with pneumoconiosis, *926*
  compensatory, *771*
  congenital lobar, 786
  infantile, *996, 997*
  low position of diaphragm, association with,
    750
  obstructive, and widening of thoracic cage, *771*
  paramediastinal, 987
  pulmonary thromboembolism and, 830
  respiratory tract obstruction and, 788
  retrolaryngeal, 789
  retrotracheal, 789
  rib notching and, 780
  roentgenologic features of, 991–993, 995
  silicosis and, *930*
  thoracic cage, changes of, 770, *771*
  thoracic deformity and, *772*
  tracheobronchiomegaly and, 794
Emphysematous gastritidies, 1659
Empyema, *897*
  circumscribed widening of pleural space and,
    761

Empyema (*Continued*)
  encapsulation of, 896
  encystment of, 896
  staphylococcal pneumonia and, 874
Encephalocele, *485, 486, 495*
Encephalitis, and intracranial calcification, 585
Enchondroma, *66*, 199, *285, 287, 288, 290, 291*
Endarteritis calcificans cerebri, 586, *587*
Endarteritis obliterans, complicating lipoid
    pneumonia, 857
Endocrine glands, bony changes associated with
    375 (table)
  radiolucent skeletal diseases and, classifica-
    tion of, 236
Endocrine osteopathy, classification of, 233
Endothelioma of bone. See *Sarcoma, Ewing's.*
Endometriosis, of colon, *1799*, 1824
  of uterus, 1420
Engelmann's disease, 191, *193*, 327, *328*, 360
  producing sclerotic changes in bone, 325, 513
Enterocolitis, necrotizing, 1814, 1831
Enterolithiasis, 1744
Enteroptosis, 1830
Eosinophilic granuloma, *635*
Ependymoma, calcification of, *467, 587*, 589
Epidermoidoma, 494, *495*
Epiglottis, 701
  displaced by carcinoma of tongue, *1527*
  in epiglottitis, 790
  inflammation of, 790
  with upper respiratory tract obstruction, 788
Epiphrenic diverticulum, *1012*
Epiphysis, 51, *275, 276, 282*, 323
  aneurysmal bone cyst and, *298*
  aseptic necrosis of steroid therapy, *414*
  chondroblastoma of, *276, 281*, 281
  classification of injuries to, *120*
  congenital stippled, 193, 199, *352*, 632
  development of, 88, 91, 199
    zones of cartilage development in epiphy-
      seal plate, *52*
  diseases affecting epiphyses primarily, 274
  dysplasia of, 193, *196*, 199, *352*
  femoral, blood supply derivation, *146*, 147
  fracture of, *120, 121*
  fracture dislocations of in knee, *150*
  in congenital syphilis, 269
  in epiphysitis (Scheuermann's disease), *635*
  in giant cell tumor of bone, *294*
  in hypothyroidism, *352*
  in Osgood-Schlatter's disease, 278
  in osteochondrosis of os calcis, 280
  in osteosarcoma of bone, *309*
  in osteosclerosis, localized, *352*
  in scurvy, *264*
  in Turner's syndrome, *219*
  in vertebral bodies, 632, *635*
  infarction of, *352*
  vessels of supply, 51, *54*
Epiphysiolysis, *118*
Epispadias, 1419
Eraserophagia, 1832
Erect position, definition of, 40
Erythema multiforme, coccidioidomycosis of
    lungs and, 847
  mycoplasma pneumonia and, 857
Erythema nodosum, 933
  coccidioidomycosis and, 847
Erythroblastosis fetalis, 255, 1873, 1874
  Deuel's halo sign and, 1870

Erythroblastosis fetalis (*Continued*)
  technique for transuterine infusion of red
    cells, 1880
Erythroid hyperplasia, 484
Erythropenia, and thymic pathology, 1034
Esophagram, 736, *942*
  in diagnosis of megaesophagus, 1057
  in differentiation of mediastinal lesion, 1030
  in examination of heart, 1067, *1069, 1070,
    1071, 1094*
  in lateral view of chest, *948*
  indentations shown by, 1023
Esophagus, *731, 734, 942, 1020, 1021, 1022, 1024,
    1025*
  abnormalities, in architecture and contour, 1565
    congenital causes of, *1551*
    in density, 1559
    in function, 1573
    in position, 1558
    in number, 1557
    in size, 1549
  achalasia, 1549, *1551, 1554,* 1555
    and congenital hypertrophic pulmonary
      stenosis, 1621
  anatomic relationships, *1537*
    to azygos venous system, *943*
    to diaphragm, *1537*
    to left atrium, *942*
    to mediastinal lymph nodes, 1026
    to mediastinum, of lesions, 1013
    to portal circulation and azygos venous
      circulation, *1539*
    to trachea and bronchi, *941*
    to tracheobronchial lymph nodes, *720*
  atresia of, 794, 1549, *1550*
  barium study of, with pulmonary sequestration,
    914
    in delineation of chest features, *942*
  bronchogenic carcinoma and, 901
    appearance of metastatic spread to lung, *922*
  carcinoma of, 1573, *1574, 1575*
  chalasia of, 1555, *1556*
  compression, by intrathoracic goiter, *1032,
    1561*
    secondary to vascular bands, *1562*
  congenital anomalies of, 794, 1549, *1550*
  constriction, 1047
    sites of, 1538
  corrosion of, *1557*
  curling of, *1558,* 1567
  deflection of, *1197, 1198, 1562*
  displacement, by parathyroid adenoma, *237*
    by thyroid, 1031
    from aneurysms, *1120, 1121, 1562*
    from left atrial enlargement, *1098, 1099*
    of trachea and, 794
    secondary to hiatal hernia, 1563
    with mitral valvular disease, 1102
  distance from tracheobronchial tree, 901, *903*
    with bronchogenic carcinoma, 911
  diverticulum of, *733,* 1053, 1565, *1566*
    epiphrenic, 1032, 1053
  duplication of, 1053, *1551*
  dynamic disorders of, 1555
  elevator esophagus, 1557
  esophageal lip, 1530, *1539*
  esophageal web, in iron deficiency anemias,
    255
  esophagitis, *1567,* 1568

Esophagus (*Continued*)
  examination technique, 1543
  filling defects in, *1571*
  film study of, *1546*
  fistula and, 1566
    and mediastinitis, 1046
  fluoroscopy of, 1543
  foreign bodies, impaction of, 1570
    ingestion, method of study, 1544
    tracheal displacement, as cause of, 794
  gas production in, 1028
  hernia(s) (classification of), 755
    congenital short esophagus and, 1563
    diagrammatic representation, *1564*
    hiatal
      incidence of, 757
      paraesophageal type, *757,* 1563
      symptoms of, 757
    sliding type, *757, 758,* 1563
  hernias involving stomach and, *1610*
  hiatus of, 755, 757, 758
    of stomach through, *757*
  Hodgkin's disease and, 1036
  indentations, with abnormalities of aortic
      arch, *1199*
    adenoma of parathyroid, *237, 238*
    metastatic carcinoma, *1572*
  inflammation of, 1542, 1567
    short esophagus and, *757*
    tracheal displacement as cause of, 794
  lateral chest view, *709, 948,* 1015
  leukoplakia of, 1555
  lower end, anatomic concepts of, *1540*
  lymphatic drainage of, 1026
  mediastinal, *1014*
  mediastinal tumor as cause of, 1053
  megaesophagus, *1029,* 1053, *1056,* 1555
    in mediastinal compartment, *1012*
    production of gas and, 1028
  muscular hypertrophy, *1558,* 1567
  peristaltic activity of, *1543*
  presbyesophagus, 1567, *1575, 1576*
  radiographic examination of, 729, *1591*
  radiographs of, *1545, 1546, 1547*
  reflux esophagitis, 1542
  roentgen signs of abnormality, 1548
  rupture of, 1566
  Schatzki's ring, *1565*
  scleroderma of, *863, 1576,* 1576
  "short esophagus," *757*
  shortened (congenital), *1551*
  spasm of, 1555, 1557, 1567
  tumors of, *1012,* 1053, 1570, 1572
  ulceration of, 1568
    peptic, 1542, *1552, 1553*
  varices of, *1569,* 1570
  venous drainage of, 1570
  web formation, 1535, *1535*
Exanthemas, acute, with finely granular lung
    shadows, 933
  with respiratory tract obstruction, 788
Exostoses, 199
  hereditary multiple cartilaginous, 360, 361
  on superior margin of ribs, 775
Exudate, of lung, 894
Exudative enteropathy, 1814
Exophthalmos, in Hand-Schüller-Christian dis-
    ease, 506
Eye, involvement in sarcoid, 1042

Facial bones, diseases of, 533
    fractures of, 542
    increased density of, 540
    roentgen pathology of, 533
Face, position drawings, *533*
Facets, articular, congenital absence of, 622, 624
Fallopian tube. See *Oviduct.*
Falx cerebri, calcification of, *582*
Familial dysautonomia, 970, 1536
Farber's disease, 222
Farmer's lung, *928, 929*
Fat
    absence of, in lipoatrophic diabetes mellitus,
        332
    Cushing's disease, 236, 1030
    differentiation, of abdominal organs, 1265
        of mediastinal lesions, 1028
    elbow, changes in fat plane, *131, 132*
        fat pad sign, 411
    epicardial fat line, 1036, 1042
    "fetal fat line," normal, 1864
    in renal hamartoma, 1443
    in renal pelvis with kidney atrophy, 1339
    intramural lipid granuloma, 1285
    kidney, distribution in, 1363
    plane overlying pronator quadratus, changes
        in trauma, 142
    retroperitoneal, relationship to paracolonic
        gutter, *1304*
    stomach and duodenum, fat-containing lesions
        of, 1659
Femur, dysgenesis of proximal, 221
    fractures of upper end, classification of, 148,
        149
    head, transitory demineralization of, 281
    neck, avulsion fracture of, *149*
        blood supply of, *146*
    shaft, axial relationships of, *383*
        fractures of, classification, 151
Ferric oxide, 929
Fetography, 1880
Fetus
    abnormalities of, 1871, 1873
    age determination, 1864, *1866*
    extrauterine, 1881
    head diameter, determination of, 1865
    length, determination of, 1864
    maturity, prediction of, 1866
    multiple fetuses, determination of, 1864
    normalcy, determination of, 1864
    presentation of, 1876
        breech, *1881*
        diagrams of, *1877*
    roentgenologic signs of death, *1870*
    skeleton in utero, determination of, 1864
    skull, measurement in cephalopelvic dispro-
        portion, *1899*
    viability or death, determination of, 1868
Fibrin bodies, as pseudotumors of pleural
        space, 761
    associated with pleura, 769
Fibroid, submucous, 1899
Fibroma(s), 1030
    of pleura, 768
    nonosteogenic, of Lichtenstein and Jaffe, *297*
    ossifying, of face and skull, 551
Fibromuscular hyperplasia of arteries, renal,
    1463, 1464
Fibrosarcoma, of bone, 311, 318, *319*
    parosteal, 320

Fibrosarcoma (*Continued*)
    simulating giant cell tumor of bone, 309
Fibrosis, 1047
Fibrous dysplasia, 251, 260, *286, 287,* 288, 295,
        506
    lucency and sclerosis of spine, association
        with, 633
    of mandible, *552*
    of skull, *507*
    of vertebra, *634*
    simulating enchondroma, *292*
    spinal involvement, 661
Fibroxanthoma, *286, 288, 778*
    nonossifying fibroma of Jaffe, 297
Fibula, fractures of shaft, 155
Filling defect, definition of, 40
Films, comparison, definition of, 40
    serial, definition of, 40
Fischgold's biventor line, *449*
Fish lung, horizontal fissure, 971
Fissure(s)
    bronchogenic carcinoma and, *898*
    inferior orbital, special views for, *575*
    interlobar, 718
    pulmonary, *1021*
        with bronchogenic carcinoma, 901, 905
        with pulmonary gangrene, 875
    nasopharyngeal angiofibroma, and enlargement
        of, 795
    superior orbital, special view for, *575*
Fistula
    bronchopleural, *896, 987*
        with actinomycosis, 844
        with pneumatocele, 874
        with staphylococcal pneumonia, 874
    Crohn's disease of small intestine and, 1717
    diverticula of bowel and, *1826*
    enterovaginal, 1910
    esophagopleural, with actinomycosis, 844
    esophagus and, 1566
    gastrocolic, 1646, *1794*
    of lung, multiple arteriovenous, 925
    rectoperineal, 1815
    rectovesical, 1815
    regional enteritis and, 1717
    retrourethral, 1815
    tracheoesophageal, *1551*
        associated with respiratory tract obstruction,
            788
    urethral, 1418
    with mediastinitis, 1046
Fistula formation
    actinomycosis of colon and, 1837
    colon and, 1790
    gastrointestinal disease and, 1839
    granulomatous colitis (redundant) and, 1799
    lymphogranuloma venereum and, 1839
    secondary to radiation, 1824
    ulcerative colitis and, 1836
Flail chest, 770, 775
Flat foot, congenital, 198
Fleischner's lines, 939
Fleischner's platelike atelectasis, producing
        linear markings of lung, 970
Fluid level, definition of, 40
Fluoride poisoning, 638
    as cause of sclerotic lesions of spine, 632
Fluorine poisoning, 327, 328
    associated with sclerosis of skull bones, 513
    producing osteosclerosis of bone, *325*

Fluoroscopy, in study of heart and mediastinum, 729
  of mediastinum, 1026
    identification of mediastinal lesions, 1028, 1030
  safety recommendations for, 28
Fluorosis, 59, *61*
Foramen, at base of skull, 498, 499
  magnum, deformities of, 619
    normal measurements of, 471 (table)
  of Bochdalek, 755, *756, 758*
  of Morgagni, 755, *755,* 758, 1036
    herniation through, *1012*
  of Winslow, paraduodenal hernia through, 1701
Fontanelle, in cleidocranial dysostosis, *186*
Foot, dislocations of, *164*
  fractures and dislocations of, 160
Foreign body
  aspiration, with respiratory tract obstruction, 788
  in bronchus, 988
  ingestion, procedure in study of esophagus, 1544
  intraocular and intraorbital, localization of, 577
Fracture(s). See also individual bones.
  analysis of radiographs, 116
  avulsion or chip type, 117, *118*
  Barton's, 135, *137*
  Bennett's, 135, 143
  bone grafts, 180
  bone remodeling, *171*
  callus, osseous primary, *170*
    secondary, *170*
  cervical spine, 653
  Chauffeur's, 135, *137*
  Colles', 135, *136*
  comminuted, *118*
  complications of, 167–181
  congenital insensitivity to pain, association with, 175, *175*
  epiphysiolysis and epiphyseal injuries, 117, *120, 121*
  extremities, 116–181
    diagrammatic representation of, *118,* 119
    lower, most frequent sites of, *146*
    upper, most frequent sites of, 119, *122*
  electrical injury and, 119
  fatigue, 117, *118*
  fixation devices, 180
  Galeazzi's, 135, *136*
  greenstick, *118*
  healing, histologic steps in, 167
    sequence of, *168*
  hematoma formation, *169*
  histologic changes, correlation with radiographic appearances, 167, 171
  hyperemia, organization of fibrous callus, *169*
  immobilization of, 178
  impacted, *118*
  insufficiency, 117
  longitudinal, *118*
  march type, 117
  metaphyseal injury, *121*
  Milkman's syndrome, 269
  oblique, spiral or screwlike, 117
  orthopedic fixation devices, *178, 179*
  pathogenesis of delayed union, 171
  pathologic, *118,* 119, 172
    hyperparathyroidism, 489
    of femur, *296*

Fracture(s) (*Continued*)
  radiographic analysis of, 172
  skull, depressed type, 486
    radiographic appearance, *487*
  Smith, 135, *136*
  stress, 117
    of metatarsal bones, 162
  study of, 116
  thoracic spine, 653
  timed sequence for film study, 117, 172
  treatment, methods of, summary of, *176, 177*
    principles of, responsibility of radiologist, 180
  types, classified, 117
Fracture healing, complications from fractures, and methods of treatment from the radiologic standpoint, 167–181
Fragilitas ossium, 209
Freiberg-Koehler's disease, *277*
Friedreich's disease, and myocardiopathy, 1158
Frontal bones, "bossing" of, 481
Frontoethmoidal region, fractures of, 548
Fungal disease, and longitudinal sclerotic changes of bone, *338*
  of stomach, 1621
Fungal lesion, causing spotted lucency of spine, 632
  of lung parenchyma, demonstrating webbing and honeycombing, 976

Gallbladder
  abnormalities, 1506
    of architecture, 1501
    of density, 1492
    of function, 1501
    of number, 1489
    of position, 1491
    of shape, 1491
  adenomyoma of, *1495, 1496*
    extraluminal, *1497*
  adenomyomatosis and, *1494*
  calcification of, 1499, *1500*
  carcinoma of, 1502
  cholecystectomy, changes following, *1507, 1508*
  cholesterolosis, 1492, *1493*
  diverticula of, *1494*
  measurements of, 1515
  nonvisualization of, 1501, 1506
  papilloma of, 1492, *1493*
  perforation of, as cause of subdiaphragmatic abscess, 759
  phrygian cap, *1489·*
  polyps, *1493*
    cholesterol, 1495
  radiographic signs of abnormality, 1488
  removal, changes following, *1508*
  visualization, in angiography, 1515
Gallstones, *1490, 1491*
  carcinoma, relationship to, 1502
  crowfoot sign, 1492
  impaction with production of ileus, 1265, *1266*
Ganglia, interosseous, and juxta-articular cystic lesions of bone, 417
  sympathetic, tumors of, and bone destruction, 1028
Ganglioneuromas, 1030
Gargoylism, 205, 208, *553*
Gas, as sign of gangrenous appendicitis, 1849

Gas (*Continued*)
  in fetal circulatory system, as sign of fetal death, 1869, *1872*
  in maternal uterus, as sign of gas-producing organism, 1870
  in mediastinal abscess, 1028
  in mediastinum, classification of causes, 1028
  in pregnant uterus, 1871
Gas patterns of bowel, 1233
  abnormalities, in architectural appearance, 1269
    in contour of loops, 1257
      intestines, 1257
      stomach, 1257
    in density in, 1267
      fluid levels, 1267
      speckled gas appearance with feces or meconium, 1267
    in plain abdominal films, classification of, 1235
    in position, 1260
      intestines, 1260–1263
      of gas related to stomach, 1260
  absence of gas in pelvis, *1248*
    with strangulation, *1253*
  ascariasis infestation and, 1271–1272
  colon, 1233
    cut-off sign, of transverse colon, 1238
    isolated distention of small portions, 1257
  displacement of, related to stomach, *1262*
  distention, isolated, of small intestinal loops, 1253
    of duodenum, with superior mesenteric artery syndrome, *1243*
    of small intestine, coiled spring appearance, 1243
    of small intestine and proximal part of colon, 1250
    secondary to toxic ulcerative colitis, *1242*
  duodenal atresia and, 1242
  duodenum, variations in, 1240
  extraluminal, classification of, *1271*
    gas, beneath diaphragm, 1269
    gas, producing free air beneath diaphragm, *1270*
    in position, in biliary tract, *1272*
  fluid levels within, *1252, 1253*
  hepatodiaphragmatic interposition, 1263
  herringbone appearance, of small intestine, *1247*
  Hirschsprung's disease, *1239*
  ileus, meconium in newborn, *1268*
    secondary to gallstone impaction, 1265, *1266, 1267*
  imperforate anus, *1237*
  in intussusception, 1255
  intraluminal, due to worm infestation, 1279
  mesenteric thrombosis, changes with, *1240, 1241*
  newborn, 1233, *1236*
  overdistention, of large intestine, 1250
  pyloric obstruction, *1237*
  rectum, 1234
  roentgen signs of abnormalities, in plain film of abdomen, 1233, 1235
  sigmoid, 1234
  simulation by dermoid cyst, *1269*
  small intestine, 1233
  stepladder appearance, *1241*
  stomach, 1233
    changes in contour of, *1258*

Gas patterns of bowel (*Continued*)
  stomach, displacement from external causes, *1258*
    variations in, 1240
  volvulus, of cecum, with, *1238*
    of sigmoid, *1256*
    of small intestine, 1255
    of stomach, 1260
Gastroenteritis, allergic, 1739
Gastrointestinal tract, malformations of, *1699*
Gastroschisis, 1304
Gaucher's disease, *66, 247, 248, 260, 287,* 360, 508
  skull, changes in, 484, 506
  spinal malalignment and, *673*
Genital tract, female, carcinoma of, *922*
Genitography, 1910, 1911
Giant cell tumor, causing spotted lucency of spine, 632
Giant osteoid osteoma. See *Osteoblastoma, benign.*
Giardiasis, of small intestine, 1737
Gibbus, definition of, 669
  formation of, and lipochondrodystrophy, *648*
Gigantism, generalized pituitary. See *Acromegaly.*
  hemigigantism, congenital hemihypertrophy, 222
  localized, 62
  partial, 222
Glands
  lacrimal, involvement in sarcoid, 1042
  salivary, involvement in sarcoid, 1042
  suprarenal, *1024*
  thyroid, *1024*
Glands of Cowper, inflammation of, 1419
Glands of Lieberkühn, *1765*
Glioblastoma multiforme, *590*
  calcification within, 589
Glomerulonephritis, *1365*
Glycogen storage diseases, and myocardiopathy, 1158
Goodpasture's syndrome, *809, 877, 878, 879*
Gout, pathology and radiographic characteristics, *416, 417*
Granuloma, abdominal, 1233
  amebic, 1836
  bone, 250
  eosinophilic, 248, *287,* 508
    "button" sequestrum and, 512
    linear changes in lung, 970
    radiographic features, 305, 306
    simulating Ewing's tumor of bone, 313
    simulating osteochondrosis, *277*
    skull, 506, *510*
    spotted lucency of spine, as cause of, 632
    vertebra, appearance of, *635*
  infectious, 876
    of lung, and linear shadows, 939
  lipoid, abdominal, 1285
    of lung, 918, *919*
  lung, 846, 848, 894, 895, 891, 915, 921
    alveolar cell carcinoma, resemblance to, 908
    calcification and, *893, 921*
    linear markings, association with, 939, 970, *973,* 975
  mycoses, of lung, 876
  pleural, 761
  sarcoidosis, 864, 1042
  secondary to histoplasmosis, 845
  small intestine, 1707

Granuloma (*Continued*)
tuberculous, of lung, 876
Wegener's, *803*, 811, *812*, *862*, 864, 867, 873, 875, 920
Granulomatoses, lipoid, and radiolucency of bone, 241, 247, 248
of lung, 740
Granulomatous colitis, 1799, *1802*, *1808*, 1834, 1835
Granulomatous disease, involving mediastinum, 1031
of childhood, chronic, 846
Graphite, 929
Gumma, luetic, and intracranial calcification, 585
Gynecography. See also *Pneumoperitoneum, pelvis.*
definition, 1908
demonstration of abnormal pelvic pathology, *1909*
Gynecologic radiology, 1894
Gynecomastia, and mediastinal choriocarcinoma, 1030

Habenular calcification, *582*
localization on skull, *452*
Habenular commissure, displacement in increased intracranial pressure, 581
Hamartoma, of kidney, 1442, 1443
of lung, *891*, 894
"popcorn-like" calcification and, 1028
Hamman-Rich disease, 260
honeycombing or web formation and, 976
interstitial pneumonia and, 977
Hand-Schüller-Christian disease, 247, 248
Haustral sacculations, 1754
Head, measurements of, in American children, *443* (table)
Heart
anatomic relationships of, lateral view, *709, 948, 1015*
left anterior oblique view, *709*
postero-anterior view, *731*
right anterior oblique view, *710*
right postero-anterior oblique view, *734*
aneurysm, 1013
angiography, in relationship to, 1026
aortic insufficiency, changes in, 1105, 1158
aortic valve, calcification in, 1105
calcific stenosis of, 1103, 1105, *1191*
atrium, *1015*, 1091, 1095
left, relationship to esophagus, *942*
right, in postero-anterior view, *942*
calcification in, *1073–1075*, 1126, *1129, 1130, 1131*
atrial, left, *1078*
coronary arteries, 1078, *1134, 1136*
mitral valves, *1136*
sites of occurrence, 1072
chamber enlargement, associated disease states, 1152, 1155, 1157
pitfalls in evaluation, 1116
specific signs (classification), 1091
chambers, in congenital heart disease, 1194
changes with, age of patient, 1089
body build, 1089
congenital heart lesions, *1169*
pregnancy, *1090*
pulmonary atelectasis, *819*

Heart (*Continued*)
combined valvular lesions, 1111, *1115*
congenital defects, Hughes-Stovin syndrome, 960
tetralogy of Fallot, 957
congenital disease of. See *Congenital heart disease.*
contour, 1088
changes with, associated aortic pathology, *1104, 1117*
congenital heart lesions, *1170*
left atrial enlargement, 1098, *1099*
left ventricular hypertrophy, *1092, 1093*
right atrial enlargement, *1100, 1101*
right ventricular dilatation, *1096, 1097*
right ventricular hypertrophy, 1096
tricuspid regurgitation, *1114*
coronary circulation, calcification in, *1128*
coronary heart disease, 1151
cor pulmonale, contour changes, *1156*
in pneumoconiosis, *926*
decrease in size of pulmonary veins secondary to heart failure, 956
dilatation of, changes in contour and, *1092*
left heart failure and, 960
"drop" or "pendulum," and bilateral low position of diaphragm, *753*
endocarditis, and valvular involvement, 1155
enlargement of
asphyxiating thoracic dystrophy of newborn and, 773
chronic passive hyperemia and, 958
collagen diseases and, 867
congenital rubella syndrome and, *268*
evaluation of, 1143, 1148
measurement of, *1079–1088*
fluoroscopic study of, 1067–1076
frontal area, *1087*
hanging drop appearance, 993
Hodgkin's disease and, 1036
hypertensive heart disease, 1153, *1154*
hypertrophy of, and left heart failure, 960
in mediastinum, *1012, 1014*
infundibulum (stenosis), and decrease in size of pulmonary veins, *945*, 957
left auricular appendage of, *942*
lymphoma in mediastinum and, *1037, 1038*
mensuration of, *1080, 1081*
microcardia, and malnutrition, 1091
mitral valve, abnormalities, classification of, 1102, 1103
disease of, contour changes accompanying, *1106, 1107*
insufficiency, 1105, *1108*, 1111
venous pulmonary signs, 1110
stenosis, 1105, 1111
pulmonary hypertension and, 952
pulmonary calcification and, 923
pulmonary vascular changes and, *1112*
myocardial infarction, 866
myocardiopathies, classification of, *1158* (table)
outline. See *Heart, contour.*
pericardium, roentgen signs of abnormality, 1139
plain film and fluoroscopic study, 1076
relationships to, pleural mediastinal reflection, *974*
position, in relation to elevation of diaphragm, *749*
postoperative complications, 1149

Heart (*Continued*)
  pulmonary agenesis and, 771
  pulmonary infarction, appearance with, *832*
  pulmonary pathology, appearance secondary
    to, *938*
  pulmonary valve, abnormalities, classification
    of, 1103
    and decrease in size of pulmonary veins, 957
    lesions, 1111
    stenosis, hemodynamic changes in lungs, *945*
  radiology of (exclusive of congenital heart
    disease), 1067–1164
  retrocardiac clear space, *732, 948*
  rheumatic heart disease, 1153
  roentgen signs of abnormality, classification
    of, 1089
  roentgenologic examination, purposes of, 1067
  rotation of, and scoliosis, *772*
  shunts, extracardiac, and abnormalities of pul-
    monary veins, 956
      and changes in aortic pulmonary window,
        956
    intracardiac, and abnormalities of pulmo-
      nary veins, 956
  size, 1088, 1089
    in pulmonary edema, 867
  specialized cardiovascular investigations, 1078
  syphilitic heart disease, 1157
  teleroentgenogram, 1067
  thyrotoxicosis, appearance with, 1159, *1159*
  toxic causes of myocardiopathy, 1158
  tricuspid valvular disease, 1103, 1111
  truncus arteriosus, and decrease in size of
    pulmonary veins, 957
  tumor of, 1013
    atrial myxoma associated with pulmonary
      hypertension, 952
  valves of
    abnormalities, classification of, 1102, 1103
    mitral, and accentuated septate or lymphatic
      lines, 971
      calcified mitral ring, *1076*
      stenosis and pulmonary hypertension, *951*
    projection in routine positions in radiog-
      raphy, *1077*
    subaortic stenosis, *1191*
    tricuspid atresia associated with decrease in
      size of pulmonary veins, 957
  valvular lesions, 1103
  veins of, *1135*
  ventricle, left,
    aneurysm, 1095, *1152*
    (apex), *942*
    enlargement, signs of, 1091, 1094
    estimation of size in cardiac fluoroscopy,
      1072
    lateral view of chest, *948*
  ventricle, right, *1015*
    enlargement, signs of, 1091, 1095
      with pulmonary hypertension, 956
    lateral view of chest, *948*
  volume, determination in infants, 1079, 1084,
    1085
    normal in children, 1087 (table)
    prediction by nomogram, *1086*
Heart disease, congenital. See *Congenital heart
  disease.*
Heavy metal poisoning, and metaphyseal trans-
    verse bands, *334*
  and sclerotic transverse bands in metaphyses,
    333

Heel-pad thickness, 365, 366
Hemangiectatic hypertrophy, 222
Hemangioma
  bone, *66, 287,* 311, 315, *316, 317*
  gastrointestinal tract, calcification in, 1831
  skull, 496, *496*
  spine, 657, *661*
  vertical lucency and sclerosis of, 633
Hematoma, lung, *1002*
  mediastinal, 1013
  paraspinous, *1012*
Hematopoiesis, extramedullary, 912, *1012,* 1013,
    1053
  with blood dyscrasias, 1030
Hemicolectomy, *1809*
Hemifacial microsomia, 221
Hemiplegia, infantile, and intracranial calcifica-
    tion, 585
Hemochromatosis, and myocardiopathy, 1158
  idiopathic, and osteoarthropathy, 413
Hemomediastinum, 1031
Hemophilia, as cause of intestinal hemorrhage,
    1718
  in small intestine, 1738
Hemorrhage, cerebral, and intracranial calci-
    fication, 586
  retroperitoneal, causes of, 1290
Hemorrhagic telangiectasia, hereditary, 925
Hemosiderosis, of lung, 877, 879, 970, 971, 977
Hemothorax, and nonpenetrating injuries of
    thoracic aorta, 1052
Henoch's purpura, as cause of intestinal hemor-
    rhage, 1717
Hepatic duct, common, *1509*
Hernia
  bowel obstruction from, 1706, 1818
  congenital short esophagus and, 1563
  diaphragm, *1564,* 1830
    widening of thoracic cage and, 771
  foramen of Bochdalek, 1013, 1031
  foramina of Morgagni, 1013, 1031
  herniagram, inguinal, 1696
  hiatal, *1012,* 1013, 1053, *1568*
    displacing esophagus, 1563
    examination of, 1591 (table)
    simulating mediastinal tumor, 1057
    sliding, *1059, 1541,* 1563
  incisional ventral, *1254*
  intra-abdominal, *1244, 1253,* 1255
  mediastinal, 1028, 1031
  of colon, 1794, *1795,* 1830
  of intervertebral disk, 681
  of stomach through diaphragm, 1260
  omental, greater, 1036, *1253,* 1796
    lesser, *1253, 1704*
  paraduodenal, *1253,* 1701, 1737
  paraesophageal, 1563
    hiatal, *1261*
  pericecal, *1253*
  sigmoidal, *1253*
  transmesenteric, 1255
Heroin intoxication, associated findings, 866
Hexamethonium toxicity, and pulmonary
    fibrosis, 980
Hilus
  arteriovenous aneurysm, connection with, 895
  arteriovenous angle, appearance of, 911
    reversal of, *903*
  bronchogenic carcinoma, appearance with,
    901, *902*
    elevation in, 911

Hilus (*Continued*)
  pulmonary carcinoma, 895, *905*
  Pancoast tumor, 909
Hip, malum coxae senilis, *396*
Hip joint, measurements of iliac and acetabular
    angles, *427*
Hirschsprung's disease, *1239*, 1250, 1780, *1781*,
    1782, 1807, 1808, 1812, 1814
  colonic calculi and, 1288
  volvulus and, 1257
Histiocytosis of lung, 260, *510*, 970, *976*, 980,
    981
Histiocytosis X, 260
  affecting bones, *246*
  interstitial fibrosis of lungs, 978
  of skull, 506
  orbital changes in, 577
Histoplasmosis
  mediastinitis, chronic, resulting from, 1046
  of ileocecal region, 1838
  of lung, 844, 845, 846, 895
    calcification of, 845, 921
Hodgkin's disease
  adrenal gland, 1036
  atelectasis, 1036
  bones, *243*, 1036
  central nervous system, 1036
  gastrointestinal tract, 1036
  genitourinary tract, 1036
  omentum, 1036
  pancreas, 1036
  pulmonary lesions, roentgenographic changes
    of, classification, 1035
  simulating osteochondrosis, *277*
  skin, 1036
  small intestine, *1737*
  spinal malalignment, *673*
  thorax, associated pathology, 1036
Homocystinuria, 191
Hormones, effects on skeletal system, classi-
    fication of, 234
Hourglass chest, 770, 775
Humerus
  axial relationships of upper end, *381*
  epiphyseal displacements of lower end, 125
  fractures, of greater tuberosity, *124*
    of lower end, *126, 127*
    of shaft, 125
    of supracondyloid process, 125, 126
  proximal, *125*
Hurler's disease, 627
  myocardiopathy and, 1158
  spinal curvature and, 668
  thoracic kyphosis and, 674
Hyaline membrane, and pneumatoceles, *882*
Hyaline membrane disease, of lung, *818*
  of newborn, 877
Hydatid cysts, *1000*
  in lung, calcification in, 923
Hydatid disease, involving lung, *802*
Hydrarthrosis, 386, 387, *388*
Hydrocephalus, 464, *466*
  craniolacunia, differentiation of, 466
  diseases associated with, 471
  nonpressure type, 464
  pathogenesis and classification, 464
  pressure type, 464
  sella turcica, changes in, 531
Hydrocephaly, 1873, 1876
Hydrocarbon, 994

Hydromyelia, 674
Hydronephrosis, *1363*, 1440
  excretory urography, grading by, *1442*
  roentgen examination of, 1441
Hydropneumothorax, and esophageal rupture,
    1566
  and mediastinitis, 1046
Hydrosalpinx, *1905*, 1907
  and circumscribed widening of pleural space,
    761
Hypercalcemia, idiopathic, 59, 1375
  infantile idiopathic, 223, *332, 337*
    boxlike sclerosis and, 633
    causing sclerotic lesions of spine, 632
    osteosclerosis and, *325*
    radiologic manifestations in spine, 640
    sclerotic transverse bands in
      metaphyses and, 333
Hyperlucency, of bone, definition of, 40
Hyperostosis frontalis interna, 353, *516*, 517
Hyperparathyroidism, 59, 61, 232, 233, 236, 548
  articular cartilage calcification, 418
  bones, changes in, *237, 239, 240*
  calcification, in kidney, *1365*
  chest deformity and, *773*
  "fish" vertebra and, *648*
  phalangeal changes, *62*
  rib notching, 780
  simulating osteochondrosis, *277*
  skull, changes in, 236, 489, *492, 508*
  spine, 632, *635*
    malalignment of, *673*
  superior marginal rib defects, 775
Hyperphalangism, 222
Hyperphosphatasemia, 59
Hypertelorism, 223, *447, 540*
  classification of causes, 538
  metaphyseal dysplasia and, 514
Hypertension, pulmonary, *1109*
  with Goodpasture's syndrome, 879
Hypertrophic pulmonary osteoarthropathy, clini-
    cal findings and radiographic features, 340,
    342
  longitudinal sclerotic lines of bone and, 337,
    338
  thyroid acropathy, differentiation from, 341
Hypervitaminosis A, metaphyseal changes and,
    260, *262*
  radiographic findings, *330*
  spine, changes in, 682
Hypervitaminoses A and D, osteosclerotic
    changes in bone, *325*
  transverse bands in metaphysis and, *332*, 333
Hypervitaminosis D. See also *Hypercalcemia,
    infantile idiopathic.*
  diagrammatic changes in, *330*
  involving metaphysis, *262*
Hypoalbuminemia, of small intestine, *1722*
Hypoparathyroidism, 59, 329
  ribs, bony changes in, *778*
  skull, changes in, 509, 586
  osteosclerotic changes in bone, *325*
Hypopharynx, functional disorders of, 1536
  roentgenologic findings with croup, 790
Hypophosphatasia, 59, 223, 266
  metaphyseal changes, 260, *261*
  radiographic findings in spine, 632, 633
Hypophosphatemia, infantile familial or
    hereditary, 200
Hypophyseal fossa, 524

Hypophysis
  adenomas of, 526, 527, *532, 587*
    basophilic, 527
    chromophobe, 527
    eosinophilic, 527
    sella turcica, changes in, 528
  prediction of size, *525*
Hypospadias, 1419, 1911
Hypothyroidism, 94
  epiphysis, involvement of, *352*
  radiographic changes in spine, 630, *631*
Hypovitaminosis D. See also *Hypercalcemia,*
    infantile idiopathic, and *Rickets.*
  metaphysis of bone, *262*
  superior marginal rib defects, 775
Hysterography, 1883
  following caesarean section, 1901
  identifying position of contraceptive
    device, 1894
Hysterosalpingography, 1896
  abnormal uterine findings, 1899
  complications of, 1909
  contraindications, 1899
  identification of pathology, 1897
  normal roentgen findings, 1896, 1898, 1899
  purposes of study, 1896
  technique of examination, 1896

Ileocecal junction, *1691, 1692*
Ileocecal region, roentgenologic changes in
  barium-filled bowel, *1804, 1805*
Ileocecal valve. See *Valve, ileocecal.*
Ileus
  adynamic or paralytic, 1706, 1818
  gallstones, 1265, *1266,* 1706, 1743, *1744*
  mechanical obstruction, 1245, 1706, 1818
    absence of gas in pelvis minor, *1252*
    associated hernia, 1251
  meconium, 1245, *1268,* 1807, 1820, 1831
    in infants, 1744
  of colon, 1818
  reflex, 1243
  secondary, to impacted gallstones, *1267*
    to myxedema, 1818
  "sentinel loop," associated with acute
    appendicitis, 1848
  small intestinal, associated with absence of
    gas, *1253*
  subdiaphragmatic abscess and, 759
  volvulus, 1246
Iliac angle, *213* (table)
Ilium, fracture of, 145
  hypoplastic, with asphyxiating thoracic dys-
    trophy of newborn, 773
  stress fracture of superior ramus, *145*
Immunological disorders, and myocardiopathy,
  1158
Imperforate anus, *1237*
Index, acetabular, 427, *428*
Infant mobilization device, *32*
Infantile cortical hyperostosis, 59, 337, 340,
  781, *783*
Infarction, of bone, 61, *257, 353, 354*
  of kidney, *1393, 1398*
    tramline calcification, *1366,* 1391
  of lung, 744, *802,* 829, 894, 939, 970, 971, *973,*
    974

Infarction (*Continued*)
  of lung, complicated by gangrene, 875
    "reverse comma" sign, 955
  of small intestine, *1810*
Iniencephaly, 1876
Insecticides, 929
Intercostal spaces, appearance with emphysema,
  993, 995
  pulmonary agenesis and, 771
Intercostal vessels, in mediastinum, *1014*
International radiological classification of
  pneumoconiosis, 931
Intervertebral disk
  anatomic relationships, *687*
  herniation of, 681
  infections of, 681
  injuries to, 681
  myelogram of, *688*
  radiographic manifestations of disease, 681
  vacuum phenomenon, 682
Intestine, large. See *Colon.*
Intestine, small, 1689–1753. See also *Duodenum.*
  abnormalities
    in architecture in disease states, 1736
    in architecture, size, contour, and function,
      1707
    in density, 1743
    in function, 1746
    in number (congenital), 1699
    in position, 1699
    in size, 1706
  amyloidosis of, 1735
  angiography of, 1696
  architectural disruption, 1723
  blind loop syndrome, 1734, *1734*
  carcinoid tumors of, *1719, 1736, 1743*
  carcinoma of, 1741, *1742*
  cobweb or lacelike reticulation, 1732
  coiled spring appearance with intestinal ob-
    struction, *1705*
  common mesentery deformity, *1704*
  differences, between jejunum, ileum, colon,
    1690
    in roentgen appearance from large
      intestine, *1757*
  displacement by urinary bladder, *1706*
  distribution, *1690*
  diverticula of, 1712, *1713,* 1737
  dysgammaglobulinemia of, 1739
  edema of intestinal walls, 1732
  enema examination, 1693
  enterogenous cysts, 1699
  eosinophilic (allergic) gastroenteritis, 1739
  foreign bodies in, 1743
  hemangioma of, 1743
  hemorrhage of, *1810*
    intramural, 1716, *1720*
  herringbone appearance with distended
    intestine, *1705*
  hypoalbuminemia, scattering and clumping
    of barium, *1722*
  in protein-losing enteropathy, *1710*
  infarction of, *1810*
  internal anatomy of, 1689
  intestinal biopsy techniques, 1696
  intubation technique, 1695
  intussusception of, 1735
  jejunal pattern in protein-losing enteropathy,
    1711

Intestine (*Continued*)
  lymphangiectasia of, 1736
  lymphomatous involvement of, *1726*
  lymphosarcoma of, *1727*, 1739, *1741*
  malignant lymphoma, *1740*
  Menetrier's disease, 1712
  metastatic carcinoma, 1741
  mucosal changes (roentgen signs), classification of, 1707
    clumping, 1712
    fistulation, 1714
    longitudinal or transverse streaking, 1714
    "moulage" accumulations, 1712
    "picket fence" appearance, 1716
    punctate spiculation, 1716
    roentgenographic appearances, 1712, 1714, 1716
    sausagelike, 1712
    sawtoothing, *1716*
    scattering, 1712
    segmentation, 1712
    "stacked coins," 1716
  normal pattern, in infant, *1694*
    in child, *1696*
  normal series, 1693
    study with water soluble iodinated contrast media, *1695*
  normal variations with age, 1697
  obstruction (mechanical), *1728, 1730*
    most frequent causes in adults, 1706 (table)
    most frequent causes in neonates, 1707
  paralytic ileus, 1706
  pattern in Zollinger-Ellison syndrome, *1733*
  peristaltic movements of, 1692
  radiation enteropathy of, 1721, *1723*
  regional enteritis, *1715*, 1717, *1719, 1720, 1721, 1724, 1733*
  related anatomy, 1689
  roentgen signs of abnormality, 1698
  roentgenologic examination in infants and children, 1695
  scleroderma of, 1713, 1715
  skip areas of involvement, 1723
  sprue, appearance in, *1708, 1709*
  stepladder appearance associated with obstruction, *1705*
  string test for bleeding, *1697*
  technique of examination, 1692
  tumors, benign, 1725
  volvulus of, 1735, 1737
  Whipple's disease, 1725, *1729*
  worm infestation of, *1732*
Intussusception, 1255, 1737, 1807, 1821, 1822
  cause of small bowel obstruction, 1706, 1735
  classification of types, 1822
    enterocolic, *1798*
    enterogenous cyst formation, 1699
    ileocolic, *1822*
    jejunogastric, *1666*
Involucrum, 249, *301*
Ischium, avulsion of tuberosity of, *145*
  in cleidocranial dysostosis, *186*
Isoamylacetate, 929
IVP. See *Urinary tract, IVP.*

Jejunum, atresia of, *1761*
  carcinoma of, *1742*

Joint(s), 380–432
  amphyarthrodial, *380*
  ankle
    anatomy, 155
    axial relationships, *161, 385*
    classification of injuries, 155
    dislocations of, 155, *160, 164*
    fractures, and ligamentous tears, *157, 159, 160*
      eversion, *158*
      inversion, 155, *156*
  arthritis involvement. See *Arthritis.*
  Charcot, *400*
  chondromatosis of, 386
  classification(s) of, 380, 427, 429
  diarthrodial, *380*
  disease of, radiologic classification, 385, 386
  elbow, axial relationships of, *382*
  glenohumeral, in rheumatoid arthritis, 784
  hip, axial relationships of, 149, *383*
    congenital dislocation, criteria for, *384*
    dislocation of, classification, 147, *147*
    fractures of, 148, *148*
    malum coxae senilis, *396*, 397
  hydrarthrosis of. See *Hydrarthrosis.*
  idiopathic capsulitis of the. See *Capsule, joint, idiopathic capsulitis.*
  inflammation of, in migratory polyarthritis, 386
  knee
    axial relationships of, *384*
    dislocations of, *151*
    fractures, classification of, *150*, 151
    ligamentous tears of, *153*
  loose bodies in, 386
  pyogenic infection of, 386
  radiocarpal (wrist), *137, 139, 140*
  radiographic analysis of, 381, *386*
  radiology of, 380–432
  radioulnar, varieties of fractures, 134, 135, *136*
  rheumatic fever associated, 386
  sacroiliac, dislocation of, 145
    obliteration associated with ulcerative colitis, *1808*
    radiological abnormalities of, 678
  shoulder, axial relationships of, *381*
  spine, abnormalities of, 677, 678
    anatomy of, 678
  subtalar, 160
  synarthrodial, *380*
  temporomandibular, position drawings, *534*
    radiographic pathology of, 551
  tuberculosis, 305
  wrist, axial relationships of, *382*
Juvenile kyphosis dorsalis. See *Vertebrae, epiphysitis.*

Kaposi's sarcoma, 1743
Kartagener's triad, 1206
Kerley's A lines, 866, 947, 957, 971
  in rheumatic heart disease, 1153
  with left heart failure, 960
Kerley's B lines, 901, *906, 939*, 947, 957, 971, *1112*
  in rheumatic heart disease, 1153
  with left heart failure, 960
  with mass lesion suggesting bronchogenic carcinoma, 901
  with pulmonary carcinoma, 908, 911

Kidney(s)
  abscess of, 1353, 1454, *1455*
  adenocarcinoma, *1356*
  anatomic and physiologic concepts sum-
    marized, 1350
  angiography, 1461
  angulation of, 1345
  arterial abnormalities, 1461, *1464*
  arterial supply, segmental distribution, 1349,
    1349
  arteriography of, *1329, 1449*
  calcification in, *1365, 1366, 1367, 1368,* 1371,
    1372, 1374, 1375, 1376
    categories of, 1378
    in children, 1378
    tramline, 1450
  calculus (staghorn), *1388*
  calyces of, *1357*
    abscess of, *1381*
    architecture, changes in, *1386*
    cicatricial changes of, *1360*
    clubbing, *1360, 1380*
    contour, alterations in, *1360, 1387*
    diverticulum, *1381, 1382*
    edge pattern, changes in, *1380*
    fraying, *1380*
    irregular filling of, *1360*
    lucencies in, (classification), 1386
    papillary necrosis, *1381*
    papilloma in, *1404*
    pyelocaliectasis, changes in, *1379*
    pyelonephritis, changes in, *1380*
    renal cyst, changes with, *1362, 1432*
    renovascular hypertension, appearance in,
      1394
    tuberculosis, changes with, *1407*
    tumor, changes with, *1361*
  carcinoma of, *1368*
    appearance of secondary metastatic spread
      to lung, 925
  collecting system (including calyces), abnor-
    malities in architecture, 1378, 1382
  contour, abnormalities of, 1334, 1353
    infantile renal lobulation, *1356*
    lobulation, 1345
    with disease states, *1359*
  cortex, *1346*
    necrosis, bilateral, 1460
  cystic disease of, *1438*
    classification, 1437
    congenital, 1436
    roentgenographic findings, 1437
  cysts of, 1353, *1362*
    classification, 1434
    peripelvic, 1436
    roentgenographic findings, *1380,* 1435
    vs. neoplasm, 1327, 1445 (table)
  density, changes in, 1358
  destructive or degenerative lesions associated
    with dystrophic calcification, 1377 (table)
  displacement, by psoas mass, *1354*
    by suprarenal tumor, *1354*
  "dromedary," 1353
  duplex, 1439
  edge pattern of, 1346
  enlargement of, classification of causes, 1434
  examination, methods of, *1340*
  fibromuscular defects of renal artery, *1397,*
    1463
  function, impairment of, 1389

Kidney(s) (*Continued*)
  horseshoe, *1354, 1355*
  hydrocele of, 1450
  hydronephrosis, 1440
    grading by excretory urography, *1442*
    roentgenographic appearance of, 1441
  hypertension, renovascular, *1389,* 1460, 1461
  infarction of, 1390, *1393, 1398*
  infections of, *1455*
  internal architecture of, 1346
  leukemic infiltration of, 1446
  longitudinal section through, *1346*
  lymphoma of, 1447
  malrotation of, *1354*
  masses in pediatric age group, 1447 (table)
  measurements of, 1342 (table)
    normal in adults and children, *1343*
  medulla of, *1346*
  medullary sponge, 1438
    pyelotubular backflow, *1381*
    roentgenologic features of, 1439
  number, variations in, 1352, *1353*
  papillary necrosis of, *1383,* 1457, *1458*
    roentgenologic features, *1459,* 1460
  pararenal pseudocyst, 1439, 1440
  pararenal pseudotumor, 1439
  pelvis of, alteration in contour, *1357*
    architectural changes, *1386*
    filling defects in, 1358
    lucencies in (classification), 1386
    roentgenographic appearance with pathology,
      1379
  physiology of, 1350, *1351*
  polycystic disease of, *1357, 1379, 1380,* 1382,
    1438
  position of, 1342, 1352, *1354*
  pseudotumor, 1353
  pyelectasis, 1440
  pyelogram, confusing appearances of, *1385*
    filling defect of pelvis, *1386*
    rapid sequence or minute, 1387
    test of renal function, 1387
  pyelointerstitial backflow, *1381, 1384*
  pyelolymphatic backflow, *1381*
  pyelonephrosis, *1379, 1380*
    chronic, 1384
  pyelotubular backflow, *1381, 1384*
  relationship to vertebrae, *1344*
  roentgen examination during surgical
    exposure, 1332
  roentgen signs of abnormality (summary),
    1352
  rupture of, *1362*
  size, variations in, 1342, 1352, *1353*
    with renovascular hypertension, *1390*
  thrombosis of renal vein, 1395, 1398
  trauma of, 1447, *1448,* 1450
    classification, 1447, 1448 (table)
  tuberculosis of, 1360, *1367, 1406,* 1453, *1455,*
    1457
    changes in calyces, *1380*
    roentgen findings in, summary, 1409, 1455
  tumor of, *1373,* 1441
    adenocarcinoma, 1443
    adenoma, 1442
    carcinoma vs. cyst, *1444,* 1445 (table)
    classification, 1441
    hamartoma, 1442, 1443
    radiographic changes, *1361*
    Wilms', *1356,* 1446

Klippel-Feil deformity, 618, 620
  and abnormality of position in relation to
    skull, 668
  in childhood, 257
Knee
  ligamentous tears of, *153*
  osseous changes with age in male and
    female, *88*
  osteochondritis dissecans, *276, 281*
KUB film, in examination of biliary system,
  1479, 1480
Kymography, 729, 736
Kyphosis, barrel chest and, 774
  basal, *449*
  definition of, 669
  in Morquio's disease, 627
  juvenile, in osteochondrosis, 279
  secondary to pulmonary hypertension, 954
  secondary to steroid therapy, 413

Ladd's bands, with malposition cecum, 1745
Lambert, channel of, *801*
Lamina dura, *548*
  hyperparathyroidism, changes in, *238, 240, 508*
Laryngogram, anatomy demonstration, *1534*
  carcinoma of tongue, study of, *1527*
  pathology demonstration, *1534*
  phonation and respiration, demonstration
    of, *1532*
Laryngomalacia, with upper respiratory tract
  obstruction, 788
Laryngopharynx, abnormalities in architecture,
  1532, 1533
  methods of study, 1524
  neoplasms of, 1535
  roentgen signs of abnormality, 1533
Larynx, 701, 706, 707, 731, 794
  abnormalities of function, 789
  anatomy of, 705
  carcinoma of, 794, 795
  radiographic study of, 702
  structure of, 702
  tuberculosis with, 839
Laterality, definition of, 39
Law of Bergionér and Tribondeau, 25
Law's position, 551, *556*
  in identification of cholesteatoma, *570*
Lead osteopathy, 333
Lead poisoning, *334*
Leiomyoma, 1030
  of stomach, 1647
  of stomach-duodenum, *1649*
Leontiasis ossei, 353, 506, 513, 519
Leri's pleonostosis, 223
Letterer-Siwe disease, 248, 508
  in skull, 506
  in spine, *246*
Leukemia, 94
  bone changes associated with, 257, 258, 259,
    331, 337, 338
  bowel, associated involvement of, 1838
  metaphyseal involvement, 260, *261*
    transverse bands in, *332,* 333
  pulmonary involvement, *900, 922*
  spinal malalignment, *673*
Leukoplakia, of esophagus, 1555
  renal, 1358
Lichen planus, with pharyngeal pathology, 1535

Ligaments
  ankle joint, tears of, *155, 157, 158, 159*
  deltoid, 155
  knee joint, tears of, *153*
  lateral collateral, 155
  medial collateral, of knee, calcification of, 387,
    424
    of tarsal navicular, 155
  petroclinoid, calcification of, 532, *583*
  tibiofibula, 155
Ligamentum arteriosum, causing compression of
  esophagus, *1560*
Ligneous perityphlitis of cecum, 1047
Lindau-von Hippel disease, 1446
Line
  anterior mediastinal, 1016
  arcuate, in acetabular dysplasia, 213
    in congenital dislocation of the hip, 213
  Chamberlain's, *449, 488, 490, 652*
  fetal fat, 1864
  Fischgold's bimastoid, *449, 488*
  Fischgold's biventor, *488*
  McGregor's, *449, 488, 490*
  of petrous ridge, *449, 488*
  posterior mediastinal, 1016
  pubococcygeal, in imperforate anus, 1814
  Reid's base line, *434*
  Shenton's, *383*
  Skinner's, *383*
  tuberculo-occipital protuberance, *449, 488*
  white line of Frankel (scurvy), *264*
Linitis plastica
  of colon, 1843
    producing localized constriction, 1824
  of sigmoid colon, *1844*
  simulated by, fungal disease, 1621
    gastric sarcoid, 1621
    syphilis, 1621
  stomach, 1624
  with carcinoma of stomach, *1626*
  with tuberculosis, 1621
Lipochondrodystrophy, bony changes with, *774*
  Moquio-Brailsford type, with wedging of
    vertebrae, *648*
  Pfaundler-Hurler type, 64
    with wedged vertebrae, 648
  wedged vertebrae, *648*
Lipoid dysplasia, *287*
Lipoid storage disease, of lung, with fibrotic disease of parenchyma, 977
Lipomas, 786, 1030
  distribution in gastrointestinal tract, 1842
  identification by water enema, 1778
  in mediastinum, *1012,* 1035
  of cauda equina, 627
  of chest wall, 786
  of colon, 1799
  of corpus callosum, *595*
  respiratory change in mediastinal and sub-
    pleural, 769
  subpleural, 769
  with endocrine ulcer syndrome, 1646
Liposkeletogenic modulation. See *Diabetes,
  lipoatrophic mellitus.*
Lipping of bone, definition of, 40
Liver
  calcification of, 1295
  cysts of, nonparasitic, 1296
  determination of volume, 1297
  engorgement secondary to left heart failure, 960
  enlargement of, displacing adjacent organs,
    1293

Liver (*Continued*)
  enlargement of, in granulomatous disease of
      childhood, 846
    roentgen signs of, 1292
  examination, techniques of, 1292
  findings in neighboring organs with liver
      pathology, 1296
  function studies in diagnosis of jaundice,
      1516 (table)
  gas accumulation in, 1295
  Hodgkin's disease, involvement in, 1035
  identification of masses in, 1296, 1297
  increased density in, 1295
  left lobe of, 1294
  methods of study, 1294
  mucoviscidosis, involvement with, 969
  roentgen signs of abnormality, 1295
  traumatic laceration of, as cause of sub-
      diaphragmatic abscess, 759
  with diaphragmatic elevation, 750
Liver disease, as cause of respiratory obstruc-
    tion, 786
Lobstein's disease, 209
Lobulation, of kidney, 1345
Loepp's projection, *575*
Lordosis, definition of, 669
Lowe's disease, 236
Luckenschädel, 505
Lunate bone, dislocations of, 135
  dorsal, *142*
  dorsal perilunar, *142*
  perilunate, 135
  radiograph of, *143*
  volar, *142*
  volar perilunar, *142*
Lung(s)
  abscess, 811, 894, *896, 897, 920*, 988
    as complication of aspiration pneumonia, 857
    causes of, 896
    cavitation in, *1001, 1004*
    differential features of, 896
    in connection with pleura, 895
    significance of air within cavity, 895
    with mucous plug impaction, *968*
    with mucoviscidosis, 969
    with pulmonary meniscus sign, 912
  accentuation of bronchial pattern due to
      mucoid impactions, 961
  accessory lobes of, 721, *724*
  acinar involvement, 706, 877
  actinomycosis, 844
  adenomatosis, *900*
  adhesions between pleura and rib cage, *762*
  agenesis of, 771
    leafless tree bronchographic sign, 883
  alveolar carcinoma, classification of ap-
      pearances, 906
    radiographic aspects of, 908, 909
    site of metastases, 909
    with finely granular shadows, 932
  alveolar duct, 706
  alveolar pores (of Kohn), 707
  alveolar proteinosis, 807
    histopathology of, *806*
  alveolar sac, *799*
  amyloidosis, with finely granular shadows, 932
  anatomy, normal roentgen, 939
  angioma of, 912
  apical region, in chronic passive hyperemia,
      958
    with increase in linear markings, *938*
  aplasia of, 771

Lung(s) (*Continued*)
  arterial hypertension, *944, 952*, 993
  arterial supply, pulmonary artery throm-
      bosis, 988
  arterial vasculature, with pulmonary
      hyperplasia, 771
  arteriolar endarteritis, 932
  arteriovenous aneurysm of, 894, 912, *913*
    changes with respiration, *913*
    radiographic features of, 912
    with linear extension to hilus, 895
  arteriovenous angle, *940*
    measurements of, *719, 1147*
  arteriovenous fistulae, edge pattern of, 925
  artery(ies), pulmonary, *719, 942*
    accentuation of, 951
    anterior segmental, in relation to right
        apical vein, *940*
    apical, *942*
      tapering in pulmonary hypertension, *953*
    as linear or reticular markings, 939
    bronchial, 941
    changes in congenital heart disease, *1169*
    changes in pulmonary hypertension, 951
    changes with hemodynamic states, *944, 945*
    diffuse dilatation with congenital heart dis-
        ease, 951
    distention of, *950, 953*
    ectopia of, 1207, 1209
    enlargement in mediastinum, *1012*
    in arterial hypertension, *952*
    in lateral view of chest, *948*
    interlobar, right, *942*
    measurements of, *940*, 947
      in children, *940*
    multiple pulmonary aneurysms of, 913
    peripheral aneurysm of, 954
    pressure changes in pulmonary hyperten-
        sion, 956
    relationship to trachea and major
        bronchus, *941*
    relationship to tracheobronchial air
        column, 947
    relationship to tracheobronchial tree, 719
    with miliary nodulation, 955
    with thromboembolic disease, 955
    within mediastinum, *1014*
  asbestosis, with fibrotic disease, 977
    with webbing or honeycombing, 976
  aspergillosis, *1000*
  aspiration of oily substances, 917
  aspiration pneumonitis, classification of, 917
  asthma, accentuation of bronchial pattern,
      961, 965
    with increased chest radiolucency, 987
    with pneumomediastinum, 1048
  atelectasis, 920, *939*, 961, 970, 971, *973*, 975
      See also *Atelectasis.*
    changes in lupus erythematosus, 858
    with bronchial asthma, 965
    with bronchiectasis, 966
    with bronchiolitis fibrosi obliterans, 962
    with bronchogenic carcinoma, *898, 899*
    with esophageal rupture, 1566
    with mucoviscidosis, 969
    with subdiaphragmatic abscess, 759
    with tracheobronchitis, 962
  atria, 706, *799*
  bandlike shadows producing linear markings,
      970
  berylliosis, *928*
  beryllium poisoning, 970, 977

Lung(s) (*Continued*)
  bleb formation with hydrocarbon ingestion, 995
  blood flow of, 944, *944, 945, 946*
    cephalization, 946
    changes in pulmonary capillary pressure, 947
  bone formation in, as sign of mitral stenosis, 1110
  bronchi, *799, 942*
    chronic bronchitis of, 961, 991, *992*
    in muscular sclerosis, 981
    mucoid impaction of, 966, 968, *968*
  bronchial asthma, with mucoid impaction, 965
  bronchial distribution of, *712*
  bronchial pattern, 961
  bronchial tree, normal, *713, 714, 715*
  bronchiectasis, *897*, 961. See also *Bronchiectasis.*
    cavitation with, *1004*
    identification by bronchography, 966
    roentgenographic findings, *964, 965,* 966
    with congenital heart disease, 1206
    with Kartagener's syndrome, 968
    with mucoviscidosis, 969
    with scimitar syndrome, 961, *962*
  bronchiolectasis with muscular hyperplasia, 981
  bronchioles, respiratory, 706, *799*
    appearance in emphysema, 993
    terminal, 706
  bronchiolitis, acute, 987, 988, *989*
    with acute exanthemas of childhood, 871
  bronchiolitis obliterans, 977
  bronchitis (chronic), and chronic obstructive pulmonary disease, *954*
    causing accentuation of bronchial pattern, 961
    dirty chest appearance with, 965
    emphysema accompanying, 965
    secondary to pulmonary hypertension, *954*
  bronchogenic carcinoma, 883, 894
    cavitary lesions, *1004*
    cavitation with, *897,* 911
    chronic lung disease and, 911
    classification, pathologic, 911
    lymphangitis spread and, *923*
    Morton's S curve, *906*
    pneumonia and, *907*
    pulmonary meniscus sign and, 912
    radiographic features of, 911
    simulating aspiration of oily substance, 917
  bronchogenic cyst of, 1045
  bronchogenic tumor of, superior pulmonary sulcus (pancoast tumor), 909
  bronchogram, air, 961
    demonstrating bronchiectasis, *967*
  bronchopneumonia, 835
    as sequel to amebiasis, 835
    caused by parasitic flat worm infestation, 835
    of viral origin, 835
    radiologic appearances, 835
  bronchopulmonary dysplasia, 877, 880, *978, 979,* 980
    causing linear changes in lung parenchyma, 970
    causing respiratory obstruction, 786
    resemblance to Wilson-Mikity syndrome, 879
  bronchus, 942, *942, 948*
    air column relationships, 948 (table)
    asthma, 965
    bronchial adenoma, 988
    changes with left atrial enlargement, 1095

Lung(s) (*Continued*)
  bronchus, changes with mitral stenosis, *1106*
    check valve obstruction of, 988
    dilatation of, 961
    mucoid impaction, with asthma, 968
      with bronchitis, 968
      with mucoviscidosis, 968
    peribronchial fibrosis, 961
    relationship to pulmonary artery, 941
  brown induration of, secondary to left heart failure, 960
  bullae, 988
    and blebs, 981
  calcification of, 744, *893,* 894, 895
    appearance in pathological conditions, 917
    bronchogenic, 895
    granulomas (conglomerate), 895
    hamartoma, 895
    histoplasmoma, 895
    neoplasm, appearance with, 923
    osteogenic sarcoma metastasis, 895
    tuberculoma of, 895
    with infectious granulomas, 921
    with metastatic neoplastic disease, 921
    with microlithiasis, 921
    with pneumoconiosis, 921, 923
    with silicosis, 921
  carcinoma, alveolar cell, 883, 906
    histopathology of, *810*
    bronchogenic, radiographic signs of, 900
      901
    cavities in, 896
    miliary finely granular shadows with, 932
    with indrawn pleural sign, 975
    with muscular sclerosis, 981
    with rheumatoid disease, 859
  carcinomatosis (lymphangitic), as cause of septate or accentuated lymphatic lines, 971
  caseation, tuberculosis with, 895
  cavitary lesions, *839, 1004*
  cavitation of, 894
    differential diagnosis, *897*
    fluid level in cavity, significance of, 923
    incidence with metastatic spread, 925
    secondary to metastatic melanocarcinomatosis, *924*
    thin walls of cavities, significance of, 923
    with bronchogenic carcinoma, *899,* 901
    with infarction, 988
    with lung pathology, 917
    with metastases, 1004, *1005*
    with pneumoconiosis, 925, *926*
    with pulmonary hematoma, *916*
    with tuberculosis, 923
    with Wegener's granulomatosis, 925
  cavity of, air-meniscus level, *896*
    differentiation between those caused by mycobacteria and those caused by tuberculosis, 841
  Ceelen Gellerstedt syndrome, 977
  chemical poisoning of, 740
  cholesterol pneumonitis, nonobstructive, 917
  chronic bronchitis, 966
    with bronchogenic carcinoma, 901
  chronic obstructive pulmonary disease, radiographic appearance, 995
  chronic passive hyperemia of, *938*
  chronicity and disease, 744
  cinéradiography, in demonstration of bronchiectasis, 966

Lung(s) (*Continued*)
  coccidioidomycosis, *846, 1000*
    classification of, 847
    roentgenologic appearance of, 847, 848
  coin lesions of, *891,* 894
  collagen disease, changes in, tabulation of, 860
    with fibrotic disease of parenchyma, 977
  collapse of. See also *Atelectasis.*
    as cause of linear or reticular markings,
      939, 971
    with pneumothorax, *762*
  congenital absence of, 771
  congenital heart lesions, changes in
    parenchyma with, *1169*
  congenital pulmonary lymphangiectasis, roent-
    genographic appearance, 993
  congenital stenosis, left upper lobe, 988
  correlation of history and laboratory studies with
    roentgen appearance, 744
  cyst formation, congenital, *1000*
    with hydrocarbon ingestion, 995
  cystic disease of, cavitation with, *897*
    diagrammatic representation, *1004*
    with widening of thoracic cage, *771*
  cysts of, 762, 895, *920*
    classification, 999, 1003
    congenital, 896
    diagrammatic differentiation, *1000*
    roentgenologic features, 1003
    simulating pneumothorax, 1003
    thin-walled cavities, significance of, 923
    with histiocytosis, 981
  densities, poorly defined, homogeneous,
    scattered, 835
  dermatomyositis of, 877
  diffuse, poorly defined homogeneous shadows
    of parenchyma, 799–889
  dysmaturity as cause of respiratory obstruc-
    tion, 876
  echinococcus granulosis (pulmonary hydatid
    disease), 836
  edema of, *718,* 803
    air bronchogram sign with, 824
    interstitial, *803*
    producing linear changes, 970, 971
  edge pattern, significance of, 925
  effusion, pleural, with Q fever pneumonia, 857
    resemblance to atelectasis, *822*
  emphysema, 741, 988, *992, 996*
    absence in bronchial asthma, 965
    alpha-1 antitrypsin deficiency and, 1005
    alveolar carcinoma and, 909
    atelectasis and, 817, *817*
    barrel-shaped chest, 775
    bronchiectasis, 966
    bronchogenic carcinoma, *898*
    bronchogram, demonstration by, *967*
    bronchopulmonary dysplasia and, 880
    bullous, *1003*
    congenital, 762
    deformity of thorax, 772
    histiocytosis and, 981
    infantile, *996*
    interstitial, contributing to lucent lesions of
      chest wall, 987
    MacLeod's syndrome and, 966
    mucoviscidosis, 970
    pathologic classification, 990
    photomicrograph, *991*

Lung(s) (*Continued*)
  emphysema, pneumoconiosis and, *926*
    pneumothorax and, 762
    pulmonary fibrosis and, 980
    pulmonary hypertension, 952
    roentgenologic appearance of, 990
    Swyer-James syndrome and, 966
  empyema, cavitation associated with, *1004*
  exanthemas, acute, of childhood, radio-
    graphic findings, 871
  fibrosis of, *979*
    causing esophageal displacement, 1559
    classification of, 970
    diseases associated with, 980
    secondary to left heart failure, 960
    with circumscribed widening of pleural
      space, 761
    with obliterative pulmonary hypertension,
      952
    with tracheobronchiomegaly, 794
  fibrotic disease of, classification, 977
  finely granular shadows of, 929
    differentiation of, 933
    radiologic classification of, 932
  fissures of, 718
    accentuation, with bronchogenic carci-
      noma, 911
    accessory, 721, 971
    azygos, 722, 971, *973*
    bronchogenic carcinoma, appearance with,
      901, *904, 905*
    displacement with atelectasis, 814, 817
    interlobar, 721
      radiographic change with accumulation of
        fluid, 947
      with bronchogenic carcinoma, *898*
    movement with atelectasis, *822*
    oblique, 971
      in associated accessory diaphragm, 758
    related to linear shadows, 971
    three dimensional concept of, *723*
    with pulmonary gangrene, 875
  fistula of, changes in appearance during
    Valsalva and Mueller procedures, 925
  Fleischner's lines of, *973*
  fluoroscopy of, pulsations in multiple pulmo-
    nary artery aneurysms, 913
  fungus infections of, 844
    actinomycosis, 845
    aspergillosis, 844, 850
    blastomycosis, 845
    histoplasmosis, 845
    nocardiosis, 844, 845
  gangrene of, roentgenographic appearance
    of, 875
  granuloma of, 894
    caused by aspiration of oily substances, 917
    infectious, causing linear shadows, 971, *973*
    lipoid, 918, *918,* 919
    producing line shadows, 970, 975
    site of involvement, 921
  granulomatous disease of, 846
  hamartomas, 894, 911
    and calcification, 923
    radiographic features of, *910,* 911
  Hamman-Rich syndrome, 976, 977
  haziness of lung fields, with increase in linear
    markings, *938*
  hemangioma (sclerosing), 912

Lung(s) (*Continued*)

hematoma of, 811, *834,* 873
  roentgenographic appearances of, 915, *916,*
    1002
  with pulmonary meniscus sign, 912
hemithorax, 723
hemorrhage of, 877, 880
  as cause of respiratory obstruction, 786
  radiographic appearance of, 880
hemosiderosis, idiopathic pulmonary, and
    fibrotic disease, 977
  secondary to left heart failure, 960
hilar glands, connecting with peripheral
    nodular lesion, *975*
hilar region, changes in sarcoidosis, 955
hilus(i)
  appearance in lung disease characterized by
    linear markings, *938*
  arteriovenous aneurysm, appearance with,
    913
  associated findings of, 925
  bronchogenic carcinoma and, *898*
    enlargement with, *898*
  connection between lung nodules, *893*
  distention in chronic passive hyperemia,
    958
  idiopathic unilateral hyperlucent lung,
    appearance with, *998*
  relationship to mediastinal lymph nodes,
    1026
histiocytosis of, classification of pathological
    features, 980
  radiographic features of, 981
histiocytosis X, and honeycomb appearance,
    976
histoplasmosis of, 933
  calcification in, *847,* 921
  radiographic appearance of, 846
honeycombing appearance, 988
  classification of, 980
  producing linear shadows, 970
  with berylliosis, 980
  with biliary sclerosis, 980
  with giant cell pneumonia, 980
  with interstitial fibrosis of lung, 978
  with interstitial pneumonia, 977
  with mesenchymomatosis, 980
  with pulmonary adenomatosis, 980
  with pulmonary histiocytosis, 981
  with pulmonary myomatosis, 980
  with sarcoid, 980
  with scleroderma, 980
  with thromboangiitis obliterans, 980
  with tuberculosis, 980
  with tuberous sclerosis, 980
hyaline membrane disease of, *813, 818,* 880,
    881, 980
  as cause of respiratory obstruction, 786
  comparison with congenital pulmonary
    lymphangiectasis, 994
  in newborn, 877
  pathogenesis, 880
  radiographic appearance of, 880
hydatid disease of, *1000*
  and pulmonary meniscus sign, 912
hyperemia, active, *938,* 950, *950*
  chronic passive, 944, *958*
hyperlucency, with pulmonary thrombo-
    embolism, 830

Lung(s) (*Continued*)

hypertension, *1109*
  classification of types, 951, 952, 954, 1109
  high altitude, *954*
  hyperdynamic, 951, *951*
  obliterative, 952
  primary idiopathic, 954
  radiographic appearance of, *954, 955, 956,*
    959
  vasoconstrictive, 952
  with fibrotic disease, 977
  with increased radiolucency of chest, 988
  with mitral stenosis, *951*
  with "pruned branch" appearance, 952
  with pulmonary fibrosis, 980
  with thromboembolic disease, 952
hypogenesis or aplasia of, with narrow hemi-
    thorax, *771*
hypoplasia, with bronchiectasis, 771
  with scimitar syndrome, 961
idiopathic unilateral hyperlucent, *998, 999*
infarction of, 829, *832,* 894
  as cause of linear markings, 939, 970, 971,
    973, 974
  elevation of diaphragm accompanying, 832
  frequency of, *832*
  pathological changes of, 829
  pulmonary hypertension and, 952
  resolution stages, *833*
  roentgenographic appearance of, 830, *831*
  secondary to schistosomiasis, 835
infiltration of, with subphrenic abscess, 759
inflammation of, with "fuzzy" external edge, 925
internal architecture, pathology of, 925
international classification of pneumoconioses,
    931
international radiological classification of
    chest films, *931* (table)
interstitial edema, 877
interstitial fibrosis, classification, 978
  with fibrotic disease of parenchyma, 977
  with webbing or honeycombing, 976
interstitial involvement, 877
interstitial pneumonia reticuloendothelioses,
    877
interstitial tissue, 947
Kerley's B lines, 901, 908, 911, *1112*
lesions of, 873, 938, *938*
  occurring primarily in lung apices, classifica-
    tion of, 836
  single nodular, classification of, 894
  solitary, distinguishing features of, 917
linear, changes of parenchyma, 955
  density, 744
  markings of, 969, *973*
    Kerley's A and B lines, *973*
  shadows, 744, 939, 971, *973, 974*
    following pulmonary infarction, 833
    of parenchyma, 970
  streaking, with scleroderma, 955
lingular portion of, 721
lipoid dyscrasias of, 932, 933
lipoid storage diseases, 970, 977
lobar or segmental distribution of pathology,
    814
lobes of, *723*
  azygos, 721
  herniation with atelectasis, *822*
  right lower, inferior accessory fissure of, 721

Lung(s) (*Continued*)
lobule of, *717*
primary, 706
lymph nodes of, with eggshell calcification, *926*
lymphadenopathy, with muscular sclerosis, 981
lymphangiectasis of, 786, *938*
congenital pulmonary, 993
lymphatic drainage of, *720*
lymphatic supply, thickening with pneumoconiosis, *926*
lymphatics of, 711, 939, 947, 970, *972*
lymphoid distribution, *972*
lymphomas of, as cause of septate or accentuated lymphatic lines, 971
malignancy of, alveolar, *900*
bronchogenic carcinoma, *899*
carcinoma resembling pneumonia, *899*
lymphangitic type, *900*
Pancoast tumor, *899*
small (oat) cell, *900*
malignant tumors of, adenocarcinoma, 897
alveolar epithelial carcinoma, 897
bronchogenic carcinoma, 897, *898*
lymphangitic spread, *898*
sites of metastases, *900*
squamous cell carcinoma, 897
melioidosis, *802*
metastases in, cavitation of, 923, 1004
lymphangitic type, *922*
miliary type, *922*
metastatic involvement vs. primary lung
disease, 920
metastatic spread, coarse nodular type, *922*
"golfball" type, *922*
pneumonic and peribronchial type, *922*
subpleural type, *922*
metastatic tumors of, *922*
method of study, bronchography, 966
microlithiasis of, 921
migratory type of involvement, 810
miliary carcinosis of, time-sequence, 933
miliary dissemination, with histoplasmosis, 846
miliary distribution of pathology, 876
mitral stenosis, pulmonary arterial pressure
changes, *1113*
with left heart failure, bone formation
associated with, 960
moniliasis, 846
mucoid impaction, with asthma, 961
with mucoviscidosis, 961
mucous plugs, *854*
mucoviscidosis, 855, *855*, 968, *969*
multiple nodular lesions of parenchyma, 919
multiple pulmonary arterial aneurysm,
simulating lymphoma, 913
simulating sarcoidosis, 913
simulating tuberculosis, 913
muscular hyperplasia of, 981
muscular sclerosis of, 981
mycoses, *802*
arrested, 933
calcification and, 921, 933
causing finely granular shadows, 932
cavitation in, *897, 1004*
differentiation of, 933
infections of, 844
site of involvement, 921
necrosis of, following trauma, *834*
necrotizing vasculitides, changes with, 864

Lung(s) (*Continued*)
neoplasms of, 883
and increased radiolucency, 988
nodular lesions, 890
classification, *891*
of parenchyma, 890
with linear shadows towards the pleura, 975
nodular shadows, 744
in diseases with increased linear markings,
938
nodulation in, *893*
cavitation, significance of presence or
absence of, 923
classification of, 890
conglomerate appearance of, *930*
connecting with hilar lesion, 975
diagnosis by polytomography, *892*
by tomography, *892, 893*
with alveolar cell carcinoma, 908
with rheumatoid disease, 858
normal arteriogram, *1112*
obliterative pulmonary hypertension, with
sarcoidosis, 952
osteoarthropathy, with actinomycosis, 844
oxygen toxicity, with fibrosis, 980
Pancoast tumor of, clinical features, 909
parenchyma
bandlike shadows connecting with pleura,
976
classification, 745
of lesions greater than 3 cm., 894
of radiographic appearances, 741
differentiation from pleural effusion, *764*
haziness due to chronic passive hyperemia,
958
lesions larger than 3 cm., 894
poorly defined diffuse homogeneous densities
of, *802, 803*
classification of, 802
parenchymal shadows, diagrammatic appearance of roentgenologic types, *920*
differentiation by size and shape, 920, *920*
location with regard to possible cause, 921
minute nodular, with pulmonary hyperemia,
958
poorly defined homogeneous, classification
of, *742*
single mass shadows larger than 3 cm. in
diameter, 895
passive hyperemia, and appearance of pulmonary arteriovenous angle, *940*
pathology, differentiation of, study of
sequential films, 933
limited to inner two-thirds, 864
of apices or subapical regions, 808
of basilar distribution, 810
with abscess formation, 811
with acinar involvement, 812
with interstitial involvement, 812
with miliary pattern of distribution, 876
with miliary spread, 812
with pneumatocele formation, 811
with suppuration, 811
periarteritis nodosa of, pulmonary hypertension changes with, 952
peribronchial fibrosis in, *938*
physiology of, in roentgen diagnosis, 739–741
pleura, as cause of linear shadows, 971
relationship to mediastinum, *1013*

Lung(s) (*Continued*)
  pneumatoceles and, 811, 896
  pneumoconiosis
    calcification with, *926*
    causing finely granular shadows of, 932
    causing line shadows of, 970
    classification of reactions induced, 929 (table)
    classification of roentgenologic appearance, 925
    fibrotic changes in parenchyma in, 977
    increased radiolucency with, 988
    linear markings with, 939, 975
    rate of progress of, 933
    vs. calcific changes, 921
    with pulmonary hypertension, 952
    with rheumatoid arthritis, *932*
  pneumonia of, *802, 803,* 825. See also *Pneumonia.*
    and mucoviscidosis, 969
    and pneumomediastinum, 1048
    interstitial, classification of, 977
    with webbing or honeycombing, 976
  pneumonitis, 961
    aspiration, 917
    caused by aspiration of oily substances, 917
    chemical, due to silo filler's disease, 962
    congenital, as cause of respiratory obstruction, 786
    hydrocarbon, 994
    interstitial, with pneumocystis carinii, 871
    obstructive, 897
    postradiation, causing linear changes in lung, 970
    with acute beryllium poisoning, 925
    with lupus erythematosus, 858
    with mucoviscidosis, 970
    with rheumatoid disease, 858
    with sarcoidosis, 1042
  pneumothorax, clear space in, *762*
    encystment of, 896
    with histiocytosis, 981
  postradiation changes, with fibrotic disease, 977
  primary infection, 836
  primary lobule of, *716, 799*
  pseudocysts, 988, *990*
    with pulmonary fibrosis, 980
  pseudolymphoma, 829
  Pseudomonas pseudomallei, 850, *853*
  pulmonary function tests, diagrammatic basis for, *741*
  radiolucent abnormalities of, 744, 746
  reticuloendothelial disease of, 976
  reticulonodular disease, *976*
  rheumatoid arthritis of, with pneumoconiosis, *932*
    with webbing or honeycomb appearance, 976
  rheumatoid changes in, with pneumoconiosis, 927
  rheumatoid disease of, 858
    with linear density, 955
    with pulmonary hypertension, 952
  roentgenographic investigation of, bronchograms, 962
  role of physiologist and radiologist compared, *739, 740*
  sarcoidosis of, 955
    appearance with aspiration of oily substances, 917

Lung(s) (*Continued*)
  sarcoidosis of, clinical progress of, 933
    finely granular shadows in, 932
    with fibrotic lung disease, 977
    with increased radiolucency, 988
    with pulmonary hypertension, 955
  scar formation, following trauma, *834*
    causing linear shadows, 971
    with changes of thorax, *771*
    with pulmonary infarction, 833
  scimitar sign, *962*
  scleroderma, changes in, *863, 864*
    with interstitial fibrosis of parenchyma, 978
    with pulmonary hypertension, 952
  secondary lobule of, *716, 717, 799, 799, 800*
    histologic appearance, *801, 805*
  segments of, *722, 725, 726, 727*
  septate or accentuated lymphatic lines, 971
  sequestration of, 771, 895, 913, *914,* 915
    cystic changes with, *914*
    extralobar, radiographic appearances of, 915
    intralobar vs. extralobar forms, 915
  shadows of
    bandlike, 939
    homogeneous, classification, 745
    honeycombing, 939, 975
    linear or reticular, caused by pleura, 971, classification, 745, *973*
    nodular, single or multiple, classification, 745
    parenchymal, occurring in any situation, 808
    scattered ill-defined irregular, *742, 743*
    segmental, 744, 804
      classification, 745
    single, irregular, mass, categories of, *895*
    weblike, 939, *973, 975*
  silicosis of, 740
    radiographic appearances, *926*
  transient tachypnea of newborn, 877, 880
  traumatic contusion of, 833
  thromboembolism, 830
  toxoplasmosis, 850
  tracheobronchial tree, *719*
    lymph nodes of, *720*
    relationship to pulmonary artery, *719*
    separation from esophagus with bronchogenic carcinoma, 911
  tuberculosis of, *802,* 836–844, 894, *920, 1000,* 1003
    adult reinfection type, 838, *840*
    atelectasis with, *838*
    atypical form of, 843, 844
    bronchitic type, 839
    calcification, *838, 841*
    cavitation, 896, *897, 1001, 1004*
    clinical classification by Amer. Thoracic Society, 842, 843
    effusion with, *838*
    endobronchial type, 838
    Ghon's focus, *838*
    miliary type (hematogenous), *839, 932, 933*
    primary (childhood) type, *838, 839*
    Ranke complex, 836, *837*
    resembling granuloma owing to aspiration of oily substances, 917
    simulating neoplasm, *839*
    site of involvement, 921
  tumor metastases of lymphangitic type, *924*
  tumorlets, 909

Lung(s) (*Continued*)
tumors of, 894
hamartomas, *910*
linear shadows and, 939, 970, 975
with widening of thoracic cage, *771*
vanishing lung disease, 1003
varicosities of, 912
vascular flow, cephalization, 710
vascular markings of, in lung disease with increase in linear markings, *938*
intensification in chronic passive hyperemia, *958*
loss of definition in left heart failure, 960
vascular supply, azygos vein, 721, *724*
hilar elevation in anonymous micro-bacteria, 841
measurements of, *719*
role of radiologist in, *740*
vascular system, 707, 711
vasculature of, as index of systemic pulmonic shunting, 1182
in congenital heart disease, 1167, *1169*, 1170, 1171, 1172, 1173, 1174, 1201, 1204
veins, 941, *942*, 947
abnormalities of, 956
accounting for linear or reticular markings, 939
anomalous, 957, 961
associated with arteriovenous malformations, 957
associated with pulmonary sequestration, 957
scimitar syndrome, 957
apical, *940, 942*
azygos, 941, *943*
basal, of right lower lobe (measurement of), *940*
bronchial, 941
central, diameter of, 941
changes in hemodynamic states, *944, 945*
changes with left heart failure, 960
hemiazygos, 941
in lateral view of chest, *948*
measurements, in children, *940*
with venous hypertension, 957
postcapillary pulmonary hypertension, classified, 957
relationship to left atrium and right pulmonary artery, 947
relationship to pulmonary arteries and bronchi, 941
secondary to massive thrombosis of main pulmonary artery, 957
size, variations in, 956, 957
classification of causes of decrease in, 957–961
decrease in, 956, 957
increase in diameter in pulmonary hypertension, *953*
thrombosis of, with linear shadows, 975
varices of, 956
solitary pulmonary varix, 961
varicosities of, 957, 961
venous engorgement, with pulmonary varicosity, 956
venous hypertension, *944, 952,* 961
postulate by Simon, 957
vessels of, differential changes with post-capillary pulmonary hypertension, 957
enlargement with emphysema, 993
measurement of, *940*

Lung(s) (*Continued*)
xanthomatosis, with honeycomb appearance, 980
Lupus erythematosus, 859, *859*
of lung, *802*
principal site of involvement, 921
roentgen changes in, 858
Lymphangiectasia, of small intestine, 1738
Lymphangiectasis, congenital pulmonary, 993
Lymphangiography, in chest, 736
in chest and mediastinum, 729
Lymphangioma, involving bone, 315
Lymph glands, enlargement in mediastinum, *1012*
lymphadenopathy, roentgenographic aspects in mediastinum, 1042
paratracheal, in mediastinal compartment, *1012*
Lymph nodes, carinal, involved with bronchogenic carcinoma, 901
eggshell calcification, with pneumoconiosis, *926*
enlargement, hilar, with acute exanthemas of childhood, 871
with pneumoconiosis, *926*
with tularemia, 872
with varicella pneumonia, 876
mediastinal, 1013
pulmonary, with psittacosis, 877
hilar and perihilar, eggshell calcification of, 925
mediastinal, identification by radioisotopic technique, 1027
with histoplasmosis, 845
of bronchopulmonary tree, secondary to sarcoidosis, 955
of tracheobronchial tree, 1025
peribronchial, right hilar mass obstruction, *721*
Lymphatic tissues in nasopharynx, absence in neutrophil dysfunction syndrome, 1034
Lymphatic trunk, *1024*
Lymphatic vessels, of esophagus, 1026
of mediastinum, *1024*
tumors of, *1012*
Lymphogranuloma venereum, *1785, 1839*
as cause of colon constriction, 1824
Lymphoid circulation, as occurs in lung, *972*
Lymphoid tissue, lymphoid hyperplasia of colon in children, 1846
Lymphoma
accentuation of pericardial fat pad, 1143
as cause of abdominal mass in childhood, 1290
as cause of intussusception in childhood, 1290
as cause of sclerotic lesions of spine, 632
deforming renal vein, 1331
demonstration in retropharynx, *1534*
esophageal displacement and, 1559
in bone, appearance with, *61*
longitudinal sclerotic changes, 337, *338*
radiographic findings, 344
in lung, *900, 922*
pleura, association with, 768
radiographic appearance, 920
with septate or accentuated lymphatic lines, 971
in mediastinum, 1013, 1031, *1037, 1039*
causing displacement of pleural stripe, 1016
in pancreatic bed, *1726*
in protein-losing enteropathies, 1712
in small intestine, *1718, 1740*
in spine, lucency and sclerosis of, 633
radiographic changes, 655
wedging of vertebra, *642*
in vertebral body, 634

Lymphoma (*Continued*)
  producing osteosclerosis, *325*
  respiratory tract obstruction and, 788
Lymphosarcoma, of cecum, *1805*
  of colon, 1843
  of lung, *922*
  of small intestine, *1727, 1739, 1741*

Madelung's deformity, *197*
Magnification, in estimation of cephalopelvic
  disproportion, 1885
Malacoplakia of urinary tract, 1451
Mandible, fibrous dysplasia of, *552*
  fractures of, 545
  position drawings, *534*
  radiographic pathology of, 551
Mandibular hypoplasia, 211
Mandibulofacial dysostosis, 211
Manganese, 929
Manubrium, in lateral view of chest, *948*
Marble bone disease, 59, *61, 192,* 327, 360, 1873.
  See also *Osteopetrosis.*
Marfan's defect, 954
  cardiac myocardiopathy and, 1158
  marginal rib defects and, 775
Marie-Strümpell's disease. See *Ankylosing
  spondylitis.*
Marrow disorders, 59
Mastectomy, radiographic appearances of, 781
  of axilla with, *787*
Mastocytosis (urticaria pigmentosa), *346,* 1653
  involving small intestine, 1738
  producing osteosclerotic changes in bone, *325*
  radiographic changes of, 328, 329
    in spine, 640
      sclerotic lesions of, *632, 633*
Mastoid bone, 551
  abnormalities in density of, 555
  development, arrested, 555, *566*
  examination, standard positions for, 551, *553*
  inflammation of (mastoiditis), 555
    sclerotic, *567*
    suppurative, *566, 567*
      with destruction of temporal bone, 568
  mastoid tip, radiograph of, *557*
  radiographic appearance in disease states, 555,
    566
  radiopacity of, increased, 566
  sclerotic reaction of air cells, *566*
Maxilla, fractures of (classification), *544*
Mayer's projection, 551, *554, 564*
McGregor's line, 449
Meconium, aspiration of, *760*
Meconium peritonitis, *1286*
Mediastinum, 729, 1011–1066
  abscess and production of gas, 1028
  air within, *760*
  anatomic compartments of, 1011, *1012*
    pathologic states associated, *1013* (table)
    sites productive of lesion, 1031
    structures in, *1014*
  anterior clear space of, *732,* 739
    accentuation with emphysema, 993
    measurements of, 993, 1018
    obliteration with bronchogenic carcinoma,
      901, 911
    pulmonary hypertension, changes in, 954,
      956
    radiolucency increased, *989, 992*

Mediastinum (*Continued*)
  bronchogenic cyst of, *1044,* 1045, *1045*
  bronchography, use of, 1027
  calcification in, 1026
    classification of, *1029*
  chorioepitheliomas of, 1031
  Cushing's disease, increase in fat in, 1030
  cystic abnormalities of, 1031
  cysts, congenital, 1606
    enteric, 1558
  deflection, with atelectasis, *827*
    with infrapulmonary effusion, *754*
    with scoliosis, *772*
  dermoid of, *1033*
  displacement, with atelectasis, 814, 822
  emphysema of, 987, *1046*
    with esophageal rupture, 1566
    with hydrocarbon ingestion, 995
  examination, radiologic technique of, 729, 1026
  fibrosis of, 1047
  fluoroscopic study, 1068
  hematoma of, *1012,* 1031
  hemomediastinum, 1031
  histoplasmosis, involvement with, 845
  Hodgkin's disease, involvement with, 1035
  infection of, 1046, *1046*
  inflammation of, 1013, 1031
    in anatomic compartments, *1012*
    secondary to chest trauma, 1031
    with rib notching, 780
  lateral view of chest, 739
    left lateral view, *1015*
  lesions, changes with time, 1031
    diseases associated, 1030
    most frequent sites of, *1012*
  lipomas in, 1035
  lymph nodes of, 1026
    enlargement, as cause of respiratory tract
      obstruction, 788
      with childhood exanthemas, *803*
      with cholesterol pneumonitis, 917
      with tularemic pneumonia, *803*
  lymphatic vessels in, *1024*
  lymphomatous involvement, *1037, 1039*
  myelograms in identification of disease, 1027
  neoplasms of, 883
  neurofibroma and, *1050*
  nonpenetrating injuries to thoracic aorta and,
    1052
  paramediastinal radiolucent line, obliteration
    with bronchogenic carcinoma, *904,* 911
  parathyroid adenomas in, 1035
  pneumomediastinography in identification of
    disease, 1027
  pneumomediastinum, 1031
    in infancy, 1048
  pneumothorax and, *762*
  position contrasted in pneumonia and
    atelectasis, *764*
  posterior mediastinal stripe, 1559, *1563*
  posterior pleural line and, *974*
  radiographic appearance, glossary of lesions,
    1031
  radiology of, 1011–1066
  relationship, of visceral and parietal pleura to
    vertebral column, *609*
    to azygos vein, 941
    to pleural lines, 971, *1016*
  roentgen signs, classification of, 1028
    of abnormality, 1027, *1029*
  sarcoid involvement of, *1040*

Mediastinum (*Continued*)
  seminomas of, 1031
  shift, with atelectasis, *764, 816*
    with change in shape of thoracic cage, *771*
    with expiration and inspiration, *754, 755*
    with pneumothorax, 761
    with unilateral low position of diaphragm,
      754
  teratomas of, 1031, 1032
  thymoma, *1034*
  tracheobronchiomegaly, 794
  tuberculosis, involvement with, 839
  tumors of, differentiation from lung, 1028
    identification in lateral chest film, 739
    with widening of thoracic cage, *771*
Medulla, normal appearance of, *61*
Medullary sponge kidney, *1365*
Medulloblastoma, 532
  calcification of, *467, 587, 589*
Megacolon, 1812. See also *Hirschsprung's
  disease.*
  idiopathic symptomatic, 1811
  toxic with ulcerative colitis, 1833
Megaesophagus, 1030, *1056*, 1555
Melioidosis, 850, 853
  of lung, *851*
Melorheostosis leri, *61, 222, 337, 338*
Membrane, interosseous, in forearm, *132,* 133
  changes accompanying injury, 134
Menetrier's disease, 1634, 1636, 1712
Meninges, coronal section, *502*
Meningioma, 353
  calcification of, *590, 592*
  of skull, 518, 519, *593, 594*
  sites of occurrence, *517, 591*
Meningocele, 486, 1030
  in mediastinum, 1012, 1013, 1053
Meniscus, traumatic laceration, *152*
Mercury, as cause of interstitial pneumonia, 977
Mesenchymomas, 1030
Mesenchymomatosis, 980
Mesenteric thrombosis, as cause of small bowel
  obstruction, 1706
Mesentery, common mesentery deformity, 1616
  normal fixation, *1745*
Mesomelic dwarfism, 205
Mesotheliomas, 1030
  of pleura, 768, *769*
Metacarpal fractures, 143
Metaphysis, 51
  aneurysmal bone cyst and, *298*
  appearance in, congenital rubella syndrome, *268*
    congenital syphilis, 269
    giant cell tumor of bone, *294*
    leukemia, *258, 259*
    neurotrophic osteopathy, *283*
    osteomyelitis, 249
    phenylketonuria, 266
    scurvy, *264*
  diabetic osteopathy, changes in, 282
  diseases of bone, changes with, *261*
  dysplasia, familial, 200
    metaphyseal, 223, 513
  Ewing's tumor of bone and, 313
  fracture of, *121*
  giant cell tumor of, *296*
  indiscrimate patchy foci of lucency or
    sclerosis, 323
  intraosseous ganglia and, 417
  lead poisoning, changes with, 333

Metaphysis (*Continued*)
  maldevelopment of, 199
  osteomyelitis, acute, early changes in, 304
  osteosclerosis, localized, *353*
  radiolucent changes, 260, *286*
  radiolucent diseases (without marginal
    sclerosis), *300*
    bone diseases, 282
  radiolucent lesions of, *275*
    with marginal sclerosis, *285, 288*
    without marginal sclerosis, 300
  transverse bands, 323, *332*
    of osteosclerosis, classification, 333
    of sclerosis, 336, *337*
  transverse striations in cretinism, 336
  traumatic cupping, 119
  vessels of supply, 51, *54*
Metastatic bone tumors. See *Tumors, metastatic
  to bone.*
Metastatic spread of carcinoma involving lung,
  differentiation from bronchogenic spread, 921
Metastatic tumor, in pleura, 761
  roentgen appearances in colon, 1846
Metatarsal bones, 162
  fractures of, 162
Metatropic dwarfism, 205
Methylbromide, 929
Methylchloride, 929
Methysergid, as cause of sclerosing mediastini-
  tis, 1047
Mica, 929
Milkman's disease, 311
Mongolism, 515
  clinical features, 215
  dysphagia with, 1559
  Klinefelter's syndrome and, 219
  roentgenologic features, *216, 217, 218*
  scoliosis and, 674
  segmentation of sternum with, 774
  spinal curvature and, 668
Moniliasis, of lung, 844, 988
Mononucleosis, finely granular lung shadows
  with, 933
Morquio-Brailsford disease, *672*
  and malalignment of spine, *673*
Morquio's disease, 203
  Hurler's disease and Morquio-Ullrich disease,
    differences from, 203
  spinal curvature and, 668
  thoracic cage, changes in, 770
  radiologic appearances of, 775
Morquio-Ullrich disease, 203
Morton's S curve, 901
  with bronchogenic carcinoma, *906*
Mounier-Kuhn syndrome, with upper respiratory
  tract obstruction, 788
Mucocele, *543*
  of frontal sinus, 540
Mucormycosis, 549, 850
Mucoviscidosis, *803, 852, 853, 855*
  in infants, 1744
  of colon, *1809*
  of lung, 968, 969
    linear changes in lung shadows, 970
    mucoid impaction with, 961
    respiratory tract obstruction with, 788
Multangular, greater, fractures of, 142
Multiple myeloma, *66, 241, 244, 270, 287, 346*
  circumscribed patchy radiolucency resulting
    from, 241

Multiple myeloma (*Continued*)
  clinical features, 242
  extrapleural sign with, 781
  metastatic malignancy, differentiation from, 781
  of skull, 512
  of spine, 644
    changes in, 637
    radiolucency of, 632
    spotted lucency of, 632
  radiographic appearances of, *245*
  radiolucency of bone with, 241
  risk of IVP, 1339
Muscle, anterior papillary, *1022*
  atrophy of, with Cushing's syndrome, 236
  hip disease in children, manifestation of, 426, 427
  iliopsoas, hypertrophy of, 1405
  papillary of ventricle, *1022*
  pectinati, *1022*
  pectoral, 781
    absence following mastectomy, *787*
    pectoralis major, 738, *1002, 1021*
  pronator quadratus, trauma with overlying fat plane, 142
  psoas, causing displacement of ureter, *1404*
    mass, displacing kidney, 1354
    shadow, in abdominal examination, *1219, 1224, 1226, 1228, 1229*
      with calcification in abdomen, *1284*
  scalenus anterior, *1024*
  sternocleidomastoid, 781
  sternomastoid, *787*
Muscular sclerosis of the lung, 981
Myasthenia gravis, 1030, *1034*
Mycelia, and increased radiolucency of lung, 988
Mycoplasma infections, as cause of interstitial pneumonia, 977
Mycosis, *803*
  cavities with, 895, 896, *897*
    thin walled cavities, 923
  cyst occurrence, *920*
  of lung, 836
    causing finely granular shadows, 932
    location of, 921
    with cavitation, 1004
    with extrapleural sign, 781
Myeloencephalogram, 498
Myelofibrosis, producing sclerosis of bone, *325*
Myelography, 682
  definition and technique, 685
  indications for use, 685
  mediastinal disease, identification of, 1027, 1051
  meningocele, differentiation of, 1053
  methods of distinguishing lesions of spinal canal and cord, *682*
  of foramen magnum clivus and, *685, 686*
  pathology, identification of, 686, 687
  position of patient, *683*
  radiographic examples, *684*
Myomatosis, pulmonary, 980
Myositis ossificans, *64*
  progessiva, *214*
    with spinal malalignment, *673*

Nasopharynx, 702
  aplasia of, 702

Nasopharynx (*Continued*)
  approximation of soft palate with posterior wall of, *1531*
  chordoma of, *1530*
  hemangiofibroma of, *1525*
    arteriogram of, *1526*
  malignant tumors of, 498
  masses in, with respiratory tract obstruction, 788
  measurement of, 702, 703
  neoplasia of, 702
  structure of, 702
  with Wegener's granuloma, 862
Nasopolyposis, with Kartagener's syndrome, 968
Navicular carpal bone (scaphoid), blood supply of, *141*
  classification of fractures, *141*
Navicular tarsal bone, 162
Neck, soft tissue abnormalities of, 1523, *1523*
  measurements of soft tissue spaces, 704
Necrosis, aseptic, from steroid therapy, *235*
Neoarthrosis, 171
Neonatal atelectasis, as cause of respiratory obstruction, 786
Nephrocalcinosis, 237, *1367, 1370*
  associated lesions, 1375 (table)
  clinical conditions causing, 1375 (table)
  in children, 1378
Nephrolithiasis, *1373*
  in childhood, 1378
Nephroptosis, *1354*
Nephrosis, with pericardial effusion, 1139
Nephrotomography, 1321, 1341, 1358
  cyst and neoplasm, differentiation between, 1327
  renal fat, demonstration of, 1339
Nerve(s)
  laryngeal, left recurrent, *1020, 1021*
  phrenic, *1020, 1021,* 1022, *1022, 1024*
    in mediastinum, *1014*
  splanchnic, *1023*
    greater splanchnic, in mediastinum, *1014*
    relationship to azygos venous system, *943*
  vagus, *1020, 1021,* 1022, *1025*
    in mediastinum, *1014*
    recurrent vagus, *1025*
    relationship to esophagus, *1537*
Neurilemomas, 1030
Neuroblastoma, 353, 1030, 1429, 1433
  longitudinal osteosclerotic changes of, *338*
  rib and skull, changes in, *493*
  roentgenologic features of, *313, 314,* 490, 1051
Neurofibroma, 314, 315, 786, 1030
  compression of sigmoid and, *1828*
  of mediastinum, *1050,* 1051
  of skull, *470*
  of superior rib margin, 775
  vertebral erosion and, 1052
Neurofibromatosis, involving colon (simulating congenital megacolon), 1814
  radiograph of, *314*
  with meningocele, 1053
  with rib notching, 780
Neurogenic arthropathy, sites of occurrence, *399*
Neuromuscular atrophy, with chest wall lucency, 987
Neuronoma, of phrenic nerve, 1013
  of vagus, 1013
Neuropathic arthropathy, of spine, 680
Neuropathy, hereditary sensory radicular, 283
Neurotrophic osteopathy, 283

Neurovisceral storage disease, 223
Niche, definition of, 40
Niemann-Pick disease, 247, 248, 508
  of skull, 506
Nitrofurantoin lung disease, 970, 980
Nitrous fumes, 929
Nocardiosis, involving lung, 845
Nose, dermoid cyst of, 549
  fractures of bones and cartilages of, 545
  position drawings, 535
Notch, greater sciatic, 1892
  sacrosciatic, 1891
Nuclei pulposi, 782

Obesity, and elevation of diaphragm, 750
Obliquity, definition of, 39
Obstetrics and gynecology, 1863–1915
Obstruction, mechanical, of bowel, causes of,
  1818
Ochronosis 633, 680
  of spine, 425, 679, 679, 680
  pathology and radiographic findings, 425
Ocular hypertelorism, 447
Odontoid process, fracture of base of, 656
  involvement with rheumatoid arthritis, 410
Odontoma. See Cyst, dentigerous.
Oligodactylia, 221
Oligodendroglioma, 589, 590
Ollier's disease, 199, 361
Omentum, herniations of, 1036
  sac of, 1253
  lesser sac of, 1245, 1703
Omphalocele, 1304
Optic nerve glioma, 578, 579
Orbit, alterations in density, 577
  asymmetry of, 576
  blow-out fractures of, 546, 547, 548
  histiocytosis X, changes with, 577
  hypertelorism. See Hypertelorism.
  interorbital distance, in mongols, 450 (table)
    measurements at various ages, 450 (table)
    normal, 451
  method of examination, 572, 573
    special techniques for, 575
  roentgen signs of abnormality, 573, 574
  routine study of, 574
Ornithosis, 876, 877
Orodigitofacial dysostosis, 223
Oropharynx, abnormalities of function, 1523
  carcinoma of, in lung, 922
  masses in, with respiratory tract obstruction,
    788
  radiographic methods of examination, 1522
  soft tissues, abnormalities in size, 1523
    of neck, 1524
  tonsillitis, radiographic appearance in, 1529
Osmium, 929
Ossification, ectopic, 57
  enchondral, sequence of, 49
  in prediction of fetal maturity, 1866
Ossification centers
  age at appearance, 90 (table), 91, 112 (table)
  appearances, in foot, 84, 85, 86, 87
    in hands, 78, 79, 80, 81, 82, 83
  bone age sampling method, 111
  determination of fetal maturity, 1869 (table)
  distribution according to sex, race, and birth
    weight, 109 (table)

Ossification centers (Continued)
  in females, 68, 69, 70, 71, 72, 110
  in males, 74, 75, 76, 77, 110
  major, 73
  number of, at different months of age, 108
Ossifying fibroma, 353
Osteitis, radiation, 301, 310
Osteitis condensans ilii, 353, 355
Osteitis fibrosa cystica, 66, 287
Osteoarthritis. See Arthritis, hypertrophic.
Osteoarthropathy, in idiopathic hemochromato-
  sis, 413
Osteoblastic activity, with decreased or deficient
  bone formation, classification, 775
Osteoblastoma, 288
  benign, 299, 299
  simulating enchondroma, 291
Osteochondritis, syphilitic, 1873
  with Wilson's disease, 266
Osteochondritis dissecans, 281, 386, 421
Osteochondrodystrophy, 635, 672
Osteochondroma, 200, 200, 358, 359, 360, 361,
  778
  multiple. See Exostoses, hereditary multiple
    cartilaginous.
  of skull, 514
Osteochondromatosis, 358
Osteochondroses, 274, 276, 352
  anatomic sites involved, 277
  pathogenesis, 276, 278, 280
  with spinal malalignment, 673
Osteoclastic activity, with increased bone resorption, classification, 775
Osteogenesis imperfecta, 94, 209, 1873
  clinical types, 489
  homogeneous radiolucency of spine, resulting
    from, 632
  marginal rib defects and, 775
  vertebrae, effect on, 629
Osteogenic fibroma. See Osteoblastoma, benign.
Osteogenic sarcoma, calcification metastatic to
  lung, 895, 921
Osteoid osteoma, 357
  radiographic findings and clinical features,
    358
  with localized sclerosis of spine, 633
Osteolysis, 282
  familial, 221
Osteoma, 353
  of calvarium, sites of occurrence, 515
  of frontal sinus, 541
  of skull, 483, 486, 514, 515
    sites of distribution, 483
  osteoid, of spine, 656
    giant, of vertebrae, 645, 646
      causing spotted lucency of spine, 632
  radiographic appearance, 359
Osteomalacia, 59, 60, 63, 232
  definition of, 40
  fish vertebra, 648
  Milkman's syndrome and, 269
  skeleton, radiographic appearance of, 261
  spine, changes in, 636, 636
    homogeneous radiolucency of, 632
    malalignment of, 673, 674
Osteomalacic disorders, 260
Osteomatoses, 421
Osteomyelitis, 241
  brucellar, 307
  causing spotted radiolucency of bone, 632

Osteomyelitis (*Continued*)
  chronic fungus, 337, 344
  chronic, of skull, *505*
  familial acro-osteolysis and, *284*
  involving extremities, *251*
  mycotic, 344
  nocardial, 305
  nonsuppurative, 304
  of facial bones, 549
  of Garré, 352, 353, *355, 374*
  of skull, 494
  of spine, difference between tuberculous and
    nontuberculous lesions, 641 (table)
  radiographic appearance of, 249, *250, 301, 311*
  roentgen changes in acute form, 304
  secondary, 316, *318*
  simulating Ewing's tumor, 313
  tuberculous, *302,* 304, 305
  ulcer (tropical), 356
  widely disseminated, 249
Osteonecrosis, 345
Osteopathia striata, 222, *346,* 659
  vertical lucency and sclerosis of spine, 633
Osteopetrosis (marble bone disease), 59, *192,*
  360, 1873
  clinical features, 191, *192*
  radiographic appearance of, *326,* 327, 638
  sclerotic bone changes, 325
    in skull, 513
Osteopoikilosis, 222, 346
  and spotted sclerosis of spine, 632
Osteoporosis, *60, 61*
  causing multiple diseases, 59
  circumscripta, and Paget's disease of skull,
    348, 479
  definition of, 40
  fish vertebra, *648*
  hyperparathyroidism and, 237
    motheaten, 237
  in spine, *636*
    malalignment, *673*
    sclerotic lesions of, 632
  with Cushing's syndrome, 236
Osteosarcoma, 61, 301
  chondrosarcoma, comparison with, *363*
  radiographic findings, *308, 309,* 310, *359*
  simulating Ewing's tumor, 313
Osteosclerosis, 59, *60*
  affecting several extremities, *325*
  distribution of, in bone, *346*
  longitudinal sclerotic lines, 337, *339*
  radiographic changes, diseases producing signs,
    324, 325, 325
  radiographic diagnosis, 569
  transverse bands in metaphyses, 333
Ovaries, atrophic, *1909*
  cysts of, 1885
  in Hodgkin's disease, 1036
  measurement of, 1907
  polycystic, 1907
Oviduct, abnormalities of, 1901
  diagrammatic tracing of hysterosalpingograms,
    1904
  diverticulosis of, 1901
  hydrosalpinx, *1905,* 1907
  polyps associated, 1907
Oxalosis, calcification in kidney, *1365*
  with radiolucency of bone, 241
Oxycephaly, 223

Oxygen toxicity, 880
  roentgenograph of lung, *882*
  with bronchopulmonary dysplasia, *979*

Paget's disease, 59, 60, 61, 345, *346*
  boxlike sclerosis in vertebra, 633, *634*
  histology and radiologic classification, 346, 347
  of skull, 478, *479*
    "cotton ball" appearance, 479
  of spine, 659
    malalignment of, *673*
  osteosclerotic changes in bone, *325*
  radiographic appearance, *348, 349*
Palate, soft, *1531*
  bulbar, with upper respiratory tract obstruc-
    tion, 788
    pseudobulbar, 788
  causing respiratory obstruction, 786
  laryngeal, recurrent, with bronchogenic car-
    cinoma, 901
  phonation studies of, *1531*
Pancoast tumor, of pulmonary apex, 909
Pancreas, 1670–1681
  angiographic study, 1675
  annular, 1624, *1627*
  calcification in, 1670
  carcinoma, in stomach-duodenum, 1672
    metastatic appearance in lung, *900, 922*
    roentgen signs of, 1673
  cystic fibrosis of, with barrel-shaped chest, 775
    with respiratory tract obstruction, 788
  cysts, in relation to, *1674*
  inflammation of, causing subdiaphragmatic
    abscess, 759
    with colon cutoff sign, *1241*
  mucoviscidosis of, 969, 1679
  pathology affecting stomach-duodenum, *1613,*
    1614, 1615, 1616
  pseudocysts of, in mediastinum, 1031
  technique of examination and roentgen signs,
    1670
Pancreatography, direct, 1678
Pancytopenia, 1030
  and thymic pathology, 1034
Pannus formation, 402, *404,* 407
Papillary necrosis, *1365*
  of kidney, 1371, 1457, *1458, 1459*
Papilloma, of gallbladder, *1493*
Paracolonic gutter, *1304*
Paraganglioma, 1051
Paraganglioneuroma, 1030
Paragonimiasis, and bronchopneumonia, 835
Paralysis, of chest or larynx as cause of
  respiratory obstruction, 786
Paraplegia, and neuroarthropathy, 681
  bone, joint, and soft tissue changes, 425
  secondary to seat belt fracture, 675
Pararenal pseudocyst, 1439, 1440
  pseudotumor, 1439
Parathyroid, adenoma of, *1012,* 1030, 1035
  measurements, 1035
  osteosclerosis, 345, *346,* 350
  skull, changes in, *509*
  hormone, 56
Parietal bones, "bossing" of, 481
  types of defects, *501*
Parietography, 1602

Parkinson's disease, and pseudobulbar palsy, *1528*
Parosteal osteoid sarcoma, 362
Patella, bipartite, *154*
    fracture, typical, 154
Patent ductus arteriosus, and increase in radio-
    lucency of chest, 988, 999
    and increase in size of pulmonary veins, 956
Payr-Strauss focal contraction of colon, *1762*
Pectoral girdle, radiology of, 781
Pectus carinatum, 773
Pectus excavatum, 773
Pedicle, congenital absence of, 622, 624
Pellegrini-Stieda disease, 387, 424
Pelvicephalometry, *1888*
Pelvis, angiography of, 1910
    architecture of, *1892*
    auto type, *397, 1894*
    bony, fractures of, *144,* 145
        most frequent sites of, *146*
    in neonatal and congenital diseases of
        bone, 211, *212*
    metastases from carcinoma of breast, *243*
    gynecoid, *1891*
    inlet, *1890, 1891, 1892*
        measurements of, *1888*
    measurement of, with cephalopelvic dispropor-
        tion, 1887, *1887*
    median section demonstrating anatomy, *1702*
    neoplasms of, 1885
    of kidney, 1347
        pyelectasis, 1440
    pneumogram of, 1907
    small, with asphyxiating thoracic dystrophy of
        newborn, 773
    walls of (convergence), *1892,* 1894
Pemphigus, with pharyngeal pathology, 1535
Periarteritis nodosa, 859
    appearance of chest, *865*
    involving lung, *803,* 921
    radiographic manifestations of, 867
    with pulmonary hypertension, 952
Pericardium, *1022*
    calcification of, *1137, 1146*
    cavity in, *1022*
    congenital absence of, *1146,* 1210
    cysts of, 1030, *1041*
    effusion, *1144*
        in collagen diseases, 867
        in Hodgkin's disease, 1036
        in rheumatic heart disease, 1153
        special procedure for examination, 1067
    esophagus, relationship to, *1537*
    fat pads, 1143, *1147*
    inflammation of (pericarditis), *1145*
        constrictive, 845
    involvement with anonymous mycobacteria,
        841
    roentgen signs of abnormality, 1139, 1141,
        1143
    within mediastinal compartment, *1012, 1014*
Pericecal, *1226*
Perichondrium, 48
Pericystitis, plastica, 1404
Periodontoplasia, *548*
Periosteum
    classification of roentgenologic changes, *231*
    differentiation of bone tumors, 370
    elevation, in Hodgkin's disease, 344
        secondary to exudate, 275

Periosteum (*Continued*)
    in acromegaly, 365
    in bone pathology, 59
    in Codman's triangle, *275, 311, 312, 374*
        in osteosarcoma, *309*
    in congenital syphilis, *267*
    in diabetic osteopathy, 282
    in Ewing's tumor, *275*
    in fibrosarcoma of bone, 318, *319*
    in hydrocephalus, 466, 468
    in hypertrophic pulmonary osteoarthropathy,
        342
    in hypervitaminosis A, *330*
    in infection, *300*
    in juvenile syphilis, *374*
    in leukemia, 257
        acute, 269
    in neuroblastoma, 490
    in neurofibroma, *374*
    in osteitis deformans, *374*
    in osteogenic sarcoma, *374*
    in osteoid osteoma, *374*
    in osteomyelitis of Garré, 352, *374*
    in osteosarcoma, *308*
    in scurvy, *264, 374*
    in skull, in neuroblastoma, *493*
        with sickle cell anemia, 481
    in thalassemia major in skull, *468,* 481
    in thyroid acropachy, 341
    injury with associated fracture, 172
    lacelike appearance in skull infection, 370, *504*
    onion skin appearance, *311,* 370, *374*
        in Ewing's tumor of bone, *312*
    periostitis, of skull, *504*
        traumatic, *311, 353*
    reaction, in Gaucher's disease, 249
        in malignant tumor of bone, *373*
        in reticulum cell sarcoma of bone, *343*
        in secondary osteomyelitis, 318
        varieties of, *374*
    sclerotic changes in, *324, 338*
    sun ray appearance, 370
        in anemias, 371
        in sickle cell anemia, *374*
    tropical ulcer, changes secondary to, 356
    vessels of supply, 51, *54*
Perirenal air insufflation, *1334,* 1337
Peritachlorophenol, 929
Peritendinitis calcarea, 387
    pathologic and radiologic features, 424
Peritoneum, inflammation of (peritonitis),
        meconium, *1286*
    separation of bowel loops, *1246*
Perodactylia, 197
Peromelia, 197
Perthes' disease, *276*
Pertussis, and lymph node enlargement, 788
Petrous bone, erosion from acoustic neurilemo-
    ma, *573*
    tumors of, classification, 569
Pfaundler-Hurler disease, *206, 207,* 208
    with spinal malalignment, *673*
Phalanges, dislocations and fracture dislocations,
    143
    fractures, 144
Pharmacoradiology, in evaluation of gastroin-
    testinal disease, 1600
Pharyngocele, 1535
Pharynx, 706
    anatomy of, 705

Pharynx (*Continued*)
  communications of, 701
  diverticulum of, *1533*, 1534
  laryngeal, 701
  paresis, cause of, 790
Phenylketonuria, 266
  and metaphyseal changes, 260, *261*
Pheochromocytoma, 1030, 1051, *1430, 1433*
  of mediastinum, 1013, 1051
  roentgenologic aspects of, 1051
Phlebectasia, 1406
  of small intestine, 1725
Phlebography, in diagnosis of superior vena
      caval syndrome, 1047
  portal, 1294
  renal, 1331
Phleboliths, 1831
  in bowel wall (hemangioma of small in-
      testine), 1743
  in mediastinal hemangioma, 1028
Phonation, abnormalities of, *1536*
Phosphatase, in bone growth, 56
Phosphorus osteopathy, and sclerotic bands in
      metaphyses, 333
Phosphorus poisoning, *334*
Photomicrograph, correlation with radiograph,
      57, *58*
Phrenic nerve, palsy or paralysis of, *771*
Phrygian cap, *1489*
Pineal gland, calcification of, 580, *582*
  displacement with increased intracranial
      pressure, 581
  localization of, *451*, 456
Pinealoma, calcification in, *467, 587, 589*
Pituitary. See *Hypophysis.*
Pituitary gigantism, 360
Placenta, abnormal implantations of, *1878*
  calcification in, 1287
  enlargement of, 1879
  measurements of, 1878
  methods for study, 1877
  placenta previa, *1878, 1879*
  premature separation of, 1879
  retained, demonstration by hysterosal-
      pingography, *1900*
  roentgen study of, *1878*
  site within uterine cavity, 1878
Plagiocephaly, *462*
Platinum, 929
Platybasia, *447, 449*
  clinical and roentgenographic changes, 486
  malalignment between cervical spine and
      skull, 668
  roentgen criteria for, *488*
Pleuroperitoneal hiatus, 755
Pleura, 761–770
  abnormalities of, *764*
    configuration and size, 761
    density, 761
  adhesions, *762, 767, 768,* 971
    fibrous, 761
  and actinomycosis, 844
  and anonymous mycobacteria, 841
  and autoimmune disease, 921
  and bronchogenic carcinoma, *898,* 901, *903*
  and Hodgkin's disease, 1035, 1036
  and Kerley's B lines, *906*
  and lung abscess, 895
  and lupus erythematosus, 858, 859
  and pneumoconioses, 925

Pleura (*Continued*)
  and pneumothorax, 896
  and pseudomonas aeruginosa pneumonia, 829,
      874
  and scar formation with change in thorax, *771*
  and sickle cell disease, 255
  and staphylococcal pneumonia, 874
  angle, cardiophrenic, 718
    costophrenic, 718
  anterior and posterior mediastinal, *1017*
    posterior, *974*
  apical, *735*
  bandlike linear shadow associated with, *973,*
      976
  calcification of, 761, 767, *767,* 921, 925
    with asbestosis, 927
  cavity of, *1020, 1021*
  circumscribed effusions of, classification, 766
  costal, 943, *1023*
  demarcation zones of, *722*
  diseases of, radiographic classification, 761
  effusion of, *749,* 763, *766, 802*
    circumscribed, 766
    classification of, 763
    differentiation, from atelectasis, *816*
      from parenchymal infiltrate, *764*
      from pneumonia and atelectasis, 763, *764*
    massive, 763
    minimal detectable, *764*
    with abnormalities of density, 761
    with alveolar cell carcinoma of lung, 908
    with atypical measles, 871
    with chronic passive hyperemia of lung, *958*
    with collagen diseases, 867
    with diaphragmatic elevation, *749*
    with esophageal rupture, 1566
    with Hodgkin's disease, 1036
    with hydrocarbon ingestion, 995
    with left heart failure, 960
    with mediastinal disease, 1030
    with mesothelioma, 769
    with mycobacterial infection, 841
    with pneumothorax, *762*
    with pulmonary edema, 867
    with nonpenetrating chest injuries, 1053
    with rheumatoid disease of, 858
    with subdiaphragmatic abscess, 759
    with subphrenic abscess, 759
    with viral pneumonia, 835
    with widening of thoracic cage, *771*
  empyema of, 896, *897*
    with cavitation, *1004*
  fibrin bodies, 769
  fibrosis, with pneumoconioses, 925, *926*
  granulomas of, 761
  interlobar circumscribed disease, *765*
  line shadows, appearance with, 939, 970, 971,
      973, 975
  lymphatic drainage of, *720*
  malignancy of, 768
    metastatic appearance in lung, *922*
  mesothelioma of, 768, 769, *769*
  neoplasm of, with circumscribed widening of
      pleural space, 761
  nodulations of, 761
    with rheumatoid disease, 858
  paramediastinal, *1029*
  paravertebral mediastinal, 1016
  plaques, *767, 768*
  radiographic identification of, 738

Pleura (*Continued*)
  relationship, of visceral and parietal to verte-
    bral column, *609*
    to azygos vein, 943
    to lung abscess, *896*
  secondary involvement with staphylococcal
    pneumonia, *873*
  stripe of, 761
    identification of, *738*
  subpleural lipoma, classification of, 769
  technique for examination of, 761
  tumors of, 894
    characteristics of fluid associated with, 768
    classification, 768
    metastatic, 768
    pancoast, of lung, 909
  visceral outline in pneumothorax, *762*
Pneumatocele, of lung, differentiation from
  other cavities, 896
  with pleural involvement, *803*
  with staphylococcal pneumonia, *873*
Pneumatosis coli, 1831
Pneumatosis cystoides intestinalis, 1744, *1812*
Pneumatosis intestinalis, 1277
Pneumaturia, 1410, 1420
Pneumoconiosis, 260, *809*, 810, 859, 988
  classification of, 929
  international classification of chest films, 931
  of chest, *926*
  of lung, 925, *926*, 927
    fibrotic changes of parenchyma, 977
    finely granular shadows of parenchyma, 932
    hypertension, 954
    increased linear markings, 939, 970, 975
Pneumocystis carinii, *803*
Pneumoencephalography, 498
  identification of intracranial space-occupying
    lesions, 579
Pneumography, retroperitoneal, *1334, 1335*, 1337,
  1426
Pneumomediastinum, *997*, 1031, *1047*, 1053
  air within, *1047*
    comparison with pneumothorax, 762, 763
  in infancy, 1048
  with aspiration of meconium, *760*
  with nonpenetrating injuries to thoracic aorta,
    1052
  with respiratory obstruction, 786
Pneumonia, *764*, 802. See also
  Bronchopneumonia.
  aerobacter, *803*, 873
  allergic, with finely granular shadows of
    parenchyma, 932
    Loeffler's syndrome, 836
  aspiration, *803*, 810, 852, 857
    chronic, 857, 858
  atypical, *803*, 877
  bacteroides, *803*, 852, 855, 873
  basilar distribution, 852
  bronchopneumonia, histopathology of, *807*
  chemical, *803*, 876, 877
  cholesterol and, 977
  clinical features of, 825
  cytomegalovirus, 876
  Eaton agent, 857
  giant cell, 978, 980
  hemophilis influenzae, *803*, 873, 875
    causing finely granular shadows of lung, 932
  histopathology of alveoli, *805*
  hypostatic, *803*, 852

Pneumonia (*Continued*)
  interstitial, *868*, 978
    accompanying neutrophil dysfunction syn-
     drome, 1034
    caused by pneumocystis carinii, 871
    desquamative, 977
    honeycombing or weblike appearance, 976
    lymphocytic, 970
    lymphoid, 978
  Klebsiella and aerobacter species
    (Friedländer's), *803*, 873, 874, 875
  lipid, 810
  lipoid, *856, 857*, 894, 915
  liverlike appearance (specimen), *828*
  Loeffler's, *803*, 859, 876, 933
  lymphogenous, 864
  migratory, 858
  mycoplasma, 852, 856, 877
    Stevens-Johnson syndrome, 857
  pathogenesis, 825
  pneumocystis carinii, 864, 871
  primary atypical, 932
  primary viral, with finely granular lung
    shadows, 933
  Pseudomonas aeruginosa, 874
    vs. staphylococcal, 874
  Q Fever, 852, 857
  radiographic features of, *828*, 829
  renal transplantation, *803*, 876, 877
    with diplococcus pneumonia, 877
    with Friedländer's bacillus, 877
    with pneumocystis carinii, 877
    with pseudomonas infection, 877
    with staphylococcus aureus, 877
  rheumatoid, 877
  sarcoidosis, 864
  scleroderma, 877
  staphylococcal, *803*, 873, *873*, 874, 1003
  tuberculous, *838*
  tularemic, *803*, 864
  varicella, *803*, 876
  viral, 835, 852, 856
    clinical evidence of, 856
  with atypical measles, 871
  with bronchial asthma, 966
  with bronchiectasis, 810
  with bronchogenic carcinoma, *907*
  with coccidioidomycosis, 848
  with exanthemas, acute, 864
    of childhood, 871
  with Hodgkin's disease, 1036
  with mucoviscidosis, 969
  with sickle cell disease, 255
Pneumonitis, 994
  aspiration, causing respiratory obstruction,
    786
  bronchiectasis and, 961
  hydrocarbon, 995
  interstitial, of cholesterol type, 915
  lipoid, 915
  miliary granulomatous, with finely granular
    lung shadows, 933
Pneumopericardium, 729, 762, 987, 1048
  diagnostic, 736
Pneumoperitoneum, 1048, 1277
  delineation of the diaphragm, 766
    secondary effects on, 755
  identification of mediastinal disease, 769, 1027
  pelvic, *1905*, 1907
  radiologic technique, *1908*

Pneumopyelograms, 1337
Pneumothorax, 736, 761–762, *762*, 987, *997, 1047*, 1048, 1053
  and bilateral low position of diaphragm, 750
  and check valve mechanism, 761
  and circumscribed widening of pleural space, 761
  and density of pleural space, 761
  and fibrin bodies, 769
  and hydrocarbon ingestion, 995
  and injuries to thoracic aorta, 1052
  and mediastinal shift, 761
  and mediastinitis, 1046
  and rheumatoid disease, 859
  and staphylococcal pneumonia, 874
  and subphrenic abscess, 759
  and widening of thoracic cage, *771*
  causing respiratory obstruction, 786
  comparison with pneumomediastinum, 762
  definition of, 761
  diagnostic, 729, 761
  encystment, 896
  identification of mediastinal disease, 1027
  radiographic signs of, 761, *762*
  simulating pulmonary cysts, 1003
Poison, effect on stomach, 1621
Polymyositis, linear changes in lung, 970
Polyostotic fibrous dysplasia, 241, *252*
Polyposis, familial, *1801*, 1840, *1841*
  of small intestine, 1737
Polyps
  cholesterol of gallbladder, *1493*, 1495
  filling defects in maxillary antrum, *543*
  in gastrointestine, 1647
  in oviduct, 1907
  in stomach, *1648*
  intrauterine, *1902*
  involving colon, 1799, *1800*
    adenomatous pedunculated, 1840
    relationship to malignancy, 1840
  with ulcerative colitis, *1790, 1803*
Polytomography, in diagnosis of pulmonary nodule, *892*
Polytopic enchondral dysostosis, 206. See also *Morquio-Brailsford disease* and *Osteochondrodystrophy*.
  Morquio type, *206*
  Morquio-Brailsford type, *207*
  Pfaundler-Hurler's disease, *206, 207*, 208
Portal circulation, relationship to esophageal circulation, *1539*
Posteroanterior view, definition of, 39
Postradiation damage, to lung parenchyma, 977
Potter-Bucky diaphragm, 10
Pregnancy, cardiac size and, *1090, 1091*
  diaphragmatic elevation and, 750
  extrauterine, 1882, *1882*, 1883
    fetus, 1881
  pelvic masses, *1884*
  protection of fetus, 31
  tubal, 1881
Premature synostosis of cranial sutures, *462, 463, 465*
Proctosigmoidoscopy, 1774
Progeria, 211
Prognathism, *449*
  in cleidocranial dysostosis, 489
  mandibular, *447*
  maxillary, *447*

Progressive diaphyseal dysplasia. See *Engelmann's disease.*
Progressive systemic sclerosis, calcinosis with, 1713
Prone position, definition of, 40
Prostate, calcification in, *1370*
  carcinoma of, metastases to bone, 331
    metastases to lung, *922*
    metastases to vertebra, *634*
  inflammation of, 1418
  malignancy of, in lung, *900*
Protective measures in x-ray diagnosis, 21–38
  effect of shielding, 25
  of patient, 28, *29, 30*
  of personnel, *31, 33, 34, 35*
  of public, 34
  safety recommendations, 31
Protein deficiency osteopathy, *232*
Protein-losing enteropathies, 1712, 1738
  exudative enteropathy of Golden, 1712
Psammoma bodies, 795
Pseudoarthrosis, *168*, 171
  congenital, clavicle, 781
Pseudodiverticula, 1825
  of colon, *1809*
  of scleroderma, 1721, 1790
Pseudogout, 387, 417, 421
Pseudohypoparathyroidism, *63, 64, 329*
Pseudomonas, 836
Pseudomonas pseudomallei, 836, *853*
  of lung, 850, *851, 852*
Pseudopolypi, and mucoviscidosis, *1809*
  in ulcerative colitis, 1833
Pseudospondylolisthesis, 654, *659*
  abnormalities of vertebral alignment, 668
  spotted lucency of spine, 632
Pseudotumor of orbit, 1047
Pseudovolvulus, 1807
  cause of mechanical bowel obstruction, 1823
Psittacosis, 876, 877
Pubic bone, disruption of interpubic ligaments, *145*
  fracture of superior ramus, 145
  subpubic angle, *1892, 1894*
  subpubic arch, variations in size and shape, *1890*
  symphysis of, diastasis, *145*, 1894
Pulmonary. See also *Lungs.*
Pulmonary arteriovenous angle, measurements of, *1147*
Pulmonary arteries, *708, 709*
Pulmonary conus, *735*
Pulmonary edema, *718, 803, 804*, 864, *868, 920*
  acute interstitial, 866
  air bronchogram sign, 824
  aspiration pneumonia and, 857
  blood transfusion and, 867
  causation of, 866
  classification of, 864, 866
  clinical aspects, 864
  exanthemas, acute, of childhood, 871
  heroin intoxication and, 866
  histopathology of, *806*
  linear changes in lung, 970, 971
  morphological types, 864
  pulmonary thromboembolism, 830
  secondary lobules, mulberry-like appearance, *869*

Pulmonary edema (*Continued*)
  subarachnoid hemorrhage, 867
  uremia, *867*
    secondary to, accompanying lupus erythematosus, 858
Pulmonary hypertension, 830
  and pneumoconiosis, 954
Pulmonary melioidosis, *853*
Pulmonary renal syndrome, *803*
Pyelitis, 1451
Pyelogram, intravenous (IVP) vs. retrograde, 1338
  rapid sequence and washout, 1340, 1341
Pyelonephritis, 1450, *1452*
  of pregnancy, 1451
  tumefactive xanthogranulomas, 1451, *1453*
Pyeloureterectasis, 1451
Pyle's disease, 199, 222, 333. See also *Metaphyseal dysplasia.*
Pylorus
  antrum, S deformity of, 1627
  deformity, secondary to adhesions, 1624, 1627
  displacement with congenitally short esophagus, *757*
  eccentricity of, 1619
  elongated canal, 1621, *1625*
  hypertrophic stenosis in infant, 1621, *1622, 1623*
  narrowness, with fungal diseases, 1621
    with gastric sarcoid, 1621
    with syphilis, 1621
    with tuberculosis, 1621
  obstruction of, *1237,* 1646
Pyogenic infection, causing spotted lucency of spine, 632
Pyonephrosis, *1452*
Pyriform sinuses, gaseous distinction of, 789

Rachitic rosary, 775
Rad, definition of, *22,* 23
Radiation dosage
  cellular effects, 25
  effects in pregnancy, 26
  genetic aberrations and sterility, 26
  hematopoietic injury, 25
  injuries to skin, 25
  reduction in life span, 27
  systemic effect, 24
  to skin and gonads in radiographic examinations, 24
  variability of tissue or organ effects, 25
Radiation effects, and superior marginal rib defects, 775
  button sequestrum as, 512
  calcification of skull as, 586
  injury to bowel as, 1824, *1825*
  on bones, 301, 310, 336
  on vertebrae, 633, 662
Radiation hazard, in pregnancy, 1864
  pelvicephalography, evaluation of, 1886
Radioactive dust, 929
  scattered, 6
Radiographic pathology
  description of, 42
    architecture, 43, 44
    contour, 45
  integration with other clinical data, 45
  sequence of study, 42

Radiography
  background fundamentals, 3–20
  body section, *12*
  general terms and concepts, 39–46
  historical review, 3
  sequence of study, 41, *43*
  spot film, 13
  stereoscopic accessories, 12
Radioisotopic scanning
  in identification of intracranial space-occupying lesions, 579
    myelocisternoencephalo photograms, 580
  in identification of mediastinal lesions, 1027
  in identification of pericardial disease, 1143
  in lung, following thromboembolic disorders, 833
  in pancreas, 1678
Radiolucency, increased, definition of, 39
Radiopacity, increased, definition of, 39
Radius, fracture sites, *133*
  fractures of, lower end, *136*
    head and neck, 128
    proximal third, 134
Raynaud's disease, *232*
RBE (relative biological effectiveness), definition of, 24
Red blood cell aplasia, 1030
Recumbency, definition of, 40
Rectosigmoid junction, *1770*
Refrigerants, 929
  pulmonary involvement, 877
Regional enteritis, 1737, 1834. See also *Granulomatous colitis.*
  roentgenologic features of, 1835
Rem, definition of, *22,* 23
Renal. See also *Kidney(s).*
Renal osteodystrophy, 94
Renal osteitis fibrosa cystica, *234*
Renal transplantation pneumonia, 877
Reproductive system, male, anatomy of, *1336*
  roentgenologic appearance, *1336*
Respiratory distress syndrome, *881*
Respiratory obstruction, 786–788
  clinical manifestations of, 788
  in newborn and young infant, classification of, 786
  intestinal atresia as cause, 786
  methods of study, 786
  radiographic appearances of, classified, 788
Reticuloendothelioses, *803*. See also *Granulomatoses, lipoid.*
  causing spotted lucency of spine, 632
  of lung, *803*, 877
  of skull, 506, 511
  vertebra, appearance of, *635*
Reticuloses. See *Granulomatoses, lipoid.*
Retrocardiac clear space, *1015, 1018*
Retroperitoneal fibrosis, 1403
  involving colon, 1824, 1825
Retroperitoneal gaseous insufflation, 1678
Retroperitoneal space, increased fatty content of, 1030
Retropneumoperitoneum, 1678
Rheumatic fever, 864
  differentiation from juvenile rheumatoid arthritis, 407
  joint involvement, diagram of characteristic features, *392*
Rheumatic heart disease, and venous hypertension, 961

Rheumatoid arthritis, and interstitial
    pneumonia, 977
  and spur formation, 633
  and superior rib erosion, 779
  closure of manubriosternal synchondrosis,
    774
  in glenohumeral joint, *784*
  in lung fields, *785, 859, 860, 861, 864*
    contrasted with scleroderma, *863*
    site of involvement, 921
  in small joints of hands, *785*
  in spine, differentiation from ankylosing
    spondylitis, 663, 665
    cervical, roentgenologic diagnosis, 663
  juvenile, in spine, 668, 680
  phalangeal changes, *62, 63*
  resorption of distal clavicle, 781, *783*
Rheumatoid disease, of lung, 877
  linear markings of, *861*
  pulmonary hypertension and, 952
  pulmonary nodules and, 859
  radiological manifestations of, 403
Rheumatoid nodules, resembling pulmonary
    appearance with pneumoconioses, 929
Ribs, 774–781
  abnormalities, classification of, 770
    in number, 662, 770
    with achondroplasia, 770
    with chondrodystrophy, 770
    with fibrous dysplasia, 777
    with hyperparathyroidism, *776*
    with neurofibromatosis, *776*
    with scurvy, *777*
    with thalassemia major, *777*
  acute bronchiolitis, appearance with, *989*
  barrel chest and, 774
  changes owing to abnormal vessels, *776*
  changes, bony, with achondroplasia, *774*
  configuration with bronchogenic carcinoma,
    898
  contour changes with paralytic poliomyelitis,
    779
  costochondral junctions, splaying with
    asphyxiating thoracic dystrophy of newborn,
    773
  destruction of, with actinomycosis, 844
    with histiocytosis, 981
    with Pancoast tumor, *899*
  dilatation of, with scurvy, *774*
  erosion of, 909
    with rheumatoid arthritis, 779
    with scleroderma, 779
  fibroxanthoma of, *778*
  fractures, pathologic, with changes in
    shape of thorax, *773*
  hypoplasia or aplasia of, 770
  interspaces, narrowed with atelectasis,
    814, *816*
    widened with atelectasis, *817*
  metaphyses, widening of, with asphyxiating
    thoracic dystrophy of the newborn, 773
  metastatic tumor of, with extrapleural sign, 781
  narrowness of head and neck, with
    lipochondrodystrophy, *774*
  notching, 770, 775, 780
    with coarctation of aorta, *1202*
    with congenital heart disease, 1195
  osteochondroma of, 778

Ribs (*Continued*)
  periostitis of (extrapleural sign), 781
    caused by actinomycosis, 844
  scurvy, compared with rickets, *774*
  superior marginal defects, with collagen
    diseases, 775
    with localized pressure, 775
    with paralytic poliomyelitis, 775
Rickets, 59, *61*, 94
  bony changes of scurvy, comparison with,
    774, 777
  causing homogeneous radiolucency of spine,
    632
  changes in thoracic cage and, 770
  cystine storage disease, 236
  Fanconi's syndrome and, 236
  hypervitaminosis D or vitamin D resistant, 59
  hypophosphatemic vitamin D refractory,
    232, 236
  involving chest, 775
  metaphyseal changes, 260, *261, 262, 263*
  periosteal reaction, *374*
  renal, 94, 232, *234*
    clinical features, 233, *234*
    metaphyseal changes with, 260
  ribs, appearance of (rachitic rosary), *263*
  skeleton, radiographic appearance of, 261
  spine, radiographic changes in, 637
Riedel's struma, 1047
Roentgen, definition of, 22, *22*
Rotation of midgut, *1700*
Runström's position, 551, 553, *563, 569*
  in diagnosis of cholesteatoma of middle ear,
    570

Sacrum, 1891
  curvature, variations of, *1892*
  hypoplasia of, 221
  special lateral view of, *616*
Salpingitis, tuberculous, *1902*
Salpingography, and abnormalities of uterus,
    1900
Salpingolithiasis, 1885
Sarcoid disease, 980, 988
  and linear densities of lung, 955
  involving mediastinum, 1042
    causing mediastinitis, 1046
  of bone, 301, 308
    in hand, *307, 418*
  of joints, 386
  of lung, 740
    with interstitial fibrosis of, 977, 978
  of stomach, 1621
  of vertebral column, 662
  pathology and roentgenologic findings, 419
  phalangeal changes, *62*
  producing calcification of kidney, *1367*
  producing pulmonary fibrosis, 970
  resemblance to tuberous sclerosis of bone, 260
Sarcoma
  Ewing's, in spine, 632, 637
  metastatic spread to lung, 925
  of joint synovium, 386
  of pleural space, 768
  osteogenic, periosteal changes in, *374*

Sarcoma (*Continued*)
  parosteal osteoid, 362
  reticulum cell, 241, *343*
    periosteal reaction, *374*
    simulating Ewing's tumor, 313
  with Paget's disease, 347
Scaphocephaly, *462*
Scaphoid (navicular carpal bone), blood supply
    of, *141*
  fractures of, 135
    classification of, 141
Scapula, apophyses of, as anatomic variations,
    781
  infantile cortical hyperostosis, *783*
  pseudoforamina of, 781
Schatzki's ring, *1565*
Scheuermann's disease, 279
Schistosomiasis, with bronchopneumonia, 835
  mansoni, 1845
Schmorl's node, *676*
Scleroderma, *859, 863,* 980
  of colon, diverticulum formation in, 1827
    radiographic appearance, *1793*
  of esophagus, *863,* 1576
    congenital short esophagus, 757
  of hands, *863*
  of lung, 740, *863, 864, 877*
    and interstitial fibrosis of, 978
    linear changes in, 970
  phalangeal changes in, *62*
  producing pulmonary fibrosis, 970
  with interstitial pneumonia, 977
  with pulmonary hypertension, 952
  with superior rib erosion, 779
Sclerotic bone islands, 655
  of spine, 633, *660*
Scoliosis, 772
  definition of, 669
  determination of primary and secondary
    curvatures, *613*
  measurement of, *613, 668, 669, 670*
  method for positioning patient, *613*
  of Down's syndrome, 629
  secondary to Turner's syndrome, 629
  with syringomyelia, 674
Scurvy, 94
  bony changes in, *264*
  changes in rickets, comparison with, *774, 777*
  metaphyseal changes in, 260, *261*
    sclerotic transverse bands, 333
  periosteum, appearance of, *374*
  radiographic appearances of, *264, 265*
  ribs, changes in, *777*
Sella turcica
  anatomy and measurements of, *456, 458,
    524, 525, 525, 526*
  calcification in, *587*
  changes with, expanded lesions, 528
    increased intracranial pressure, *530, 531,
      580, 581*
    diseases causing destruction, of base,
      classification of, 532
    of sphenoid bone, 532
  hydrocephalus, appearance in, 466
  infantile form, *528*
  intrasellar, *467*
  normal, tracings of, *457*
    variations of, 527, *529*
  optic nerve glioma, appearance in, 579

Sella turcica (*Continued*)
  plain skull film, value of, 526
  synchondroses, parasellar, *528*
  volume of, *458, 525*
Seminal vesicle, calcification in, *1370*
Seminal vesiculography, 1337
Seminomas, of mediastinum, 1031
  pulmonary metastases, appearance of, *922*
Semirecumbent position, definition of, 40
Sensitivity disorders, with myocardiopathy,
    1158
Sequestration, 249, *802*
  of lung, 895
  with tuberculosis of bone, 403
Sequestrum, *301*
  "button" type, 512
  in fibrous dysplasia, 345
Sesamoid bones, developmental variations of,
    163
  fractures of, roentgen criteria, 164
  of foot and ankle, *163, 164*
  peroneal, 162
Sever's disease, 280
Sex, intersex, classification of, 1911
Sex determination, prenatal, 1880
Shadows, of breast (female), 781
  of nipple, 781
  of lung parenchyma, weblike, 970, 975
  psoas, obliteration in appendicitis, 1848
  pulmonary, nodular, *920*
Shoulder, dislocations of, 122, *123*
    recurrent, *124*
  fracture-dislocation of, *124*
Sickle cell anemia, with bony infarction, *257*
Siderosis, 929
Sign
  air bronchogram, 824, *825*
  air dome, *1275,* 1277
  barium wall, in infected cavity, 912
  bat-wing flare of thymus, *1047*
  "beaten brass" of skull owing to premature
    synostosis, *462*
  "bite," of osteonecrosis, 345
  boot-shaped contour of heart, *1191*
  bowing of the pterygopalatine fossa and canal,
    in juvenile nasopharyngeal fibroma, *792*
  blister of bone, in aneurysmal bone cyst, 298
  Buddha, in fetal death, 1873, *1875*
  bull's eye, in bowel, 1728, 1846
    with melanoma, 1847
    with ulcerating polypoid metastasis, *1731*
  Carman-Kirklin meniscus, in gastric ulceration,
    1641
  cartwheel configuration, in stomach-duodenal
    ulcer, 1638
  Case's pad sign, *1612*
  cluster of grapes, with mucoid impaction of
    bronchi, 966
  cobblestone, of colon, 1801, *1808*
    classification of causes in diseases of small
      intestine, 1723
    in ulcerative colitis, 1833
  cobra head, *1401, 1402*
  coeur en sabot (wooden shoe), 1096, *1194*
  coiled linear streaking, 1728
    due to intestinal worms, 1728
  colon cut-off, 1241
    in connection with pancreatic disease, 1257
    of transverse colon, 1238

Sign (*Continued*)
comma, of intraluminal diverticulum, 1713
common duct, 1618
    dilated, *1617*
corkscrew, 1819
"cotton ball," in Paget's disease, *348*
crowfoot, *1492*
Deuel's "halo," 1870, *1875*
    as sign of fetal death, *1872*
    in erythroblastosis fetalis, *1874*
dirty chest appearance, with bronchitis, 965
double bubble in duodenal atresia, *1242*
doughnut, with coccidioidomycosis, *920*
dunce cap, 1427
elevator, of esophagus, 1557
empty mediastinum, 1034
extrapleural air, 781
    classification of causes, 781
    with aspiration of meconium, *760*
    with pneumomediastinum, 761
Felson's cervicothoracic, 1028
figure eight, *1174*
fingerprint, of lymphoma or linitis plastica,
    1654
fleck, in stomach-duodenal ulceration, 1638
Fleischner's "pointed ileum," *1792*
floating tooth, in eosinophilic granuloma
        of bone, 306
    in Hand-Schüller-Christian disease, 508
    in histiocytosis, 306
    in reticuloendotheliosis, *511*
football, *1275, 1277, 1931*
Frostberg's inverted 3, *1612*
gloved finger shadow of Simon, 961
gluteus medius, *426, 1227*
H bomb, 1634
hanging drop, 993
hilum convergence of Felson, 1028
Horner-Spalding, of fetal death, 1869, 1870
iceberg, of Felson, 1030
ileopsoas, *426, 1227*
indrawn pleural, 975
inverse comma of right pulmonary artery,
    1128
inverted S, with bronchogenic carcinoma, *898*
inverted 3, 1614, 1674
inverted U, in volvulus of sigmoid, 1256, *1787*
ischial varus, 427
Kerley's B lines, with bronchogenic carcinoma,
    911
leafless tree bronchographic, 883
leather bottle, in linitis plastica, 1624
molar tooth, *565*
Morton's S Curve, with bronchogenic
    carcinoma, 901, *906,* 911
obturator, *426,* 427, *1227*
omega, of gallbladder, *1495*
onion peel, in tropical ulcer, *356*
onion skin, of periosteum, *374*
Pelken's, in scurvy, *264*
pipestem, in ulcerative colitis, 1233
positive elbow fat pad, in rheumatoid
    arthritis, 411
positive metacarpal, in Turner's syndrome,
    219
positive "rim," in shoulder fracture, 122, 125
pruned branch, 952, 1128
pseudotumor, of Frimann-Dahl, 1255
    of vascular occlusion of colon, 1845
pubic, 427

Sign (*Continued*)
pulmonary meniscus, 912
pyloric string sign, 1621
reverse comma, 955
Rigler notch, 901, 911
    with bronchogenic carcinoma, 908
rim, of osteonecrosis, 345
rugger jersey, *634, 636*
    in agnogenic myeloid metaplasia, 332
S deformity of antrum, 1627
sail, of thymus, 1028, 1029
sandwich appearance, in agnogenic myeloid
    metaplasia, 332
sawtooth appearance in ulcerative colitis,
    1789, 1800, *1803, 1833*
scimitar, 771, *962, 963*
"Scotty dog," of spondylolisthesis, *618*
"shaggy heart," 871
sigmoid elevator, 1847
"sign of the duct," 1656
Silhouette, 820, *823*
snake head, in small intestinal obstruction,
    1730
snowman, 1174
spider web appearance, with obstructive
    pulmonary emphysema, *967*
spidering, of bronchi, 991
    of bronchioles with emphysema, 993
"squeeze," of lipoma, 1842
stacked coin, *1810*
Stierlin's, in tuberculosis of colon,
    1792, 1837
stovepipe, of ulcerative colitis, 1786, 1833
string, *1732*
    of elongated pylorus, *1625*
    of small intestine, 1738
"tacked down," in metastatic carcinoma to gut,
    1741
tear drop, 427, 1028, *1029*
tethered cord, with meningoceles of spine, *628*
thick walls, 1435
thumbprinting of colon, 1845
    in ischemic colitis, 1820
thymic sail, with pneumothorax, 762
tit, with pyloric sphincter hypertrophy, 1621
tramline, 991, *992*
    in chronic bronchitis, 962
trapped air, 1627
tumor track, with malignant neoplasm of lung,
    975
twisted taper, 1819
ulcer collar, of stomach-duodenal ulcer, 1638
ulcer mound, 1638
V sign of Neclario, 1566
vallecular, with pharyngeal paresis, 790
wasp-waist, 622
    of congenitally fused vertebral bodies, 622
wide mouth diverticula, of scleroderma, 1827
wooden shoe, with right ventricular
    hypertrophy, 1096
Silicates, 929
Silicatosis, producing changes in lung, 970
Silicosis, 740, 859, 929
    eggshell calcification in hilus, *927*
    of lung, 927, 970
    roentgenologic changes, *926, 930*
        classification of, 927
    with mediastinitis, 1046
    with rheumatoid arthritis, 927
Sillimanite, 929

Silo filler's disease, 877, 929, 962
Simon's postulate, 957
Sinus(es)
    coronary, *1022*
    of Valsalva, aneurysms of, 1127
    paranasal, Caldwell's view, *536*
        density, changes in (classification), 540
            diminished, 549
            increased, entities responsible for, *541*
        diseases of, 533
        lateral view of, *537*
        roentgen pathology of, 533
        routine views for study of, *535, 536*
        Water's view, *536*
    pericardial, oblique view, *1022*
    pyriform, in laryngogram of carcinoma of
        tongue, *1527*
        with Parkinson's disease and pseudobulbar
            palsy, 1528
Sinus pericranii, 496, 581
Sinusitis, acute and chronic, 538, 540, *541, 543*
    with Kartagener's syndrome, 968
Situs inversus viscerum, 968, 1606
Skeletal maturation, 88
    abnormalities of, 93 (table)
        Fels Research Institute technique, 99
    indicators of, *89*
    methods of estimating, 98
        Oxford method, 99
        recommended, 89
        Tanner-Whitehouse method, 99
    usefulness of studies, 98
Skeleton, traumatic lesions of, 174
Skull. See also *Cranium.*
    abnormalities of, contour, 481
        density, 488
    alterations in shape due to premature
        synostosis of sutures, *462*
    anemias, changes in, 481, *481, 482,* 484
    angiogram, 498
    angioma of (Sturge-Weber) calcification of,
        590
    Arnold-Chiari malformation, *448*
    basilar impression, *449*
    brachycephalic, 445, 446
    calcification in, *582*
    contracting skull, 460, 461
    convolutional pattern, accentuated, *469*
    demarcated areas of radiolucency, 492
    diseases manifest by diffuse increase in
        radiopacity, 513
    diseases manifest by multiple demarcated
        areas of radiopacity, 514
    dolichocephalic, 445, *446, 447*
    enlargement of, classification of causes, 461
    erosion of secondary to intracranial tumors,
        593
    fractures of, 486, *487*
    growth and age changes in, 440, *441, 442, 443*
        in newborn, *442*
        measurements at different age levels,
            441 (table)
    habenular calcification, localization of, *452*
    infections of, *504, 505*
    internal aspect of base, *500*
    lacunar (luckenschädel), 505
    lining diagrams, *434, 449*
        illustrating platybasia and basilar impression,
            488
    localized depressions of, 486
    macrocephaly, 445

Skull (*Continued*)
    measurements of, 445
        in children, 444 (table)
    method of study, 434
    microcephaly, 445
    multiple areas of demarcated radiolucency
        foramina in base of skull, 498
    osteoporosis of bones with increase in
        intracranial pressure, 581
    pineal gland, localization of, *451*
    posterior fossa, changes in, 595
    roentgen signs of abnormality, 459
    roentgenology of, 433–523
        special areas and space-occupying lesions
            within cranium, 524–601
    routine of study, *433*
        axial view (verticosubmental), *439*
        Caldwell's projection, *435*
        lateral view, *438*
        postero-anterior view, *436*
        Towne's projection, *437*
    scaphocephaly, 445, *447*
    single or confluent demarcated areas of
        sclerosis, 514
    size, evaluation of, in children, 445
    small, classification of causes, 461
    submentovertical view, *558*
    temporal bone, Chamberlain-Towne's view,
        561
        Mayer's projection, *564*
        Runström's view, *563*
        Stenver's view, *560*
        submentovertical view, *562*
    turricephaly, 445, *447*
    types of, *446*
    vascular grooves, abnormal, with increased
        intracranial pressure, 581
    view from below, *501*
Small intestine. See *Duodenum* and
    Intestine, small.
Soft palate, 701, 702
Soft tissue
    acromegaly, increased width of heel in, *364*
    nasopharyngeal angiofibromas and, 795
    of aryepiglottic folds, *788*
    of neck, measurements of, *1524*
        roentgenology of, 1523, *1523*
    of thoracic cage, 787
    pretracheal, appearance in epiglottitis, 790
    retropharyngeal, appearance in epiglottitis,
        790
    widening with hypothyroidism, 795
    retrotracheal, emphysema of, 789
    rupture of achilles tendon, changes with, 160
    supraclavicular, 781, *787*
    tracheobronchiomegaly and, 794
    width, variations of, 789
Soft tissue space, between rectum and sacrum,
    1775
    retropharyngeal, sagittal measurements of, 607,
        651
    retrorectal, 1834
        measurements of, 1234
    rectosacral, *1829*
        measurements of, 1776
            in ulcerative colitis, 1834
    retrotracheal, sagittal measurements of,
        607, 651
Soft tissue swelling, of thoracic chest wall
    due to actinomycosis, 844
Soft tissue tumor, of chest wall, 786

Spherocytosis, hereditary, 253
Spina bifida, 1873
Spina ventosa (of tuberculosis), *303*
Spinal cord, relationship of medulla and dura, *943*
Spine
  abnormalities, classification of, 607
    of shape and size, 622
  anterior superior iliac, avulsion of, *145*
  bamboo, in ankylosing spondylitis, 410
  cervical, congenital fusions of, 622
    posterior indentations due to nuclei pulposi impressions, *782*
    roentgenologic examination of, *602, 604, 605, 606, 608*
  fracture of (hematoma), causing displacement of pleural stripe, 1016
  hemangioma of, *661*
  ischial, 1891
    variations of, *1892*
    with parturition, 1894
  joint abnormalities of, 677, 678
  kyphosis of. See *Kyphosis.*
  lumbar, routine positions for examination of, *603*
    special views for detection of mobility of, *603*
  lumbarization of, 622, *623*
  lumbosacral, *614, 615, 617*
  malalignment of, diseases responsible for, *673*
  neoplasms of, causing displacement of pleural stripe, 1016
  normal curvature of, 669
  osteomyelitis of, 641
    causing displacement of pleural stripe, 1016
  pedicles, interpedicular distance, *619*
  rugger jersey, *634*
    in Fanconi's pancytopenia, *636*
  sacralization, 622, *623*
  scoliosis. See *Scoliosis.*
  thoracic, *610, 611*
    routine positions for examination, *602*
  tuberculosis of, 305
  tuberculous abscess of, 403
  tuberculous osteomyelitis of, 304
  vertebra, cross-sectional view, *1020*
Spinous processes, cleft, 624
Spleen
  abscess of, caused by perforation, 759
  as seen on postero-anterior film of abdomen, 1298
  calcified tubercles of phleboliths in, 1298
  enlargement of, with granulomatous disease of childhood, 846
    with primary myeloid metaplasia, 923
  examination, techniques of, 1297, 1298
  in Hodgkin's disease, 1035
  measurement of splenic shadow, 1300
  roentgen signs of abnormality, 1300
  roentgenographic methods, 1299
  rupture, radiographic signs of, *1301, 1302,* 1303, *1303*
Splenoportography, 1675
Spondylisthesis, reverse, 654
Spondylitis, ankylosing, 663, *666*
  deformans, 662
  paratyphoid, *643*
  pyogenic vs. tuberculous, 643 (table)
  rheumatoid, 663

Spondylitis (*Continued*)
  syphilitic, 641, 663
  tuberculous vs. pyogenic, 643 (table)
Spondyloepiphyseal dysplasia tarda, 205, 627
Spondylolisthesis, *618,* 654
  abnormalities of vertebral alignment and, 668
  causing spotted lucency of spine, 632
  instability, method of measuring, *658*
  radiographic analysis and method of lining, *658*
  reverse type, causing spotted lucency of spine, 632
  with abnormalities of vertebral alignment, 668
Spondylolysis, 654
  causing spotted lucency of spine, 632
Spondylosis deformans, with spur formation of spine, 633
Spongioblastoma polare, calcification in, 589
Sporotrichosis, involving bone, 344
  of lung, 844
Sprengel's deformity, 213, *214,* 781
Sprue (nontropical), scattering and clumping of barium, *1722*
Stannosis, 929
Stature, small, disorders accompanying, 92, *184*
Stature, large, disorders accompanying, 92
Stenver's view, 551, 553, *556*
  in cholesteatoma, *570*
  in diagnosis of acoustic neuroma, *572*
Sternocleidomastoid, radiographic identification of, 738
Sternum, *732, 772, 1015, 1018*
  abnormalities of, 773, 774
  barrel chest and, 774
  bony changes, classification of, 770
  clefts or notches, 770, 774
  in lateral view of chest, *948*
  manubriosternal synchondrosis, closure in rheumatoid arthritis, 774
  manubrium of, *731, 1015, 1018*
  pectus carinatum, 770, *772*
  pectus excavatum, 770, *772*
  pulmonary hypertension, changes with, 954
  relationship to vertebral spaces, 1025
Stomach. See also *Stomach and duodenum.*
  abnormalities, of contour, *1586, 1587*
    of position and shape, 1609
      owing to extragastric displacement, *1262*
    of size, with foreign bodies, *1629*
  adenoma of, with duodenal ulcer, 1646
    villous, *1654*
  carcinoma of, *1626, 1650, 1652, 1652*
    metastatic appearance in lung, *900, 922*
    of fundus, *1654*
    recurrence following resection, *1668*
    roentgen appearance, *1651, 1653*
    with "fingerprint" sign, *1654*
  cascade, *1608, 1609*
  congenital anomalies of, 1606
  dilatation of, classification of causes, 1603
    with pyloric obstruction, *1605*
  displacement of, *1258*
  distance from diaphragm, 738
  diverticulum of, *1630*
  duplication of, 1606
  eosinophilic granuloma of, 1653
  foramen of Morgagni, appearance with, 758
  fundoplication, 1661, 1665
  gastrogenic cysts, 1606
  glands (fundus), histology of, *1589*

Stomach (*Continued*)
  herniation of, 1609, *1610*
  hypertrophic gastritis, *1624*
  hypertrophic rugation, *1637*
  inflammation of (gastritis), 1632
    classification of, 1634
    hypertrophic hypersecretory gastropathy,
      1636
    Menetrier's disease, 1636
    roentgenographic appearance, 1634, 1635
    with diabetes, *1638*
  intrathoracic, *1551*
  lymphoma of, 1653
    with fingerprint sign, *1654*
  lymphosarcoma of, *1655, 1656*
  magenblase, *731, 735*
    relation to diaphragm, 766
  mucosa of, prolapse into base of duodenal
    bulb, 1621
  necrosis, from poisoning, 1621
  normal rugal pattern, 1585
  organoaxial rotation of, 1260, 1606, *1608,*
    1796, *1797*
  physiological considerations, 1587
  polyp, *1622*
  polypoid lesions of, in eosinophilic
    granuloma, 306
  postoperative, afferent loop syndrome, *1667*
    antral remnant syndrome, *1668*
    complications, 1662
    dumping syndrome, 1669
    examination, method of, 1660
    gastrojejunoscopy, varieties of, *1662*
    technique for utilization of small bowel
      series, 1695
    terminology and radiographic appearance,
      1660, *1663, 1664*
  stricture associated with poisoning, 1621
  tumors, benign, 1647
  ulceration of, *1628, 1644*
    benign vs. malignant, *1642*
    giant benign gastric, *1641*
    hourglass deformity, *1628*
    in geriatric age group, 1643
    in hyperparathyroidism, *239*
    in infancy and childhood, 1644
    incisura formation, 1627
    malignant, roentgen signs of, 1641
    marginal, following resection, *1643*
    perforation of, as cause of subdiaphragmatic
      abscess, 759
    response to treatment, 1641
    significance of site, 1642
    with Menetrier's disease, 1646
    Zollinger-Ellison syndrome, involving
      pancreas, 1644
      roentgenologic signs of, 1646
      sites of, *1668*
  volvulus of, 1260, *1608,* 1606, 1609
Stomach and duodenum, 1582–1669. See also
  Duodenum.
  abnormalities, of architecture, 1628
    of contour, 1585, 1617
    of density, 1659
    of number, 1606
    of position and shape, 1585, 1606, *1607,*
      1611, *1611, 1612*
    of size, 1602
  anatomic relationships of, 1582, 1583, *1584*
  Crohn's disease of, 1647
  diverticula of, 1631, *1631*

Stomach and duodenum (*Continued*)
  evacuation of, 1588
  foreign bodies in, classification, 1628
  gastrectomy and gastroduodenoscopy, *1661*
  hemorrhage, examination for, 1597
  pancreatic pathology, effects of, *1612, 1613,*
    1614, 1615, 1616, 1672
  peristalsis, 1588
  physiology of, *1588, 1590*
  polyp of pyloric antrum, *1657*
  postoperative stomach, 1660
  pseudodiverticula, 1631
  roentgenologic examination of, *1591, 1594,*
    1595, 1596, 1597, 1598, 1599, 1600, 1601
    fluoroscopy, *1592*
    methods of, 1590
    spot film study of duodenal bulb, *1593*
  rugal pattern of, 1585
  secretion, glandular, *1588*
  tone, 1588
  ulceration of, *1618,* 1638
    benign vs. malignant, 1639
    complications of, 1646
    incidence of, *1618, 1640*
    prepyloric vs. pyloric, *1639*
    roentgen signs of benign, 1638
Stress incontinence, 1421
Steroid therapy, secondary effects on bones,
  235
Stripe, pleural, displacement of, 1016
  posterior mediastinal, *1017,* 1559, *1563*
  superior and inferior esophageal-pleural, 1016
Subdiaphragmatic abscess, 749, 759, *759*
Subdural hematoma, as cause of respiratory
  obstruction, 786
  calcification of, *467*
  intracranial calcification of, 586, *587*
Submento-vertical view, *558*
Sudeck's atrophy, 172
Sulphuric fumes, 929
Supine position, definition of, 40
Suprarenal gland, 1423–1433
  abnormalities, of architecture, 1429
    of contour, 1427
    of density, 1428
    of function, 1429
    of position, 1429
  adenoma of, *1428, 1430*
  anatomy of, 1423
  blood supply of, 1425
  calcification of, 1428, 1429, 1431, *1432*
  cysts of, *1432,* 1433
  dimensions of, 1425
  displacement of kidney, *1354*
  examination, methods of, 1425
  mass, demonstration of, *1906*
  metastases to, 1433
  pheochromocytoma of, 1429, 1430, *1431*
  roentgen signs of abnormalities of, 1426
Surgery, radical mastectomy, 781
  resections, with chest wall lucency, 987
Suture, coronal, diastasis of, *487*
  diastasis of, secondary to hydrocephalus, 466
    secondary to increased intracranial pressure,
      578, 580
    with neuroblastoma, *493*
  of skull, vs. fracture lines, 486, *487*
Swallowing function, study by cineradiography,
  1524, 1542
Sympathetic chain, cervical, involved with
  Pancoast tumor, 909

Sympathetic ganglia, *1023*
  mediastinum, *1014*
Sympathetic trunk, *1023*
  mediastinum, *1014*
  relationship to azygos venous system, *943*
Syndactylia, 197
Syndrome
  absent patella-fingernail, 185
  adrenogenital, 1433
  afferent loop, *1667*
  aglossia-adactylia, 222
  Albright's, 1375
  alveolar capillary block, with fibrotic disease
    of lung parenchyma, 977
  Apert's, 210
  Asherman, *1903*
  "battered child," 174, *174*
  "blind loop," 1734, *1734*, 1737
  Borhoeve, 1566
  Brachmann-DeLang, 222
  Caplan's, 859, 927, 932
  Carcinoid, 1743, 1842
    producing sclerotic changes in bone, 325
    with bronchial adenoma, 824
  Ceelen Gellerstedt, with fibrotic disease of
    parenchyma, 977
  cerebrohepatorenal, 1435
  congenital rubella, 267, *268*
    with metaphyseal changes, 260
  Costen's, 551
  Cushing's, 1429, 1433
    causing generalized radiolucency of bone,
      233
    causing increased radiolucency of spine, 632
    roentgenographic changes in spine, 629, 630
    roentgenographic findings in infancy, 236
    secondary to steroid therapy, 236
    with spinal malalignment, *673*
    with thymic pathology, 1034
  Dandy-Walker, appearance of posterior fossa,
    448, 595
    radiographic findings, 473, *474*
  Down's. See *Mongolism.*
  dumping, *1669*
  endocrine ulcer, 1646
  Ehlers-Danlos, 175, 191, 210
  Fanconi's, *232*
    with rickets, 236
  Felty's, 411
  Franceschetti's, 211
  Freeman-Sheldon, 222
  Gardner, 1841
  Goldenhar's, 221
  Goodpasture's, *809*, 810, 877, *878*, 879
    causing linear changes in lung, 970
  Hamman-Rich, 977
    causing linear changes in lung, 970
  hand-foot-uterus, 222
  Hanhart's, 211
  Holt-Oram, 223
  Hughes-Stovin, 960
  Hutchinson-Gilford, 223
  intestinal knot, 1819
  intestinal lipodystrophy, 1725
  Ivemark, 1235, 1263, *1296*, 1606
    and right-sided heart, *1200*
  Jaffe-Lichtenstein, 251, *252*
  Kartagener's, 968
  Klinefelter's, 216
  Klippel-Feil, 190

Syndrome (*Continued*)
  Larsen's, 223
  Leriche, 1288
  Loeffler's, 810, 836, 859
  MacLeod's, 966, 988, 999
  Maffucci's, 200
  malabsorption, 1711
  Mallory-Weiss, 1542
  Manhart's, 222
  Marchesani, 221
  Marfan's, 191, 208, 629
  meconium plug syndrome, 1820, 1821
  Mikulicz, 1042
  Milkman's, 119, 269, 636
    with spinal malalignment, *673*
  Moebius, 211, 222
  Mounier-Kuhn, 788, 794
  nephrotic, intermittent mediastinal widening,
    1048, *1049*
  neutrophil dysfunction, 1034
  otopalata-digital, 223
  ovarian vein (right), 1406
  Pancoast, 909
  Peutz-Jeghers, *1729*, 1841
  Plummer-Vinson, 1536
  polyostotic fibrous dysplasia of Albright,
    296
  pseudogout, 421
  pseudo-Turner, 220
  pulmonary renal, *803*
  Reiter's, 412, 413, 680
  respiratory distress, *881*
  Riley-Day, 970
  Klippel-Trenaunay-Weber, 222
  Robin's, 211
  scrimitar, compared with bandlike shadows
      between lung and pleura, 976
    with anomalous pulmonary veins, 956, 961
  Silver's, 222
  Sjögren's, 411, *412*, 970
  Stein-Leventhal, *1905, 1909*
    demonstration by pneumoperitoneum, 1907
  Stevens-Johnson, 857
  Stewart-Morel-Moore, 517
  straight back, 677
  Sturge-Weber, calcification of, *588, 590*
    intracranial, 586
  superior mesenteric artery, with duodenal
    distention, *1243*
  superior vena caval, with idiopathic fibrosis
    of mediastinum, 1047
  Swyer-James, 966, 988, 999, 1139
  Thibierge-Weissenbach, 1713
  Tietze's, *779*
  trapped air, *992, 993*
  Treacher-Collins, 211
  Turcot, 1841, 1842
  Turner's, 210, *219*, 220
    appearance of vertebrae, *635*
    radiographic changes in spine, *220*, 629
    with scoliosis, 674
    with spinal curvature, 668
  Van der Hoeve's, 209
  Van der Woode's, 223
  Wegener's, *862*
  whistling face, 222
  Wilson-Mikity, *803*, 873, 877, 879, *879*
  Zollinger-Ellison, 1644
    small intestinal pattern, 1732, *1733*
Synovial chondrometaplasia, 348

Synovioma, 419, *420*

Synoviosarcoma, 386, 419

Syphilis, congenital, 94, 269, *306,* 307
   bony changes in, *266*
   metaphyseal changes of heart and vessels, 260, 333
   periosteal reaction, *374*
   in skull with acquired form, *504*
   involving metaphysis, *261*
   juvenile or tertiary, causing longitudinal sclerosis of bone, 337
     causing osteosclerosis of bone, *325, 338*
     periosteal changes in, *374*
   of bone, 306
   of spine, causing spotted lucency, 632
   of stomach, 1621
   with intracranial calcification, 585

Syphilitic spondylitis, with spur formation, 633

Syringomyelia, roentgenologic findings, 674

Tachypnea, transient, as cause of respiratory obstruction, 786

Taeniae coli, 1754

Talus, fractures of, 160, *161*
   classification, 160

Talus (vertical), 198

Tannic acid, as component of barium enema, 1769, 1773

Tarsal coalition, 198

Tear drop distance, 278, *279*

Teleroentgenograms, 17
   in cardiac examination, 1067
   in cephalopelvic disproportion, 1886

Temporal bone, 551
   anatomy of (diagram), *559*
   destruction, pathogenesis of, 568
   Mayer projection, *564*
   radiographic abnormalities of (classification), 555
   routine used, *556*
   Runström's view, *563*
   standard positions for radiography, 551, *553*
   Stenver's view, *560*
   submentovertical view, *562*

Tendon, Achilles, spontaneous rupture of, 160

Teratoma, 1873
   mediastinal, *1012,* 1013, 1031, 1032
   presacral, 1290
   retroperitoneal, 1290
     containing calcium, 1288
   sacrococcygeal, 645
     causing spotted lucency of spine, 632

Test, "tilt," in dorsal scoliosis, *670*

Tetralogy of Fallot, 1137

Thalassemia, of spine, 632, 638

Thalassemia anemia, as cause of extramedullary hematopoiesis, 1053

Thalassemia major, bony changes in, 255
   in skull, 481

Thalassemia minor, extramedullary foci of hematopoiesis, 912

Thanatophoric dwarf, 202, *202,* 204

Thiemann's disease, *277*

Thoracic cage, 770–786
   abnormalities of, bone (classification), 770
     soft tissues (classification), 770
   asymmetrical changes of, 770

Thoracic cage (*Continued*)
   barrel chest, 774
     accompanying allergies, 775
     accompanying pertussis, 774
     with acute exanthemas, 775
     with cystic fibrosis of pancreas, 775
     with emphysema, 775
   bony changes associated with lipochondrodystrophy, 774
   collapse as sign of fetal death, 1870, *1872*
   fibrothorax, 845
   flail chest, 775
   hourglass chest, 775
   interspace variation with pneumonia, effusion, and atelectasis, *764*
   narrowing of, 771, *771*
   neurofibroma of chest wall, 786
   roentgen signs of abnormality (classification), 770
   scurvy and, 774
   soft tissues of, *787*
     classification, 781
   symmetrical changes of, 770
   tumors of, 894
   widening of, 771, *771*

Thoracic duct, *1020,* 1021, *1021, 1022, 1024*
   anatomic description, 1025

Thoracoplasty, 770
   with narrowing of thorax, *771*

Thorax, contour, abnormalities of, *772, 773*
   narrowing with asphyxiating thoracic dystrophy of newborn, 773

Thresher's disease, 929

Thromboangiitis obliterans, 980

Thrombocytopenic purpura, idiopathic, as cause of intestinal hemorrhage, 1717

Thrombosis, of cavernous sinus caused by mucormycosis, 850
   of mesenteric artery, as cause of small bowel obstruction, 1706

Thumb, absent, hypoplastic, or supernumerary, in hypoplastic anemias, 256
   fracture (Bennett's), 143
   fracture dislocation of carpometacarpal joint, *144*

Thymus, 1013, *1021*
   atrophy of, in Cushing's syndrome, 236
   cysts of, 1032
   hyperplasia, as response to steroid test, 1031
   outline, changes in infants, *1088*
   thymoma of, *1012,* 1030, 1032, 1034
     clinical features, 1030
     localization by radioisotopic techniques, 1027
     roentgenologic aspects of, 1034, *1034*

Thyroid, *1024*
   acropathy and, 340, *341*
   calcification in, 795
   carcinoma, and calcification, 1028
     metastatic appearance in lung, 921, *922*
   displacement of esophagus by, 1558
   enlargement into mediastinum, 1030, 1031
   in fetus, 1873
     tumors, 1874
   intrathoracic extension of, 1032
   intrathoracic goiter, *1032*
   relationship between enlargement and mediastinal compartment, *1012*

Thyroid (*Continued*)
  substernal extension, 1559
  thyrotoxic heart, *1159*
  tumors of, in mediastinum, 1013
    identification by radioisotopic techniques, 1027
  with Hodgkin's disease, 1036
Tibia, condyle, fractures of, *152, 153*
  plateau, fractures of, *153*
  shaft, fractures of, 155
  T or Y fractures of, 153
Tin, in lung following inhalation, 923
Toe, fractures of, 162
Tomogram, in demonstration of giant osteoid osteoma of vertebra, *646*
  in demonstration of petrous erosion, *573*
  in diagnosis of pulmonary nodule, *892, 893*
  in differentiation of mediastinal and pulmonary masses, 1028
  in elucidation of destruction of temporal bone, 568
  in identification of mediastinal lesions, 1028
  in occipitalization of atlas, *621*
Tonsillitis, *1529*
Torticollis, congenital, definition and radiographic manifestations, 672
  with spinal curvature, 668
Torulosis, of lung, 850
  with intracranial calcification, 585
Total body opacification, 1316
Touhy needle, 1881
Towne's position, 553, *557*
  in demonstration of acoustic neuroma, *571*
  in demonstration of cholesteatoma of middle ear, *570*
  in diagnosis of petrous erosion, *573*
Toxoplasmosis, of lung, 850
  with intracranial calcification, 585
Trabeculi of medulla, with bone pathology, 59
Trachea, 702, *941*, 947, *1014, 1015, 1018, 1020, 1021, 1024*
  abnormal architecture of, 789
  air column relationships, 948
  anatomic relationship to esophagus, *1538*
  angle of bifurcation, 702
  collapse secondary to croup, *789*
  compression of, *1560*
    by intrathoracic goiter, *1032*
  croup, appearance in, 790
  deflection, with atelectasis, *817, 827*
    with vascular anomalies of aortic arch, *1198*
  deviation, with nonpenetrating injuries to thoracic aorta, 1052
  displacement of, 789, 794
    by aneurysm of arch of aorta, *1120*
    by thyroid, 1031
    by tracheoesophageal fistula, *1551*
  epiglottitis, appearance in, 790
  in lateral view of chest, 948, *1018*
  indentation, by arch of aorta, 1025, *1199*
    with arterial anomalies, 1207
  narrowness of, 794
    with polychondritis, 794
  paratracheal structures, rigidity in epiglottitis, 790
  polychondritis of, 791
  position of, in pneumonia, pleural effusion, and atelectasis, *764*

Trachea (*Continued*)
  positional changes in atelectasis, 824
    with chronic tuberculosis, *840*
  relationship, to azygos venous system, *943*
    to mediastinal lymph nodes, 1026
  shift with atelectasis, *816*
  size, variations in, 789
    with tracheobronchiomegaly, 794
    with tracheomalacia, 790
  tumor of, *1012*, 1013
  Wegener's syndrome, appearance with, 862
  with associated carcinoma of tongue, *1527*
  with bronchogenic cyst, 1045
    with pseudobulbar palsy, *1528*
    with pulmonary agenesis, 771
Tracheobronchial tree, *708*. See also *Trachea and Bronchus(i)*.
  constriction with mediastinal fibrosis, 1047
  distance from esophagus, measurements of, 901
    with bronchogenic carcinoma, *903*
  fistulation with mediastinitis, 1046
  lymph nodes adjacent to, 1025
  mucoviscidosis, involvement with, 969
  relationship to pulmonary artery, *708*
  variations in size, 789
Tracheobronchiomegaly, 794
  with upper respiratory tract obstruction, 788
Tracheobronchitis, 962, *962*
Tracheomalacia, 790, 791, *791*
  with upper respiratory tract obstruction, 788
  vs. croup, 790
Transfusion, intrauterine fetal, 1880
Transient tachypnea of newborn, *803*
Transposition of viscera (situs inversus), 1606
Trapezium, fractures of, 142
Trauma, as cause of respiratory obstruction, 786
  with asymmetrical changes in chest, 770
Trendelenburg position, in differentiation between mediastinal lipomas and subpleural lipomas, 769
Trichinosis, with intracranial calcification, 585
Triquetrum, fractures of, 142
Trisomy 21, 215. See also *Mongolism*.
Trousseau's phenomenon, 1678
Truemmerfeld zone in scurvy, *264*
Tuberculoma, calcification in, *467*
  intracranial calcification of, 585, *587*
  of lung, 895
Tuberculosis, *803*, 873, 980
  apical, 836
  as cause of colon constriction, 1824
  as cause of extrapleural sign, 781
  as cause of mediastinitis, 1046
  cavitation and, *1000*
  chronic fibroid of lung, 877
  chronic, vs. tumorlet of lung, 909
  Dunham's fan and, 895
  miliary, *803*, 932, *933*
  of bone, 305
  of colon, *1792*, 1837
  of diaphysis, 304
  of fallopian tube, *1902*
  of kidney, *1407*, 1409, *1455, 1456, 1457*
    producing calcification, *1367*, 1399
  of lung, *808*, 894, *897*, 920
    calcification and, 921
    location of, 921
    webbing and honeycombing, 976

Tuberculosis (*Continued*)
  of oviduct, *1904*
  of skull, with "button" sequestrum, 512
  of spine, causing displacement of pleural
      stripe, 1016
    simulating mediastinal tumor, 1057
    vs. pyogenic osteomyelitis, 641 (table)
  of stomach, 1621
  of ureter, *1370*
  of vertebral column, with "wedging" of
      vertebral bodies, *650*
  pulmonary type, with cavitation, 1004
  tuberculous meningitis, calcification of,
      585, *587*
  tuberculous sicca, 403
  vs. aspergillosis and moniliasis, 850
  with wedging of vertebra, *642*
Tuberculum sellae, 524
Tuberous sclerosis, 980
  causing spotted sclerosis of spine, 633
  of bone, 260
  of hand, *589*
  of lung, with webbing and honeycombing, 976
  of skull, calcification in, 585, *589*
  of spine, radiologic changes in, 655
  with interstitial fibrosis of lung, 978
Tularemia, *803*
  oculoglandular form, 872
  pulmonary form, 872
  radiographic appearance, 872
  typhoidal form, 872
  ulceroglandular form, 872
Tumors
  benign, affecting joints, 419
    of cranial nerves, 498
  bone, age of occurrence, *372* (table)
    and cartilage, in mediastinal compartment,
        1012
    benign vs. malignant, 369, *372*
    malignant, *373*
    primary, classification of, 366, 367
      relative radiosensitivity of, 375 (table)
  bone neoplasms, prevailing sites, *370*
  carcinoma, of colon, 1843
    of esophagus, *1574, 1575*
    of jejunum, *1742*
    of kidney, 1443
      differentiation from cyst, 1445
    of maxillary antrum, *543*
  Ewing's, 241, 311, *311, 312,* 313
    onion skin effect, *275*
    osteosclerotic changes from, *338*
    periosteal reaction, *374*
    sites for metastatic spread, 512
  giant cell, of bone, *287, 294, 295, 296,*
      301, *309*
    of vertebra, 645
  glioma of optic nerve, *578, 579*
  glomus jugularis, 571
  in joints, xanthomatous giant cell tumors, 419
  intracranial, calcification in, *588–592*
  mesenchymal, 1013
  metastatic to bone, 241, 242, *287,* 301,
      368, 369
    carcinoma of breast, 350
    carcinoma of prostate, 325, *325,* 331, 350,
        350
    osteosclerotic, 345, *346,* 350
    radiographic appearance of, *243*
    resembling hyperparathyroid disease, 509
  metastatic to lung, *1005*

Tumors (*Continued*)
  metastatic to skeleton, 242
  metastatic to skull, 510, 514
    with "button" sequestrum, 512
  metastatic to spine, 644, 662
    with spotty radiolucency, 632
    with spotty sclerosis, 633
    with wedging of vertebrae, *642*
  nasopharyngeal, 675
    with abnormalities of alignment in relation
        to skull, 668
  neurogenic, of mediastinum, *1012,* 1048
  of adrenal gland, 1433
  of apex of petrous bone, 569
  of blood vessels, in mediastinum, *1012*
  of esophagus, 1572
  of facial bones and paranasal sinuses, 549
  of heart, 1013
  of joints, 386. See also names of individual
      tumors.
  of kidney, *1368*
  of lung, with linear shadows, 939, 975
    with "tumor track," 975
  of lymph vessels, *1012*
  of nerve, ganglioneuroma of mediastinum, 1051
    neuroblastoma, 1051
    neurofibromas, 1051
  of skull, 498
    with osteolytic foci, *511*
  of thyroid gland, 1013
  of trachea, 1013
  orbital, 577
  paraspinal, in mediastinal compartments, *1012*
  parathyroid, 1013
  pericardial, 1013
  primary bone, classification of, 366, 367
  Wilms', 1287, *1291*
    as cause of abdominal mass in infancy, 1290
Turricephaly, *462*
Typhlitis, 1838

Ulcer
  Barrett's, 1570
  esophageal, *1568*
    complicating achalasia, 1555
    peptic, *1153, 1552*
  gastric. See *Stomach.*
  Hunner's, 1410, 1414
Ulcerative colitis, 1799, *1808, 1811,* 1823
  idiopathic, anatomic distribution of, 1833
    comparison with granulomatous colitis, 1835
  in children, 1834
  polypoid mass in, *1790, 1803*
  radiographic signs, *1783, 1785, 1789*
  resemblance to mesenteric thrombosis, 1251
  rupture of bowel following barium enema, 1776
  spinal effects, 680
  ulceration, longitudinal, *1811*
  with arthritis, 412
  with carcinoma, 1799
Ulna, coronoid process, fractures of, 127, *129*
  olecranon process, fractures of, 128, *129*
Upper respiratory tract obstruction, 788
Ureter, 1348
  abnormalities, in architecture, 1405
    in density, 1407
    in function, 1409
    in position, 1404
  achalasia of, 1403

Ureter (*Continued*)
  beading as sign in tuberculosis, 1407
  calcification in, 1407
  caliectasis, localized, 1403
  carcinoma of, *1401*
  gas in fascial planes surrounding, *1408*
  megaureter, 1403
  obstruction of, 1403
  polyp, *1402*
  pseudovalves, 1407, *1408*
  retrocaval, 1404, *1405*
  roentgen signs of abnormality, 1399
  tuberculosis of, *1370*, 1399, *1406*
  ureterectasis, 1400, *1400, 1401*
  ureterocele, *1401, 1414*
    in child, *1402*
Ureteritis cystica, *1388*, 1399, 1405, 1451
Urethra, 1348
  calculus in, *1370*
  diverticulum of, 1419
  fistula of, 1418
  male, anatomy of, *1319*
  roentgen signs of abnormality, classification of, 1410
  valve, anterior, 1466
    congenital, *1465*
    posterior, *1418*
Urethrogram, 1316, *1319, 1419*
  female, *1319*
  pyelogram, rapid sequence dehydrated excretory, 1320
Urinary bladder, 1348
  pneumograms of, 1337
  triple contrast study of, *1332, 1333*
Urinary tract, 1310–1476
  anatomy of, *1347*
  angiography of, contrast media used, 1314–1315 (table)
  calculi in, *1370*, 1421
  IVP, analysis of film studies, 1339
    changes with renal infarction, *1398*
    in child, *1317*
    radiographic demonstration, *1312, 1392*
    time sequence of films, 1313
  KUB film, *1311*
    analysis of, 1339
  malacoplakia, 1451
  pyelogram, confusing appearances, 1423, 1424
    in diagnosis of hypertension, 1320
    infusion excretory, 1318
      advantages of, 1339
      IVP, *1340*
        ectopic kidney, *1355*
      "minute," 1321
      rapid sequence intravenous, 1321
        combined with hydrated pyelogram, 1320
      retrograde, 1322, *1322, 1392*
        demonstrating adenocarcinoma, *1356*
        demonstrating horseshoe kidney, *1355*
        washout test for renovascular hypertension, 1352
  radiologic methods of study, 1310, 1313
  stress incontinence, roentgen techniques, *1328*
  total body opacification, 1316
  tuberculosis of, roentgenologic features, *1406, 1407, 1455, 1456*
Urogram, excretory. See *Urinary tract, IVP.*
Urography, infusion excretory, 1318
  changes in pyelocaliectasis, *1379*
Urticaria pigmentosa (mastocytosis), *346*, 1653
  involving small intestine, 1738

Urticaria pigmentosa (mastocytosis) (*Continued*)
  producing osteosclerotic changes in bone, *325*
  radiographic changes of, 328, 329
    in spine, 640
    sclerotic lesions, 632, 633
Uterus
  abnormal roentgen findings in hysterosalpingography, *1900*
  adenomyosis, 1897, 1899
  arcuatus, *1903*
  carcinoma of, *1902*
  cervix, abnormalities of canal, 1901
  endometrial hyperplasia, 1897
  fibroid, submucous, 1899
  fibromyoma of, 1885
  filling defects, of uterine cavity, 1901
  myoma of, *1903*
  rupture of, *1883, 1884*
  sinus tracts of, 1901
  synechiae, 1897, *1900*, 1901, *1903*
  uterine axis factor, *1892*
  uterine cavity, variations of, as seen by hysterosalpingograph, *1902*
  uterus didelphys, *1903*
  variations in cavity with hysterosalpingography, *1903*
Utricle, 1419

Vacuum phenomenon, 679
Vaginography, barium, 1910
Valleculae, carcinoma of tongue and, *1527*
  gaseous distinction of, 789
  Parkinson's disease and, *1528*
Valsalva maneuver, in examination of the chest, 730, 1089
Valve(s)
  aortic, classification of roentgenologic signs, 1102
  ileocecal, *1758, 1759*
    cathartic colon, appearance in, 1808
    differentiation from prolapse, *1691*
    normal anatomy of, 1754
  mitral, *1022*
    roentgenologic features, classification of, 1102, 1103
  of heart, classification of pathology, 1102–1103
    in routine positions, *1077*
  of inferior vena cava, *1022*
  of Kerchring, 1689
  pulmonary, 1103
    cusp of, *1022*
  tricuspid, *1022*
    roentgenologic findings, classification of, 1103
  valvular lesions, combined, 1103
Vanadium, 929
Varices, esophageal, *1569, 1570, 1650*
  of stomach, *1650*
  pulmonary, solitary, 961
Vascular anomalies, calcification in abdomen, 1288
  mesenteric vascular occlusion, 1251
  tracheal displacement or narrowness, 794
Vascular disease, with abnormal gas pattern in plain film of abdomen, 1246
Vein(s)
  abdominal connection with esophageal varices, *1569*

Vein(s) (*Continued*)
  azygos, *943, 1022, 1024*
    and tributaries, *1023*
    aneurysm of (varix), *1061*
    azygography, 1026
    detection in cardiac esophagram, 1069
    enlargement of, in mediastinum, *1012*
        1013
    in mediastinum, *1014*
    knob, *943*
    relationship to esophagus, 1537
  azygos venous system, relationship to
      esophagus and portal circulation, *1539*
  brachiocephalic, *948, 1014*
  dural sinuses, thrombosis with
      Hughes-Stovin syndrome, 960
  hemiazygos, *943, 1023*
    accessory, in mediastinum, *1014*
    inferior, *1024*
    superior, *1022, 1024*
  hepatic, opening into right atrium, *1022*
  inferior vena cava, *732, 942, 948, 1015, 1018,*
      1024, 1330, 1331
    calcification of thrombus in, 1287
    in Hodgkin's disease, 1036
    in mediastinum, *1014*
    valve of, *1022*
    with anomalous venous drainage, *962*
  innominate, *943, 1020, 1023*
  intercostal, *1020, 1024*
    relationship to azygos venous system, *943*
  internal jugular, *943, 1023, 1024*
  internal mammary, *943, 1023*
  lumbar, *1024*
  of Galen, aneurysm of, 586
    calcification of, characteristic findings, 588
  of heart, *1135*
  paravertebral, *1330*
  peripheral, thrombosis in Hughes-Stovin
      syndrome, 960
  pulmonary, *1014, 1015, 1018, 1022*
    constriction in mediastinal fibrosis, 1047
    identification by angiography, 1026
    measurement of, *1147*
    thrombosis, appearance with, 975
    venogram associated with thrombotic state,
        1141
  renal, *1024*
    thrombosis of, 1389, *1398*
  subclavian, *943, 1023*
  superior vena cava, *731, 942, 1021, 1022*
    chronic adhesive pericarditis, appearance
        with, *1145*
    dilated, 1013
    enlargement within mediastinum, *1012,*
        1014
    relationship to aneurysm of azygos vein,
        1061
    relationship to azygos vein, 943
    rib notching associated with, 780
  venous thrombosis of abdomen, 1251
Vena cavography, 1026
Venography, demonstrating kidney, *1330, 1331*
  of dural sinus, in investigation of
      intracranial space-occupying lesions, 579
Ventricle, left, *1015*
  changes with dilatation, *1092*
  changes with hypertrophy, *1092, 1093*
  diagnosis of enlargement, 1095
  laryngeal, 702
  measurement of, *1094*
  right, infundibulum of, *1022*

Ventriculogram, in identification of
    intracranial space-occupying lesions, 579
Vertebra(e)
  abnormalities in number, 609
  block, 618, *620*
  butterfly, *620, 626*
  change in shape and size secondary to
        aortic aneurysm, 631
    secondary to aneurysm of vertebral artery,
        632
  clefts of, 622
  collapsed bodies with steroid therapy, 413
  congenital abnormalities of, *620*
  Cushing's syndrome, changes in, 630
  destruction of, secondary to actinomycosis,
      844
  endplates, changes with cretinism, *335*
    in osteochondrosis, *277,* 279
    in rheumatoid arthritis, 410
    indentations due to nuclei pulposi, 782
  epiphysitis (Scheuermann's disease), causing
      spotted lucency of spine, 632
    radiographic appearance, 647
    with spinal curvature, 668
  erosion, caused by aneurysm of descending
      thoracic aorta, *1121*
    radiologic differences between aneurysm
        and tumor, *630*
    with Pancoast tumor, *899*
  fibrous dysplasia, 353
  "fish," 254, *648*
    in sickle cell anemia, 254
  hemangioma, involvement with, 315
  hemivertebra, *649, 675, 676*
    and abnormalities of alignment, 668
  intervertebral disks, relationship to azygos
      venous system, *943*
  "ivory," radiographic appearance of, 638
  notched, *620*
  occipital, abnormalities of fusion, 619
    malalignment between cervical spine and
        skull, 668, 675
  plana, *635*
    and spinal malalignment, *673*
  radiation effects on, 633
  radiology of, 602–697
  relationship to kidney, *1334*
  sickle cell anemia, appearance in, *256*
  thoracic, erosion of pedicles with Pancoast
      tumor, 909
  transverse bands, in lipoatrophic diabetes
      mellitus, 332
  vascular notches of, in sickle cell disease,
      255
Vertebral bodies
  abnormalities of metabolic origin, 627
  alignment of C-1 and C-2, *652*
  clefts of, 624
    coronal, 624, *625*
    sagittal, 624
  congenital abnormalities of, 627
  dimensions of, *782*
  erosion with meningocele, 1053
  spur formation, displacement of esophagus,
      1558
  wedging of, *642, 648, 649*
    congenital in origin, *649*
    neoplastic in origin, *650*
    pyogenic in origin, *650*
    secondary to ischemic necrosis, *648*
    secondary to tuberculosis, *650*
    traumatic in origin, *649*

Vertebral column. See also *Spine*.
  abnormalities, of contour and alignment, 668, 669
    of curvature, 668, 669. See also *Scoliosis*.
    of radiodensity and architecture, classification, 632, 633
  cervical spine, abnormalities of alignment in relation to skull, *652,* 668
    fractures of, *656, 657*
      classification of, 653
      spur formation, 664
  congenital anomalies of, *676*
  fractures and dislocations, with malalignment of vertebrae, 675
    with spinal curvature, 668
  fractures of, seat belt, 675
  kyphosis. See *Kyphosis*.
  radiation effects on, 662
  relationship of visceral and parietal pleura, *609*
  roentgen changes in architecture, *634, 635*
  thoracic spine, fractures of, 653
  traumatic changes, 632, 647
    arthropathy, 681
    involving cervical spine, *651*
    with malalignment, 668, 677
    with seat belt injuries, *654*
Villonodular synovitis. See *Xanthomatous giant cell tumor*.
Virchow, plane of, *554*
Virus infection, as cause of interstitial pneumonia, 977
Vitamin D, in bone formation, 57
  intoxication, 59
Vocal cords, 702
  abnormalities in contour of, 789
Volkmann's ischemic contracture, with fracture of humerus, 126
Volvulus, as cause of small bowel obstruction, 1706
  involvement of enterogenous cyst, 1699
  of colon, *1786, 1787, 1807,* 1818
  of small intestine, 1255, 1735, 1737
  of stomach, 1260, 1606, *1608,* 1609
  roentgenologic findings, 1819

Waldenström's macroglobulinemia, producing linear changes in lung, 970
Water test, in assessment of esophageal function, 1544
Water-siphonage test of De Carvalho, 1544
Water's projection, *535*
Web formation of esophagus, *1535*
Wegener's syndrome, *862*
Wheat dust, 929
Whiplash injury, 653
Whipple's disease, 1725
  and protein-losing enteropathy, 1712
  in small intestine, *1729,* 1738
  pathology of, 1725
  roentgen signs of, 1725
Wilson's disease, 266, 270
Wilson-Mikity syndrome, *803,* 873, 877, 879
  as cause of respiratory obstruction, 786

Wilson-Mikity syndrome (*Continued*)
  radiographic appearance of, 879, *879,* 880
Worm infestations, involving lung, *802*

Xanthoma, 386
Xanthomatosis, 980
Xanthomatous giant cell tumor, 420, *421*
X-ray(s)
  accessories for recording, 8
  body section radiographic equipment, 8
  cassette, 8, *9*
    care of, *9*
  contrast media, 8
  control panel of x-ray machine, 30
  distortion, 17, *19*
  film, 8
  fluoroscope, 8, 12, *14*
    equipment, *15*
  grids, stationary and moving, 8, 10
  hard cathode rays, *21*
  image, accessories necessary for, 8
    amplification of, electronic, 13
    amplifier, 8, *14*
    formation, geometry of, 17
    production of, cut-off effect by anode heel, *19*
    projection, use of, *19*
  infant immobilization device, *32*
  magnification, 14, *16,* 17, *19*
    accessories, 8
    effect of focal object distance and object film distance on, *18*
  penetrability, relationship to body tissues, *7*
  penumbra formation, 17, *18*
  Potter-Bucky diaphragm, 8
  production of, 3
  properties of, fluorescence effect, *7*
    penetrability of tissue, *6*
    photographic effect of, *6*
  rapid sequence film changes, 14
  "remnant rays," radiolucent, intermediate, and radiopaque types, *7*
  soft, 21
  spot film radiography, 8
  stereoscopic radiographic accessories, 8
  stereoscopy, principles of, *13*
  television use, in fluoroscopy, *15*
    in radiology, 13
  toning devices, 11
  tube, 3
    anodes "stationary or rotating," *4*
    components of, *4*
    focal spot, *5*
    focusing cup, 5, *5*
    heat dissipation from, *5*
    target, *4*
    tungsten filament of, *4*

Zygoma, fractures of, 545